Micronutrients in Health and in Disease Prevention

Micronutrients in Health and in Disease Prevention

edited by

Adrianne Bendich
Hoffmann-La Roche Inc.
Nutley, New Jersey

C. E. Butterworth, Jr.
University of Alabama at Birmingham
Birmingham, Alabama

Marcel Dekker, Inc.   New York • Basel • Hong Kong

Library of Congress Cataloging-in-Publication Data

Micronutrients in health and in disease prevention / edited by
    Adrianne Bendich, C. E. Butterworth, Jr.
            p.   cm.
    Includes bibliographical references and index.
    ISBN 0-8247-8539-8
    1. Trace elements in nutrition. 2. Trace element deficiency
diseases. 3. Health. I. Bendich, Adrianne. II. Butterworth, C.
E. (Charles Edwin)
    [DNLM: 1. Health. 2. Preventive Medicine. 3. Trace Elements-
-physiology. 4. Vitamins--physiology.   QU 130 M6258]
QP534.M52   1991
613.2--dc20
DNLM/DLC
for Library of Congress   91-20099
                                                                  CIP

This book is printed on acid-free paper.

MARCEL DEKKER, INC.
270 Madison Avenue, New York, New York 10016

Current printing (last digit):
10   9   8   7   6   5   4   3   2   1

PRINTED IN THE UNITED STATES OF AMERICA

To my husband and best friend, David Kafkewitz; my children, Jorden and Debra; my parents, Joseph and Lillian Bendich; and my sister, Elaine, for their unending faith and encouragement.

—A. B.

To my patient and understanding wife, Joyce.

—C. E. B.

Foreword

Epidemiologists have been telling us for some time that unbalanced diets are major contributors to heart disease and cancer and are likely to be as important as smoking, which causes 30% of cancer and 25% of heart disease. The main dietary imbalances appear to be too few fruits and vegetables and too much fat. Patterson and Block indicate in their NHANES II survey (Chapter 18), for example, that 91% of the population does not eat enough fruit and vegetables; almost half the population ate no fruit or vegetables on the day of their study. Many Americans appear to be choosing judiciously from among the five major food groups: sugar, salt, grease, alcohol, and coffee.

Particular substances in fruit and vegetables that we know are important in disease prevention are antioxidants (carotenoids, tocopherols, ascorbate) and folic acid, but many other vitamins and essential minerals may play a large role in countering disease. The body is a very complex machine that has a variety of defenses to combat the degenerative biochemical processes that are natural consequences of metabolism. Micronutrients are required for the functioning of these defenses, and optimizing micronutrient levels is critical if we wish to minimize degenerative processes. Thus, as this book so persuasively argues, optimizing micronutrient intake must be a major component of our efforts to prevent disease.

We have been particularly interested in antioxidants (Stocker and Ames, 1987; Stocker et al., 1987a,b; Frei et al., 1988, 1989, 1990) because our studies show that daily endogenous oxidative DNA damage is enormous (Ames, 1989; Fraga et al., 1990; Degan et al., 1991; Adelman et al., 1988; Ames et al., 1991). A normal young rat cell has about 10^6 oxidative adducts, and this number increases with age. About 10^5 new oxidative adducts per cell are formed every day, most of which are repaired. These are the same type of adducts that are produced by radiation, an oxidative mutagen. We conclude that endogenous oxidative damage is a major factor in aging. Thus, there are good theoretical reasons to support the clinical findings that antioxidants are important in the prevention of the degenerative diseases associated with aging, such as cancer, heart disease, and cataracts. The role of the different antioxidants, such as ubiquinol (Frei et al., 1990), in different tissues and cell compartments still needs clarification.

White blood cells defend the body against bacteria and viruses in part by bombarding them with large amounts of NO, O_2^-, H_2O_2, and OCl^-. The downside of this defense is that healthy cells are also damaged by all these oxidants, which can contribute to aging and cancer. Oxidants are not only mutagens, but are also stimulants for increased cell division (wound healing). Chronic mitogenesis (cell division), e.g., from chronic inflammation, is an important risk factor for carcinogenesis (Ames and Gold, 1990); thus antioxidants are important anticarcinogens because they are both antimutagens and antimitogens.

Work showing that caffeine interacts with folate deficiency to enhance chromosome breakage (MacGregor et al., 1990) reinforces the large literature covered in this volume indicating that folate deficiency is an important cause of cancer and birth defects. A sizable proportion of the population (30% or more) may be ingesting insufficient levels of folate.

A major area of research in the quest to delay aging and to prevent cancer and heart disease is determining the level of each micronutrient that is optimal for long-term health. The Recommended Daily Allowance (RDA) is based on the level to prevent an immediate pathological effect, but optimal levels may be different. The great genetic variability of the human species makes it highly likely that many people will require a higher-than-average optimal level of particular micronutrients, as discussed by R. J. Williams, Linus Pauling, and others. Furthermore, a variety of stresses ranging from pregnancy to infections are likely to increase micronutrient requirements. This variability will require the development of in vivo short-term assays that measure specific determinants of micronutrient deficiency on an individual basis. Our own interest is to develop such assays for DNA damage (Degan et al., 1991; Ames et al., 1991; MacGregor et al., 1990).

Epidemiology is a major key to uncovering the causes of disease, as can be seen from the many studies discussed in this book. Epidemiology, particularly studies involving dietary factors, is difficult and not terribly useful for assessing small effects, so epidemiological results must be reinforced by animal studies that elucidate the basic mechanisms of disease. The combination of these approaches is leading to a basic understanding of how to prevent disease and minimize the degenerative processes associated with aging. Thus there is every reason to think that our ever-increasing average life expectancy will continue to increase in the next decades. This book is one milestone on this path.

Bruce N. Ames, Ph.D.
Professor of Biochemistry
and Molecular Biology
University of California, Berkeley
Berkeley, California

REFERENCES

Adelman R, Saul RL, Ames, BN. Oxidative damage to DNA: Relation to species metabolic rate and life span. Proc Natl Acad Sci USA 1988; 85:2706–2708.

Ames BN. Endogenous oxidative DNA damage, aging, and cancer. Free Rad Res Comms 1989; 7:121–128.

Ames BN, Gold LS. Chemical carcinogenesis: Too many rodent carcinogens. Proc Natl Acad Sci USA 1990; 87:7772–7776.

Ames BN, Shigenaga MK, Park E-M. DNA damage by endogenous oxidants as a cause of aging and cancer, in: Oxidative Damage and Repair: Chemical, Biological and Medical Aspects (Proceedings of the International Society for Free Radical Research Conference, Nov. 14–20, 1990) Pergamon Press, New York, 1991 (in press).

Degan P, Shigenaga MK, Park E-M, Alperin P, Ames BN. Immunoaffinity isolation of urinary 8-hydroxy-2'-deoxyguanosine and 8-hydroxyguanine and quantitation of 8-hydroxy-2'-deoxyguanosine in DNA by polyclonal antibodies. Carcinogenesis, 1991 (in press).

Fraga CG, Shigenaga MK, Park J-W, Degan P, Ames BN. Oxidative damage to DNA during aging: 8-hydroxy-2'-deoxyguanosine in rat organ DNA and urine. Proc Natl Acad Sci USA 1990; 87:4533–4537.

Frei B, Stocker R, Ames BN. Antioxidant defenses and lipid peroxidation in human blood plasma. Proc Natl Acad Sci USA 1988; 85:9748–9752.

Frei B, England L, Ames BN. Ascorbate is an outstanding antioxidant in human blood plasma. Proc Natl Acad Sci USA 1989; 86:6377–6381.

Frei B, Kim MC, Ames BN. Ubiquinol-10 is an effective lipid-soluble antioxidant at physiological concentrations. Proc Natl Acad Sci USA 1990; 87:4879–4883.

MacGregor JT, Schlegel R, Wehr CM, Alperin P, Ames BN. Cytogenetic damage induced by folate deficiency in mice is enhanced by caffeine. Proc Natl Acad Sci USA 1990; 87:9962–9965.

Stocker R, Ames BN. Potential role of conjugated bilirubin and copper in the metabolism of lipid peroxides in bile. Proc Natl Acad Sci USA 1987; 84:8130–8134.

Stocker R, Glazer AN, Ames BN. Antioxidant activity of albumin-bound bilirubin. Proc Natl Acad Sci USA 1987a; 84:5918–5922.

Stocker R, Yamamoto Y, McDonagh AF, Glazer AN, Ames BN. Bilirubin is an antioxidant of possible physiological importance. Science 1987b; 235:1043–1046.

Preface

The full importance of vitamins and minerals as micronutrients in the prevention of disease is just beginning to be appreciated by health scientists. In addition to their established roles in human nutrition, previously unsuspected relationships have come to light in recent years. The objective of this book, therefore, is to serve as a key reference to some of the most widely accepted current research linking essential dietary micronutrients to critical health issues, including cancer, cardiovascular disease, arthritis, immunity, birth defects, cataracts, and certain other acute and chronic illnesses.

In organizing the book, we have included chapters written by internationally recognized authorities who have reviewed recent research findings, emphasizing their impact on disease prevention. The volume is organized according to physiological functions, disease states, and broad-based health issues. The chapters are fully referenced and include tables, graphs, and figures that enhance the understanding of the contents of the volume. In addition to research-oriented chapters, a careful analysis of what Americans are and are not eating has been included; also, important information has been compiled on programs of nutrition education currently available in medical schools, as well as the most frequently utilized sources of nutrition information for physicians. The critical area of vitamin safety has been included as a separate chapter.

The volume is intended as a source of information for nutritionists and dietitians, primary care physicians, internists, geriatricians, pediatricians, obstetricians, oncologists, pharmacists, epidemiologists, public health authorities, molecular and cellular biologists, biochemists, toxicologists, and physiologists. The book can also be used as a supplement for graduate courses in nutrition or dietetics.

The editors gratefully acknowledge the efforts of Paul Dolgert and Elaine Grohman at Marcel Dekker, Inc. in bringing this volume to fruition. In addition, each of us is grateful to family members who were most tolerant of the added time and effort involved in this project, and we appreciate the support of our colleagues, especially Dr. Lawrence J. Machlin, for critical review of certain chapters.

Adrianne Bendich
C. E. Butterworth, Jr.

Contents

NEUROLOGICAL FUNCTIONS

BIRTH DEFECTS

IMMUNOLOGICAL FUNCTIONS

POPULATION GROUPS AND PREVENTIVE NUTRITION

Contributors

Joseph E. Baggott Division of Nutritional Biochemistry, Department of Nutrition Sciences, University of Alabama at Birmingham, Birmingham, Alabama

Adrianne Bendich Department of Clinical Nutrition, Hoffmann-La Roche Inc., Nutley, New Jersey

David Benton Department of Psychology, University College, Swansea, Wales, United Kingdom

Gladys Block Division of Cancer Prevention and Control, Clinical and Diagnostic Trials Section, Biometry Branch, National Cancer Institute, National Institutes of Health, Bethesda, Maryland

Jeffrey B. Blumberg Department of Nutritional Immunology and Toxicology, U.S. Department of Agriculture Human Nutrition Research Center on Aging, Tufts University, Boston, Massachusetts

C. E. Butterworth, Jr. Department of Nutrition Sciences, University of Alabama at Birmingham, Birmingham, Alabama

Harinder Garewal Department of Medicine, University of Arizona Cancer Center and Veterans Affairs Medical Center, Tucson, Arizona

Donald H. Gemson   Division of Sociomedical Sciences, Columbia University School of Public Health, New York, New York

Joanne F. Guthrie   Nutrition Education Division, Human Nutrition Information Service, U.S. Department of Agriculture, Hyattsville, Maryland

John N. Hathcock   Experimental Nutrition Branch, Food and Drug Administration, Washington, D.C.

Jean H. Humphrey   Dana Center for Preventive Ophthalmology, Wilmer Eye Institute, Baltimore, Maryland

Paul F. Jacques   U.S. Department of Agriculture Human Nutrition Research Center on Aging, Tufts University, Boston, Massachusetts

Paul Knekt   Research Institute for Social Security, Social Insurance Institution, Helsinki, Finland

William E. M. Lands   Department of Biological Chemistry, University of Illinois at Chicago, Chicago, Illinois

Lillian Langseth   Division of Environmental Sciences, Columbia University School of Public Health, New York, New York

Kilmer S. McCully   Laboratory Service, Veterans Affairs Medical Center, Providence, Rhode Island

Simin Nikbin Meydani   Department of Nutritional Immunology, U.S. Department of Agriculture Human Nutrition Research Center on Aging, Tufts University, Boston, Massachusetts

Sarah L. Morgan   Division of Clinical Nutrition, Departments of Nutrition Science and Internal Medicine, University of Alabama at Birmingham, Birmingham, Alabama

Blossom H. Patterson   Division of Cancer Prevention and Control, Clinical and Diagnostic Trials Section, Biometry Branch, National Cancer Institute, National Institutes of Health, Bethesda, Maryland

Howerde E. Sauberlich   Department of Nutrition Sciences, University of Alabama at Birmingham, Birmingham, Alabama

Christopher J. Schorah   Department of Clinical Pathology and Immunology, University of Leeds, Leeds, England

Glenn J. Shamdas   Section of Hematology-Oncology, Department of Internal Medicine, University of Arizona Cancer Center, Tucson, Arizona

Richard W. Smithells   Department of Pediatrics and Child Health, University of Leeds, Leeds, England

Manfred Steiner   Division of Hematology, Department of Medicine, Memorial Hospital of Rhode Island, Providence, Rhode Island

Amy F. Subar   Applied Research Branch, Surveillance Program, Division of Cancer Prevention and Control, National Cancer Institute, National Institutes of Health, Bethesda, Maryland

Allen Taylor   U.S. Department of Agriculture Human Nutrition Research Center on Aging, Tufts University, Boston, Massachusetts

Susan Welsh   Nutrition Education Division, Human Nutrition Information Service, U.S. Department of Agriculture, Hyattsville, Maryland

Keith P. West, Jr.   Dana Center for Preventive Ophthalmology, Wilmer Eye Institute, Baltimore, Maryland

Regina G. Ziegler   Environmental Epidemiology Branch, Epidemiology and Biostatistics Program, Division of Cancer Etiology, National Cancer Institute, National Institutes of Health, Bethesda, Maryland

1

Introduction

C. E. Butterworth, Jr.

University of Alabama at Birmingham, Birmingham, Alabama

Adrianne Bendich

Hoffmann-La Roche Inc., Nutley, New Jersey

The relationship between micronutrient status and disease prevention is becoming so well recognized that preventive nutritional guidelines (i.e., eat more fruits and vegetables) are commonly heard in everyday conversation. The major objective of this volume is to present evidence that optimal levels of micronutrient intake are associated with lowered risk of many chronic diseases. It will be seen that in many cases marginal or deficient intakes may not be recognized by ordinary standards and yet may lead to pathological tissue changes months or years later. Thus, it may be necessary to reexamine the methods used to establish recommended levels of nutrient consumption. It is becoming apparent that major physiological events link micronutrient status to the maintenance of health and the prevention of disease. It remains necessary to determine what is meant by ''optimal intake'' and to define goals and end points. But it is becoming clear that numerous situations exist in which micronutrient intake at higher levels than those currently recommended could prevent or delay the onset of certain chronic degenerative diseases.

INTERMEDIATE END POINTS

During the evolution of knowledge about disease, it often becomes possible to identify a precursor stage which can be eradicated prior to the onset of full-blown pathological manifestations. Many of the achievements in modern cancer surgery, chemotherapy, preventive medicine, and indeed nutrition science can be attributed to early recognition of disease. Thus, it is not necessary to wait for pelvic invasion to occur before making a diagnosis of cervical cancer; carcinoma in situ can be identified by a Pap smear and eradicated as an "intermediate end point."

In recent years the term "intermediate end points" has become popular in medical jargon in connection with research on the progressive stages of chronic disease. In spite of the fact that the phrase is something of an oxymoron, i.e., the juxtaposition of incongruous, incompatible, or contradictory words, it serves a useful purpose and merits further evaluation. When a health-related problem has enormous dimensions (as, for example, nutrition and cancer), it simply makes good sense to identify the early steps and intermediate stages that precede a more serious situation. Not only is it logical to equate the earliest manifestation of a disease with the disease itself ("things equal to the same thing are equal to each other"), it is often more efficient and less complicated, in terms of resource management, to deal with an early or asymptomatic phase of an illness. This approach offers a cost-effective means to achieve beneficial results for the greatest number of people.

Similarly, dietary intake patterns and biochemical indices of nutritional status can detect marginal deficiencies before gross clinical manifestations are evident. However, subtle and important nutritionally related intermediate end points not associated with deficiency states have been overlooked. For example, it now seems appropriate to take a fresh look at the role of specific individual dietary nutrients in relation to present day global issues such as (1) environmental pollution, (2) new infectious diseases such as HIV and HPV, (3) aging, (4) chronic diseases, as well as (5) genetic defects and (6) new therapeutic regimens, including antibiotics, hormones, and enzyme inhibitors. It is now possible to identify specific early stages in many health-related phenomena in which micronutrients have an important but previously unsuspected role.

MAJOR CLINICAL END POINTS

In past years micronutrient requirements have been based primarily on amounts needed to prevent clinical manifestations of deficiency disease. For example, end points have included pathological fractures of bone, visible and palpable thyroid enlargement (goiter), corneal clouding, skin lesions, joint swelling, and mortality rates. This approach has been the classical foundation for investigating vitamin, mineral, and other essential nutrient deficiencies in experimental animals and in many clinical studies involving humans. In other situations little attention has been given to states of mild chronic deficiency, or to the effects of recurrent periods of transitory inadequacy or excess of intake. Likewise, there has been little effort to link biochemical indices of nutritional status and nutrient metabolism (other than lipids) with common chronic diseases. This book has been designed to address some of these issues and, by describing the functional role of micronutrients, to identify areas in which good nutrition may prevent illness.

NEW RESEARCH FINDINGS OF UNCONVENTIONAL ASSOCIATIONS

Entirely aside from intermediate stages which may precede the onset of "classical" manifestations of a deficiency syndrome, more and more epidemiological studies tend to link long-term consumption of higher than standard levels of certain micronutrients with lowered risk of seemingly unrelated diseases. Some examples of this phenomenon include the association of high intakes of beta-carotene with reduced risk of lung cancer; high intakes of vitamin C and E and decreased incidence of senile cataracts; and low intakes of folate and greater risk of certain forms of cancer as well as birth defects. Recently, in a large intervention study, those who had angina and were taking beta-carotene supplements had significantly lower risk of death than the placebo group. Each of these examples seems to reflect a protective function of the nutrient which might not have been anticipated from data available at the time of its original discovery. Also, each seems to depend on exposure to secondary risk factors which may or may not occur in all individuals. The dietary intake requirement may be quite different in persons exposed to a given risk as compared to those not exposed.

ANTIOXIDANTS

Some of the most exciting research today involves the identification of biochemical markers of degenerative disease. Products of lipid peroxidation, the same compounds that cause fats to become rancid, have been linked to several adverse effects such as depressed immune responses, increased inflammation, and cataract formation. The compounds which generate oxygen-containing free radicals have been shown to alter DNA and thus may be critical in the carcinogenic process.

A number of the molecules that protect against oxidative damage are essential micronutrients such as vitamin E, vitamin C, and beta-carotene. In addition, minerals such as zinc, selenium, copper, and manganese are essential to the functioning of the antioxidant enzymes. There is a growing appreciation that as life expectancy increases the cumulative oxidative damage may outweight the antioxidant protective mechanisms. In fact, the concentration of antioxidant vitamins required to balance the peroxidative events can be well above that required to prevent nutritional deficiencies and cannot easily be attained through diet. Fortunately, the antioxidant vitamins have very high safety margins, and supplementation with high doses has not been shown to cause clinically relevant adverse effects.

It has also been found that prevention of many other ills of aging, such as cataracts is strongly associated with long-term high intake of the antioxidant micronutrients. This is really the goal of preventive nutrition—to educate the public to appreciate the importance of years of good nutrient intake to increase the chances for healthy living, especially with increasing age.

WOMEN OF CHILDBEARING POTENTIAL

One population group that can benefit from preventive nutrition is women of childbearing potential. There are data clearly showing that the prepregnancy weight of the mother predicts the weight of the newborn. Moreover, research begun almost 30 years ago strongly suggested that low micronutrient status, especially that of folic acid is implicated in the incidence of serious malformations such as neural tube defects. Current evidence indicates that maternal undernutrition may have adverse effects on the developing fetus even before the mother is aware of the pregnancy. Thus, it is important that young women be made aware of the importance of good nutrition before conception so that dietary modification and nutritional supplementation can commence prior to the embryonic formation of tissues and organs such as the fetal neural tube. The potential for lowering the risk of birth defects becomes even more appealing when one realizes that the use of a single U.S. RDA level multivitamin-mineral supplement daily, which has no known adverse effects associated with its use, has been found to reduce the risk of congenital neural tube defects. Recent studies would strongly suggest that the medical community and the medical insurance firms instruct women contemplating pregnancy to visit a family-planning clinic prior to, rather than after, missing even one menstrual period.

INCREASED VITAMIN NEEDS DUE TO INFECTION

There has never been a question of vitamin supplementation when overt signs of deficiency are found. The widespread practice of vitamin A supplementation for children in third world countries with ophthalmic signs of deficiency is an excellent example of the importance of supplementation with a single vitamin to prevent blindness. Vitamin A supplementation has also been shown to lower the risk of measles-associated mortality in overtly deficient children. Yet there is growing evidence that even marginal deficiency of vitamin A in children is directly linked to increases in measles-associated deaths and mortality. The administration of vitamin A supplements to such children in hospitals overseas significantly lowered death rates. Thus, recognition of the intermediate end point (mild vitamin A deficiency) makes it possible to avert more disastrous consequences.

The intake of vitamin A for women and children at the poverty level in the United States is reported to be less than one-third the recommended intake levels, and there has been a recent increase in measles in young children in the United States. Based on compelling recent evidence of significant benefit and no harm, vitamin A supplementation of U.S. children with measles should not be dismissed out of hand. U.S. children could benefit as much as third world children.

THE BASIS OF DETERMINING OPTIMAL DIETARY RECOMMENDATIONS

During periods of experimentally induced single deficiencies, it becomes obvious that certain tissues maintain higher concentrations of the essential nutrient than others; for instance, during vitamin E depletion the serum level may be undetectable, while the level in the brain remains quite high, especially in the cerebellum. Similarly, apparently selenium-deficient male rodents having no detectable circulating levels have selenium in the testes, the last organ to be depleted of this essential element. Experimental studies of depletion and repletion have consistently shown that tissues and organs have distinctive rates of uptake and loss of essential micronutrients, and that these are also distinct for different micronutrients. Thus, the dietary intake of a specific micronutrient required to saturate tissue stores of one tissue may not be sufficient to meet the requirements of another. For instance, the level of dietary vitamin E sufficient to prevent testicular degeneration, muscle wasting, and hemolysis in rats has been found to be significantly ($2-10 \times$) less than that required for optimal responses of the immune system. Enhancement of immune function has also been observed when healthy, elderly humans were given over 25 times the U.S. RDA(800 IU/day) of vitamin E for 1 month, suggesting a higher requirement of this vitamin for optimal immunity.

It is possible that immune function is not the only sensitive indicator of micronutrient requirements. For certain vitamins, it may be that neurological functions or DNA protection require the highest intakes for the optimal level of protection. These requirements are probably affected by age, lifestyle, genetic predisposition, work environment, economic and other factors. The issue of determining requirements may seem overwhelming when viewed in its entirety, yet a dynamic process based on new research can only help improve the overall understanding of nutritional needs. If requirements are based on the most sensitive index currently known, the needs of the general population can be better served.

PREVENTIVE NUTRITION: DEFINITION

Preventive nutrition can be defined as the use of dietary measures to prevent the development of acute or chronic disease states and to decrease morbidity and mortality associated with such conditions. Successful preventive nutrition programs which are familiar to the medical and lay public include the lowering of intake of cholesterol by those with high circulating cholesterol levels and the curtailment of salt intake by salt-sensitive hypertensives. The consistent association of high dietary intakes of high-soluble-fiber diets with lowered risk of colon cancer has also been accepted as an important preventive strategy.

It seems clear that we are entering an era in which dietary requirements need to be defined in the broadest general terms. Ultimately it may become necessary for a new generation or a new breed of clinical scientist to identify a series of nutritional risk factors and intermediate end points. It will probably be necessary to characterize populations with regard to such matters as occupation, lifestyle, environmental quality, medical history, genetic background, existing disease states, lifestyle habits, such as smoking/drinking/drug use, and even some sort of automated laboratory profile for the biochemical assessment of nutritional status. The latter is a formidable matter but may be feasible at least for representatives of selected population groups.

The chapters that follow are concerned with a wide range of essential micronutrients, their metabolic effects, and the effects of various patterns of intake. In many cases, the data are based on intermediate end points of disease status. There is often a concerted effort to identify risks that can be used in search of desirable patterns of micronutrient intake to prevent disease and maintain health. It is hoped that this volume has highlighted the importance of micronutrients in human health and stimulates further research on the study of intermediate end points and nutrient-related risk factors.

CARDIOVASCULAR FUNCTION

2

Polyunsaturated Fatty Acid Effects on Cellular Interactions

William E. M. Lands

University of Illinois at Chicago
Chicago, Illinois

CRITERIA FOR NUTRITIONAL ADEQUACY AND INADEQUACY

Much of the important nutritional research on the essential fatty acids was completed before we knew of their biosynthetic conversion to the highly potent hormone-like compounds called eicosanoids (which include prostaglandins, thromboxane, leukotrienes, and fatty acid epoxides). Now the curent awareness of the importance of prostaglandins and leukotrienes as signaling agents mediating the actions of polyunsaturated fatty acids in mammalian physiology makes it important to reexamine the early evidence for the need for the essential fatty acids and reevaluate the appropriate limits of the term ''deficiency'' in the context of preventive nutrition. The different types of polyunsaturated fatty acids (see Fig. 1) are known to have competitive interactions in biochemical processes that influence eicosanoid-mediated events. To detect and interpret important competitive interactions between the n-3 and n-6 types of fatty acids, we need to identify physiological criteria for designating when either of these types of fatty acid might be in either inadequate or excessive supply. The purpose of this chapter is to examine the limits of the evidence for human needs in the context of the probable physiological mechanisms involved and to provide a basis for selecting the proportions of dietary n-3 and n-6 polyunsaturated fatty acids suitable for attaining goals in preventive nutrition.

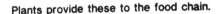

Plants provide these to the food chain.

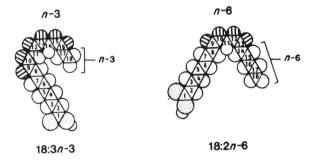

Humans can make these independently.

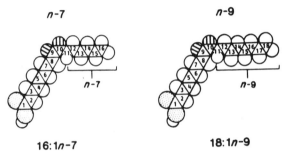

Figure 1 Four different types of unsaturated fatty acid. Each structure represents a common fatty acid that can be elongated and desaturated to long-chain highly unsaturated forms. The location of the last double bond in each acid is described in reference to the "*nth*" carbon (the terminal methyl carbon). (Reprinted from *Fish and Human Health* with permission of Academic Press.)

Description of Physiological Manifestations

The signs of a deficiency that convinced Burr and Burr (1929) that there was such a thing as an essential fatty acid (EFA) included scaly condition of the skin, necrosis of the tail, and degeneration of the kidneys. A 1930 paper added several more signs: growth clearly depended on the presence of highly unsaturated fatty acids in tissue phospholipids; deficient rats drank twice as much water that was not lost in the urine; ovulation was irregular and litters were small in number; males could not sire litters (and many did not even mate); and dietary protein exacerbated the renal degeneration. Reviewing the existing information on fatty acids in tissue phospholipids, those authors (1930) deduced that warm-blooded animals cannot synthesize appreciable quantities of linoleic acid although they can synthesize oleic acid. Therefore linoleic (18:2n-6) and linolenic (18:3n-3) came to be regarded as essential fatty acids.

Later, a valuable clue to the mechanism of action of essential fatty acids came from the observation that either oral linoleate or injected chorionic gonadotropin could restore to normal the weight of testes, prostate, and seminal vesicles in animals made deficient in essential fatty acids (Greenberg and Ershoff, 1951). Apparently, the needed fatty acids were mediating the release of important pituitary hormones that were not adequately supplied in the absence of the essential fatty acids. This concept was extended with the observation that hypophysectomized rats exhibited poor growth and scaly skin characteristic of EFA-deficient animals (Jensen and Privett, 1969; Haeffner and Privett, 1973) even though the animals had typically normal tissue levels of the essential acid 18:2n-6. An interdependency between pituitary function and prostaglandin biosynthesis may also involve a requirement for pituitary hormones to maintain the activity of prostaglandin synthase in peripheral tissues (Privett et al., 1972) as well as the requirement for essential fatty acids in prostaglandin formation that mediates the release of hormones from the hypothalamus and pituitary.

Reviews of the role of prostaglandins in hypothalamic function (Ojeda et al., 1979, 1981) have summarized the important mediating actions of prostaglandins. These actions include releasing adrenocorticotropic hormone (ACTH) from the pituitary [perhaps by increasing corticotropin-releasing hormone (CRH) from the hypothalamus]; enhancing the response of thyroid tissue to thyroid-stimulating hormone (TSH); stimulating growth hormone (GH) release from pituitary by stimulating release of growth hormone-releasing hormone (GRH) from the hypothalamus; promoting prolactin (PRL) release by decreasing the release from the hypothalamus of the prolactin-inhibiting factor (PIF) and increasing the prolactin-releasing factor (PRF); and stimulating the release of gonadotropins [leuteinizing hormone (LH) and follicle-stimulating hormone (FSH)] by stimulating the release of leuteinizing hormone-releasing hormone (LHRH) from the hypothalamus (although PGI_2 decreased LHRH and PGE_2 increased LHRH; Ottlecz and McCann, 1988).

Synthesis of leukotrienes C_4, D_4, and E_4 in appreciable amounts was reported to occur in the hypothalamus and median eminence (Lindgren et al., 1984), and the synthesizing cells also appeared to have significant LHRH content (Hulting et al., 1985). In response to added leukotriene C_4, anterior pituitary cells in culture released LH (but not GH) (Hulting et al., 1985). Incubation of pieces of rat median eminence with LTC_4 and LTD_4 stimulated release of the LHRH (Gerozissis et al., 1987). Thus we now must consider selective eicosanoid modulations of hypothalamic-pituitary function by both prostaglandins and leukotrienes, and we must also consider that the eicosanoids may be synthesized from either the n-3 or n-6 fatty acids.

The pivotal role of hypothalamic function in modulating the release of pituitary hormones and in influencing hunger, sex, and aggression provides a profound area of inquiry regarding the impact of essential fatty acids on the quality of human life, and it creates inescapable consequences from our choices of selecting dietary supplies of the n-3 and n-6 polyunsaturated fatty acids.

Comparisons of Different Acids

Further work by Burr et al. (1932) showed that both linoleic and linolenic (but not oleic) improved the growth of rats suffering from EFA deficiency. Subsequent studies confirmed that linolenic acid (18:3n-3) as well as cod liver oil (with 20:5n-3 and 22:6n-3) gave good growth of rats, but these acids had little effect in preventing the skin abnormality of EFA deficiency (Burr et al., 1940). Thus the polyunsaturated fatty acids could no longer be considered as an interchangeable group, but each individual acid must be evaluated in terms of specific physiological dysfunctions. This distinction was also emphasized by Turpeinen (1937) who showed that some polyunsaturated acids (18:2n-6, 18:3n-3, and 20:4n-6) were effective for growth, whereas the polyunsaturated acid 9, 11, 13–18:3 was inactive. In fact, 20:4n-6 was several fold better than 18:2n-6. Hume et al. (1938) reported that the methyl ester of 22:6n-3 improved weight gain but failed to cure the skin lesions. These authors noted that the principal symptoms described by Burr et al. were reproduced but argued for the importance of using some criterion other than weight increase (which was not necessarily associated with healing skin lesions).

Unfortunately, the diverse physiological dysfunctions associated with a deficit of essential polyunsaturated fatty acids has prevented the development of a constructive consensus even to this date. Three excellent reviews of essential fatty acids (Aaes-Jorgensen, 1961; Holman, 1968; Rosenthal, 1987) describe many of these diverse phenomena, and this chapter focuses on only a few. Holman (1958) once summarized the status of the field with the overview that only the n-6 acids should be regarded as "essential" since they alone were able to prevent both dermal signs and poor weight gain (in contrast to the n-3 acids). The contrast between the n-6 and n-3 acids was also emphasized by Privett et al. (1958), who noted that the growth-promoting activity of the n-3 acids in tuna oil was not accompanied with an ability to prevent dermal symptoms. Clearly, the mediators of growth were not identical to those affecting dermal integrity. Sinclair (1981) emphasized that both n-3 and n-6 types of fatty acid had some essential function, and he objected to restrictive interpretations that permitted only acids with unique features to be assigned as essential fatty acids. Little came from the protest. A major conceptual barrier to forming a constructive consensus seems to be in deciding whether or not we can include as essential an acid that has some—but not all—of the desired qualities.

This uncertainty was apparent in a number of almost bittersweet reports of the search for a requirement for n-3 fatty acids which failed to show that the n-3 acids were needed for any function that *could not be met by 18:2n-6* (Tinoco et al., 1971, 1978; Leat, 1981). For this reason, irrespective of the actions of the n-3 fatty acids in supporting many physiological processes, these acids are often regarded as "not essential." Tinoco et al. (1978) considered that before the question of essentiality can be answered, a *specific* function for the n-3 fatty acids should be conceived and demonstrated. Such a criterion of uniqueness was protested unsuccessfully by Sinclair (1981). Ironically, the inability of the n-3 acids to function as vigorously as n-6 acids in eicosanoid function may actually provide some benefits (see "Formation of Eicosanoids"and "History of Recommendations" below).

Inadequate reproduction paralleled dermal lesions (acrodynia) in being cured by 18:2n-6 or 20:4n-6 (Quackenbush et al., 1942) but not by 18:3n-3. Subsequently, a study of gestation and parturition in rats (Leat and Northrup, 1981) showed that 18:3n-3 was comparable to 18:2n-6 in satisfying the requirements for growth, development, and gestation in the rat but was inadequate for normal parturition. Apparently, the mediators of parturition are not identical to those affecting growth.

The high concentration of highly unsaturated n-3 fatty acids in the retina led to a report that docosahexaenoic acid (22:6n-3) is "involved in the transduction process of visual excitation" (Benolken et al., 1973). This was further studied by Neuringer et al. (1984, 1986) who concluded that dietary n-3 fatty acids are essential for normal prenatal and postnatal development of retina and brain. Such a conclusion also seems related to the report that the learning ability of young rats in a Y maze appeared to be better when the diet contained moderate amounts of n-3 acids (Lamptey and Walker, 1976). In this regard, recent work by Yamamoto et al. (1987) showed that correct response ratios for rats in a brightness discrimination learning test were higher for rats receiving high dietary ratios of n-3/n-6 acids than for those receiving very low ratios of n-3/n-6 acids.

Poor growth on diets containing no polyunsaturated fats was noted for rainbow trout (Castell et al., 1972), and added 18:3n-3 consistently aided growth whereas 18:2n-6 gave erratic results with lower overall average growth. An added behavioral phenomenon with the trout was fainting, or shock syndrome, which occurred when the diets had low ratios of n-3/n-6 fatty acids. More research is needed to determine whether the syndrome represents a response to excessive amounts of n-6 eicosanoid metabolites or to too few n-3 eicosanoid metabolites. The section "Formation of Eicosanoids" considers the possibilities of whether the beneficial function of n-3 acids might be in providing eicosanoids in diminished amounts with diminished function relative to the vigorous action of the n-6 eicosanoids derived from 20:4n-6.

Quantitative Estimates of Need

With several different physiological dysfunctions to evaluate in terms of the actions of essential fatty acids, we might expect that a variety of different levels of requirement would evolve from the many research reports. Unfortunately, few quantitative indices of the physiological requirement for essential fatty acids have been developed to assess the status under controlled conditions, and growth has been the principal quantitative index. For example, growth curves indicating the effectiveness of a fatty acid supplement were used in quantitative comparisons of different fatty acids (Turpeinen, 1937; Greenberg et al., 1950). Growth of young male rats increased proportionally to added linoleate in the range of 5–50 mg/animal/day (~0–0.7% of total dietary calories, i.e., 0–0.7 en%), whereas for female rats the range was only from 0 to 10 mg/animal/day (Greenberg et al., 1950). These authors (working in California) noted that growth with added 18:3n-3 alone was markedly inferior to that with 18:3n-3 combined with 18:2n-6. The results contrasted with the good growth-promoting activity of both acids reported earlier by Burr et al. (1940) (from Minnesota). Apparently, low humidity can increase the requirement for essential fatty acids and can enhance subtle differences between the n-3 and n-6 fatty acids. Thus a modified method for quantitating essential fatty acids was developed with limited drinking water by means of a water-rationing apparatus (Thomassen, 1953). This new method measured growth in a way that placed great importance on the role of water balance when estimating the ability of a supplemental fatty acid to support normal physiology, and it clearly permitted only the n-6 fatty acids to be effective "essential fatty acids" (Thomassen, 1962).

Improvement of gas chromatography and radioisotope techniques in the 1950s permitted a successful test of the hypothesis that 20:3n-9 was formed from 18:1n-9 in the fat-deficient rat (Fulco and Mead, 1959). (Less frequently discussed was the demonstration of a parallel synthesis and accumulation of 20:3n-7 from 16:1n-7 and 18:1n-7.) Many reports indicate a competitive interaction of the four types of unsaturated fatty acids for the elongation and desaturation enzymes (Fig. 2). The disappearance of these triene acids when polyunsaturated fats are included in the diet led Holman (1960) to correlate dietary linoleate with dermal scores and with plasma triene/tetraene ratios, and he suggested the use of that ratio as an alternate index of the EFA status of animals and humans. Dermal scores were significant for animals eating 0.14% of total dietary calories (0.14 en%) as 18:2n-6 but were negligible for animals receiving 0.56 to 20.2 en% 18:2n-6. The transition from 0.14 to 0.56 en% was associated with a change of triene/tetraene ratio from 1.35 to 0.51, indicating that normal physiology could be associated with triene/tetraene ratios greater than 0.5 and less than 1.3.

The most extensive quantitative study of fatty acid requirements in the rat was reported in a series of papers by Mohrhauer and Holman (1963a,b, 1967a,b).

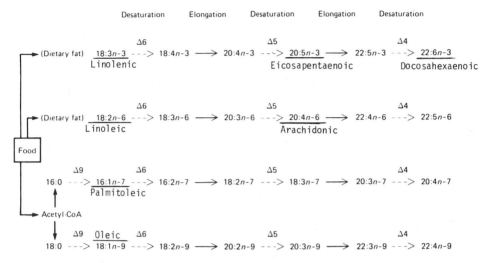

Figure 2 Pathways for forming highly unsaturated fatty acids from simple precursors. (Reprinted from *Fish and Human Health* with permission of Academic Press.)

Extensive data indicated that growth responded proportionally to supplements of 18:2n-6, 18:3n-3, and 20:4n-6, with near-optimal growth when the n-6 acids reached 0.5 en% (Mohrhauer and Holman, 1963a). A subsequent series of 18 diets containing 0.08, 0.3, or 0.6 en% 18:2n-6 (Mohrhauer and Holman, 1963b) produced no severe deficiency symptoms, although mild dermatitis was detected with rats receiving only 0.08 en% 18:2n-6. Thus, the amount of dietary 18:2n-6 that prevented dermal symptoms of EFA deficiency in rats on a sucrose-rich diet was somewhat more than 0.08 and less than 0.3 en% 18:2n-6. Ratios of 20:3n-9/20:4n-6 in liver lipids for the animals on the marginal diets (with mild dermatitis) ranged from 0.8 to 1.9, whereas ratios for the animals free of deficiency symptoms ranged from 0.18 to 0.94. It seems evident from the data (Mohrhauer and Holman, 1963b) that the threshold condition for detecting dermal defects, the most sensitive indicator of physiological deficiency in rats, was associated with about 0.2 en% dietary 18:2n-6 and with a ratio of about 1 for 20:3n-9/20:4n-6 in plasma lipids.

A study of 66 swine on low-fat diets with glucose and/or lactose as the principal carbohydrate (Hill et al., 1961) showed no physiological symptoms (either dermatitis or aortic lesions) even though many animals had liver lipids with triene/tetraene ratios ranging from 1 to 4. The absence of any physiological aberation did not prevent the authors from indicating their belief that the high triene/tetraene ratio was a biochemical "lesion" that should take precedence over the lack of dermatitis in judging EFA deficiency. In another attempt to observe essential fatty acid deficiency in pigs, no difference in growth rate or food conversion was noted for dietary 18:2n-6 in the range of 0.07 to 3.5 en% (Leat, 1962). The diets were rich in starch (rather than sucrose used in most rat studies), and perhaps the stored 18:2n-6 might be effectively redistributed among tissues under these dietary conditions (see Section "Effects of Sugars and Insulin" below). The apparent dietary requirement of pigs for less than 0.07 en% 18:2n-6 in a starch-rich diet was confirmed later by Christensen (1985), who noted no deficiency symptoms with such diets. Clearly, small amounts of 18:2n-6 can meet the needs of these animals. In this regard, the sucrose-rich diet containing 0.08 en% 18:2n-6 was only marginally inadequate in preventing physiological symptoms in rats (Mohrhauer and Holman, 1963a,b). It would be instructive to learn whether 0.07 en% would be adequate in rats with a starch-rich diet that might have less tendency to elevate insulin levels and suppress fat mobilization.

METABOLIC EVENTS INVOLVED

The diverse set of physiological functions affected by the presence or absence of polyunsaturated fatty acids provides a serious challenge to identify a unifying concept of the role for essential fatty acids. One concept that was commonly held 30 years ago considered membrane integrity to be the basis for "essentiality." This concept was based on reports that emphasized the occurrence of mito-chondrial abnormalities (especially partially uncoupled respiration), and it was encouraged by a renaissance in membrane biochemistry at that time. Unfortu-nately, the mechanism for the membrane defect was as poorly defined as the physiological dysfunctions, and there was no clear causal linkage between the apparent membrane defects and the observed physiological defects. Nevertheless, there remain some good reasons to continue to examine membrane biochemistry for additional clues to essential functions of polyunsaturated fatty acids. This chapter regards the important action of essential fatty acids to be in forming eicosanoids with a secondary (but still important) action in ensuring adequate membrane biogenesis.

Formation of Eicosanoids

Several historic events define the rapid, dramatic progress in our understanding of the eicosanoids. The isolation and characterization of the prostaglandins in the period 1950–1960 laid the basis for the discovery (Bergstrom et al., 1964) that these bioactive compounds are biosynthesized from the essential fatty acid, arachidonic acid (20:4n-6). Then a powerful tactic evolved from the discovery of Vane (1971) that the biosynthesis of prostaglandins by cyclooxygenase was blocked by aspirin, indomethacin, and other nonsteroidal anti-inflammatory drugs. This discovery permitted biomedical researchers to test for the modulating role of prostaglandins in a wide range of physiological events by determining whether or not the drugs could modify the physiological outcome. As more research progressed on the biosynthetic intermediates to prostaglandins (see Fig. 3), Hamberg and Samuelsson (1974) were able to identify the metabolic intermediate, PGH_2, and show (1975) its conversion to the short-lived potent agent that mediated platelet aggregation and thrombosis, thromboxane A (TXA_2). Subsequently, Gryglewski et al. (1976) characterized a different metabolite of PGH_2 which was formed by vascular endothelium, the potent antiaggregatory prostacyclin, PGI_2. The two materials, TXA_2 and PGI_2, constitute a significant control system for regulating intracellular levels of cAMP and calcium, thereby affecting the interactions of platelets (and other cells) with the walls of blood vessels.

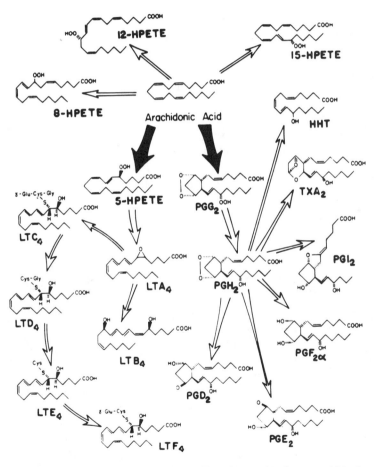

Figure 3 Pathways for forming the major eicosanoids from arachidonic acid (20:4n–6). (Reprinted from *Biochemistry of Arachidonic Acid Metabolism* with permission of Martinus Nijhoff.)

Additional control systems related to immune-inflammatory responses of cells became better understood with the discovery of the leukotrienes, LTB, LTC, and LTD (Murphy et al., 1979). These materials are formed by way of a lipoxygenase activity (rather than the cyclooxygenase), but few therapeutic inhibitors are available to test for the participation of leukotrienes in the way that succeeded so well for prostaglandins with the nonsteroidal anti-inflammatory agents. At this time, nearly every tissue is recognized to have cells that participate in an important physiological or pathophysiological response mediated by either prostaglandins or leukotrienes.

One important factor influencing the action of an eicosanoid is the concentration of the active agent at specific cellular receptors that transduce the signal into cellular responses. The eicosanoids (prostaglandins, thromboxanes, and leukotrienes) are rapidly inactivated by catabolic enzymes, and the evidence suggests that active material is not stored (Crowshaw, 1969; Jouvenaz et al., 1970), but is only formed occasionally in small amounts in response to physiological signaling. These occasional small amounts are rapidly inactivated so that most of the time in normal tissues there is normally not much eicosanoid signaling. In fact, pathophysiology is generally associated with rates of eicosanoid biosynthesis that are greater than normal, and a major effort of the pharmaceutical industry is to provide antagonists to the production of eicosanoids and to their action at specific cellular receptors. Excessive formation and function of eicosanoids are implicated in thrombosis, vasospasm, atherogenesis, arthritis, asthma, headache, dysmenorrhea, immune-inflammatory disorders, and some metastatic processes. This wide variety of disorders provides many interesting opportunities for preventive medicine (Lands, 1986) to accompany the many vigorous therapeutic approaches now available.

The amount of precursor 20:4n-6 for eicosanoid biosynthesis is generally abundant in tissue esters, although the amount of nonesterified substrate may be limiting (Lands and Samuelsson, 1968). Certainly, a severe dietary deficiency of essential fatty acids seems likely to limit the rate of eicosanoid biosynthesis and thereby alter physiological responses. When eicosanoids are formed slowly, they tend to be metabolically inactivated before they can fully occupy the receptor. In this way any event that slows the *rate* of eicosanoid biosynthesis can markedly diminish receptor-mediated signals, even though the same overall amount of eicosanoid is eventually synthesized (and metabolized). The well-recognized competition between the n-3 and n-6 types of polyunsaturated fatty acids can slow the rate of formation of n-6 eicosanoids and thereby diminish the abundance of active material at cellular receptors. There are two indirect tactics for examining the role of n-6 eicosanoids in physiology in a manner achieved with nonsteroidal anti-inflammatory agents by Vane (1971): relating altered physiological responses in EFA-deficient animals, and relating altered responses when the n-3/n-6 abundances have been altered.

A major difference in reaction rate with the n-3 and n-6 fatty acids was noted for cyclooxygenase with 20:5n-3 forming prostaglandin at a negligible rate under conditions in which 20:4n-6 reacted rapidly (Lands et al., 1973). The lower synthetic rate with 20:5n-3 is especially sensitive to the inhibition by peroxidases that remove the hydroperoxide activators essential for fatty acid oxygenase action (Lands and Pendleton, 1988). In addition, the active forms of the eicosanoids from 20:5n-3 are often less active than those from 20:4n-6 at receptors (Needleman et al., 1979; Lee et al., 1985). Thus, lower rates of formation and function of eicosanoids can be expected when increased amounts of n-3 fats are included in the diet. This phenomenon was evident with decreased experimental myocardial infarction in dogs fed fish oil (Culp et al., 1980). Concern for marginal statistical differences for platelet function in humans ingesting fish oil was partially resolved by demonstrating the nonlinear relation between thromboxane synthetic capacity and the observed percent aggregation (Lands et al., 1985). Many individuals produced much more thromboxane than was needed for full aggregation, so that many responses were not in the linear dose-response range.

The rate of biosynthesis of eicosanoids from 20:4n-6 clearly affects platelet signaling (via thromboxane) and it may also be important in modulating the activity of alpha-adrenergic receptors that mediate arrhythmias (Reibel et al., 1988; McLennan et al., 1988) and vasospasm (Lockette et al., 1982). The actions of dietary n-3 fatty acids in reducing myocardial ischemic damage (Hock et al., 1987) may be in antagonizing the formation and/or function of n-6 leukotrienes that appear to mediate the ventricular vulnerability to fibrillation (Cooper et al., 1988) and may enhance the hypoxia-induced increase in alpha-adrenergic receptor levels (Heathers et al., 1987). Also, ingesting fish oil, with its n-3 fatty acids, diminished the vascular hyperresponsiveness in patients with Reynaud's phenomenon (DiGiacomo et al., 1989). In this regard, Berry and Hirsch (1986) reported that the content of 18:3n-3 in adipose tissue (but not 18:2n-6) was significantly related to lower blood pressure in humans. Clearly there is much information to justify a vigorous examination of the possible benefits of increased dietary ratios of n-3/n-6 polyunsaturated fatty acids.

Formation of Membrane Lipoproteins

During the growth and differentiation of a cell there are many occasions for the alteration of cellular membranes, and an inadequate supply of membrane lipid precursors might cause inadequate assembly and inadequate subsequent physiological responses. The need for an adequate supply of an essential fatty acid is readily observed during in vitro culture conditions when the synthesis of certain types of fatty acids that are needed for cell integrity may not occur. For example, cultured cells that cannot synthesize unsaturated fatty acids are dependent on an exogenous supply of these acids to maintain growth, cell division, and proper physiology (Henning et al., 1969; Keith et al., 1969). Because mammalian cells cannot synthesize de novo either the n-3 or the n-6 type of polyunsaturated fatty acids, they might exhibit inadequate physiological functions if the n-3 and/or n-6 types of fatty acids were preferred for biosynthesis and were not adequately available. Investigators have reported little difference among 18:1n-9, 18:2n-6, and 18:3n-3 in modifying the behavior of single cells in culture (e.g., Rosenthal, 1987). However, a single-cell culture system does not express the many important intercellular interactions with other adjacent cell types that are vital to integrated physiological behavior. Thus the essential phenomena that must be monitored may be subtle and difficult to measure in cell culture.

In the absence of any clear cellular requirement for either an n-3 or an n-6 polyunsaturated fatty acid, it may be helpful to review the development and differentiation of eukaryotic cells faced with a deficit of an unsaturated fatty acid that cannot be synthesized. In the assembly of the mitochondrial membrane, there is a time period during which a supply of certain unsaturated fatty acids is needed to give functional respiratory units (Walenga and Lands, 1975a,b). The preexisting esterified fatty acids in other membranes of the cells are not able to replace the need for fresh supplies during the assembly of new membranes. In the absence of fresh supplies, the cells failed to develop adequate respiratory membranes under conditions that usually would induce functional respiratory membrane units. An additional model of the consequences of cellular requirements is in assembling a new nucleic acid–membrane complex for the replication and segregation of the mitochondrial gene, which seems more demanding than nuclear genes in requiring an adequate supply of certain unsaturated fatty acids (Graff et al., 1983). As a result, cellular division could be maintained with nutrient fatty acid supplies that did not permit adequate replication of the mitochondrial gene, and a large percentage of the daughter cells (not receiving the mitochondrial gene) were permanently unable to develop functional respiratory units, irrespective of later "adequate" supplies of the needed fatty acids.

These examples illustrate that even a transient inadequate supply of a needed fatty acid can impair the subsequent development of a needed function if it occurs at a time of rapid membrane assembly. Such a situation might occur during the rapid fetal and postnatal development of neural and retinal membranes that contain large amounts of 22-carbon polyunsaturated fatty acids. The 22-carbon acid derivatives seem preferred by the CDP ethanolamine:diacylglycerol ethanolaminephosphotransferase (Kanoh and Ohno, 1974; Masuzawa et al., 1982, 1986). Factors that limit the availability of highly unsaturated 22-carbon acids (which cannot be synthesized de novo) during a time of differentiation and development might impair the subsequent physiology of the cells. It seems possible that the facile elongation and desaturation of n-3 acids (see Lands, 1989) may ensure adequate supplies of C-22 acids at perinatal stages of rapid neural development.

Alteration of Liver Lipoprotein Formation

For many years, biomedical researchers have been aware of the ability of polyunsaturated fatty acids to decrease fatty acid biosynthesis and the secretion of lipoproteins by liver. Unfortunately, the mechanism of this suppression has not yet been elucidated. For example, elevated rates of fatty acid biosynthesis in rats fed high-sucrose, EFA-deficient diets returned to control values in 4 days after supplementation with 18:2n-6, 20:4n-6, or 18:3n-3 (Chu et al., 1969). The proportion of 18:2 in lipids did not seem to be a critical factor since dietary 18:3n-3 and 20:4n-6 decreased synthetase while tissue contents of 18:2n-6 remained unchanged. Another report (Flick et al., 1977) appeared to eliminate signaling by prostaglandins as the mechanism for this effect of polyunsaturated fatty acids when similar reductions in fatty acid synthesis were observed in either the presence or absence of the prostaglandin endoperoxide synthase inhibitor indomethacin. Subsequent work has shown 20:5n-3 to decrease lipoprotein secretion under conditions in which 18:1n-9 stimulated secretion (Nestel et al., 1984). Recently, a report (Williams et al., 1989) noted that 18:3n-3, 20:4n-6, or 22:6n-3 (but not 18:1n-9) reduced hepatic triglyceride secretion in vivo. These reports have significance for preventive nutrition in relation to other reports noting a selective lowering of plasma triglyceride by dietary fish oils for humans (Nestel et al., 1984; Sanders et al., 1985). Hopefully, we can identify advisable tactics to prevent unreasonable rates of fatty acid biosynthesis without depending solely on the suppressive action of elevated dietary polyunsaturated fatty acids (by what is still an unknown mechanism). Continued attention to the triglyceride and cholesterol contents of plasma lipoproteins seems certain to lead researchers to an eventual elucidation of the mechanism for this interesting phenomenon.

DIETARY INTAKE, BIOAVAILABILITY, AND TURNOVER RATES

Extracellular and Intracellular NEFA

Early research on prostaglandin biosynthesis noted that the abundant phospholipid reservoir of arachidonate was not directly oxygenated to form prostaglandins, but that the oxidative biosynthesis occurred with the nonesterified fatty acid (Lands and Samuelsson, 1968). Since that time much attention has been placed on a need for phospholipase action to provide sufficient quantities of substrate for sustained biosynthesis of appreciable quantities of the active hormone-like derivatives. Unfortunately, a significant sustained biosynthesis may be pathological, so that attention has been on the composition of the esterified precursors with too little attention on the composition of the actual precursor pool, the nonesterified fatty acids (NEFA). It is the composition of the NEFA that most probably controls the transient rates of biosynthesis of the eicosanoids (see Fig. 4).

A simple illustration of the dynamic impact that can be made by fatty acids in the NEFA pool is in the rapidly fatal consequence of injecting 20:4n-6 (but *not* 18:1, 18:2, 20:5, etc.) into rabbits (Silver et al., 1974). A less severe, but related, phenomenon occurs when feeding the ethyl ester of 20:4n-6 to healthy male volunteers; platelet aggregability with ADP became so enhanced that two of the four volunteers were removed from the protocol (Seyberth et al., 1975). Alternatively, the rapid entry of antagonists into the NEFA pool underlies the successful therapeutic use of ibuprofen, a competitive inhibitor ($K_i = \sim 2\ \mu M$) of arachidonate binding to the prostaglandin synthase (Rome and Lands, 1975). The rapid acceptance of this agent after its commercial introduction indicates the relief that can be provided in diminishing overrapid biosynthesis of prostaglandins with an inhibitory fatty acid analog. Ingesting 1 mmol of ibuprofen leads to elevated plasma levels of about 100 μM within an hour (Kaiser and Van Geissen, 1974), which then fall to about 10 μM by about 5 hr as the material is steadily cleared into the urine. The rapid entry of this 13-carbon fatty acid analog into cellular NEFA permits it to antagonize prostaglandin biosynthesis. It then tends to remain in the extracellular and intracellular NEFA pools because it has an alpha-methyl branched chain that prevents reaction with CoA and precludes incorporation into cellular lipids.

Other fatty acids have been shown to antagonize arachidonate conversion to prostaglandins (such as 20:5n-3 and 22:6n-3; $K_i = \sim 2\ \mu M$; Lands et al., 1973), but their increased concentration in the NEFA pool is counteracted by activation to CoA esters and esterification into cellular lipids in a manner similar to that of 20:4n-6. Nevertheless, during times when dietary n-3 acids are moving through the NEFA pool, a suppression of the rate of synthesis of n-6 eicosanoids seems inevitable, and decreased receptor occupancy is the consequence.

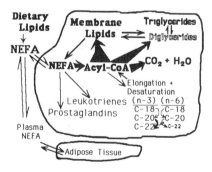

Figure 4 Flow of nutrient acids into cellular metabolic processes.

A major concern for the possible risk from too much dietary polyunsaturated fatty acid comes from its positive association with increased proliferation of mammary (Carroll and Braden, 1985; Hubbard and Erickson, 1987), colon (Reddy and Maruyama, 1986) and pancreatic (O'Connor et al., 1989) tumors in experimental animal models. The increased proliferation appears to be mediated by n-6 eicosanoids since it can be antagonized by antiprostaglandin drugs (Narisawa et al., 1981; Kollmorgen et al., 1983) and also by dietary n-3 fatty acids (Carroll and Braden, 1985; Reddy and Maruyama, 1986; O'Connor et al., 1989; Nelson et al., 1988). Thus, it seems not to be a general effect of polyunsaturated fatty acids per se, but is another aspect of eicosanoid signaling among cells that is facilitated by greater supplies of n-6 substrate and diminished by greater supplies of the n-3 analogs.

An important, detailed dose-response study (lp et al., 1985) employed eight carefully controlled diets containing varied amounts of 18:2n-6 that ranged from 1 en% to 23 en%. The number of breast tumors in the rats after treatment with dimethylbenzanthracene was greater with increased amounts of dietary 18:2n-6: 2/1 en%; 9/2.2 en%; 11/4.4 en%; 17/11.5 en%. The results indicated no "safe" lower limit below which there was no risk of tumor enhancement. As a result, a concern for preventive nutrition must raise the question of whether there is any merit in ingesting more of the n-6 precursors of the eicosanoids than the minimum demonstrated to be needed for young growing mammals (~0.3–0.5 en%). Because serious tumors in humans tend to occur only long after growth has ceased, the question about intakes of 18:2n-6 greater than needed takes on even more importance in light of the absence of any clear physiological evidence of a dietary need by free-living adults. Clearly, we need better evidence before one could designate upper and lower thresholds for a safe "permissible" dietary range of 18:2n-6. The evidence suggests that for Americans ingesting 7–10 en% 18:2n-6 (20-fold greater than evident need!), much more arachidonate may be available in the tissues than is desirable for rational preventive nutrition.

Effects of Sugars and Insulin

The inability to create the symptoms of essential fatty deficiency in adult animals may be most easily attributed to the accumulation of adipose tissue stores of linoleate. For example, the average content of 18:2n-6 in human adipose tissue fat is about 12% of total fatty acids. This would represent 1.5 kg of 18:2n-6 in a 70-kg male with 18% body fat or 1.65 kg in a 55-kg female with 25% body fat; a formidable reservoir of essential fatty acids!

The first description of a clinical deficiency in an adult human (Collins et al., 1971) occurred when a dry, scaly rash developed on the face and chest following more than 60 days of fat-free intravenous therapy. This sensitive indicator of a deficiency of n-6 fatty acids (but not n-3 fatty acids) disappeared after fat was administered, reappeared after a month of fat-free infusion, and then disappeared when fat was again added to the infusion. The appearance of dermal symptoms only occurred several weeks after the level of 20:3n-9 in plasma phospholipids became greater than that for 20:4n-6. The detailed report of Collins et al. (1971) provided the first clear evidence that the threshold for the biochemical index of an essential fatty acid deficiency (a sustained ratio of 20:3n-9/20:4n-6 greater than 1) correlated to the clinical signs in an adult human. This value of about 1 was also obtained for liver lipids in rats on the marginally deficient diet that produced a mild dermatitis (Mohrhauer and Holman, 1963b). Apparently the continuous infusion of glucose prevented the mobilization of the adipose reservoir of 18:2n-6. Further study of parenteral feeding (Wene et al., 1975) showed that healthy, well-nourished adult humans had elevated levels of 20:3n-9/20:4n-6 in serum lipids within a few days of being infused continuously with a fat-free diet that contains glucose. There was a drop in 18:2n-6 to about 2.3% of phospholipid fatty acids [one-tenth of the baseline level of 23%] while 20:3n-9 rose to about 3% of fatty acids, giving a ratio of 20:3n-9/20:4n-6 greater than 1. Fasting, which decreases circulating insulin levels and leads to mobilization of adipose fatty acids, can cause a rise in plasma linoleate as the total circulating NEFA rises (Connor, 1975). The alternate fasting and feeding that occurs in a typical day's activities usually leads to twofold changes in circulating NEFA, and it seems likely that the vast reserves of adipose 18:2n-6 can be available to free-living individuals without any concern for a functional deficiency as occurred with continuous, prolonged parenteral feeding. The possibility that dietary n-3 acids may alter the degree of induction of lipid-synthesizing enzymes (Flick et al., 1977; Johnson and Berdanier, 1987) has opened new initiatives for evaluating the impact of dietary n-3/n-6 ratios.

RECOMMENDED DIETARY SUPPLEMENTS FOR HUMANS

History of Recommendations

Two important nutrient thresholds must be regarded: one below which it is inadvisable to ingest less because of the risk of a deficiency, and another above which it is inadvisable to ingest more because of the risk of overreactions. Between these two thresholds there may be a wide range of permissible levels which an individual may select in accord with individual priorities. Biomedical research is needed to define the physiological criteria that indicate those thresholds and to help interpret the consequences of choices made in the permissible range.

Physiological or clinical evidence of a deficient state in humans is rarely obtained, and ethical considerations make it unlikely that much future evidence will ever be available under controlled conditions. Thus, the demonstration of deficiency symptoms in rats has provided the principal type of experimental evidence to support the concept of a requirement of "essential fatty acids" by mammals. Fortunately, the results with rats have many close parallels with those from humans, but unfortunately the limited quantitative evidence for a requirement has not been treated rigorously or consistently, and the historic process of interpreting recommended levels of intake for humans needs careful reexamination. Two official reports placed the n-3 and n-6 fatty acids in a recommended status for humans: in 1958, the Food and Nutrition Board of the NAS/NRC declared that "judging from animal experiments," 1 or 2 en% 18:2n-6 "should be adequate"; and in 1978, the Food and Agriculture Organization of the United Nations recommended that linolenic acid (n-3 fatty acids) be "included in human diets." This section examines the quantitative clinical evidence of fatty acid requirements for humans.

An early report of therapeutic use of dietary polyunsaturated fatty acids with infantile eczema (Hansen, 1933) noted an improvement in skin appearance as the iodine value of the serum lipids rose in treated infants. A subsequent report (Hansen, 1937) noted that some relationship existed between eczema and a disturbance in lipid metabolism, but there was no indication that the diet accounted for the low degree of unsaturation of serum lipids of breast-fed eczematous infants. Hansen (1937) noted that an uncertainty as to proper criteria for diagnosis, together with the danger of confusion due to a characteristic tendency to spontaneous remissions and recurrences, should make one cautious in drawing rigid conclusions about eczema and polyunsaturated fats. Two decades later, he joined Wiese et al. (1958) in describing several infants who had mild attacks of diarrhea when receiving skim milk; some infants had drying of the skin, which appeared to be related to a low intake of essential fatty acids. Serum fatty acid levels of 10.5% diene, 2.7% triene, and 7.4% tetraene were associated with 1 en% dietary 18:2n-6 (somewhat arbitrarily described as "minimum normal" conditions), whereas different levels (23.7% diene, 0.6% triene, and 10% tetraene) were noted for 4 en% 18:2n-6 (described as "optimum"). Hansen et al. (1958) also provided a preliminary report of 27 infants whose parents approved having them on a low-fat regimen for periods from 2 weeks to 12 months. The results showed that young healthy infants may develop dermal symptoms within a relatively short time, and these can be reversed with small amounts of added linoleate.

This report was followed by a clinical observation (Combes et al., 1962) of 71 infants ingesting for a period of 40 days one of three diets containing either 0.01, 0.5, or 4.5 en% 18:2n-6. During the study, the infants showed no unusual skin changes and no significant difference in weight gain; however, the serum lipids showed clear differences that reflected the dietary supply of 18:2n-6 in a manner parallel to that seen for rats on experimental diets. As the dietary 18:2n-6 rose, the dienoic and tetraenoic acids also rose: from 0.01 (6 and 4%) to 0.5 (11 and 5%) to 4.5 en% (23 and 12%). Thus, a wide range of fatty acid compositions may occur in individuals with apparently normal clinical status. However, it will be important to evaluate the consequence of having the abundance of the tetraene eicosanoid precursor increasing several fold. However, the authors, reaffirming the need for caution in interpreting the evidence, noted that diets containing from 0.4 to 0.9 en% of dietary essential fatty acids had produced thousands of well-grown infants without any clinical evidence of nutritional deficiency. The diet with 0.5 en% 18:2n-6 led to a ratio of about 1 for triene/tetraene acids in serum (Combes et al., 1962). A recalculation and reappraisal of these results (Cuthbertson, 1976) indicated that the amount of dietary linoleate needed to prevent symptoms in infants was probably less than 0.5 en%.

The most comprehensive report of the need for essential fatty acids by infants involved 428 infants studied over a 4-year period (Hansen et al., 1963). The study involved five different feeding formulas that contained different levels of linoleate: 0.04, 0.07, 1.3, 2.8, and 7.3 en% 18:2n-6. In the first 3 months of life, many infants (21 of 32; 66%) receiving the first diet had loose stools, whereas only 29 of 65 (45%) on the second diet had that condition, and the other diets produced no dose-related effect (7 of 103; 7 of 116; and 9 of 112). Similarly, 100% of the full-term infants receiving the first diet (0.04 en% 18:2n-6) showed dryness of skin, desquamation, and redness, whereas only 40% of those receiving the second diet (0.07 en% 18:2n-6) showed these signs. The latter group had an average serum ratio for triene/tetraene acids of about 1.4 whereas infants ingesting 1.3 en% 18:2n-6 (and free of deficiency symptoms) had an average ratio of 0.3. Unfortunately, the study included no diets in the important range of 0.1–0.5 en% 18:2n-6, leaving unexplored an important range that would define the lower threshold for preventive nutrition. The range of 0.1–0.5 en% 18:2n-6 (with 20:3n-9/20:4n-6 ratios near 1) was also the range in which experimental studies with rats showed no further signs of essential fatty acid deficiency (see "Quantitative Estimates of Need" above).

By 1981, the lack of direct evidence for a unique essential role for n-3 fatty acids that could not be fulfilled by n-6 fatty acids left the 1978 FAO/UN recommendation of dietary n-3 fatty acids in an uncertain status. That status changed with the report (Holman et al., 1982) of neurological symptoms in a 6-year-old girl (undergoing long-term total parenteral feeding) which diminished a few months after the regimen was changed to include 18:3n-3. Five years later, two reports of possible deficiencies of 18:3n-3 (Bjerve et al., 1987 a,b) described a scaly dermatitis in patients on long-term gastric tube nutrition which cleared with essential fatty acid supplementation. In critically reviewing the evidence, Anderson and Connor (1989) argued against the likelihood that skin lesions were suitable evidence of an n-3 deficiency, and they reemphasized a concern for the tendency of continuous glucose infusion to block the release of essential fatty acids from adipose stores. At this time, there remains very little clear evidence for a unique role for n-3 acids that cannot be met by n-6 fatty acids. Nevertheless, the probable importance of the n-3 fatty acids in forming the membrane lipids of retinal and neural tissues (and other tissues) supports retaining the 1978 recommendation of the FAO/UN for including some n-3 polyunsaturated fatty acids in the diet.

Possible Alternative Recommendations

Twenty years ago, when little was known about prostaglandins (and thromboxane, prostacyclins, and leukotrienes had not been discovered), medical researchers encouraged the consumption of greater amounts of n-6 polyunsaturated fatty acids in an attempt to lower serum triglycerides and cholesterol, which are risk factors for thrombosis and atherosclerosis linked to excessive dietary saturated fats. Much attention was placed on increasing the P/S ratio by increasing the dietary polyunsaturated fat (with predominantly n-6 fats!). Although greatly reduced intakes of saturated fats would probably have produced better results in reducing those risk factors, the increased use of n-6 fats prevailed. In the absence of any clear rationale for harm, more and more fats rich in n-6 acids were included in the diet until our average national intake may be 20 times more than our need. Now we know that excessive formation and function of n-6 eicosanoids is associated with a wide variety of chronic disorders, and we have reason to ask, "What level of n-6 ingestion is too much to avoid overreactions?" Clear answers are not easily obtained, but some compelling clues are available (see "Extracellular and Intracellular NEFA" above). Certainly the evidence accumulated in the past few years withdraws support for an earlier hypothesis (Lands, 1986) that megadoses of 18:2n-6 might usefully diminish n-6 eicosanoid signaling.

Now biomedical researchers are increasingly exploring the benefits of including more n-3 fatty acids in the diet to antagonize the excessive formation and function of n-6 eicosanoids. It seems timely to consider whether or not decreased intakes of n-6 fats might provide better general health than ingesting large amounts of n-3 fats (Lands, 1986). As benefits appear to derive from the antagonistic actions of n-3 fatty acids from the diet, there is an obvious need to answer the question, "What ratio of n-3/n-6 will eventually cause a threshold deficit in n-6 function?" Although the n-6-mediated functions leading to thrombosis, arthritis, and metastasis seem greater than desired, we do not yet have a sound philosophical basis for deciding whether our hypothalamic and pituitary functions tend to be greater or less than desired. The scientific community has a full palette and an unprecedented opportunity to paint a picture of the nutrition and physiology of human health and disease with broad strokes and also with finer detail. The primary need is for focused research that will provide quantitative descriptions of physiological parameters in terms of upper and lower threshold transitions.

While waiting for better physiological and clinical evidence, some dietary choices may still be possible with the existing information. Evidence for the existence of low thresholds for n-6 fats would lead to inclusion of only 0.5 en%

18:2n-6 and 0.5 en% n-3 fatty acids to ensure meeting essential needs. Individuals could monitor the relative proportions of dietary n-3/n-6 by the occurrence of both n-3 and n-6 fatty acids in plasma lipids. Also, the question of excessive intake of dietary polyunsaturated fatty acids might be monitored by the level of 20:3n-9 in plasma lipid, with excessive intakes correlating with a suppression of 20:3n-9 below detectable levels.

Although some monoenoic acid (18:1n-9) might be included to increase the caloric density, there is insufficient evidence that this type of fatty acid can appreciably diminish any tendency for excessive induction of fatty acid biosynthetic enzymes in the liver with its concomitant overproduction of secreted triglycerides.

There appears to be no physiological requirement for any saturated fat, and its only apparent role is in increasing caloric density; useful for active, growing children, but not a very necessary feature for sedentary adults. In addition, there is no clear requirement for total fat calories per se. Above 20 en% as fat, the amount of physical activity and the desired caloric density of the diet will influence choices, and there is a generally increasing tendency to discourage ingesting total fat above the 30 en% level. To monitor their status in this regard, individuals could probably use indices of ''ideal'' weight maintainance as a physiological index for diet decisions.

Thus individuals have a wide range of ''permissible,'' discretionary fat intake from about 4 en% to 20 en%. In this range, individuals may benefit from knowing that the minimum threshold of 1 en% of combined n-3 and n-6 nutrient polyunsaturated fatty acids will be met by almost any mixture of foods that are available. Attention can then turn away from concern for the lower threshold and be placed on attaining desired ratios of n-3/n-6 fatty acids and deciding how to establish personal goals for the upper thresholds of permissible intake. In the absence of a major reduction in dietary n-6 fats, individuals may wish to obtain the moderating effects of dietary n-3 fats.

REFERENCES

Aaes-Jorgensen E. Essential fatty acids. Physiol Rev 1961; 41:2–46.

Anderson GJ, Connor WE. On the demonstration of n-3 essential-fatty-acid deficiency in humans. Am J Clin Nutr 1989; 49:585–587.

Benolken RM, Anderson RE, Wheeler TG. Membrane fatty acids associated with the electrical response in visual excitation. Science 1973; 182:1253–1254.

Bergstrom S, Danielsson H, Klenberg D, Samuelsson B. The enzymatic conversion of essential fatty acids into prostaglandins. J Biol Chem 1964; 239:4006.

Berry EM, Hirsch J. Does dietary linolenic acid influence blood pressure? Am J Clin Nutr 1986; 44:336–340.

Bjerve KS, Mostad IL, Thoresen L. Alpha-linolenic acid deficiency in patients on long-term gastric-tube feeding: Estimation of linolenic acid and long-chain unsaturated n-3 fatty acid requirement in man. Am J Clin Nutr 1987a; 45:66–77.

Bjerve KS, Fischer S, Alme K. Alpha-linolenic acid deficiency in man: Effect of ethyl linolenate on plasma and erythrocyte fatty acid composition and biosynthesis of prostanoids. Am J Clin Nutr 1987b; 46:570–576.

Burr GO, Burr MM. A new deficiency disease produced by rigid exclusion of fat from the diet. J Biol Chem 1929; 82:345–367.

Burr GO, Burr MM. On the nature and role of the fatty acids essential in nutrition. J Biol Chem 1930; 86:587–620.

Burr GO, Burr MM, Miller ES. On the fatty acids essential in nutrition. III. J Biol Chem 1932; 97:1–9.

Burr GO, Brown JB, Kass JP, Lundberg WO. Comparative curative values of unsaturated fatty acids in fat deficiency. PSEBM 1940; 44:242–245.

Carroll KK, Braden LM. Dietary fat and mammary cancer. Nutr Cancer 1985; 6:254–259.

Castell JD, Sinnhuber RO, Wales JH, Lee DJ. Essential fatty acids in the diet of rainbow trout (Salmo gairdneri): Growth, feed conversion and some gross deficiency symptoms. J Nutr 1972; 102:77–86.

Christensen K. Determination of linoleic acid requirements in slaughter pigs. Report from the National Institute of Animal Science, Denmark, Copenhagen.

Chu L-C, McIntosh DJ, Hincenbergs I, Williams MA. Dietary unsaturated fatty acids and liver fatty acid synthetase in rats. Biochim Biophys Acta 1969; 187:573–575.

Collins FD, Sinclair AJ, Royle JP, Coats DA, Maynard AT, Leonard RF. Plasma lipids in human linoleic acid deficiency. Nutr Metabol 1971; 13:150–167.

Combes MA, Pratt EL, Wiese HF. Essential fatty acids in premature infant feeding. Pediatrics 1962; 30:136–144.

Connor WE. Pathogenesis and frequency of essential fatty acid deficiency during total parenteral nutrition. Ann Int Med 1975; 83:895–896.

Cooper DR, Kelliher GJ, Kowey PR. Modulation of arachidonic acid metabolites and vulnerability to ventricular fibrillation during myocardial ischemia in the cat. Am Heart J 1988; 116:1194–1200.

Crowshaw K. Biosynthesis of renal prostaglandins. Fed Proc 1969; 28:845.

Culp BR, Lands WEM, Lucchesi BR, Pitt B, Romson J. The effect of dietary supplementation of fish oil on experimental myocardial infarction. Prostaglandins 1980; 20:1021–1031.

Cuthbertson WFJ. Essential fatty acid requirements in infancy. Am J Clin Nutr 1976; 29:559–568.

DiGiacomo RA, Kremer JM, Shah DJ. Fish-oil dietary supplementation in patients with Raynaud's phenomenon: A double blind, controlled, prospective study. Am J Med 1989; 86:158–164.

Flick PK, Chen J, Vagelos PR. Effect of dietary linoleate on synthesis and degradation of fatty acid synthetase from rat liver. J Biol Chem 1977; 252:4242–4249.

Food and Agriculture Organization of the United Nations. Dietary fats and oils in human nutrition. FAO Food and Nutrition Paper 1978; 3, p. 19, FAO, Rome, Italy.

Food and Nutrition Board Report. Natl Acad Sci/Nat Res Council Publ 575, 1958.

Fulco AJ, Mead JF. Metabolism of essential fatty acids. 8. Origin of 5,8,11-eicosatrienoic acid in the fat-deficient rat. J Biol Chem 1959; 234:1411–1416.

Gerozissis K, Saadi M, Dray F. Leukotrienes C4 and D4 stimulate the release of leutinizing hormone-releasing hormone from rat median eminence in vitro. Brain Res 1987; 416:54–58.

Graff G, Sauter J, Lands WEM. Selective mutational loss of mitochondrial function can be caused by certain unsaturated fatty acids. Arch Biochem Biophys 1983; 224:342–350.

Greenberg SM, Calbert CE, Savage EE, Deuel HJ, Jr. The effect of fat level of the diet on general nutrition. J Nutr 1950; 41:473-486.

Greenberg SM, Ershoff BH. Effects of chorionic gonadotropin on sex organs of male rats deficient in essential fatty acids. Proc Soc Expt Biol Med 1951; 78:552–554.

Gryglewski RJ, Bunting S, Moncada S, Flower RJ, Vane JR. Arterial walls are protected against deposition of platelet thrombi by a substance (prostaglandin X) which they make from prostaglandin endoperoxides. Prostaglandins 1976; 12:685–713.

Haeffner EW, Privett OS. Development of dermal symptoms resembling those of an essential fatty acid deficiency in immature hypophysectomized rats. J Nutr 1973; 103:74–79.

Hamberg M, Samuelsson B. Prostaglandin endoperoxides. VII. Novel transformations of arachidonic acid in guinea pig lung. Biochem Biophys Res Commun 1974; 61:942.

Hamberg M, Samuelsson B. Thromboxanes: A new group of biologically active compounds derived from prostaglandin endoperoxides. Proc Natl Acad Sci USA 1975; 72:2994–2999.

Hansen AE. Serum lipid changes and therapeutic effects of various oils in infantile eczema. PSEBM 1933; 31:160–161.

Hansen AE. Serum lipids in eczema and in other pathologic conditions. Am J Dis Child 1937; 53:933–946.

Hansen AE, Haggard ME, Boelsche AN, Adam DJD, Wiese HF. Essential fatty acids in infant nutrition. III. Clinical manifestations of linoleic acid deficiency. J Nutr 1958; 66:565–576.

Hansen AE, Wiese HF, Boelsche AN, Haggard ME, Adam DJD, Davis H. Role of linoleic acid in infant nutrition. Clinical and chemical study of 428 infants fed on milk mixtures varying in kind and amount of fat. Pediatrics 1963; 31:171–192.

Heathers GP, Yamada KA, Kanter EM, Corr PB. Long-chain acylcarnitines mediate the hypoxia-induced increase in al-adrenergic receptors on adult canine myocytes. Circ Res 1987; 61:735–746.

Henning U, Dennert G, Rehn K, Deppe G. Effects of oleate starvation in a fatty acid auxotroph of Escherichia coli K-12. J Bacteriol 1969; 98:784–796.

Hill EG, Warmenen EL, Silbernick CL, Holman RT. Essential fatty acid requirement in swine. 1. Linoleate requirement estimated from triene:tetraene ratio of tissue lipids. J Nutr 1961; 74:335–341.

Hock CE, Holahan MA, Reibel DK. Effect of dietary fish oil on myocardial phospholipids and myocardial ischaemic damage. Am J Physiol 1987; 21:H554–H560.

Holman RT. Essential fatty acids. Nutr Rev 1958; 16:33–35.

Holman RT. The ratio of trienoic: Tetraenoic Acids in tissue lipids as a measure of essential fatty acid requirement. J Nutr 1960; 70:405–410.

Holman RT. Essential fatty acid deficiency. Prog Chem Fats Lipids 1968; 9:275–348.

Holman RT, Johnson SB, Hatch TF. A case of human linolenic acid deficiency involving neurological abnormalities. Am J Clin Nutr 1982; 35:617–623.

Hubbard NE, Erickson KL. Enhancement of metastasis from a transplantable mouse mammary tumor by dietary linoleic acid. Cancer Res 1987; 47:6171–6175.

Hulting A-L, Lindgren JA, Hokfelt T, Eneroth P, Werner S, Patrono C, Samuelsson B. Leukotriene C4 as a mediator of leutinizing hormone release from rat anterior pituitary cells. Proc Natl Acad Sci USA 1985; 82:3834–3838.

Hume EM, Nunn LC, Smedley-Maclean I, Smith HH. Studies of the essential unsaturated fatty acids in their relation to the fat-deficiency disease of rats. Biochem J 1938; 32:2162–2177.

Ip C, Carter CA, Ip MM. Requirement of essential fatty acid for mammary tumorigenesis in the rat. Cancer Res 1985; 45:1997–2001.

Jensen B, Privett OS. Effect of hypophysectomy on lipid composition in the immature rat. J Nutr 1968; 99:210–216.

Johnson BJ, Berdanier CD. Effect of menhaden oil on the responses of rats to starvation-refeeding. Nutr Rep Int 1987; 36:809–817.

Jouvenaz GH, Nugteren DH, Beerthuis RK, VanDorp DA. A sensitive method for the determination of prostaglandins by gas chromatography with electron-capture detection. Biochim Biophys Acta 1970; 202:231–234.

Kaiser DG, Van Geissen GJ. GLC determination of ibuprofen [(+ −)2-(p-isobutyl-phenyl)propionic acid] in plasma. J Pharm Sci 1974; 63:217–221.

Kanoh H, Ohno K. Substrate-selectivity of rat liver microsomal 1,2-diacylglycerol: CDPcholine(ethanolamine) Choline(ethanolamine)phosphotransferase in utilizing endogenous substrates. Biochim Biophys Acta 1974; 380:199–207.

Keith AD, Resnick MR, Haley AB. Fatty acid desaturase mutants of Saccharomyces cerevisiae. J Bacteriol 1969; 98:415–420.

Kollmorgen GM, King MM, Kosanke SD, Do, C. Influence of dietary fat and indomethacin on the growth of transplantable mammary tumors in rats. Cancer Res 1983; 43:4714–4719.

Lamptey MS, Walker BL. A possible essential role for dietary linolenic acid in the development of the young rat. J Nutr 1976; 106:86–93.

Lands WEM. Fish ahd human health. Orlando: Academic Press, 1986: 1–186.

Lands WEM. n-3 Fatty acids as precursors for active metabolic substances: Dissonance between expected and observed events. J Int Med 1989; 225, Suppl. 1:11–20.

Lands WEM, Samuelsson B. Phospholipid precursors of prostaglandin. Biochim Biophys Acta 1968; 164:426–429.

Lands WEM, LeTellier PR, Rome LH, Vanderhoek JY. Inhibition of prostaglandin biosynthesis. Adv Biosci 1973; 9:15–27.

Lands WEM, Culp BR, Hirai A, Gorman R. Relationship of thromboxane generation to the aggregation of platelets from humans: Effects of eicosapentaenoic acid. Prostaglandins 1985; 30:819–825.

Lands WEM, Pendleton RB. n-3 Fatty acids and hydroperoxide activation of fatty acid oxygenases. In: Simic MG, Taylor KA, Ward JF, vonSonntag C, eds, Oxygen radicals in biology and medicine. New York: Plenum Press, 1988; 675–681.

Leat WMF. Studies on pig diets containing different amounts of linoleic acid. Br J Nutr 1962; 16:559–569.

Leat WMF. Man's requirement for essential fatty acids. TIBS 1981; April: IX–X.

Leat WMF, Northrop CA. Effect of linolenic acid on gestation and parturition in the rat. Prog Lipid Res 1981; 20:819–821.

Lee TH, Hoover RL, Williams JD, Sperling RI, Ravelese JR III, Spur BW, Robinson DR, Corey EJ, Lewis RA, Austen KF. N Engl J Med 1985; 312:1217–1223.

Lindgren JA, Hokfelt T, Dahlen S-E, Patrono C, Samuelsson B. Leukotrienes in the rat central nervous system. Proc Natl Acad Sci. USA 1984; 81:6212–6216.

Lockette WE, Webb EC, Culp BR, Pitt B. Vascular reactivity and high dietary eico-sapentaenoic acid. Prostaglandins 1982; 24:631–639.

Masuzawa Y, Nakayawa, Waku K, Lands WEM. Distinctive incorporation of docosate-traenoic acid by Ehrlich ascites tumor cells. Biochem Biophys Acta 1982; 713:185–192.

Masuzawa Y, Okano S, Waku K, Sprecher H, Lands WEM. Selective incorporation of various C-22 polyunsaturated fatty acids in Ehrlich ascites tumor cells. J Lipid Res 1986; 27:1145–1153.

McLennan PL, Abeywardena MY, Charnock JS. Dietary fish oil prevents ventricular fibrillation following coronary artery occlusion and reperfusion. Am Heart J 1988; 116:709–717.

Mohrhauer H, Holman RT. The effect of dose level of essential fatty acids upon fatty acid composition of the rat liver. J Lipid Res 1963a; 4:151–159.

Mohrhauer H, Holman RT. Effect of linolenic acid upon the metabolism of linoleic acid. J Nutr 1963b; 8:67–74.

Mohrhauer H, Rahm JJ, Seufert J, Holman RT. Metabolism of linoleic acid in relation to dietary monoenoic fatty acids in the rat. J Nutr 1967a; 91:521–527.

Mohrhauer H, Holman RT. Metabolism of linoleic acid in relation to dietary saturated fatty acids in the rat. J Nutr 1967b; 91:528–534.

Murphy RC, Hammarstrom S, Samuelsson B. Leukotriene C: A slow-reacting substance from murine mastocytoma cells. Proc Natl Acad Sci USA 1979; 76:4275–4279.

Narisawa T, Sato M, Tani M, Kudo T, Takahashi T, Goto A. Jnhibition of development of methylnitrosourea-induced rat colon tumors by indomethacin treatment. Cancer Res 1981; 41:1954–1957.

Needleman P, Raz A, Minkes M, Ferrendelli JA, Sprecher H. Triene prostaglandins: prostacyclin and thromboxane biosynthesis and unique biological properties. Proc Natl Acad Sci USA 1979; 76:944–948.

Nelson RL, Tanure JC, Andianopolous G, Souza G, Lands WEM. A comparison of dietary fish oil and corn oil in experimental colorectal carcinogenesis. Nutr Cancer 1988; 11:215–220.

Nestel PJ, Connor, WE, Reardon MF, Connor S, Wong S, Boston R. Suppression by diets rich in fish oil of very low density lipoprotein production in man. J Clin Invest 1984; 74:82–89.

Neuringer M, Conner WE, Van Petten C, Barstad L. Dietary omega-3 fatty acid deficiency and visual loss in infant rhesus monkeys. J Clin Invest 1984; 73:272–276.

Neuringer M, Connor WE, Lin DS, Barstad L, Luck S. Biochemical and functional effects of prenatal and postnatal omega-3 fatty acid deficiency on retina and brain in rhesus monkeys. Proc Natl Acad Sci USA 1986; 83:4021–4025.

O'Connor TP, Roebuck BD, Peterson FJ, Lokesh B, Kinsella JE, Campbell TC. Effect of dietary omega-3 and omega-6 fatty acids on development of azaserine-induced pre-neoplastic lesions in rat pancreas. J. Natl Cancer Inst 1989; 81:858–863.

Ojeda SR, Naor Z, Negro-Vilar A. The role of prostaglandins in the control of gonadotropin and prolactin secretion. Prostagl Med 1979; 5:249–275.

Ojeda SR, Negro-Vilar A, McCann SM. Role of prostaglandins in the control of pituitary hormone secretion. In: Physiopathology of endocrine diseases and mechanisms of hormone action. New York: Alan R. Liss, 1981:229–247.

Ottlecz A, McCann SM. Concomitant inhibition of pulsatile luteinizing hormone (LH) and stimulation of prolactin release by prostacyclin (PG12) in ovariectomized (OVX) conscious rats. Life Sci 1988; 43:2077–2085.

Privett OS, Aaes-Jorgensen E, Holman RT, Lundberg WO. The effect of concentrates of polyunsaturated acids from tuna oil upon essential fatty acid deficiency. J Nutr 1958; 67:423–432.

Privett OS, Phillips F, Fukazawa, Kaltenbach CC, Sprecher HW. Studies on the relationship of the synthesis of prostaglandins to the biological activity of essential fatty acids. Biochim Biophys Acta 1972; 280:348–355.

Quackenbush FW, Kummerow FA, Steenbock H. The effectiveness of linoleic, arachidonic and linolenic acids in reproduction and lactation. J Nutr 1942; 24:213–224.

Reddy BS, Maruyama H. Effect of dietary fish oil on azoxymethane-induced colon carcinogenesis in male F344 rats. Cancer Res 1986; 46:3367–3370.

Reibel, DK, Holahan MA, Hock, CE. Effects of dietary fish oil on cardiac responsiveness to adrenoceptor stimulation. Am J Physiol 1988; 254:H494–H499.

Rome LH, Lands WEM. Structural requirements for time-dependent inhibition of prostaglandin biosynthesis by anti-inflammatory drugs. Proc Natl Acad Sci USA 1975; 72:4863–4865.

Rosenthal MD. Fatty acid metabolism of isolated mammalian cells. Prog Lipid Res 1987; 26:87–124.

Sanders TAB, Sullivan DR, Reeve J, Thompson GR. Triglyceride-lowering effect of marine polyunsaturates in patients with hypertriglyceridemia. Arteriosclerosis 1985; 5:459–465.

Seyberth HW, Oelz O, Kennedy T, Sweetman BJ, Danon A, Frolich JC, Heimberg M, Oates JA. Increased arachidonate in lipids after administration to man: effects on prostaglandin biosynthesis. Clin Pharmacol Therap 1975; 18:521–529.

Silver MJ, Hoch W, Kocsis JJ, Ingerman CM, Smith JB. Arachidonic acid causes sudden death in rabbits. Science 1974; 183:1085–1087.

Sinclair HM. The relative importance of essential fatty acids of the linoleic and linolenic families: Studies with an eskimo diet. Prog Lipid Res 1981; 20:897–899.

Tinoco J. Williams MA, Hincenbergs I, Lyman RL. Evidence for nonessentiality of linolenic acid in the diet of the rat. J Nutr 1971; 101:937–946.

Tinoco J, Babcock R, Hincenbergs I, Medwadowski B, Maljanich P, Williams MA. Linolenic acid deficiency. Lipids 1978; 14:166–171.

Thomasson HJ. Biological standardization of essential fatty acids (a new method). Int Rev of Vit Res 1953; 25:62–82.

Thomasson HJ. Essential fatty acids. Nature 1962; 194:973.

Turpeinen O. Further studies on the unsaturated fatty acids essential in nutrition. J Nutr 1937; 15:351–366.

Vane J. Inhibition of prostaglandin synthesis as a mechanism of action for aspirin-like drugs. Nature New Biol 1971; 231:232–235.

Walenga RW, Lands WEM. Effectiveness of various unsaturated fatty acids in supporting growth and respiration in Saccharomyces cerevisiae. J Biol Chem 1975a; 250:9121–9129.

Walenga RW, Lands WEM. Requirements for unsaturated fatty acids for the induction of respiration in saccharomyces cerevisiae. J Biol Chem 1975b; 250:9130–9136.

Wene JD, Connor WE, DenBesten L. The development of essential fatty acid deficiency in healthy men fed fat-free diets intravenously and orally. J. Clin Invest 1975; 56:127–134.

Wiese HF, Hansen AE, Adam DJD. Essential fatty acids in infant nutrition. J Nutr 1958; 66:345–360.

Williams MA, Tinoco J, Yang Y-T, Bird MI, Hincenbergs I. Feeding pure docosahexaenoate or arachidonate decreases plasma triacylglycerol secretion in rats. Lipids 1989; 24:753–758.

Yamamoto N, Saitoh M, Moriuchi A, Nomura M, Okuyama H. Effect of dietary a-linolenate/linoleate balance on brian lipid compositions and learning ability of rats. J Lipid Res 1987; 23:144.

3

Vitamin E Supplementation and Platelet Function

Manfred Steiner

Memorial Hospital of Rhode Island
Pawtucket, Rhode Island

INTRODUCTION

Platelets constitute one of the four main components of the hemostatic system, which protects the body from the effects of trauma and preserves the integrity of blood vessels. Platelets represent a "first-line" defense in this system, which also includes the vessel wall, and the coagulation and fibrinolytic systems. Although lacking a nucleus and thus the ability to divide, platelets are extremely complex cellular structures whose metabolic products may influence the activity of the cell wall and in turn are affected by products released from the vascular endothelium. Platelets are also essential for an optimal operation of the coagulation system. Upon activation, platelets become very sticky, adhere to a variety of surfaces and to each other, and their membrane allows rapid activation of certain coagulation factors. The stimuli that "activate" platelets are manifold and are mentioned in greater detail later in this chapter. The coagulation process involves a complex series of reactions that eventually changes the soluble plasma protein fibrinogen to an insoluble form, fibrin, which links and reinforces the platelet plug that is formed when platelets are rendered sticky. The fourth component of the hemostatic mechanism, the fibrinolytic system, is not directly linked to the platelets and subserves the prevention of an unrestrained progression of the clotting mechanism.

This sequence of events is set in motion at times under circumstances in which the continuity of the blood vessel has not been disrupted. The damage sustained

35

to the endothelium of the vascular system by atherosclerosis allows the blood to come in contact with the collagenous tissue of the subendothelium, thereby leading to platelet activation.

Platelets play an important role in the formation of thrombi, whether they occur in the arterial or the venous circulation. In arterial thrombosis the formation of a platelet plug is the indispensible initiating event, whereas in veins stasis and damage to the vascular endothelium usually precipitate thrombosis. This difference in the pathophysiological role of platelets in the initiation of thrombus formation in the different vascular trees has important implications for the therapy of these conditions. Antiplatelet agents are the agents used to prevent thromboembolic disease in the arterial circulation, whereas anticoagulants are the agents of choice to prevent venous clots.

Platelets may also have a direct role in the development of arterisoclerotic changes of blood vessels. A growth factor, platelet-derived growth factor, which is released from platelets upon activation, is a potent mitogen for mesenchymal cells, leading to the proliferation of the smooth muscle cells of blood vessels, a process that characterizes arteriosclerotic disease. In addition, platelets have receptor sites for low-density lipoproteins, important participants in the development of this disease of blood vessels. Thus, platelets occupy a central role in hemostasis, whether it occurs under physiological or pathological circumstances.

The participation of platelets, the cellular elements generated by megakaryocytes, in the initial phase of hemostasis is characterized by a sudden change of their discoid shape to a contracted, spherical form with multiple, elongated, thin projections extruding from the platelet body. The sudden alteration in the morphological appearance of the platelet upon activation by an agonist is accompanied by profound structural changes of the platelet cytoskeleton and the granular elements within. The release of nucleotides, biogenic amines, and a variety of proteins, some with enzyme activity, enriches the immediate environment of the activated platelets with substances some of which can induce similar changes in platelets that become exposed to them. There has been great progress in understanding the biochemical events and their temporal sequence that accompany the activation of platelets. A complex system of messengers, quite similar to those responsible for cellular activation of the exocrine system, produces a contractile response of the actomyosin system and extensive changes in the cytoskeleton as well as the membrane glycoproteins.

The fact that the activation of platelets is accompanied by a marked consumption of oxygen and that platelets contain a large amount of polyunsaturated fatty acids, primarily in the form of 5,8,11,14-eicosatetraenoic acid (arachidonic acid), provides a natural setting for the development of lipid peroxidation. Because of its well-known antioxidant effect, alpha-tocopherol was thought to be a potential inhibitor of platelet activation. Although this question has now been investigated for close to 15 years, there is still uncertainty as to which platelet functions are affected by this natural antioxidant and how inhibitory effects may be explained. Nonetheless, considerable progress has been made, especially in certain animal species in whom dietary intake levels of vitamin E can be drastically varied and deficiency states can be compared to different levels of tissue saturation. Some of the more recent findings on the effect of alpha-tocopherols on the adhesion of human platelets point to a new direction that research in this area may be taking. This chapter focuses an experimental findings in an effort to find common ground among the sometimes disparate results. A review of the various theories that have been advanced to explain the purported effects of alpha-tocopherol on platelet function will probably not be able to provide the reader with a simple explanation of the way vitamin E affects platelet behavior, but hopefully will convey the current thinking on this matter by the investigators involved in this research.

Finally, a note on the composition of this chapter. Each of the sections describing the effect of vitamin E on a specific platelet function has been prefaced by a brief review that delineates the nature of the platelet function and briefly reviews its relation to hemostasis. Because of space constraints, many individual references to these "general aspects" have been omitted. A large number of reviews on various aspects of platelet function, biochemistry, and morphology are available. For the interested reader, the following texts are recommended: Weiss (1975), Gerrard and White (1976), Marcus (1978), Phillips and Shuman (1986).

TOCOPHEROL LEVELS IN HUMAN PLATELETS

The measurements of tocopherol in human platelets show considerable variation. While earlier reports may have been suspect as to the accuracy of the assay method employed, more recent methodology relying primarily on high-pressure liquid chromatographic estimation shows that tocopherol assays are not as susceptible to methodological variability as the previous ones. Nevertheless, the wide variability has persisted and probably reflects far-ranging differences in individual vitamin E intake. A summary of some of the more recently published values of platelet alpha-tocopherol levels is shown in Table 1. The systematic evaluation of platelet tocopherol levels in men and women by Lehmann et al. (1988) and in a small group of men and women (unpublished data) showed no statistically significant difference. Behrens and Madere (1986) noted no distinct difference in serum vitamin E concentrations between men and women. There are only few analyses of age-dependent differences in platelet vitamin E levels. Vericel et al. (1988) and Vatassery et al. (1983) found significant age-dependent decreases in alpha- and gamma-tocopherol concentrations of platelets. Vericel et al. (1988), on the other hand, did not detect an effect of age on plasma tocopherol levels. However, a large-scale, detailed report (Behrens and Madere, 1986), in

Table 1 Platelet Tocopherol Levels

Ref.	Alpha-tocopherol[a]	Gamma-tocopherol[a]
Lehmann et al. (1988)	0.77 ± 0.02	0.20 ± 0.02
Vatassery et al. (1983a)	0.77 ± 0.004	0.23 ± 0.02
Nordoy and Strom (1975)	1.21 ± 0.534	0.18 ± 0.081
Vatassery et al. (1983b)	0.82 ± 0.03	0.24 ± 0.025
Kockmann et al. (1988)	3.25 ± 0.17	—
Jandak et al. (1989)	0.68 ± 0.03	—

[a] Mean ± SEM. All measurements of platelet tocopherol levels are reported as nmol/L × 10^9 platelets. When results were expressed per gram protein, a conversion value of 1.8 mg protein/L × 10^9 platelets was used.

which a correlation between age and alpha-tocopherol concentrations in serum was made, shows a definite tendency for levels to increase with advancing age. Most investigators found linear correlations between tocopherol levels of platelets and those in plasma (Vatassery et al., 1983a; Lehmann et al., 1988; Steiner and Anastasi, 1976).

Compared to alpha-tocopherol, gamma-tocopherol constitutes a relatively small portion of the total tocopherol concentration in the platelet (Nordoy and Strom, 1975; Vatassery et al., 1983; Lehmann et al., 1988; Vericel et al., 1988). A change in the dietary habits in the United States has resulted in soy bean oil becoming the predominant dietary fat (Bieri and Evarts, 1974a). As it contains almost eight times more gamma-tocopherol than alpha-tocopherol, the former vitamer is the most abundant tocopherol in our diet at the present time. Studies by Bieri and his associates (Peake et al., 1972; Bieri and Evarts, 1974a) have shown that its absorption from the intestinal tract equals that of alpha-tocopherol, but its concentration in plasma and in platelets, as well as in other tissues, is only one-fourth to one-tenth that of alpha-tocopherol (Nordoy and Strom, 1975; Vatassery et al., 1983a,b; Lehmann et al., 1988). A faster tissue turnover may be responsible for the markedly lower biological activity of gamma-tocopherol, approximately 10% that of alpha-tocopherol (Brubacher and Wieser, 1967; Bieri and Evarts, 1974b). A study of a large number of healthy men and women ranging in age from 19 to 70 showed that serum gamma-tocopherol did not show the age-dependent increase that was characteristic of the serum alpha-tocopherol levels (Behrens and Madere, 1986). In addition, these authors noted an inverse relation between alpha- and gamma-tocopherol levels in serum. This manifested itself especially when the diet was supplemented by increasing doses of alpha-tocopherol (Lehmann et al., 1988). As the supplementation level of vitamin E increased, a progressive rise in alpha-tocopherol levels of platelets and plasma was accompanied by a progressive decrease in gamma-tocopherol levels. Platelets appear to be the blood components most sensitive to different levels of vitamin E intake (Lehmann et al., 1988; Vatassery et al., 1983b). They are possibly the most accurate indicators of the nutritional vitamin E status of an individual.

PLATELET AGGREGATION

General Aspects

Platelet function in clinical conditions is usually evaluated by assaying platelet aggregation. The popularity of this test is probably due to the simple methodology that permits accurate quantitative measures of this platelet function (Born and Cross, 1963). Under standard conditions, platelet aggregation is evaluated by following changes in the optical transmission of a stirred plasma suspension of platelets as a function of time.

Platelets participate in the initial phase of hemostasis by adhering to exposed collagenous tissue. The shape change that is induced in platelets is accompanied by a release of a wide range of substances from three different types of subcellular granules including, among others, nucleotides, serotonin, calcium, a variety of hydrolytic enzymes when lysosomal release is part of the activation phenomenon, mitogens, e.g., platelet-derived growth factors, clotting factors, e.g., factor V, von Willebrand factor, thrombospondin, and several other proteins (Table 2). In

Table 2 Platelet Granule Contents

(Electron) dense granules	Alpha granules	Lysosomal granules
ADP	Platelet factor 4	Acid phosphatase
ATP	(heparin neutralizing factor)	Beta-glycerophosphatase
Serotonin	Beta-thromboglobulin)	Collagenase
Calcium	Platelet basic protein	Beta-N-acetylglucosaminidase
Pyrophosphate	Von Willebrand factor	Galactosidases
	Factor V	Cathepsins
	Factor VIII	Aryl sulfatase
	Thrombospondin	Fucosidases
	High molecular weight kininogen	Beta-glucuronidase
	Fibronectin	Alpha-mannosidase
	Fibrinogen	Alpha-arabinosidase
	Albumin	
	Platelet-derived growth factor (PDGF)	
	Transforming growth factor (TGF-B)	

addition, changes in the configuration, exposure, and distribution of membrane glycoproteins take place. The release of agonists into the environment of adherent platelets allows platelets in their immediate vicinity to undergo shape change and to interact by clumping with the platelets that have attached themselves to the collagenous tissue exposed by the loss of endothelial cell continuity.

A multitude of substances are known to induce activation of platelets under experimental conditions, but only a few are physiologically important platelet activators. Collagen, especially types IV and V but also I and III, provide the initiating impulse for platelet activation under physiological conditions of hemostasis. Specific receptors for this protein exist on the platelet surface and a plasma protein also present in platelets, von Willebrand factor, mediates the adherence of platelets to collagen. The nucleotide ADP propagates platelet activation by recruiting other platelets into the activation process initiated by the contact of platelets with collagen. In addition, activation-induced changes in the lipids of platelet membranes provide a matrix for the activation of certain clotting factors. The protease thrombin, an important product of the coagulation cascade, is a potent platelet-aggregating agent which causes specific changes in platelet glycoproteins and has its major function in the late stages of the hemostatic process converting the soluble plasma protein fibrinogen to the insoluble fibrin. Platelet-activating factor, a phospholipid generated by the activated platelet, is a very potent aggregating agent whose physiological role in the hemostatic process is not yet completely clear. Finally, thromboxane A_2, the end product of the oxidative conversion of arachidonic acid in stimulated platelets, is the most potent aggregating agent known at present. It too is a very important agent propagating platelet activation, being responsible for rendering the growing platelet clump incapable of dissociating again (Hamberg et al., 1975).

Platelet aggregation can be inhibited by a large number of drugs, especially those belonging to the group of nonsteroidal anti-inflammatory agents. The primary example of the latter, acetylsalicylic acid (aspirin), leads to irreversible acetylation of cyclooxygenase, the enzyme instrumental in converting arachidonic acid to biologically functional oxidative degradation products. Even though the aspirin-induced inhibition of this enzyme is complete, it does not entirely prevent platelet aggregation, thus underlining the fact that platelet activation is a multifactorial process in which the oxidative conversion of arachidonic acid is only one pathway of producing platelet-activating substances.

The highly oxidative milieu in which platelet activation takes place was responsible for the initial trials of alpha-tocopherol, a natural antioxidant agent, as a potential inhibitor of platelet activation and release.

Effect of Alpha-Tocopherol

The first to demonstrate an inhibitory effect of alpha-tocopherol on platelet aggregation were Higashi and Kikuchi (1974) who inhibited hydrogen peroxide-induced platelet clumping in vitro by addition of alpha-tocopheryl acetate or nicotinate. The formation of lipid peroxides, which rises sharply when platelets undergo the release reaction, could be inhibited in vitro by the addition of vitamin E (Steiner and Anastasi, 1976). The addition of alpha-tocopherol in concentrations of 0.9 mM, a 15- to 40-fold excess of the normal alpha-tocopherol concentration of human plasma, produced virtually complete inhibition of platelet activation induced by ADP, collagen, or epinephrine (Fig. 1). The release reaction as evaluated by the discharge of 5-hydroxytryptamine from electron-dense granules as well as by the release of *N*-acetylglucosaminidase from lysosomes was inhibited in a dose-dependent manner by in vitro addition of alpha-tocopherol (Fig. 2). The formation of malonaldehyde-yielding lipid peroxides was decreased commensurate to the amount of alpha-tocopherol added. Similar results were obtained by other investigators (Fong, 1976; White et al., 1977; Agradi et al., 1981; Srivastava, 1986). Experiments performed with platelets of various animal species also showed the effectiveness of alpha-tocopherol as an inhibitor of platelet aggregation (MacIntosh et al., 1987; Diez Marques et al., 1987; Machlin et al., 1975).

It was of considerable interest when first reported that oxidized vitamin E

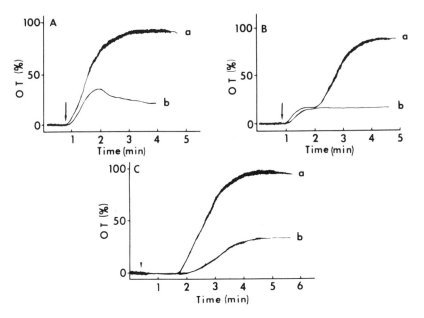

Figure 1 Alpha-tocopherol-induced inhibition of platelet aggregation promoted by 2.5 μM ADP (A), 2.5 μM epinephrine (B), and 70 μg/ml collagen (C). Curve (a) control; curve (b) 0.9 mM alpha-tocopherol. [From Steiner and Anastasi (1976).]

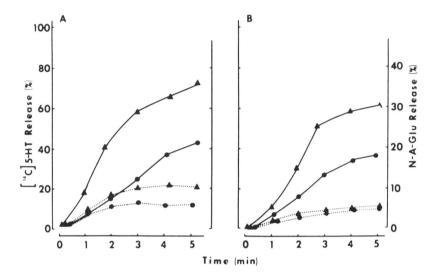

Figure 2 Inhibition by alpha-tocopherol (final concentration 1.5 mM) of the platelet release reaction. [^{14}C]5-Hydroxytryptamine release (triangles); *N*-acetylglucosaminidase release (circles). Aggregation was induced by 70 μg collagen (A) and 5 μM epinephrine (B). Solid lines, control platelets; dotted lines, vitamin E-enriched platelet suspensions. [From Steiner and Anastasi (1976).]

preparations, i.e., alpha-tocopheryl quinone, were more effective inhibitors of platelet aggregation and secretion than the alpha-tocopherol itself. However, this observation by Cox et al. (1980) was subsequently shown to be due to the byproducts of nitric acid oxidation of vitamin E which the authors used to generate the quinone (Mower and Steiner, 1982). Although tocopheryl quinone per se does not have the purported effect that Cox et al. (1980) ascribed to it, it has an antiaggregating effect on platelets that is approximately equal to that of alpha-tocopherol (Mower and Steiner, 1982). Even though the quinone is not totally lacking in antioxidant power, its equal effectiveness to the fully reduced form of vitamin E gives one pause to consider the antioxidant capability as the sole determinant for the antiplatelet activity of these substances.

Compared to normal plasma levels, the concentrations of alpha-tocopherol needed to accomplish an effective inhibition of platelet stimulation are relatively high, and difficult if not impossible to achieve under in vivo conditions. It is therefore not surprising that ex vivo experiments in subjects on vitamin E supplementation ranging from 200 to 1200 IU/day failed to show the inhibitory activity that alpha-tocopherol was able to exhibit in vitro (Steiner, 1983; Stampfer et al., 1988; Kockmann et al., 1988). A careful analysis of these results shows that the testing of the effect of alpha-tocopherol supplementation was usually not done at the threshold level of a particular platelet agonist. Thus, minor reductions in platelet aggregability, as could be seen in normal women when collagen was used to induce aggregation (Steiner, 1983), may be easily missed. Virtually all of the reports in the literature that denied an antiaggregation effect of dietary vitamin E supplementation tested platelet aggregation at some arbitrary level of platelet agonist which probably was in excess of the threshold dosage still capable of inducing complete platelet activation. There is no doubt, however, that the alpha-tocopherol levels which can be obtained with ''reasonable'' doses of vitamin E supplementation are insufficient to produce an inhibition of platelet activation of the degree that is quite readily achieved by administration of aspirin and some of the other nonsteroidal anti-inflammatory platelet agents (Weiss, 1982).

The effectiveness of alpha-tocopherol as a platelet inhibitory agent is more easily shown in animals. Comparison of vitamin E-depleted with vitamin E-replete animals clearly demonstrates a marked difference in the response of platelets to aggregating agents (Machlin et al., 1975; McIntosh et al., 1987). There is generally a marked increase of platelet responsiveness to the agonists tested in conditions of vitamin E deficiency and at least normalization or a decrease of platelet responsiveness under conditions of supplemental vitamin E intake. Machlin et al. (1975) found a markedly increased platelet number and aggregability in vitamin E-deficient Sprague–Dawley rats. Similarly, Bendich et al. (1986) demonstrated an inverse relationship between the platelet count and the plasma vitamin E level in weanling male spontaneously hypertensive rats (genetically related to the Wistar Kyoto rat). Whitin et al. (1982), on the other hand, were unable to demonstrate these effects of vitamin E deficiency in other rat strains and in mice. Therefore, species differences have to be considered in evaluating animal experiments.

McIntosh et al. (1987) examined the effect of vitamin E and linoleate, both of which are present in high concentrations in sunflower seed oil, in a group of marmoset monkeys. The two dietary components were evaluated independently for their influence on a variety of parameters including platelet reactivity. A diet marginally deficient in vitamin E compared to a supplemented one showed a significant enhancement of platelet aggregability in response to collagen. The lack of or very weak antiaggregatory activity that alpha-tocopherol supplementation produces in humans is therefore probably due to the replete vitamin E status of normal individuals. Additional supplementation, unless possibly given in extremely high doses, is thus incapable of exerting a very noticeable desensitization of platelets to agonistic stimulation.

Heightened aggregatory response of platelets has been described by a number of authors in patients suffering from diabetes mellitus (Sagel et al., 1975; Colwell et al., 1976; Davis et al., 1985). Careful assessment of their vitamin E status shows that many insulin-dependent (Type I) diabetic subjects have decreased platelet tocopherol concentrations compared to normal individuals, although the plasma levels of alpha-tocopherol were found to be normal (Karpen et al., 1985). Supplementation of their diet with vitamin E produces a normalization of alpha-tocopherol in platelets and restores their aggregability to a normal pattern (Gisinger et al., 1988; Colette et al., 1988). Similar observations were made in strepto-zotocin-induced diabetic rats (Karpen et al., 1982), which showed decreased vitamin E levels and increased platelet aggregability before vitamin E supple-mentation of their diets and normalization of these values after vitamin E sup-plementation.

An interesting relation between tissue vitamin E levels and platelet survival could be demonstrated in spontaneously hypertensive rats. The stroke-prone rat model showed significantly decreased tissue vitamin E levels compared to the normotensive, genetically related Wistar Kyoto strain. Koganemaru and Ku-ramoto (1982) reported a significant reduction of platelet survival in spontaneously hypertensive rats that were fed a regular diet, but a normal survival upon ad-ministration of a vitamin E-supplemented diet. The platelet survival of stroke-resistant spontaneously hypertensive rats was normal when these animals were fed a regular diet, but shortened when they were supplied with a vitamin E-free diet. These findings therefore suggest that deficiency of vitamin E results in a shortening of the platelet survival time. Platelet production evaluated by [^{75}Se]selenomethionine was found to be enhanced when vitamin E was deficient in these animals. In humans with hyperlipoproteinemias of types II and IV, dietary vitamin E supplementation was found to suppress evaluated concentrations of plasma lipid peroxides and produced a moderate suppressant effect on platelet aggregability (Szczeklik et al., 1985).

PLATELET PROSTANOID METABOLISM

General Aspects

Platelets are capable of synthesizing eicosanoids, a series of oxygenated products of eicosa-5,8,11,14-tetraenoic acid (ω-6), and arachidonic acid, which are gen-erated in response to the stimulation of platelets by agonists (Fig. 3). Arachidonate is released by a phospholipase A_2 that is specific for phosphatidylinositol, by the combined action of phospholipase C, which is phosphatidylinositol-specific, and diacylglycerol lipase, and possibly by a phosphatidic acid-specific phospholipase. Both phospholipase A_2 and C are calcium-dependent but the phosphatidylinositol-specific phospholipase C was shown to function in platelets at concentrations of calcium which can also be found in unstimulated platelets (Rink et al., 1982). The phosphatidylinositol polyphosphate 1,4,5-triphosphate is a potent calcium mobilizer. 1,2-Diacylglycerol, an important lipid intermediate of the phosphati-dylinositol pathway, is produced upon receptor stimulation and functions as a

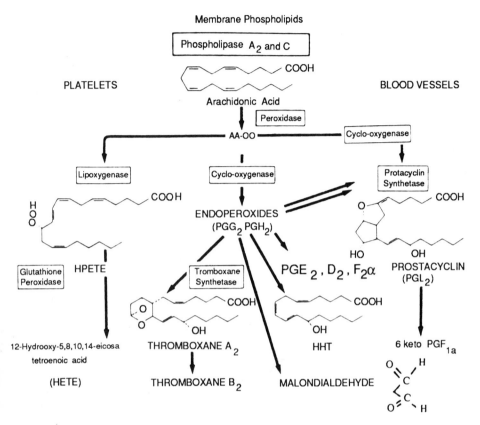

Figure 3 Oxidative conversion products of arachidonic acid in platelets and blood vessels. Enzymes active in these processes are boxed in. [Reproduced with permission from M. J. Stuart, *Prostaglandins and hemostasis: An overview,* in LA Barnes et al, eds, *Adv Pediatr* 1983; 30: 321.]

cofactor for protein kinase C, stimulating the enzyme together with calcium to promote phosphorylation of a platelet protein of MW 47,000 (Fig. 4). The overwhelming majority of arachidonic acid is contained in phosphatidyletha-nolamine and phosphatidylcholine, contributing together about 80% of the total platelet arachidonate pool. Phosphatidylinositol, on the other hand, contains only approximately 10% of the total arachidonate in platelets. Agonist-induced release of archidonate from its phospholipid carriers produces oxygenation at C-11 and C-12 of eicosa-5,8,11,14-tetraenoic acid by cyclooxygenase and at C-12 by lipoxygenase. Both of these enzymes are present in platelets and oxidative conversion of the fatty acid substrate along these two pathways leads to different end products. Lipoxygenase leads to the production of 12-hydroxy-5,8,10,14-

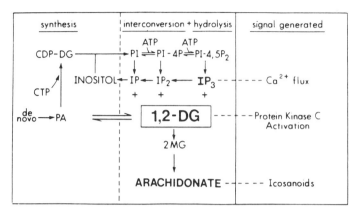

Figure 4 Phosphoinositide metabolism in platelets. Symbols shown in the figure are the following: PI = phosphatidylinositol; PI-4P = phosphatidylinositol-4-phosphate; PI-4, 5P$_2$ = phosphatidylinositol-4,5-trisphosphate; 1,2-DG = 1,2-diglyceride; 2MG = 2 monoglyceride; PA = phosphatidic acid; CTP = cytidine trisphosphate; CDP-DG = cytidine diphosphodiglyceride; IP$_3$ = inositol-1,4,5-tris phosphate; IP$_2$ = inositol-1,4-biphosphate and IP$_1$ = inositol-1-phosphate. [Reproduced with permission from PW Majerus in The molecular basis of blood diseases, G Stamatoyannopoulos et al, eds, WB Saunders, 1987.

eicosatetraenoic acid (12-HETE) whereas cyclooxygenase gives rise to 15-hydroperoxy-9,11-peroxyprosta-5,13-dienoic acid prostaglandin G$_2$ (PGG$_2$). The action of a peroxidase subsequently catalyzes the reduction of PGG$_2$ to PGH$_2$ which is finally converted to thromboxane A$_2$ (TxA$_2$) in a dismutase type of reaction. This enzyme is also responsible for the formation of 12-hydroxy-5,8,10-heptadecatrienoic acid (HHT) and malondialdehyde, the latter in almost stoichiometric amounts to TxA$_2$. Isomerases are also present in the platelet. They are responsible for the formation of PGE$_2$ and PGD$_2$ but only small amounts of these respective prostaglandins are formed in platelets. Several of these cyclooxygenase products produced by platelets have a functional effect on this cell. PGH$_2$ and TxA$_2$ both have a stimulatory effect, whereas PGD$_2$ is a potent inhibitor of platelet aggregation. HHT has been reported to be involved on chemotaxis (Goetzl and Gorman, 1978) whereas malondialdehyde is a highly reactive molecule capable of crosslinking proteins and disturbing enzyme functions.

Although prostacyclin (PGI$_2$) is not produced by platelets but only by endothelial cells, there is good evidence that the balance of TxA$_2$ and PGI$_2$ in the plasma is an important determinant of platelet reactivity. PGI$_2$, one of the most potent inhibitors of platelet aggregation, stimulates cyclic AMP production and can directly counteract the effect of TxA$_2$, a potent aggregating agent of platelets.

Effect of Tocopherols on Oxidative Conversion of Arachidonate

Effect on Cyclooxygenase

There is ample documentation in the literature that TxA_2 and malondialdehyde production is increased in vitamin E deficiency states (Karpen et al., 1981; Toivanen, 1987; Valentovic et al., 1982; Pritchard et al., 1982; Giani et al., 1986; Hamelin and Chan, 1983). The synthesis of PGE_2 showed dramatic increases in vitamin E-deficient rodents (Hope et al., 1975; Tangney and Driskell, 1981). These findings were primarily obtained in animal experiments and led to the conclusion that dietary supplementation with vitamin E could produce an inhibition of prostanoid production in platelets. Some authors were able to substantiate an inhibitory effect, albeit moderate in degree, of alpha-tocopherol on cyclooxygenase activity (Ali et al., 1980; Mower and Steiner, 1983; Kockmann et al., 1988) (Fig. 5a and b). Generally only high concentrations of the antioxidant in experiments performed in vitro were able to inhibit the activity of cyclooxygenase, even though some authors were able to show such an effect (Srivastava, 1986). As far as low or moderately high concentrations of alpha-tocopherol are concerned, especially when provided as a dietary supplement (Stampfer et al., 1988), there appears to be a consensus that this administration yields negative results. At times the effect is only recognizable by observing the relative stoichiometric ratios of arachidonic acid conversion via the two competing oxidative pathways of lipoxygenase and cyclooxygenase or the relative difference between HETE and HHT in platelets (Mower and Steiner, 1983) (Fig. 6). It should be pointed out, however, the methodological details may play an important role in the outcome of the experiments when exogenous [^{14}C]arachidonic acid is used to evaluate cyclo- and lipoxygenase pathways in the platelet. Thus, avoiding pulse labeling of platelets with arachidonic acid by addition of this fatty acid in small portions over an extended period of time and the administration of alpha-tocopherol as an emulsion instead of an ethanolic solution makes a difference in the outcome of the experiments.

Hope et al. (1975) found an inverse relationship between alpha-tocopherol and serum levels of $PGF_{2\alpha}$ and PGE_2. Tissue differences may play a role in determining whether or not an inhibitory response to tocopherol is seen. Zenser and Davis (1978) found that alpha-tocopherol in concentrations as high as 5 mM did not affect PGE_2 and $PGF_{2\alpha}$ production in the renal medulla of rats. The cyclooxygenase reaction is known to depend on the availability of hydroperoxides which are necessary for the activation of this enzyme (Hemler et al., 1979; Hemler and Lands, 1980; Taylor et al., 1983). One thus may assume that scavenging of the propagating peroxyl radicals of arachidonic acid will lead to an inhibition of the cyclooxygenase activity. This, in fact, was observed by Hemler and Lands (1980). A variety of phenolic antioxidants inhibited oxygenation rates of cyclooxygenase and extended the lag period of this heme enzyme, which could

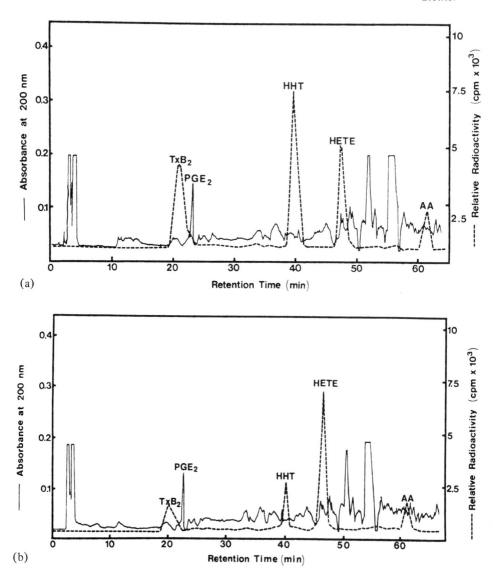

(a)

(b)

Figure 5 High-performance liquid chromatogram of arachidonic acid metabolites of normal (a) and vitamin E-pretreated (1 mM) (b) platelets, aggregated with 1 U thrombin/ml in the presence of [^{14}C]arachidonic acid. PGE$_2$ was added as an internal standard. [From Mower and Steiner (1983).]

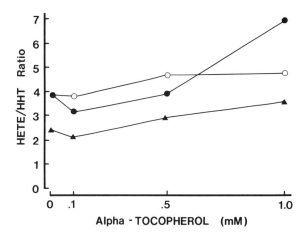

Figure 6. Changes in the difference between HETE and HHT evaluated as a function of vitamin E concentration in the incubation medium. Platelets prelabeled with [^{14}C-] arachidonic acid were preincubated with different vitamin E concentrations for 5 min prior to a 3-min aggregation induced by thrombin (1 U/ml). Each of the different symbols represents one experiment. The origin is 0. [From Mower and Steiner (1983).]

be shown to be needed for the accumulation of sufficient amounts of the hydroperoxide product activator (Hemler and Lands, 1980). Yet contrary observations were made by Seeger et al. (1988) who utilized ram vesicular gland microsomal cyclooxygenase to show that alpha-tocopherol did not inhibit the oxygen consumption accompanying the conversion of arachidonic acid by the enzyme. It is interesting and somewhat surprising that these authors also reported a stimulant activity of the carboxylic acid chromane compound of alpha-tocopherol (Trolox) on ram vesicular gland cyclooxygenase. This compound differs from alpha-tocopherol primarily in the absence of the phytyl side chain which the natural vitamin contains. This side chain is believed to facilitate the access of the chromane compound to lipid-rich compartments and to enhance the retention of vitamin E in such areas (Niki et al., 1985). A provocative and interesting hypothesis promulgated by Diplock and Lucy which will be commented upon below, may provide a possible explanation for this effect. The important role of hydroperoxides as modulators of the cyclo- and lipoxygenase pathways gives a plausible rationale to the effect of alpha-tocopherol, a well-known and potent scavenger of hydroperoxides.

Effect on Phospholipase A_2

A somewhat different explanation may underlie the effect of alpha-tocopherol on platelet phospholipase A_2 (Douglas et al., 1986). The inhibition that was produced by various forms of tocopherol, including tocol (2-methyl-2-phytyl-6-chromanol), but not by tocopheryl acetate may be not so much an indication of a general inhibitory effect of vitamin E and related compounds on the enzyme, but may rather signify an effect of tocopherol on the substrate that Douglas et al. used to measure phospholipase A_2 activity. We suspect that the particular substrate *sn*-1-palmitoyl-2-arachidonylphosphatidylcholine was responsible for the observed inhibitory effect because a special affinity exists between polyunsaturated fatty acids of the arachidonyl type and tocopherol. The physiocochemical interaction between this phospholipid and alpha-tocopherol will be further expanded below. Such an interaction is believed to be an important mechanism by which alpha-tocopherol exerts its biological function.

Effect on Lipoxygenase Enzymes

Several investigators have found a suppression of platelet 12-lipoxygenase activity by vitamin E supplementation (Pritchard et al., 1986; Gwebu et al., 1980). A more detailed analysis by Chan et al. (1986), however, showed that vitamin E can elicit a transitory increase of lipoxygenase activity while suppressing the peroxidase activity. This effect observed ex vivo in a group of normal human individuals supplemented with 400 IU vitamin E/day reversed after more than 3 weeks of dietary supplementation. The significance of such a temporary increase of 12-lipoxygenase activity is not known, but it is interesting to note that a similar response to vitamin E supplementation was observed when the 5-lipoxygenase activity of human leukocytes was measured (Goetzl, 1980). A bidirectional modulation of the neutrophil 5-lipoxygenase activity, enhancing arachidonic acid lipoxygenase at low tocopherol concentrations and decreasing it at higher ones, was identical to the effect observed in platelets (Mower and Steiner, 1983).

Summary

Although the experimental evidence describing the effect of alpha-tocopherol on prostanoid metabolism in platelets is at first confusing, there are clear indications of an interference of this vitamin with those enzyme reactions that are modulated by hydroperoxides. The inability of some investigators to obtain this evidence is probably due to testing the effect of alpha-tocopherol at a concentration at which its biphasic response profile is in the stimulant phase. Technical details of measuring the enzyme activities may also impact importantly upon the results.

DIPLOCK–LUCY HYPOTHESIS

It has been widely held that the in vivo function of alpha-tocopherol is the prevention of destructive peroxidation of polyunsaturated lipids. This theory first formulated by Tappel (1962 and 1972) continues to constitute the cornerstone of most explanations of the biological activity of alpha-tocopherol in mammalian tissues. Certain inconsistencies in this hypothesis have been pointed out by Green and Bunyan (1969) which subsequently led Diplock and Lucy (1973) to propose an alternate hypothesis for the action of alpha-tocopherol that was founded primarily on the physiocochemical interaction between the phytyl chain of the vitamin and certain polyunsaturated fatty acids. With the discovery that glutathione peroxidase, a lipid peroxide-destroying enzyme, contained selenium in its active site (Hoekstra, 1973), the biochemical rationale for the close metabolic relationship of selenium and vitamin E was clearly demonstrated. An association between vitamin E and selenium has been realized ever since the discovery by Schwarz and Foltz (1957) that traces of dietary selenium were able to prevent necrotic liver degeneration in vitamin E-deficient rats. In 1969, Thompson and Scott convincingly demonstrated that selenium was an essential trace element independent of vitamin E. Although this removed some of the perceived inconsistencies of the antioxidant hypothesis, there remains the fact that the rate of destruction of trace quantities of alpha-tocopherol in tissues of vitamin E-deficient animals is not directly related to the intake of polyunsaturated fatty acids (Green et al., 1967). Very persuasive experimental evidence has been obtained by Diplock, Lucy, and their collaborators (Diplock et al., 1977; Maggio et al., 1977; Lucy, 1978) showing that maximum "fit" was obtained between the natural alpha-tocopherol molecule containing the 15-carbon phytyl side chain and the arachidonyl portion of arachidonylphosphatidylcholine. Any change in the side chain of alpha-tocopherol, whether an increase or a decrease in the number of carbons, as well as alterations in the fatty acyl chains providing either less unsaturation or shorter chain length significantly reduced the extent of the interaction.

It is generally agreed now that the chromanol nucleus of alpha-tocopherol which is the portion of the molecule ultimately responsible for the antioxidant effect of the vitamin is believed to be oriented toward the lipid–water interface of the phospholipid bilayer (Cushley and Forrest, 1977; Fragata and Bellemare, 1980; Massey et al., 1982; Baig and Laidman, 1983; Perly et al., 1985). The hydroxyl groups of the chromanol ring are hydrogen-bonded to the carbonyl oxygens of acyl ester bonds of phospholipids. Kagan and Quinn (1988) showed that as the phytyl chain length increases, there is an increasing tendency of the chromanol ring to be drawn into the hydrophobic interior of the lipid bilayer. The same authors point out the existence of an interesting dual-distribution profile of alpha-tocopherol in lipid membranes, one of monomeric units and another one involving aggregates. Whether the latter can also form in intact biological membranes and not solely in artificially prepared liposomes remains a question.

A strong argument for the Diplock–Lucy hypothesis is the fact that alpha-tocopherol raises the threshold concentration for arachidonic acid-induced platelet aggregation. On the other hand, the chromanol nucleus without the phytyl side chain does not affect this threshold concentration of arachidonic acid (unpublished observations).

Recently, Urano et al. (1987) reported measurements of ^{13}C spin lattice relaxation times of alpha-tocopherol labeled with ^{13}C in various methyl positions on the chromanol ring as well as in the one methylene position and in the methyl locations along the phytyl side chain that was introduced into liposomes containing either no, a minimal (2.6%), or a high (19%) content of arachidonyl residues. The spin lattice relaxation time of carbon nuclei will be influenced by the overall tumbling and segmental motion of the molecule. Decrease of this parameter at a specific atom, e.g., carbon, reflects a decrease in the segmental motion of the molecule that the carbon is part of. The experiments of the above authors showed that the spin relaxation times did not correlate with the arachidonyl acid content of the liposomes. The authors reasoned that according to the Diplock–Lucy hypothesis, the segmental motion of the methyl groups in the 4' and 8' positions of the phytyl side chain of alpha-tocopherol should have been markedly reduced in liposomes containing high concentrations of arachidonyl acid residues. As this was not clearly apparent, they suggested that their results refuted the Diplock–Lucy hypothesis. It could be argued, however, that the increased mobility that may be inherent in lipid bilayers containing higher concentrations of polyunsaturated fatty acids may have mitigated any dampening effect on segmental motion of the methyl groups along the phytyl side chain of alpha-tocopherol. Whatever the explanation, the results of Urano et al. (1987) are not considered sufficiently convincing to justify a rejection of the Diplock–Lucy hypothesis.

It is interesting to note that most investigators in this area of research accept either one or the other hypothesis, i.e., the physical interaction or the antioxidant theory of alpha-tocopherol, but apparently are not willing to concede that both mechanisms may be operative when alpha-tocopherol is distributed in intact cells or tissue. Both theories are quite plausible and as far as the platelet is concerned, certain effects are better explained by the antioxidant, others by the physical interaction hypothesis.

OTHER HYPOTHESES OF ALPHA-TOCOPHEROL ACTION

Mahoney and Azzi (1988) recently reported that vitamin E can inhibit brain protein kinase C in vitro. The IC_{50} was approximately 450 μM, which is more than one order of magnitude higher than the reported plasma levels of alpha-tocopherol. It is possible, however, that local concentrations of alpha-tocopherol in certain lipid structures or membranes (Burton et al., 1983) may be high enough to inhibit the enzyme. Neither calcium, phosphatidylserine, nor phorbol esters played a role in the interaction of vitamin E with this protein kinase. Whether this inhibition of protein kinase C could be a factor in the alpha-tocopherol-induced reduction of the platelet release reaction remains to be established.

It is interesting to note that whereas calcium was not found to be a mediator of the above alpha-tocopherol effect, Butler et al. (1979) reported that vitamin E inhibited the release of calcium from a platelet membrane fraction in vitro. Whether alpha-tocopherol per se or a tocopherol-induced rise in cyclic AMP was responsible for the reduced release of calcium ions (Salganicoff and Sevy, 1985) was not established. An elevation of cyclic AMP levels, albeit modest in degree, could be expected in view of the reported inhibition of cyclic nucleotide phosphodiesterase by alpha-tocopherol (Steiner and Mower, 1982). Even though only the high K_m fraction of phosphodiesterase appears to be affected, elevations of platelet cyclic AMP could be caused by alpha-tocopherol.

PLATELET ADHESION

General Aspects

Because of the difficulty in measuring platelet adhesion as a phenomenon distinctly separate from platelet aggregation, the assessment of this platelet function has not attained the popularity of platelet aggregation. A variety of methods have been introduced over the years, many of these "static" in nature, which bring platelet suspensions in contact with an adhesive surface. The "dynamic" systems measure the adherence of platelets to surfaces that are perfused either with platelet-rich plasma or whole blood. Laminar flow chambers, especially of the Hele–Shaw type, are one of the many devices for measuring platelet adhesiveness under controlled circumstances. These chambers can be perfused at shear rates varying from high (≤ 800–900 sec^{-1}) to low (≥ 20–25 sec^{-1}) and observations may be made "snapshot-like" after a given period of perfusion or in a time-resolved manner in which adhesion measurements are taken at intervals over an extended (13–15 min) time period (Richardson et al., 1977).

Platelet adhesion denotes the attachment of platelets to a surface other than of their own kind. It represents one of the earliest steps in hemostasis and takes place physiologically whenever flowing blood containing platelets comes in contact with a collagenous surface exposed by severing the continuity of the vascular endothelial cell layer. This may also occur as a consequence of a pathological process such as that associated with the atherosclerotic changes of a blood vessel. In either case, adhesion takes place between the glycoprotein IIb/IIIa complex of the platelet and the collagen of the subendothelial tissue. Von Willebrand factor, a large-size plasma glycoprotein, which usually occurs in various multimer forms and has binding sites on platelet glycoprotein complexes Ib/IX as well as IIb/IIIa, mediates the interaction between collagen and platelets. It is now known that glycoproteins Ib and IIb belong to a group of adhesive proteins that share peculiar biochemical characteristics of structure. The tripeptide arginine-glycine-aspartic acid (RGD according to the one-letter amino acid code) forms a recognition site in several of the proteins that are commonly classified as integrins. A disulfide bridge linking a smaller to a larger polypeptide constitutes another important characteristic of these proteins.

Effect of Alpha-Tocopherol on Platelet Adhesion

As discussed above, platelet aggregation was little affected by alpha-tocopherol. The effect of alpha-tocopherol on platelet adhesion was then examined using the method of Spaet and Lejnieks (1969), a system fashioned after the turbidimetric method of platelet aggregometry. Fibrillar Achilles tendon collagen wound around a small stirring bar is agitated at the bottom of a suspension of platelet-rich plasma while changes in optical density are continuously being recorded. This system provides a kinetic element to platelet adhesion measurement that facilitates comparative evaluations. It also made it possible to obtain the first indication of an inhibitory effect of alpha-tocopherol on platelet adhesiveness (Steiner, 1983). Measurements taken with platelets obtained from individuals whose diet was

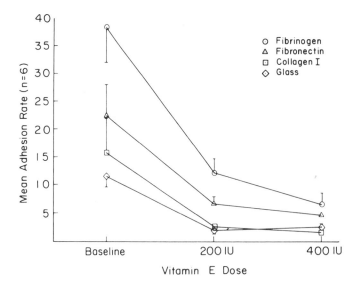

Figure 7 Adhesion trend lines for four different adhesive surfaces. Mean adhesion rates (cumulative platelet number $\times$ min^{-1}) $\pm$ SEM are shown for baseline and vitamin E-supplemented periods. Differences between baseline and 200 and 400 IU were significant at $p <$ 0.0 for fibrinogen and glass and between baseline and 400 IU for collagen I. The remaining differences in adhesion rate between baseline and vitamin E-supplemented levels were significant at the $p < 0.05$ level. [From Jandak et al. (1989).]

supplemented with a 6-week course of increasing vitamin E (400 to 1200 IU/day) showed a moderate to extensive inhibition of platelet adhesion to collagen.

Subsequently, platelet adhesiveness was investigated by a time-resolved method using a laminar flow chamber (Jandak et al., 1988, 1989). Adhesion measurements were made with collagen I, fibronectin, and fibrinogen as adhesive surfaces. Alpha-tocopherol, even in concentrations as low as those provided by 200 IU vitamin E/day, showed a highly significant inhibition of platelet adhesion to all of these adhesive surfaces (Figs. 7 and 8). At 400 IU vitamin E/day platelet adhesion was virtually completely inhibited ($\geq$85%). The time-resolved measurements of platelet adhesiveness not only showed that the total number of platelets that adhered was sharply reduced by administration of alpha-tocopherol to the platelet donor, but also gave evidence of a greatly reduced reutilization of the number of adhesion sites. Platelets from non-vitamin E-supplemented individuals have a great tendency to adhere to sites that had been visited by platelets at some time before. As adhesion measurements are made over a 13-min time period, individual adhesion sites may be revisited up to seven or eight times during the course of observation. Alpha-tocopherol supplemented platelets, on the other hand, rarely reused sites more than twice.

A reasonably good correlation was apparent between the amount of alpha-

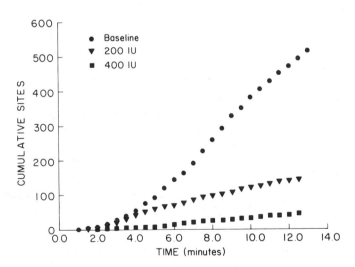

Figure 8 Cumulative number of adhesion sites over a 13-min period. Platelet adhesion to a fibrinogen-coated surface was studied at baseline (circles), after 2 weeks of 200 IU vitamin E (triangles) and after an additional 2 weeks of 400 IU vitamin E supplementation (squares). Data depicted are representative of those obtained during a typical adhesion assay. [From Jandak et al. (1989).]

tocopherol present in the platelet and the adhesiveness parameters, either total number of platelets adherent/time or number of sites revisited by platelets. Such results were obtained with all of the different adhesive surfaces used in the studies. Supplementation levels higher than 400 IU/day added little further inhibitory effect. In fact, in some individuals, vitamin E concentrations greater than 800 IU/day appeared to have less inhibitory effect than those of 400 IU/day (Jandak et al., 1988). It has yet to be determined whether this is a significant effect.

Initial experiments were obtained at relatively low shear rates, i.e., approximately 25 sec^{-1}. More recently, it was possible to show that the same observations held true at higher shear rates, i.e., greater than 650 sec^{-1}. Whereas low shear rates, sometimes even completely stagnant flow conditions, exist in rupture sites and cavities of atherosclerotic plaques, preferred sites for the initiation of coronary thrombosis (Davies and Thomas, 1981, 1985), high shear rate conditions prevail in arteries, such as the coronary arterial circulation.

These studies thus provide the first indication that vitamin E supplementation of 400 IU/day affects a platelet function that is important under physiological and pathological conditions.

SHAPE CHANGES FOLLOWING VITAMIN E SUPPLEMENTATION

Scanning electron microscopic examinations of vitamin E-replete platelets attached to the adhesive surface revealed a dearth of pseudopodia that normally adorn the platelets that are adherent to an adhesive surface (Jandak et al., 1989) (Figs. 9 and 10). However, the elongated, slender projections that protrude from the contracted spherical body of normal platelets are completely missing in platelets from vitamin E-supplemented individuals. Rounded, short projections were the only pseudopodia seen in vitamin E-replete platelets. One can easily imagine that such stubby projections would allow ready dislodging of the platelets should they adhere to the surface. These changes can be visualized in platelets of vitamin E-supplemented individuals irrespective of the adhesive surface to which they are attached. A dose-dependent progression of these changes can be seen when control platelets are compared with platelets from individuals at 200 IU and at 400 or 800 IU vitamin E/day.

The reason for these morphological changes induced by alpha-tocopherol is not clear, although several speculative interpretations can be given. At this time it is not known whether the protrusion of pseudopodia in the course of the shape change occurs at specific sites or is a random event that may take place anywhere on the platelet membrane. It is proposed that the extrusion of pseudopodial processes is destined to occur in areas of the membrane that have an inherent reduced resistance to the internal pressure developed by the agonist-induced

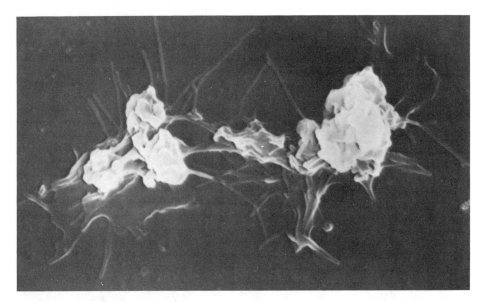

Figure 9 Scanning electron microscopic examination of normal platelets adherent to the fibronectin coated upper deck of the Hele-Shaw flow chamber. From Jandak et al. (1989).

contraction of the platelet. The existence of such sites of "lesser resistance" would presuppose discrete domains in the surface membrane indicative of incomplete miscibility of membrane components. An inhomogeneous distribution of alpha-tocopherol has been shown in multibilayer vesicles of various phosphatidylcholines and phosphatidylethanolamines (Ortiz et al., 1987). Alpha-tocopherol was found to be associated with the more fluid zones, which usually are those that contain the more unsaturated fatty acyl chains. This observation is predicted by the Diplock–Lucy hypothesis.

Membrane fluidity measurements have been widely used in recent years as a simple method to evaluate the effect of changes in lipid composition that membranes undergo when challenged by different dietary intake. Many studies of this type use steady-state fluorescence measurements of a fluorescent probe inserted into the membrane. 1,6-Diphenyl-1,3,5-hexatriene (DPH) is one of the most popular probes because of its strong quantum yield and its well-characterized location in the lipid bilayer of the membrane. Liposomes, whether produced from single phospholipids (Urano et al., 1988) or from isolated platelet membrane lipids (Steiner, 1978, 1981), enriched with alpha-tocopherol show a decrease in their fluidity as revealed by fluorescence polarization measurements of DPH (Fig.

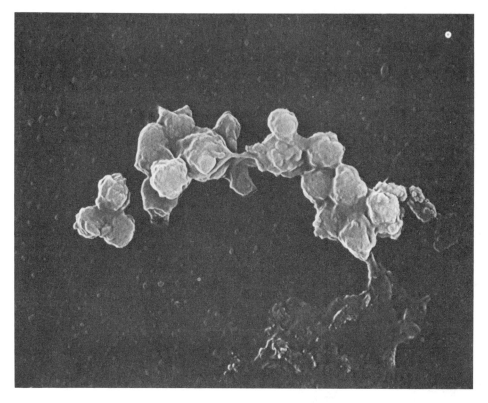

Figure 10 Scanning electron microscopic examination of platelets after 2 weeks of 200 IU vitamin E/day adherent to the fibronectin coated upper deck of the flow chamber. [From Jandak et al. (1989).]

11). A dose dependency between alpha-tocopherol and the degree of change in fluorescence polarization is readily apparent. The effect of vitamin E is predicated on its chromanol ring and its phytyl side chain (Steiner, 1978; Urano et al., 1988). A good correlation also exists between the length of the isoprenoid chain and the fluidity of the liposome vesicles. The longer the chain, the greater the decrease in fluidity. Not only the chain length but also the methyl groups of the isoprenoid chain contribute to this effect (Urano et al., 1988). In addition, the number of methyl groups on the chromanol ring affected the fluorescence polarization of DPH in liposomes. A reduction of the number of methyl groups was found to be associated with less decrease in fluidity. The effect of alpha-tocopherol on intact membranes or membrane reconstituted from platelet lipids and platelet membrane proteins is quite different, however. Evaluation of the

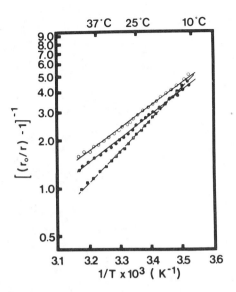

Figure 11 Temperature dependence of fluorescence polarization of diphenylhexatriene in liposomes prepared from platelet membrane lipids. Liposomes were incubated with alpha-tocopherol at a final concentration of 2 mM (open circles), 1 mM (closed circles), and without additional alpha-tocopherol (squares). Fluorescence intensities of diphenylhexatriene were measured parallel and perpendicular to the direction of a polarized excitation beam. From these measurements, the fluorescence anisotrophy r was calculated. The apparent microviscosity was approximated as described by Shinitzky and Barenholz (1978) utilizing a maximal limiting anisotropy value of $r_0 = 0.362$ for diphenylhexatriene. The ordinate is a fluorescence polarization term which relates to membrane fluidity; the abscissa is the reciprocal of the absolute temperature. [From Steiner (1981).]

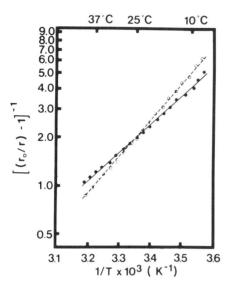

Figure 12   Temperature dependence of the fluorescence polarization of diphenylhexatriene in normal (closed circles) and 1 mM alpha-tocopherol-loaded (open circles) platelets. Fluorescence polarization was measured as described in legend to Fig. 11. [From Steiner (1981).]

fluidity over the temperature range 4–40°C shows that addition of vitamin E induces a decrease in fluidity at temperatures less than 25–27°C but increases fluidity at higher temperatures (Fig. 12). Unfortunately, measurements of fluorescence polarization give overall evaluations of the fluidity of membranes and thus fail to report on changes in discrete lipid domains.

PERSPECTIVES AND FUTURE RESEARCH

This review of our present state of knowledge of the function of vitamin E in platelets has shown up several areas of controversy. Some of these appear to be due to the belief that vitamin E should measure up favorably in terms of potency to agents such as acetylsalicylic acid if it has any chance of being accepted as a platelet inhibitory agent. The problem with such a comparison is that one is a pharmacological agent which is not normally present in the body, whereas the other is a micronutrient that is an inherent component of all cells and tissues of mammalian origin. In investigating the effect of alpha-tocopherol on platelets we are trying to define whether vitamin E supplementation above and beyond the normal level is capable of reducing platelet function. In view of the variable dietary habits and the strong correlation between vitamin E and the content of dietary polyunsaturated fatty acids, it is not surprising that plasma and platelet concentrations of this micronutrient are very variable. In vitro, under conditions whereby the concentration of alpha-tocopherol can be raised to any desired level, an inhibitory effect of vitamin E on platelet aggregation and release is quite definite. The difficulty of achieving similar concentrations by dietary supplementation in vivo may preclude the observation of an inhibitory effect of vitamin E in many individuals.

The observation that alpha-tocopherol may have a potent inhibitory effect on platelet adhesiveness, found in ex vivo studies with dietary supplementations that are within 5–10 times the recommended dietary allowance (RDA), provides a totally novel aspect of the biological function of this substance. At present, there are very few agents that have antiadhesive properties and none that constitute a normal part of the diet. A dose–response relationship between the local concentration of the antiplatelet agent and its inhibitory effect is an essential criterion for a substance that is normally present in the platelet. This could be demonstrated for the antiadhesive activity of alpha-tocopherol (Jandak et al., 1989). There is a rational basis for the effect of alpha-tocopherol which explains its inhibition of platelet aggregation and release. The mechanism of action by which vitamin E inhibits platelet adhesion, however, is still somewhat uncertain. The short, stubby pseudopodia of vitamin E-enriched platelets undergoing stimulation may explain why such platelets are less capable of adhesion than their non-vitamin E-enriched counterparts. The reason why vitamin E supplementation should bring about such drastic morphological changes remains unclear at this time. It is conceivable that tocopherol incorporated into the platelet membrane may alter the resistance of discrete areas that normally allow extrusion of pseudopodia. Plausible though this explanation is, there is little substantive evidence to support it at present.

Future research will undoubtedly explore the effect of alpha-tocopherol in individuals who are at risk of arterial thrombotic disease, basically similar clinical settings for which aspirin and other antiplatelet agents have been used. The platelet function to be followed should be adhesiveness; correlations between dose and effect should be given priority. The use of combinations of agents, e.g., alpha-tocopherol plus a nonsteroidal anti-inflammatory agent such as acetylsalicylic acid, may have great promise in the future to become a regimen that may inhibit both platelet adhesion and aggregation. Such trials may be easier to conduct than those of alpha-tocopherol as a single agent, as the use of aspirin is becoming quite pervasive in the prevention of arterial thrombotic diseases. A combination of two micronutrients that may hold considerable promise as an effective antithrombotic regimen is that of alpha-tocopherol and ascorbic acid. Already a considerable literature has accumulated which demonstrates the beneficial effect of ascorbic acid in enhancing the effectiveness of alpha-tocopherol as an anti-oxidant (Tappel, 1968; Packer et al., 1979; Niki et al., 1982; Doba et al., 1985; Mukai et al., 1987). It is possible that these two vitamins together with aspirin may provide another effective combination for preventing thrombotic disease.

Further studies of the antiadhesive effect of alpha-tocopherol will be important, not only to explain the basis of the antiadhesive effect of vitamin E, but also to provide answers to questions of the functional behavior of plasma membranes, the role of lipid soluble dietary additives in modifying membrane functions, and the distribution of membrane components in the plane of the lipid bilayer. Such investigations could be very rewarding as vitamin E has few if any side effects when given in doses of up to 3200 IU/day (Bendich and Machlin, 1988).

ACKNOWLEDGMENT

This review was partly supported by grants HL 22951 and HL 39192 of the National Heart, Lung and Blood Institute.

REFERENCES

Agradi E, Petroni A, Socini A, Galli C. In vitro effects of synthetic antioxidants and vitamin E on arachidonic acid metabolism and thromboxane formation in human platelets and on platelet aggregation. Prostaglandins 1981; 22:255.

Ali M, Gudbranson CG, McDonald JWD. Inhibition of human platelet cyclooxygenase by alpha-tocopherol. Prostaglandins and Medicine 1980; 4:79.

Baig MMA, Laidman DL. Spectrophotometric evidence for a polar interaction between alpha-tocopherol and phospholipids: The effect of different phosphatides and mineral salts. Biochem Soc Trans 1983; 11:600.

Behrens WA, Madere R. Alpha- and gamma-tocopherol concentrations in human serum. J Am Coll Nutr 1987; 5:91.

Bendich A, Machlin LJ. Safety of oral intake of vitamin E. Am J Clin Nutr 1988; 48:612.

Bendich A, Gabriel E, Machlin LJ. Dietary vitamin E requirement for optimum immune responses in the rat. J Nutr 1986; 116:675.

Bendich A, Gabriel E, Machlin LJ. Differences in vitamin E levels in tissues of the spontaneously hypertensive and Wistar-Kyoto rats. Proc Soc Exp Biol Med 1983; 172:297.

Berlin E, Shapiro SG, Friedland M. Platelet membrane fluidity and aggregation of rabbit platelets. Atherosclerosis 1984; 51:223.

Bieri JG, Evarts RP. Gamma tocopherol: Metabolism, biological activity and significance in human vitamin E nutrition. Am J Nutr 1974a; 27:980.

Bieri JG, Evarts RP. Vitamin E activity of gamma-tocopherol of the rat, chick and hamster. J Nutr 1974b; 104:850.

Born GVR, Cross MJ. The aggregation of blood platelets. J. Physiol 1963; 168:179.

Brubacher G, Weiser H. Biologische wirksamkeit von tocopherol und von antioxydation. Wiss Veroeffentl Deut Ges Ernachrung 1967; 16:50.

Burton GW, Joyce A, Ingold KU. Is vitamin E the only lipid-soluble, chain-breaking antioxidant in human blood plasma and erythrocyte membranes? Arch Biochem Biophys 1983; 221:281.

Butler AM, Gerrard JM, Peller J, Stoddard IR, Rao GHR, White JG. Vitamin E inhibits the release of calcium from a platelet membrane fraction in vitro. Prostaglandins and Medicine 1979; 2:203.

Chan AC, Raynor C, Douglas C, Patrick J, Boland M. Transitory stimulation of human platelet 12-lipoxygenase by vitamin E supplementation. Am J Clin Nutr 1986; 44:278.

Colette C, Pares-Herbute N, Monnier LH, Cartry E. Platelet function in type I diabetes: effects of supplementation with large doses of vitamin E. Am J Clin Nutr 1988; 47:256.

Colwell JA, Halushka PV, Sarji K, Levine J, Sagel J, Nair RMG. Altered platelet function in diabetes mellitus. Diabetes 1976; 25 (Suppl. 2):826.

Cox AC, Rao GHR, Gerrard JM, White JG. The influence of vitamin E quinone on platelet structure, function and biochemistry. Blood 1980; 55(6):907.

Cushley RJ, Forrest BJ. Structure and stability of Vitamin E-lecithin and phytamic acid-lecithin bilayers studied by ^{13}C and ^{31}P nuclear negative resonance. Can J Chem 1977; 55:220.

Davies MJ, Thomas T. The pathological basis and microanatomy of occlusive thrombus formation in human coronary arteries. Phil Trans R Soc London 1981; 294:255.

Davies MJ, Thomas AC. Plaque fissuring: The cause of acute myocardial infarction, sudden ischemic death, and crescendo angina. Br Heart J 1985; 53:363.

Davis TMR, Bown E, Turner RC. Platelet sensitivity in vitro to adenosine-5'-diphosphate and prostacyclin and diabetic retinopathy. Diabetologia 1985; 28:274.

Diplock AT, Lucy JA. The biochemical modes of action of vitamin E and selenium: A hypothesis. FEBS Lett 1973; 29(3):205.

Diplock AT, Lucy JA, Verrinder M, Zieleniewski A. alpha-tocopherol and the permeability to glucose and chromate of unsaturated liposomes. FEBS Lett 1977; 82(2):341.

Doba T, Burton GW, Ingold KU. Antioxidant and co-antioxidant activity of vitamin C. The effect of vitamin C, either alone or in the presence of vitamin E or a water-soluble vitamin E analogue, upon the peroxidation of aqueous multilamellar phospholipid liposomes. Biochim Biophys Acta 1985; 835:298.

Douglas CE, Chan AC, Choy PC. Vitamin E inhibits platelet phospholipase A_2. Biochim Biophys Acta 1986; 876:639.

Fong JSC. Alpha tocopherol: Its inhibition on human platelet aggregation. Experientia 1976; 32:639.

Fragata M, Bellemare F. Model of singlet oxygen scavenging by alpha-tocopherol in biomembranes. Chem Phys Lipids 1980; 27:93.

Gerrard JM, White JG. The structure and function of platelet, with emphasis on their contractile nature. Pathobiol Ann 1976; 6:31.

Giani E, Masi I, Galli C. Dietary heated fat alters and vitamin E restores the thromboxane/prostacyclin balance in the rat. Prog Lipid Res 1986; 25:239.

Gisinger C, Jeremy J, Speiser P, Mikhailidis D, Dandona P, Schernthaner G. Effect of vitamin E supplementation on platelet thromboxane A_2 production in type I diabetic patients. Diabetes 1988; 37:1260.

Goetzl EJ. Vitamin E modulates the lipoxygenation of arachidonic acid in leukocytes. Nature 1980; 288:183.

Goetzl EJ, Gorman RR. Chemotactic and chemokinetic stimulation of human eosinophil and neutrophil polymorphonuclear leukocytes by 12-L-hydroxy-5,8,10-heptadecatri-enoic acid (HHT). J Immunol 1978; 120:526–531.

Green J, Bunyan J. Vitamin E and the biological antioxidant theory. Nutr Abstr Rev 1969; 39:321.

Green J, Diplock AT, Bunyan J, McHale D, Muthy IR. Vitamin E and stress. I. Dietary unsaturated fatty acid, stress and the metabolism of alpha-tocopherol in the rat. Br J Nutr 1967; 21:69.

Gwebu ET, Trwyn RW, Cornwell DG, Panganamala RV. Vitamin E and the inhibition of platelet lipoxygenase. Res Commun Chem Pathol Pharmacol 1980; 28(2):361.

Hamberg M, Svensson J, Samuelsson B. Thromboxanes: A new group of biologically active components derived from prostaglan endoperoxides. Proc Natl Acad Sci USA 1975; 72:2994.

Hamlin SJ, Chan AC. Modulation of platelet throboxane and malonaldehyde by dietary vitamin E and linoleate. Lipids 1983; 18(3):267.

Hemler ME, Lands WEM. Evidence for a peroxide-initiated free radical mechanism of prostaglandin biosynthesis. J Biol Chem 1980; 255(13):6253.

Hemler ME, Cook HW, Lands WEM. Prostaglandin biosynthesis can be triggered by lipid peroxides. Arch Biochem Biophys 1979; 193:340.

Higashi O, Kikuchi Y. Effects of vitamin E on the aggregation and the lipid peroxidation of platelets exposed to hydrogen peroxide. Tokohu J Exp Med 1974; 112:271.

Hoekstra WG. In Hoekstra WG, Suttie JW, Ganther HE, Mertz W, eds, Trace element metabolism in animals. Baltimore: University Park Press, 1973; 61–77.

Hope WC, Dalton C, Machlin LJ, Filipski RJ, Vane FM. Influence of dietary vitamin E on prostaglandin biosynthesis in rat blood. Prostaglandins 1975; 10:557.

Jandak J, Steiner M, Richardson PD. Reduction of platelet adhesiveness by vitamin E supplementation in humans. Thromb Res 1988; 49:393.

Jandak J, Steiner M, Richardson PD. Alpha-tocopherol, an effective inhibitor of platelet adhesion. Blood 1989; 73(1):141.

Jurgens R, Deutsch E, Koller F. Effect of alpha-tocopherol administration on platelet function in man. Thromb Haemostas 1983; 49(2):73.

Kagan VE, Quinn PJ. The interaction of alpha-tocopherol and homologues with shorter hydrocarbon chains with phospholipid bilayer dispersions. Eur J Biochem 1988; 171:661.

Karpen CW, Merola AJ, Trewyn RW, Cornwell DG, Panganamala RV. Modulation of platelet thromboxane A_2 and arterial prostacyclin by dietary vitamin E. Prostaglandins 1981; 22(4):651.

Karpen CW, Pritchard KA, Harnold JH, Cornwell DG, Panganamala RV. Restoration of prostacyclin/thromboxane A_2 balance in the diabetic rat. Diabetes 1982; 31:947.

Karpen CW, Cataland S, Odorisio TM, Panganamala RV. Production of 12-hydroxyei-cosatetraenoic acid and vitamin E status in platelets from type I human diabetic subjects. Diabetes 1985; 34:526.

Kockmann V, Vericel E, Croset M, Lagarde M. Vitamin E fails to alter the aggregation and the oxygenated metabolism of arachidonic acid normal human platelets. Prosta-glandins 1988; 36(5):607.

Koganemaru S, Kuramoto A. The effect of vitamin E on platelet kinetics of stroke-prone spontaneously hypertensive rats (SHRSP). J Nutr Sci Vitaminol 1982; 28:1.

Lehmann J, Rao DD, Canary JJ, Judd JT. Vitamin E and relationships among tocopherols in human plasma, platelets, lymphocytes, and red blood cells. Am J Clin Nutr 1988; 47:470.

Lucy JA. Structural interactions between vitamin E and polyunsaturated phospholipids. In DeDuve C, Hayaishi O, eds. Tocopherol, oxygen and biomembranes. Amsterdam: Elsevier/North Holland Biomedical Press, 1978; 109.

Machlin LJ, Filipski R, Willis AL, Kuhn DC, Brin M. Influence of vitamin E on platelet aggregation and thrombocythemia in the rat. Proc Soc Exp Biol Med 1975; 149:275–277.

Maggio B, Diplock AT, Lucy JA. Interactions of tocopherols and ubiquinones with monolayers of phospholipids. Biochem J 1977; 161:111.

Mahoney CW, Azzi A. Vitamin E inhibits protein kinase C activity. Biochem Biophys Res Commun 1988; 154(2):694.

Marcus AJ. The role of lipids in platelet function: with particular reference to the arachidonic acid pathway. J Lipid Res 1978; 19:793.

Marques D, Casano L, Rodrigues PM. dl-Alpha-tocopherol acetate induces hypocoagulability and platelet hyopaggregability in rats. Int J Vit Nutr Res 1987; 57:375.

Massey JB, She HS, Pownall HJ. Interaction of vitamin E with saturated phospholipid bilayers. Biochem Biophys Res Commun 1982; 106:842.

McIntosh GH, Bulman FH, Looker JW, Russell GR, James M. The influence of linoleate and vitamin E from sunflower seed oil on platelet function and prostaglandin production in the common marmoset monkey. J Nutr Sci Vitaminol 1987; 33:299.

Mower R, Steiner M. Synthetic byproducts of tocopherol oxidation as inhibitors of platelet function. Prostaglandins 1982; 24:137.

Mower R, Steiner M. Biochemical interaction of arachidonic acid and vitamin E in human platelets. Prostaglandins Leukotrienes and Medicine 1983; 10:389.

Mukai K, Fukada K, Ishizu K, Kitamura Y. Stopped-flow investigation of the reaction between vitamin E radical and vitamin C in solution. Biochem Biophys Res Commun 1987; 146:134.

Niki E, Tsuchiya J, Tanimura R, Kamiya Y. Chem Lett 1982; 789.

Niki E, Kawakami A, Saito M, Yamamoto Y, Tsuchiya J, Kamiya Y. Effect of phytyl side chain of vitamin E on its antioxidant activity. J Biol Chem 1985; 1260:2191.

Nordoy A, Strom E. Tocopherol in human platelets. J Lipid Res 1975; 16:386.

Ortiz A, Aranda FJ, Gomez-Fernandez JC. A differential scanning calorimetry study of the interaction of alpha-tocopherol with mixtures of phospholipids. Biochim Biophys Acta 1987; 898:214.

Packer JE, Slater TF, Willson RL. Direct observation of a free radical interaction between vitamin E and vitamin C. Nature 1979; 278:737.

Peake IR, Windmueller HG, Bieri JG. A comparison of the intestinal absorption, lymph and plasma transport, and tissue uptake of alpha- and gamma-tocopherols in the rat. Biochim Biophys Acta 1972; 260:679.

Perly B, Smith ICP, Hughes L, Burton GW, Ingold KU. Estimation of the location of natural alpha-tocopherol in lipid bilayers by ^{13}C-NMR spectroscopy. Biochim Biophys Acta 1985; 819:131.

Phillips DR, Shuman MA. Biochemistry of platelets. Orlando: Academic Press, 1986.

Pritchard KA, Karpen CW, Merola AJ, Panganamala RV. Influence of dietary vitamin E on platelet thromboxane A_2 and vascular prostacyclin I_2 in rabbit. Prostaglandins Leukotrienes and Medicine 1982; 9:373.

Pritchard KA, Greco NJ, Panganamala RV. Effect of dietary vitamin E on the production of platelet 12-hydroxyeicosatetraenoic acid (12-HETE). Thromb Haemostas 1986; 55(1):6.

Richardson PD, Mohammed SF, Mason RG. Flow chamber studies of platelet adhesion at controlled spatially varied shear rates. Proc Eur Soc Artif Organs 1977; 4:175.

Rink TJ, Smith SW, Tsien RY. Cytoplasmic free Ca^{++} in human platelets: Ca^{++} thresholds and Ca^{++}-independent activation for shape change and secretion. FEBS Lett 1982; 148:21.

Sagel J, Colwell JA, Crook L, Laimins M. Increased platelet aggregation in early diabetes mellitus. Ann Intern Med 1975; 82:733.

Salganicoff L, Sevy RW. The platelet strip II. Pharmacochemical coupling in thrombin-activated human platelets. Am J Physiol 1985; 249:C288.

Schwarz K, Foltz CM. Selenium as an integral part of factor 3 against dietary necrotic liver degeneration. J Am Chem Soc 1957; 79:3292.

Seeger W, Moser U, Roka L. Effects of alpha-tocopherol, its carboxylic acid chromane compound and two novel antioxidant isoflavanones on prostaglandin H synthase activity and autodeactivation. Arch Pharmacol 1988; 338:74.

Shattil SJ, Cooper RA. Membrane microviscosity and human platelet function. Biochemistry 1976; 15(22):4832.

Shinitzky M, Barenholz Y. Fluidity parameters of lipid regions determined by fluorescence polarization. Biochim Biophys Acta 1978; 515:367.

Spaet TH, Lejnieks I. A technique for estimation of platelet-collagen adhesion. Proc Soc Exp Biol Med 1969; 132:1038.

Srivastava KC. Vitamin E exerts antiaggregatory effects without inhibiting the enzymes of the arachidonic acid cascade in platelets. Prostaglandins Leukotrienes and Medicine 1986; 21:177.

Stampfer MJ, Jakubowski JA, Faigel D, Vaillancourt R, Deykin D. Vitamin E supplementation effect on human platelet function, arachidonic acid metabolism, and plasma prostacyclin levels. Am J Clin Nutr 1988; 47:700.

Steiner M. Inhibition of platelet aggregation by alpha tocopherol. In: deDuve C, Hayaishi O, eds. Tocopherol, oxygen and biomembranes. Amsterdam: Elsevier/North Holland Biomedical Press, 1978, 143.

Steiner M. Vitamin E changes the membrane fluidity of human platelets. Biochim Biophys Acta 1981; 640:100.

Steiner M. Effect of alpha-tocopherol administration on platelet function in man. Thromb Haemostas 1983; 49:73.

Steiner M, Anastasi J. Vitamin E, an inhibitor of the platelet release reaction. J Clin Invest 1976; 57:732.

Steiner M, Mower R. Mechanism of action of vitamin E on platelet function. Ann NY Acad Sci 1982; 393:289.

Szczeklik A, Gryglewski J, Domagala B, Dworski R, Basista M. Dietary supplementation with vitamin E in hyperlipoproteinemias: Effects on plasma lipid peroxides, antioxidant activity, prostacyclin generation and platelet aggregability. Thromb Haemost 1985; 54(2):425.

Tangney CC, Driskell JA. Effects of vitamin E deficiency on the relative incorporation of ^{14}C-arachidonate into platelet lipids of rabbits. J Nutr 1981; 111:1839.

Tappel AL. Vitamin E as a biological lipid antioxidant. Vitamins and Hormones 1962; 20:493.

Tappel AL. Will antioxidant nutrients slow aging processes? Geriatrics 1968; 23:97.

Tappel AL. Vitamin E and free radical peroxidation of lipids. Ann NY Acad Sci 1972; 203:12.

Taylor L, Menconi MJ, Polgar P. The participation of hydroperoxides and oxygen radicals in the control of prostaglandin synthesis. J Biol Chem 1983; 258:6855–6857.

Thompson JN, Scott ML. Role of selenium in the nutrition of the chick. J Nutr 1969; 97:335.

Toivanen JL. Effects of selenium, vitamin E and vitamin C on human prostacyclin and thromboxane synthesis in vitro. Prostaglandins Leukotrienes and Medicine 1987; 26:265.

Urano S, Iida M, Otani I, Matsuo M. Membrane stabilization of vitamin E; Interactions of alpha-tocopherol with phospholipids in bilayer liposomes. Biochem Biophys Res Commun 1987; 146(3):1413.

Urano S, Yano K, Matsuo M. Membrane stabilizing effect of vitamin E: Effect of alpha-tocopherol and its model compounds on fluidity of lecithin liposomes. Biochem Biophys Res Commun 1988; 150: 469.

Valentovic MA, Gairola C, Lubawy WC. Lung, aorta and platelet metabolism of ^{14}C arachidonic acid in vitamin E deficient rats. Prostaglandins 1982; 24(2):215.

Vatassery G T, Krezowski AM, Eckfeldt JH. Vitamin E concentrations in human blood plasma and platelets. Am J Clin Nutr 1983a; 37:1020.

Vatassery GT, Morley JE, Kuskowski MA. Vitamin E in plasma and platelets of human diabetic patients and control subjects. Am J Clin Nutr 1983b; 37:641.

Vericel E, Croset M, Sedivy P, Courprom P, Dechavanne M, Lagarde M. Platelets and aging I-aggregation, arachidonate metabolism and antioxidant status. Thromb Res 1988; 49:331.

Weiss HJ. Platelet physiology and abnormalities of platelet function. N Eng J Med 1975; 293:531.

Weiss HJ. Platelets: Pathophysiology and antiplatelet drug therapy. New York: Alan R. Liss., 1982, 46.

White JG, Rao GHR, Gerrard JM. Effects of nitroblue tetrazolium and vitamin E on platelet ultrastructure, aggregation and secretion. Am J Pathol 1977; 88:387.

Whitin JC, Gordon RK, Corwin LM, Simons ER. The effect of vitamin E deficiency on some platelet membrane properties. J Lipid Res 1982; 23:276.

Zenser TV, Davis BB. Antioxidant inhibition of prostaglandin production by rat renal medulla. Metabolism 1978; 27:227.

4

Micronutrients, Homocysteine Metabolism, and Atherosclerosis

Kilmer S. McCully

Veterans Affairs Medical Center
Providence, Rhode Island

INTRODUCTION

In most economically developed countries, including the United States, complications of atherosclerosis are the leading cause of morbidity and mortality
within the population. The most common complications of atherosclerosis are
coronary heart disease and myocardial infarction, cerebrovascular disease and
stroke, renovascular disease, hypertension and renal failure, generalized atherosclerosis and gangrene of extremities, and atherosclerotic aortic aneurysm.

The homocysteine theory of arteriosclerosis was developed from the observation of arteriosclerotic changes in patients with hereditary deficiencies of different enzymes controlling methionine and homocysteine metabolism. The central
principle of the theory is that increased synthesis and accumulation of homocysteine from metabolism of methionine are the initiating and promoting factors
in the development of atherosclerotic plaques (McCully, 1983). Methionine, an
essential amino acid, is the only known metabolic source of homocysteine, and
the conversion of dietary methionine to homocysteine is controlled by enzyme
systems requiring the essential micronutrients pyridoxine, folate, cobalamin, and
riboflavin. In addition, the utilization of homocysteine by arterial tissues is dependent on other essential micronutrients, including ascorbate, retinoic acid, and
cobalamin. The nonessential nutrients choline and betaine are potential sources
of control of homocysteine accumulation because they serve as methyl sources
in transmethylation of homocysteine to methionine. Finally, antioxidant micro-

69

nutrients, such as ascorbate, tocopherol, glutathione, selenium, bioflavonoids, carotenoids, and polyunsaturated fatty acids, may function to control the oxidation of homocysteine to homocysteic acid and conversion to phosphoadenosine phosphosulfate, important intermediates in homocysteine utilization.

CLINICAL MANIFESTATIONS, PATHOGENESIS AND EPIDEMIOLOGY OF ATHEROSCLEROSIS

Clinical Manifestations

Atherosclerosis produces symptoms and organ failure by narrowing and occlusion of the arteries supplying the vital organs. Narrowing of arteries by atherosclerotic plaques produces ischemic changes within affected organs because of a reduction in blood flow, resulting in angina pectoris when coronary arteries are affected, transient ischemic attacks when cerebral arteries are affected, uremia and hypertension when renal arteries are affected, and intermittent claudication when peripheral arteries are affected. Sudden occlusion of an atherosclerotic artery occurs because of thrombosis at a site of narrowing or hemorrhage within an atherosclerotic plaque, resulting in myocardial, cerebral, or renal infarction, or gangrene of an extremity, depending on which artery is affected. Atherosclerosis commonly commences in the second or third decade and frequently remains asymptomatic until the fifth or sixth decade, when sudden occlusion of an artery causes an infarct of a vital organ.

Pathogenesis

The principal pathological component of atherosclerotic plaques is dense fibrous tissue. Fibrosis and prominent deposits of calcium salts within artery wall cause rigidity and sclerosis, associated with narrowing of the lumen and loss of elasticity. In fully developed plaques, called atheromas, fibrin, amorphous protein precipitate, and lipids, including crystals of cholesterol, form swollen areas covered by a fibrous cap. As these atheromas gradually increase in size, they encroach on the lumen, causing partial or total obstruction. Occlusion of the lumen may be caused by diffuse fibrocalcific plaques, by gradual accumulation of atheromas, or by sudden obstruction from thrombosis at a site of narrowing or from hemorrhage within an atherosclerotic plaque. Atherosclerotic aneurysm occurs when intraluminal blood pressure gradually expands a focal area of arterial or aortic wall, weakened by destruction of elastic fibers, loss of elasticity, and fibrosis. The distribution of atherosclerotic plaques within the arterial system generally follows areas of high pressure, angulation, turbulence of blood flow, or motion of artery wall. The most common sites for plaques are coronary artery, aorta, cerebral arteries, splenic artery, and femoral arteries.

Arteriolosclerosis, the diffuse narrowing of small arteries in many organs of the body, frequently is present in persons with atherosclerotic plaques and atheromas of the aorta and major arteries. Pathologically arteriolosclerosis is characterized by diffuse fibrous intimal plaques, frequently associated with destruction of elastica interna and deposition of glycoproteins or fibrin within arteriolar walls. Arteriolosclerosis is particularly common in the kidney, where the process causes loss of renal function by producing nephrosclerosis. Arteriolosclerosis is frequently associated with diabetes mellitus and hypertension.

Atherosclerotic plaques are generally considered to arise from a response of the cells and tissues of the artery wall to injury of the endothelial cell layer lining the intimal surface of arterial lumen (Ross, 1986). Early atherosclerotic lesions consist of hyperplastic intimal smooth muscle cells associated with deposits of extracellular matrix bound to lipoproteins, forming fatty streaks within the intimal layer. Interaction of platelets and macrophages from the bloodstream with the injured areas of endothelium is believed to cause release of polypeptide growth factors from these elements of blood which promote hyperplasia of the smooth muscle cells of atherosclerotic plaques. Intimal injury causes increased permeability of intima to the flow of plasma through the artery wall, exposes subintimal tissues to filtered plasma, and allows deposits of fibrin to form over and within the injured areas.

The hyperplastic smooth muscle cells of developing plaques synthesize collagen which becomes deposited in layers within the intima, gradually encroaching on the lumen and extending to the adjacent media. Focal splitting and destruction of elastica interna of arteries and elastic lamellae of aorta are also associated with formation of fibrous plaques. Hyperplastic smooth muscle cells synthesize an extracellular matrix which is deposited within developing plaques. Increased filtration of plasma through damaged endothelium carries lipoproteins into the plaques, where insoluble complexes are formed with sulfated glycosaminoglycans of the arterial wall matrix. Finally, calcification develops within smooth muscle and fibrous tissue; cholesterol is released from deposited lipoproteins, forming crystalline cholesterol deposits; small blood vessels and inflammatory cells form within the plaques; lipid deposits are taken up by macrophages and smooth muscle cells to form small numbers of foam cells; amorphous deposits of protein and lipids are formed; and layers of fibrin are deposited on the surface and within the developing atheroma.

Epidemiology

Epidemiological studies have shown that populations that consume a high-calorie diet rich in animal protein, animal fats, refined carbohydrates, and processed foods have a high incidence of atherosclerosis. Populations that consume a diet of reduced caloric content consisting of plant proteins, plant fats, complex carbohydrates, and fresh, unrefined foods have a low incidence of the disease (Keys, 1975). Except for certain uncommon hereditary diseases which predispose to atherosclerosis, such as hypercholesterolemia or homocystinuria, genetic factors do not explain the incidence of atherosclerosis in different population groups.

Persons of Japanese ancestry, for example, develop a much higher incidence of atherosclerosis when consuming the atherogenic diet of southern California, compared to their relatives in Japan who consume a nonatherogenic diet. The potential reversibility and protection from atherosclerosis by consumption of a diet of reduced caloric content with predominantly unrefined plant foods is shown by the dramatic decrease in the disease which was observed in northern Europe during World Wars I and II. More recently, beginning about 1965, mortality from atherosclerosis and coronary heart disease has steadily and progressively declined in the United States, but the principal factor or factors responsible for this decline have not been identified with certainty (NIH, 1979).

For many years, an increased risk of atherosclerosis has been known to be associated with increased total serum cholesterol, increased low-density lipoprotein, and lowered high-density lipoprotein in susceptible populations (Keys, 1975). Studies of atherosclerotic lesions in fatal cases have shown correlations of these lipid abnormalities, as well as cigarette smoking, with severity of disease, but no consistent association was found with obesity or physical activity (Solberg and Strong, 1983). Although the dietary and drug therapy alternatives for reducing serum lipids are controversial, there is a growing consensus that lowering serum cholesterol levels will reduce the incidence of atherosclerosis in susceptible populations (Grundy, 1986).

HOMOCYSTEINE METABOLISM AND THE PATHOGENESIS OF ATHEROSCLEROSIS

Homocystinuria and Atherosclerosis

The relation between altered homocysteine metabolism and the pathogenesis of atherosclerosis was discovered through the study of children with homocystinuria caused by different inherited enzymatic disorders (McCully, 1969). In the most common form of homocystinuria, a deficiency of cystathionine synthetase causes decreased synthesis of cystathionine from homocysteine and serine (Mudd et al., 1964). As a result of this enzyme deficiency, the serum and urine of these individuals contain homocystine, homocysteine-cysteine mixed disulfide, and small quantities of several unusual derivatives of homocysteine (Perry, 1971). The chemical structure of a number of relevant derivatives of homocysteine is illustrated in Fig. 1.* The deficiency of cystathionine synthetase also causes

---

* *Note*: The chemical structure in Fig. 1 for the complex formed from *N*-homocysteine thiolactonyl retinamide and adenosylcobalamin was determined by synthesis and spectroscopy (McCully and Vezeridis, 1989a). A definitive and detailed chemical structure of the complex remains to be established by crystallography and other methods. Current evidence suggests a structure corresponding to di-homocysteine *thio*lactonyl*retina*mido*co*byrinate, and ''thioretinaco'' is proposed as a shortened version of this name. A corresponding shortened name for *N*-homocysteine *thio*lactonyl*retinamide* (McCully and Vezeridis, 1987) is proposed to be ''thioretinamide.''

CH₃SCH₂CH₂CH(NH₂)COOH — methionine

HSCH₂CH₂CH(NH₂)COOH — homocysteine

HOOCCH(NH₂)CH₂CH₂SSCH₂CH₂CH(NH₂)COOH — homocystine

HOOCCH(NH₂)CH₂CH₂SSCH₂CH(NH₂)COOH — homocysteine cysteine disulfide

HOOCCH(NH₂)CH₂SCH₂CH₂CH(NH₂)COOH — cystathionine

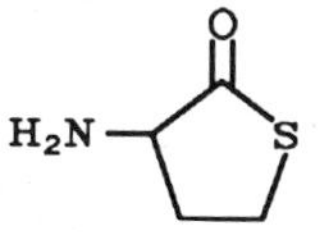

homocysteine thiolactone

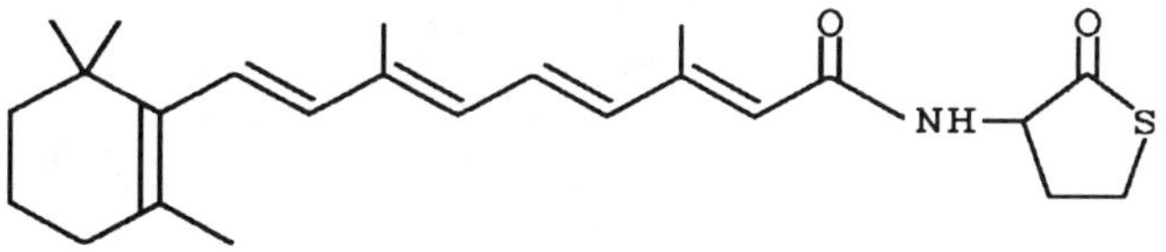

N-homocysteine thiolactonyl retinamide

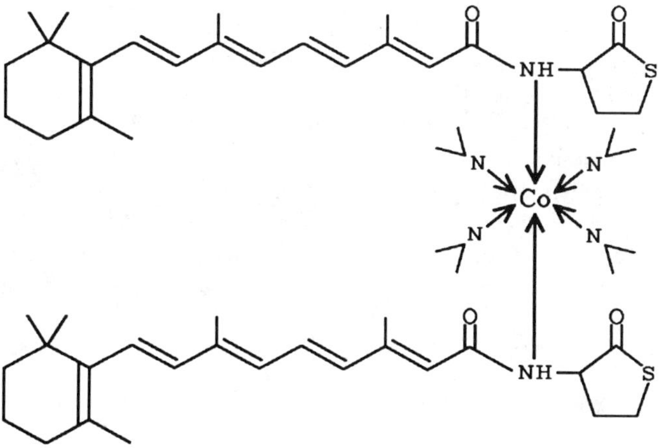

N-homocysteine thiolactonyl retinamido cobalamin

Figure 1 Chemical structures of key homocysteine compounds involved in atherogenesis are indicated. Two molecules of *N*-homocysteine thiolactonylretinamide are bound to the cobalt atom of the corrin ring of cobalamin to form *N*-homocysteine thiolactonylretinamidocobalamin.

decreased concentration of cystathionine in plasma and in tissues and increased concentration of methionine in plasma, resulting from increased methylation of homocysteine to methionine. The coenzyme which catalyzes cystathionine synthesis from homocysteine and serine is pyridoxal phosphate. About half of individuals with homocystinuria and cystathionine synthetase deficiency respond metabolically to large doses of pyridoxine by a dramatic reduction or elimination of homocysteine derivatives from plasma. Patients with homocystinuria caused by cystathionine synthetase deficiency develop arteriosclerosis in childhood with many pathological features similar to those of the atherosclerotic lesions seen in the general adult population (McCully, 1983).

In an infant with homocystinuria and cystathioninuria caused by deficiency of homocysteine methyltetrahydrofolate methyltransferase, arteriosclerotic plaques were discovered which are similar to those occurring in the arteries in cystathionine synthetase deficiency (McCully, 1969). In the plasma and urine of this child, increased concentrations of homocystine, homocysteine-cysteine mixed disulfide, cystathionine, and methylmalonic acid, and decreased concentration of methionine were found (Mudd et al., 1969). The homocysteine methyltetrahydrofolate methyltransferase enzyme requires cobalamin and methyltetrahydrofolate for optimum activity. Since elevated homocysteine was the common metabolic abnormality and cystathionine and methionine concentrations differed in these cases, the development of arteriosclerotic plaques was attributed to an atherogenic effect of homocysteine on the cells and tissues of the arteries.

A third type of homocystinuria results from deficiency of methylenetetrahydrofolate reductase, the enzyme which catalyzes methyltetrahydrofolate synthesis from methylenetetrahydrofolate (Mudd et al., 1972). The arteriosclerotic plaques which develop in this disease resemble those found in homocystinuria caused by deficiencies of cystathionine synthetase or homocysteine methyltetrahydrofolate methyltransferase (Kanwar et al., 1976), supporting the conclusion that homocysteine accumulation causes arteriosclerotic plaques in homocytinuria.

In Fig. 2 the pathways of metabolism of methionine and homocysteine are illustrated, and the three principal enzyme deficiencies which cause homocystinuria are indicated.

Homocysteine Theory of Arteriosclerosis

The observations correlating arteriosclerotic lesions with elevation of blood homocysteine in hereditary enzymatic disorders led to the development of the homocysteine theory of arteriosclerosis (McCully, 1983). The central tenet of this theory is that accumulation of homocysteine within blood is atherogenic, both in experimental animals and in persons with or without hereditary enzymatic deficiencies of homocysteine metabolism. This hypothesis has been substantiated by experimental demonstration of arteriosclerotic plaques in rabbits, baboons,

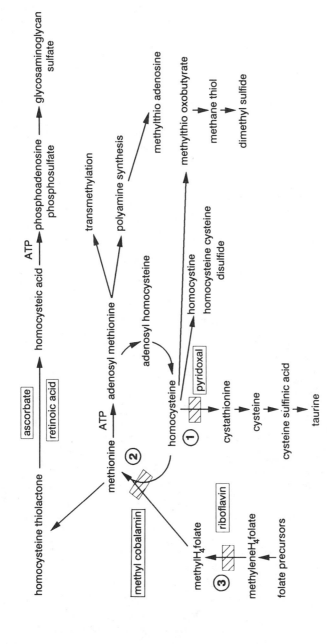

Figure 2 Three enzyme deficiencies which cause homocystinuria and arteriosclerosis are indicated by bars. 1, cystathionine synthetase; 2, homocysteine methyltetrahydrofolate methyltransferase; and 3, methylenetetrahydrofolate reductase. Coenzymes required for key reactions are circled.

rats, and pigs given homocysteine, homocystine, or homocysteine thiolactone by subcutaneous, intravenous, or alimentary routes. Furthermore, homocysteine accumulation has been demonstrated in persons with coronary, cerebral, or peripheral atherosclerosis without known hereditary disorders of homocysteine metabolism (Table 1).

The metabolic origin of homocysteine (Fig. 2) consists of demethylation of the essential amino acid methionine by a complex series of biochemical reactions involving synthesis of adenosyl methionine from methionine and ATP, demethylation of adenosyl methionine, and hydrolysis of adenosyl homocysteine. The metabolic fate of homocysteine is either remethylation by methylcobalamin to form methionine, transamination to methylthiooxobutyrate, and degradation to methanethiol and dimethylsulfide, or reaction with serine to form cystathionine, which is subsequently metabolized to cysteine, homoserine, cysteine sulfinic acid, and taurine. Methionine is also converted by demethylation to the chemically reactive anhydride homocysteine thiolactone, which forms peptide-bound homocysteinyl groups with free amino groups of proteins, nucleic acids, and glycosaminoglycans, or polymers of the cyclic dipeptide homocysteine diketopiperazine (DuVigneaud et al., 1938). Homocysteine thiolactone is oxidized in normal cells and tissues to homocysteic acid, phosphoadenosine phosphosulfate, and the sulfate esters of glycosaminoglycans (McCully, 1971).

Micronutrients and Homocysteine Metabolism

Essential micronutrients are the precursors of the coenzymes which catalyze many of the key reactions controlling homocysteine synthesis and catabolism (Fig. 2). Thus dietary adequacy of micronutrients and metabolic, hormonal, or toxic effects on the coenzymes formed from these micronutrients may inhibit or accelerate formation of atherosclerotic plaques by controlling the synthesis, catabolism, and accumulation of homocysteine in the blood.

Pyridoxine is the micronutrient precursor of pyridoxal phosphate, the coenzyme required for cystathionine synthesis from homocysteine and serine. Chronic pyridoxine deficiency causes accumulation of blood homocysteine and produces atherosclerotic plaques in monkeys and other experimental animals (Rinehart and Greenberg, 1949; Smolin et al., 1983). Experimental pyridoxine deficiency also causes both homocystine and cystathionine excretion in human volunteers (Park and Linkswiler, 1970).

N-methyltetrahydrofolate is the methyl donor leading to the formation of methyl cobalamin, which is the coenzyme for the conversion of homocysteine to methionine by the enzyme, homocysteine methyltetrahydrofolate methyltransferase. Deficiency of either folate or cobalamin, as determined by assay of human serum, is associated with increased blood homocysteine (Kang et al., 1987; Stabler et al., 1988; Chu and Hall, 1988). The methyl group precursors, choline and

Table 1 Plasma Homocysteine in Atherosclerosis

Study	Method	Site	Sex	Patients (nmol/ml)	Number (n)	Controls (nmol/ml)	Number (n)
Brattstrom et al. (1984)	Free	Cerebral	M,F	5.1 ± 0.6^a	19	3.5 ± 0.2	17
Kang et al. (1986)	Sulfhydryl	Coronary	M	5.41 ± 1.62^b	173	4.37 ± 1.09	93
			F	5.66 ± 1.93^b	68	4.16 ± 1.62	109
Israelsson et al. (1988)	Sulfhydryl	Coronary	M	16.4 ± 6.9^a	21	13.5 ± 3.6	36
Malinow et al. (1989)	Sulfhydryl	Peripheral	M	15.44 ± 5.76^a	26	10.74 ± 2.16	53
			F	17.04 ± 8.26^a	21	9.04 ± 2.16	50
Olszewski and Szostak (1988)	Peptide	Coronary	M	95.8 ± 8.4^c	26	3.8 ± 1.1	26

[a] $p < .05$.
[b] $p < 0.0005$.
[c] $p < 0.001$.

Note: Plasma homocysteine was determined in patients with atherosclerosis by three methods: chromatography of deproteinized plasma (free), plasma treated with sulfhydryl reagents and deproteinized (sulfhydryl), and plasma hydrolyzed with acid (peptide). The results for acid hydrolysis (peptide) are 10-fold lower than presented in the original report because of correction of a calculation error (Olszewski, personal communication, 1990). Data are given as mean ± SD except for Brattstrom et al., mean ± SEM.

betaine, are micronutrients which potentially counteract homocysteine accumulation by facilitating transmethylation of homocysteine to methionine through enhanced formation of methyltetrahydrofolate and methylcobalamin. Administration of betaine diminishes blood homocysteine in individuals with pyridoxine-responsive cystathionine synthetase deficiency and homocystinuria given oral methionine (Wilcken et al., 1985).

Riboflavin is the precursor of flavin adenine dinucleotide, the coenzyme for methylenetetrahydrofolate reductase, the enzyme which catalyzes the formation of methyltetrahydrofolate from methylenetetrahydrofolate. Riboflavin is also involved in the reduction of the cobalt atom of cobalamin, which accepts transfer of methyl groups from methyltetrahydrofolate to form methylcobalamin. Riboflavin deficiency has not been implicated in homocysteine accumulation and atherogenesis, except in individuals with hereditary deficiency of methylenetetrahydrofolate reductase and homocystinuria.

Metabolism of Homocysteine Thiolactone and Atherogenesis

The oxidation of homocysteine thiolactone to homocysteic acid and conversion to phosphoadenosine phosphosulfate requires ascorbate, since this reaction is inhibited in experimental scurvy (McCully, 1971). Homocysteic acid promotes growth of hypophysectomized animals through release of somatomedin (Clopath et al., 1976). Homocysteine thiolactone forms a retinamide with *trans*-retinoic acid (McCully and Vezeridis, 1987). Both *N*-homocysteine thiolactonylretinamide (thioretinamide) and its complex with cobalamin, *N*-homocysteine thiolactonylretinamidocobalamin (thioretinaco), are anticarcinogenic and antineoplastic in experimental animals (McCully and Vezeridis, 1989a,b). Retinoids have been implicated in the biochemical transformation of methionine to sulfate, and thioretinaco may be involved in this metabolic pathway. Both thioretinamide and thioretinaco facilitate atherogenesis by a synthetic diet in experimental animals (McCully et al., 1990.

Micronutrients such as ascorbate, retinoids, and cobalamin which promote oxidation of homocysteine thiolactone to phosphoadenosine phosphosulfate and sulfate esters of glycosaminoglycans may affect atherogenesis by facilitation of homocysteine utilization. Antioxidants such as tocopherol, glutathione, or troxerutin would be expected to counteract atherogenesis by inhibition of homocysteine thiolactone oxidation and utilization. Accelerated oxidation by hyperbaric oxygen or by the effects of ionizing radiation would be expected to promote atherogenesis by facilitation of oxidation and utilization of homocysteine thiolactone.

Homocysteine and Atherosclerotic Plaque Formation

Homocysteine is an important factor in initiating the cellular and macromolecular changes involved in formation of atherosclerotic plaques (McCully, 1983). Chemical injury to endothelial cells by homocysteine results in denudation of intimal surfaces, endothelemia, and adherence of platelets to the sites of injury. The free base of the anhydride of homocysteine is highly toxic to tissues of experimental animals, causing intense necrosis at the site of injection accompanied by regenerative changes of epithelial and stromal cells, with fibrosis, calcification, angiogenesis, acute and chronic inflammation, hypertrophy of ducts and nerves, acanthosis, hyperkeratosis and dysplasia of squamous epithelium, and intravascular fibrin thrombi (McCully and Vezeridis, 1989c). The free base of homocysteine thiolactone is also active at low concentration in causing aggregation and release of thromboxane and prostacyclin by platelets (McCully and Carvalho, 1987).

Following chemical injury of endothelium by homocysteine, the growth factors released from platelets and macrophages induce hyperplasia of smooth muscle cells of arterial walls. The hyperplastic smooth muscle cells of developing plaques synthesize sulfated glycosaminoglycans, principally proteochondroitin sulfate and proteodermatan sulfate, as well as tropocollagen fibrils, resulting in deposition of extracellular matrix and collagen. The sulfate groups of extracellular matrix are derived from oxidation of homocysteine thiolactone, a process correlated with cellular and tissue growth. Homocysteine is believed to produce the characteristic fragmentation and degeneration of elastica interna of the intima of developing atherosclerotic plaques by formation of tetrahydrothiazine adducts with lysyl aldehyde of tropoelastin, preventing synthesis of the desmosine and isodesmosine crosslinks of mature elastin. Calcification occurs as the result of deposition of hydroxyapatite crystals within the collagen and extracellular matrix of developing plaques by ionic bonding with sulfate and other acidic groups of the constituent macromolecules.

Homocysteine and Lipoprotein Metabolism in Atherosclerosis

The characteristic deposition of lipoproteins and cholesterol within atheromas occurs because of binding between extracellular matrix of developing plaques and lipoproteins of plasma filtered through sites of intimal injury. The insoluble lipoprotein–glycosaminoglycan sulfate complexes are degraded by tissue enzymes, such as lipoprotein lipase, proteases, and glycanases, releasing free cholesterol, which becomes deposited as crystals in advancing plaques. Some of the lipoprotein–glycosaminoglycan sulfate complexes and degraded lipids are phagocytosed by macrophages, forming the foam cells which are found in small numbers in atheromas.

There is evidence for a connection between homocysteine and lipoprotein metabolism. The sulfate groups of arterial wall sulfated glycosaminoglycans which form insoluble complexes with filtered plasma lipoproteins are derived from oxidation of homocysteine thiolactone to homocysteic acid and phosphoadenosine phosphosulfate. Homocysteic acid has growth hormone activity (Clopath et al., 1976), and growth hormone affects lipid metabolism by elevating the plasma concentration of free fatty acids (Raben and Hollenberg, 1959). Cholic acid, the oxidized form of cholesterol which is not metabolized further in human tissues (Bergstrom and Borgstrom, 1956), is excreted in the bile conjugated with taurine, a product of homocysteine metabolism by the transsulfuration pathway. The administration of homocysteine thiolactone to rabbits produces elevation of total serum cholesterol, low-density lipoproteins, triglycerides, and phospholipids, metabolic changes which are present in some individuals with atherosclerosis (Gaggi and Gianni, 1973).

Elevated plasma homocysteine is correlated with both elevated total cholesterol and elevated triglycerides in men with ischemic heart disease (Olszewski et al., 1989). Although many clinical studies have associated elevated serum cholesterol and low-density lipoprotein with increased risk of atherosclerosis, significant numbers of cases are found to have severe or fatal atherosclerosis without elevation of blood lipids. In a retrospective study of 194 consecutive autopsies, the majority of cases developed severe atherosclerosis without evidence of elevated serum cholesterol, diabetes, or hypertension (McCully, 1990). This study shows that human atherosclerosis frequently progresses to the terminal phase without elevated plasma lipoproteins. Individuals with homozygous hypercholesterolemia due to deficiency of cellular membrane receptors for low-density lipoprotein are at increased risk of fatal atherosclerosis (Brown et al., 1981). Homocysteine metabolism has not been studied in these individuals or in those with nonhereditary elevation of plasma lipoproteins.

CLINICAL STUDIES OF MICRONUTRIENTS AND HOMOCYSTEINE METABOLISM IN ATHEROSCLEROSIS

Methods of Homocysteine Analysis

Human plasma or serum from normal individuals contains small quantities (2–4 nmol/ml) of free homocystine, homocysteine-cysteine mixed disulfide, and traces of homocysteine. Slightly larger quantities of homocysteine (8–11 nmol/ml) are bound to plasma proteins by disulfide bonds, and treatment of normal plasma with reducing reagents, such as dithiothreitol, mercaptoethanol, or sodium borohydride, releases free homocysteine, which is detected by high-pressure liquid chromatography or conventional amino acid chromatography. When normal serum is subjected to acid hydrolysis, similar quantities (3.8 nmol/ml) of homocysteine are detected as homocystine and homocysteine-cysteine mixed disulfide by amino acid chromatography (Olszewski and Szostak, 1988; Olszewski, personal communication, 1990). Other methods for assay of plasma homocysteine include radioenzymatic assay, utilizing synthesis of adenosyl homocysteine from ATP and homocysteine, and gas chromatography-mass spectrometry. Attempts to isolate homocysteine thiolactone from normal serum or lipoprotein fractions by extraction and chromatography have been unsuccessful (McCully, 1989). Peptide-bound homocysteine, which is released by acid hydrolysis, is believed to originate from reaction of endogenous homocysteine thiolactone with free amino groups of plasma proteins.

Plasma Homocysteine in Atherosclerosis

Several laboratories have demonstrated that persons with coronary, cerebral, or peripheral atherosclerosis have elevated concentrations of plasma homocysteine, compared to normal controls (Table 1). In a study of 19 patients with arteriosclerotic cerebrovascular disease, the free homocysteine-cysteine mixed disulfide of deproteinized plasma was found to be 5.1 ± 0.6 nmol/ml (mean $\pm$ SEM), which is significantly higher ($p < 0.05$) than the concentration of 3.5 ± 0.2 nmol/ml found in 19 age-matched controls. Four hours after an oral methionine load, the values increased to 16.0 ± 3.6 in the patient group and 11.9 ± 1.0 nmol/ml in the control group (Brattstrom et al., 1984). Similar findings were reported in a group of 25 patients with cerebrovascular disease, and 30% of 50 patients under 50 with peripheral and cerebrovascular disease were found to be heterozygous for cystathionine synthetase deficiency, as determined by the oral methionine load test and enzymatic assay of cultured skin fibroblasts (Boers et al., 1985). In a group of 99 men with coronary heart disease, as demonstrated by angiography, the plasma free homocysteine-cysteine mixed disulfide became elevated after oral methionine in 16%, compared to 2% of the control group (Murphy-Chutorian et al., 1985). The free mixed disulfide of plasma was found to be increased in 25 patients with coronary heart disease, as demonstrated by angiography, compared to 22 controls, following oral methionine (Wilcken and Wilcken, 1976), although a later study was equivocal (Wilcken et al., 1983).

Using a method for sulfhydryl-bound homocysteine, 241 patients with coronary heart disease were found to have significantly higher ($p < 0.0005$) total homocysteine of plasma, 5.41 ± 1.62 nmol/ml (mean $\pm$ SD), than 202 controls, 4.37 ± 1.09 nmol/ml (Kang et al., 1986). Using a method for total free homocysteine plus protein disulfide-bound homocysteine, 21 men with previous myocardial infarction without other risk factors had a significantly higher ($p < 0.05$) value, 16.4 ± 6.9 (mean $\pm$ SD), than controls, 13.5 ± 3.6 nmol/ml (Israelsson et al., 1988). Using a high-performance liquid chromatography method with electrochemical detection, the total free and disulfide-bound homocysteine of plasma was found to be significantly higher ($p < 0.05$) in 47 patients with peripheral arteriosclerosis, 15.22 ± 5.76 (mean $\pm$ SD) (men) and 17.04 ± 8.26 (women) nmol/ml, compared to controls, 10.74 ± 2.16 (men) and 8.58 ± 2.82 (women) nmol/ml (Malinow et al., 1989).

The use of acid hydrolysis of serum or plasma for estimation of total blood homocysteine in atherosclerosis yields different results because homocysteine bound to amino groups of plasma proteins by peptide bonds, as well as disulfide-bound and free homocysteine, are released by this method. In a study of 26 male survivors of acute myocardial infarction, acid hydrolysis of plasma yielded 95.8 nmol/ml (mean ± SD), compared to 3.8 nmol/ml for the control group (Olszewski and Szostak, 1988; Olszewski, personal communication, 1990). These results show that the majority of blood homocysteine is carried bound to plasma proteins by acid-labile bonds, and the fraction bound by peptide bonds probably originates from reaction of endogenous homocysteine thiolactone with free amino groups of plasma proteins (McCully, 1989). Further studies are needed to determine whether the method for sulfhydryl bound homocysteine or the method for peptide bound homocysteine will prove to be the more useful.

Using the method for disulfide-bound homocysteine, normal men are found to have higher total homocysteine of plasma than women (Wilcken and Gupta, 1979a; Kang et al., 1986). For example, men under 60 have a higher ($p < 0.05$) total homocysteine, 11.18 ± 3.58 (mean ± SD), than women under 60, 8.58 ± 2.82 nmol/ml (Malinow et al., 1989). In addition, younger premenopausal women have a lower total plasma homocysteine than older postmenopausal women (Boers et al., 1983). These findings suggest that higher plasma homocysteine concentrations may explain the greater susceptibility to development of athero-sclerosis of men compared to women, and the greater susceptibility of post-menopausal women compared to premenopausal women.

Micronutrients and Homocysteine Metabolism in Atherosclerosis

Patients with chronic renal failure are at high risk for development of athero-sclerosis. These patients have increased free homocysteine and homocysteine-cysteine mixed disulfide, compared to persons with normal renal function (Wilcken and Gupta, 1979b). The elevation of homocysteine is attributed to decreased renal clearance, since plasma homocysteine is positively correlated with serum creatinine, and renal transplantation restores the homocysteine con-centration to normal. Several of the micronutrients which facilitate homocysteine catabolism were given to patients with chronic renal failure, including pyridoxine, folate, and cobalamin. Only folic acid was found to lower elevated plasma homocysteine, even in the absence of demonstrable folate deficiency (Wilcken et al., 1981, 1988). Folic acid was also found to lower the total plasma homocysteine in postmenopausal women and in healthy subjects (Brattstrom et al., 1985, 1988).

In a study of 21 patients with ischemic heart disease (Table 2), six micro-nutrients, folate, cobalamin, pyridoxine, choline, riboflavin and troxerutin, were found to lower total plasma homocysteine, as estimated by the acid hydrolysis method (Olszewski et al., 1989). Plasma levels of homocysteine were found to be correlated with total cholesterol, triglycerides, and body mass index. These

Table 2 Effect of Micronutrients for Homocysteine Catabolism on Plasma Lipid and Homocysteine Levels in Coronary Heart Disease

Plasma level	Units	Treated (n = 12)		Untreated (n = 10)	
		Before	After 21 days	Before	After 21 days
Homocysteine	nmol/ml	79.2 ± 25.8	53.9 ± 24.9[a]	81.6 ± 23.7	84.9 ± 28.6
Cholesterol	mmol/ml	6.80 ± 0.83	5.35 ± 0.83[a]	6.62 ± 1.24	6.72 ± 0.72
Triglycerides	mmol/ml	2.53 ± 1.01	1.72 ± 0.51[b]	2.33 ± 0.98	3.08 ± 0.69
LDL apoB	mmol/ml	3.56 ± 0.58	2.24 ± 0.59[a]	3.69 ± 0.83	3.50 ± 0.69
HDL cholesterol	mmol/ml	1.19 ± 0.24	1.14 ± 0.32	1.06 ± 0.15	1.22 ± 0.14

[a] $p < 0.001$.
[b] $p < 0.01$.

Note: Survivors of acute myocardial infarction were given pyridoxine, folate, cobalamin, choline, riboflavin, and troxerutin for 21 days. Results are given as mean ± SD. The results for homocysteine are 10-fold lower than presented in the original report because of correction of a calculation error (Olszewski, personal communication, 1990).

Source: Modified from Olszewski et al. (1989) with permission, copyright Elsevier Scientific Publishers Ireland, Ltd.

six micronutrients also reduced the cholesterol, triglycerides, and low-density lipoproteins to normal levels. This finding shows that lowering plasma homocysteine has a favorable influence on the abnormalities of lipoprotein metabolism found in patients with atherosclerosis. The six micronutrients all facilitate homocysteine catabolism by different biochemical pathways. Folic acid and cobalamin are precursors of the coenzymes which transfer methyl groups to the sulfhydryl groups of homocysteine, forming the nonatherogenic amino acid methionine. Choline is a source of methyl groups for transmethylation reactions, and riboflavin is a precursor of the flavoprotein reductase which converts methylenetetrahydrofolate to methyltetrahydrofolate. Troxerutin is an antioxidant which inhibits conversion of ascorbate to semidehydroascorbate, the cofactor for conversion of homocysteine to homocysteic acid and phosphoadenosine phosphosulfate.

A recent nutritional survey showed that dietary intake of vitamin B_6 is less than the RDA, 2.0 mg/day for 79% of women over 60 and less than the RDA, 2.2 mg/day, for 75% of men over 60 (Manore et al., 1989). Plasma pyridoxal phosphate was significantly low in one-third of these individuals. A study by Kok et al. (1989) of plasma pyridoxal phosphate showed a significantly lower concentration in acute myocardial infarction, 24.0 $\pm$ 2.0 nM (mean $\pm$ SEM), compared to a control group, 30.9 $\pm$ 1.6 nM ($p < 0.05$), confirming earlier reports (Serfontein et al., 1985; Vermaak et al., 1987).

Analysis of a recent nutritional survey has shown that 88% of U.S. adults consume less folate than the RDA, 0.4 mg/day (Subar et al., 1989). Low serum cobalamin values were found in 5.3% of an elderly population over 70, and atrophic gastritis and gastrectomy were found to be major contributory factors in the deficiency state (Nilsson-Ehle et al., 1989). Nutritional deficiency of pyridoxine, folate, and cobalamin among the elderly may explain the high incidence of atherosclerosis in this group because of the consequent induction of a chronic homocysteinemic state.

Genetic Factors in Homocysteine Metabolism and Atherosclerosis

Extensive investigation of homocystinuria caused by homozygous cystathionine synthetase deficiency has documented prominent vascular pathology with thromboembolic complications in these individuals (Mudd and Levy, 1983). The possibility of increased risk of atherosclerosis in heterozygotes for this disease is controversial. A study based on a questionnaire survey of 260 families concluded that there was no increased risk of atherosclerosis among obligate heterozygotes (Mudd et al., 1981). The conclusions of this study were questioned by Swift and Morrell (1982), who drew attention to increased "heart attacks" in grandmothers aged 30–44 and in fathers of probands, although the risk was only two- to threefold that of control groups and did not reach statistical significance. In a multicenter study of 629 homozygous patients with cystathionine synthetase deficiency, 71% of the 64 deaths were caused by thromboembolism, and treatment of pyridoxine-responsive patients decreased the expected incidence of thromboembolism in 120 survivors, confirming earlier studies (Mudd et al., 1985).

Heterozygotes for cystathionine synthetase deficiency are detected by a combination of plasma homocysteine elevation following oral methionine and enzyme analysis of cultured skin fibroblasts (Mudd and Levy, 1983). Using this approach, Boers et al. (1985) concluded that 30% of 50 unselected patients under the age of 50 with peripheral and cerebral atherosclerosis were heterozygous for cystathionine synthetase deficiency. Similarly, Israelsson et al. (1988) concluded that 14% of 21 men under the age of 60 with myocardial infarction were in the range for heterozygous cystathionine synthetase deficiency.

Other genetic factors involving homocysteine metabolism may also affect susceptibility to atherosclerosis. Interesting examples of thermolabile methylenetetrahydrofolate reductase deficiency were discovered in two unrelated individuals with subnormal folate and an eight- to 15-fold increase in plasma total homocysteine (Kang et al., 1986). One of these patients was found among a group with coronary heart disease and the other was found to have subnormal plasma folate.

Another example of a congenital relation to atherosclerosis is Down syndrome, in which atherosclerosis is rare or absent, and cystathionine synthetase of cultured fibroblasts is increased compared to that of controls (Brattstrom et al., 1987). Oral methionine loading resulted in decreased homocysteine accumulation in patients with Down syndrome compared to patients with other forms of mental retardation (Chadefaux et al., 1988). These findings suggest that in Down syndrome susceptibility to atherosclerosis is diminished by increased efficiency of the transsulfuration pathway of homocysteine metabolism.

EFFECTS OF DRUGS, TOXINS AND HORMONES ON MICRONUTRIENTS AND HOMOCYSTEINE METABOLISM

Azaribine, Thrombosis, and Homocysteine Metabolism

The drug azaribine, triacetyl-6-azauridine, was found to produce urinary excretion of homocystine and other amino acids in rabbits (Slavik et al., 1969). Azaribine is an antimetabolite of nucleic acid metabolism which is effective in treating patients with refractory psoriasis or mycosis fungoides (Calabresi and Turner, 1966). Treatment of psoriatic patients with azaribine resulted in an increased incidence of arterial and venous thrombosis with stroke, myocardial infarction, and peripheral gangrene, which were attributed to homocystinemia induced by the drug (Shupak, 1977). Azaribine causes depletion of pyridoxal phosphate in the serum of rabbits, and the subsequent homocystinemia is prevented by administration of pyridoxine (Slavik et al., 1982). These observations show that homocystinemia induced by azaribine exacerbates human atherosclerosis, supporting the conclusions drawn from observation of atherosclerotic lesions in hereditary disorders of homocysteine metabolism. The use of azaribine in psoriasis was discontinued by the Food and Drug Administration, which cited the atherogenic effect of induced homocystinemia as the reason for withdrawing the drug from use.

Toxins, Micronutrients, and Atherosclerosis

In a study of deaths among male workers exposed to carbon disulfide in the viscose rayon industry, a more than twofold increase in coronary heart disease mortality was discovered, compared to workers not exposed to the toxin (Tiller et al., 1968). Carbon disulfide antagonizes the action of pyridoxal phosphate, probably by combining with the pyridoxamine phosphate form of the coenzyme, forming the inactive dithiocarbamic acid derivative, and pyridoxine relieves many of the toxic effects of carbon disulfide (Calabrese, 1984). The elevation of serum cholesterol, low-density lipoprotein, triglycerides, and other lipids which was induced by experimental carbon disulfide poisoning in rats was ameliorated by pyridoxine (Petrova, 1985). Although homocysteine metabolism has not been studied in carbon disulfide toxicity, increased production of homocysteine thiolactone from methionine would be expected to produce the observed atherogenic and hyperlipemic effects.

Another important toxin which antagonizes pyridoxal phosphate is carbon monoxide, one of the principal toxic components of tobacco smoke. Cigarette smoking is a major risk factor for atherosclerosis and coronary heart disease. A survey of 106 male smokers revealed significantly lower pyridoxal phosphate concentration in plasma compared to 146 nonsmokers (Serfontein et al., 1986). The previously reported inverse relationship of plasma pyridoxal phosphate concentration with age was confirmed by a highly sensitive chromatographic method, and a correlation was found between the risk of coronary heart disease and depressed levels of pyridoxal phosphate (Serfontein et al., 1985). Thus depressed plasma pyridoxal phosphate levels are correlated with smoking, age, and susceptibility to atherosclerosis. Although homocysteine metabolism has not been studied in smokers, the atherogenic effect of carbon monoxide would be expected to result from homocysteine accumulation caused by antagonism of pyridoxal phosphate.

Hormones, Homocysteine Metabolism, and Atherosclerosis

Estrogens and oral contraceptives have been shown to antagonize the metabolic effects of pyridoxine and to lower the concentration of pyridoxal phosphate in the plasma (Bender, 1987). In experimental human pyridoxine deficiency, oral methionine results in excretion of cystathionine and homocystine (Park and Link-swiler, 1970). Arteriosclerotic lesions and increased risk of thrombosis are observed in high-dose oral contraceptive use (Irey and Norris, 1973). These complications may be related to altered homocysteine metabolism (McCully, 1975). Reduced plasma pyridoxal phosphate and small quantities of homocystine were found in the urine of oral contraceptive users before and after oral methionine (Miller et al., 1978).

Paradoxically, normal endogenous ovarian hormones protect premenopausal women against atherosclerosis, and normal or surgically induced menopause is associated with increased risk of the disease. In a study of methionine catabolism, premenopausal women were found to have increased activity of the transamination pathway for methylthiooxobutyrate formation, explaining the lower concentration of plasma homocysteine in premenopausal women compared to young men (Blom et al., 1988).

PREVENTION AND TREATMENT OF ATHEROSCLEROSIS

Dietary Prevention of Atherosclerosis

Since methionine is the only dietary source of homocysteine, the methionine content of dietary protein may be regarded as an important factor in prevention of atherosclerosis. Proteins of animal foods of all types, including meat, fish, poultry, and milk, contain approximately two to three times as much methionine as dietary plant proteins, including grains, legumes, vegetables, and fruits. Therefore, consumption of a diet composed principally of plant proteins will reduce the quantity of dietary methionine available for conversion to homocysteine. In fact, populations consuming a primarily vegetarian diet are protected against atherosclerosis, compared with those consuming a diet rich in proteins and animal sources. Furthermore, changing dietary consumption of a population from animal to plant sources dramatically reduces the incidence of atherosclerosis, as happened in the northern European populations during World Wars I and II.

Some methods of food processing and preservation are known to deplete fresh foods of their normal content of micronutrients which control homocysteine synthesis from methionine. Certain naturally occurring forms of pyridoxine, folate, and riboflavin are sensitive to heat, radiation, or chemical oxidation. Supplementation of processed foods by addition of synthetic micronutrients to the levels recommended by the National Research Council helps to restore the quantities of those micronutrients known to be destroyed in food processing. Populations which consume a diet composed principally of unprocessed, fresh foods have been found to be protected against atherosclerosis, compared with populations consuming a diet composed principally of processed foods. In fact, the decline in mortality from coronary heart disease in the United States is correlated with increased supplementation of processed foods by synthetic pyridoxine (McCully, 1983).

Consumption of a diet rich in refined carbohydrates, such as sugar and bleached white flour, increases the susceptibility of the population to atherosclerosis. Furthermore, consumption of a diet with a high content of fat increases susceptibility to atherosclerosis, particularly if the fat is rich in saturated fatty acids. Both refined carbohydrates and fats are deficient in water-soluble micronutrients, and increased consumption of these nutrients decreases consumption of the micronutrients which prevent homocysteine accumulation. The higher serum cholesterol and low-density lipoprotein levels found in populations consuming a high-refined-carbohydrate, high-fat diet may result from the metabolic effects of increased homocysteine synthesis on control of cholesterol, triglyceride, and lipoprotein formation because of decreased micronutrient consumption.

A preventive diet for atherosclerosis, designed according to the principles of the homocysteine theory of arteriosclerosis, would consist predominantly of plant protein sources, with abundant fresh, minimally processed foods, including whole grains, legumes, fresh vegetables, fruits, and a minimum of refined carbohydrates and added fats. Such a diet supplies a modest methionine intake with sufficient micronutrients to prevent homocysteine accumulation without supplementation by synthetic micronutrients. This diet is compatible with the recommendations of the U.S. Surgeon General, the American Heart Association, and the National Research Council.

Micronutrients and the Treatment of Atherosclerosis

For individuals with clinical manifestations of advanced atherosclerosis, a preventive diet may be insufficient to delay onset of further complications of the disease, and micronutrient supplementation may prove to be beneficial. Few published clinical studies have been designed to test the efficacy of this approach. A preliminary study of 17 patients with coronary heart disease and stable angina pectoris concluded that reduction of animal protein consumption to approximately one-quarter to one-half of the previous intake, combined with 100 mg of pyridoxine and B complex supplements daily, caused complete or partial relief of angina, increase in exercise tolerance, and complete or marked regression of electrocardiographic abnormalities over a period of 13 months (Suzman, 1973).

Very large doses of pyridoxine, in the range of 0.2–2 g/day, have been reported to cause peripheral neuropathy in a few individuals (Parry and Bredesen, 1985; Schaumberg et al., 1983). However, more than 1000 patients with carpal tunnel syndrome have been treated with 100–200 mg/day of pyridoxine for years without evidence of neuropathy (Ellis, 1987).

A preliminary study of nutrient intake and plasma homocysteine among 15 persons at high risk and low risk for atherosclerosis showed a negative correlation between both dietary vitamin B_6 and the vitamin B_6/protein ratio and plasma sulfhydryl-bound homocysteine (Swift and Shultz, 1986). There was also a negative correlation between plasma vitamin B_{12} and free homocysteine. The high-risk group had a significantly higher free plasma homocysteine than the low-risk group. The dietary intakes of vitamins B_6, vitamin B_{12}, and folate were somewhat higher in the low-risk than the high-risk group.

A short-term study of 15 patients with peripheral arteriosclerosis concluded that parenteral folate improved visual acuity, increased skin temperature and capillary blood flow (Kopjas, 1966). Folate reduces the free and disulfide-bound plasma homocysteine in patients with renal failure (Wilcken et al., 1988), in normal volunteers (Brattstrom et al., 1988), and in postmenopausal women (Brattstrom et al., 1985), but the possible effects on vascular disease were not determined in these studies. The efficacy of folate, pyridoxine, cobalamin, riboflavin, choline, and troxerutin in reducing plasma homocysteine and plasma lipids was demonstrated (Table 2) in a study of 21 patients with ischemic heart disease (Olszewski et al., 1989).

These preliminary studies on homocysteine metabolism, micronutrients, and atherosclerosis are promising with regard to prevention of the disease but inconclusive because of their limited scope. A prospective, long-term study is needed in a large group of patients with atherosclerosis to determine to what extent a preventive diet and supplemental micronutrients which promote homocysteine catabolism will prevent clinical manifestations of the disease.

REFERENCES

Bender DA. Oestrogens and vitamin B_6: Actions and interactions. Wld Rev Nut Diet 1987; 51:140.

Bergstrom S, Borgstrom B. Metabolism of lipids. Ann Rev Biochem 1956; 25:177.

Blom HJ, Boers GHJ, Elzen JPAM, Roessel JMF. Differences between premenopausal women and young men in the transamination pathway of methionine catabolism, and the protection against vascular disease. J Clin Invest 1988; 18:633.

Boers GHJ, Smals AG, Trijbels FJM. Unique efficiency of methionine metabolism in premenopausal women may protect against vascular disease in the reproductive years. J Clin Invest 1983; 72:1971.

Boers GHJ, Smals AGH, Trijbels FJM, Fowler B, Bakkeren JAJM, Schoonderwaldt HC, Kleijer WJ, Kloppenborg PWC. Heterozygosity for homocystinuria in premature peripheral and cerebral occlusive arterial disease, N Engl J Med 1985; 313:709.

Brattstrom LE, Hardebo JE, Hultberg BL. Moderate homocysteinemia: A possible risk factor for arteriosclerotic cerebrovascular disease. Stroke 1984; 15:1012.

Brattstrom LE, Hultberg BL, Hardebo JE. Folic acid responsive post menopausal homocysteinemia. Metabolism 1985; 34:1073.

Brattstrom LE, Englund E, Brun A. Does Down syndrome support homocysteine theory of arteriosclerosis? Lancet 1987; 1:391.

Brattstrom LE, Israelsson B, Jeppsson JO, Hultberg BL. Folic acid: An innocuous means to reduce plasma homocysteine. Scand J Clin Lab Invest 1988; 48:215.

Brown MS, Kovanen PT, and Goldstein JL. Regulation of plasma cholesterol by lipoprotein receptors. Science 1981; 212:628.

Calabrese EJ. Environmental validation of the homocystine theory of arteriosclerosis. Med Hypoth 1984; 15:361.

Calabresi P, Turner RW. Beneficial effects of triacetyl azauridine in psoriasis and mycosis fungoides. Ann Int Med 1966; 64:352.

Chadefaux B, Ceballos I, Hamet M, Conde M, Poissonnier M, Kamoun P, Allard D. Is absence of atheroma in Down syndrome due to decreased homocysteine levels? Lancet 1988; 2:741.

Chu RC, Hall CA. The total serum homocysteine as an indicator of vitamin B_{12} and folate status, Am J Clin Pathol 1988; 90:446.

Clopath P, Smith VC, McCully KS. Growth promotion by homocysteic acid. Science 1976; 192:372.

DuVigneaud V, Patterson WI, Hunt M. Opening of the ring of the thiolactone of homocysteine. J Biol Chem 1938; 126:217.

Ellis JM. Treatment of carpal tunnel syndrome with vitamin B_6. South Med J 1987; 80:882.

Gaggi R, Gianni AM. The role of homocysteine in the pathogenesis of arteriosclerosis. Proc 1st Cong Hung Pharmacol Soc 1973; 2:287.

Grundy SM. Cholesterol and coronary heart disease. A new era. J Am Med Assoc 1986; 256:2849.

Irey MS, Norris HJ. Intimal vascular lesions associated with female reproductive steroids. Arch Pathol 1973; 96:227.

Israelsson B, Brattstrom LE, Hultberg BL. Homocysteine and myocardial infarction. Atherosclerosis 1988; 71:227.

Kang SS, Wong PWK, Norusis M. Homocysteinemia due to folate deficiency. Metabolism 1987; 36:468.

Kang SS, Wong PWK, Cook HY, Norusis M, Messer JV. Protein-bound homocyst(e)ine. A possible risk factor for coronary artery disease. J Clin Invest 1986; 77:1482.

Kang SS, Zhou J, Wong PWK, Kowaliszn J, Strokosch G. Intermediate homocysteinemia: A thermolabile variant of methylenetetrahydrofolate reductase. Am J Hum Genet 1988; 43:414.

Kanwar YS, Manaligod JR, Wong PWK. Morphologic studies in a patient with homocystinuria due to 5,10-methylenetetrahydrofolate reductase deficiency. Pediatr Res 1976; 10:598.

Keys A. Coronary heart disease: The global picture. Atherosclerosis 1975; 22:149.

Kok FJ, Schrijver J, Hofman A, Witterman JCM, Kruyssen DACM, Remme WJ, Valkenburg HA. Low vitamin B_6 status in patients with acute myocardial infarction. Am J Cardiol 1989; 63:513.

Kopjas TL. Effect of folic acid on collateral circulation in diffuse chronic arteriosclerosis. J Am Geriat Soc 1966; 14:1187.

Malinow MR, Kang SS, Taylor LM, Wong PWK, Coull B, Inhara T, Mukerjee D, Sexton G, Upson B. Prevalence of hyperhomocysteinemia in patients with peripheral arterial occlusive disease. Circulation 1989; 79:1180.

Manore MM, Vaughn LA, Carroll SS, Leklem JF. Plasma pyridoxal 5'-phosphate concentration and dietary vitamin B_6 intake in free-living low income elderly people. Am J Clin Nutr 1989; 50:339.

McCully KS. Vascular pathology of homocysteinemia: Implications for the pathogenesis of arteriosclerosis. Am J Pathol 1969; 56:111.

McCully KS. Homocysteine metabolism in scurvy, growth and arteriosclerosis. Nature 1971; 231:391.

McCully KS. Homocystine, atherosclerosis, and thrombosis: Implications for oral contraceptive users. Am J Clin Nutr 1975; 28:542.

McCully KS. The homocysteine theory of arteriosclerosis: Development and current status. Atherosclerosis Rev 1983; 11:157.

McCully KS. Homocysteinemia and arteriosclerosis: Failure to isolate homocysteine thiolactone from plasma and lipoproteins. Res Commun Chem Pathol Pharmacol 1989; 63:301.

McCully KS. Atherosclerosis, serum cholesterol and the homocysteine theory: A study of 194 consecutive autopsies. Am J Med Sci 1990; 299:217.

McCully KS, Carvalho ACA. Homocysteine thiolactone, N-homocysteine thiolactonyl retinamide, and platelet aggregation. Res Commun Chem Pathol Pharmacol 1987; 56:349.

McCully KS, Vezeridis MP. Chemopreventive and antineoplastic activity of N-homocysteine thiolactonyl retinamide. Carcinogenesis 1987; 8:1559.

McCully KS, Vezeridis MP. Chemopreventive effect of N-homocysteine thiolactonyl retinamido cobalamin on carcinogenesis by ethyl carbamate in mice. Proc Soc Exp Biol Med 1989a; 191:346.

McCully KS, Tzanakakis GN, Vezeridis MP. Inhibition of neoplastic growth by N-homocysteine thiolactonyl retinamido cobalamin. Res Commun Chem Pathol Pharmacol 1989b; 66:117.

McCully KS, Vezeridis MP. Histopathological effects of homocysteine thiolactone on epithelial and stromal tissues. Exp Mol Pathol 1989c; 51:159.

McCully KS, Olszewski AJ, Vezeridis MP. Homocysteine and lipid metabolism in atherogenesis: Effect of the homocysteine thiolactonyl derivatives, thioretinaco and thioretinamide. Atherosclerosis 1990; 83:197.

Miller LT, Dow MJ, Kokkeler SC. Methionine metabolism and vitamin B_6 status in women using oral contraceptives. Am J Clin Nutr 1978; 31:619.

Mudd SH, Levy HL. Disorders of transsulfuration. In: Stanbury JB, Wyngaarden JB, Frederickson DS, Goldstein JL, Brown MS, Eds. Metabolic basis of inherited disease, 5th ed. New York: McGraw-Hill, 522.

Mudd SH, Finkelstein JD, Irrevere F, Laster L. Homocystinuria: An enzymatic defect. Science 1964; 143:1443.

Mudd SH, Levy HL, Abeles RH. A derangement in the metabolism of vitamin B_{12} leading to homocystinuria, cystathioninuria and methylmalonic aciduria. Biochem Biophys Res Commun 1969; 35:121.

Mudd SH, Uhlendorf BW, Freeman JM, Finkelstein JD, Shih VE. Homocystinuria associated with decreased methylenetetrahydrofolate reductase activity. Biochem Biophys Res Commun 1972; 46:905.

Mudd SH, Havlik R, Levy HL, McKusick VA, Feinleib M. A study of cardiovascular risk in heterozygotes for homocystinuria. Am J Hum Genet 1981; 33:883.

Mudd SH, Skovby F, Levy HL, Pettigrew KD, Wilcken B, Pyeritz RE, Andria G, Boers GHJ, Bromberg IL, Cerone R, Fowler B, Grobe H, Schmidt H, Schweitzer L. The natural history of homocystinuria due to cystathionine β-synthase deficiency. Am J Hum Genet 1985; 37:1.

Murphy-Chutorian DR, Wexman MP, Grieco AJ, Heininger JA, Glassman E, Gaull GE, Ng SKC, Feit F, Wexman K, Fox AC. Methionine intolerance: A possible risk factor for coronary artery disease. J Am Coll Cardiol 1985; 6:725.

NIH Conference on the Decline in Coronary Heart Disease Mortality. NIH Publ. No. 79–1610, 1979.

Nilson-Ehle H, Landahl S, Lindstedt G, Netterblad L, Stockbruegger R, Westin J, Ahren C. Low serum cobalamin levels in a population study of 70- and 75-year old subjects. Dig Dis Sci 1989; 34:716.

Olszewski AJ, Szostak WB. Homocysteine content of plasma proteins in ischemic heart disease. Atherosclerosis 1988; 69:109.

Olszewski AJ, Szostak WB, Bialkowska M, Rudnicki S, McCully KS. Reduction of plasma lipid and homocysteine levels by pyridoxine, folate, cobalamin, choline, riboflavin and troxerutin in atherosclerosis. Atherosclerosis 1989; 75:1.

Park YK, Linkswiler H. Effect of vitamin B_6 depletion in adult man on the excretion of cystathionine and other methionine metabolites. J Nutr 1970; 100:110.

Parry GJ, Bredesen DE. Sensory neuropathy with low dose pyridoxine. Neurology 1985; 35:1466.

Perry TL. Unusual sulphur-containing amino acids in homocystinuria. In: Carson NJ, Raine DN, Eds. Inherited disorders of sulphur metabolism. Edinburgh: Churchill Livingstone, 224.

Petrova S. (The action of pyridoxine on lipid metabolism in rats with carbon disulfide poisoning.) Vopr Pitan 1985; 5:43.

Raben MS, Hollenberg CH. Effect of growth hormone on plasma fatty acids. J Clin Invest 1959; 38:484.

Rinehart JF, Greenberg LD. Arteriosclerotic lesions in pyridoxine deficient monkeys. Am J Pathol 1949; 25:481.

Ross R. The pathogenesis of atherosclerosis: An update. N Engl J Med 1986; 314:488.

Schaumberg H, Kaplan J, Windebank A, Vick N, Rasmus S, Pleasure D, Brown MJ. Sensory neuropathy from pyridoxine abuse. N Engl J Med 1983; 309:445.

Shupack JL, Grieco AJ, Epstein AM, Sansaricq C, Synderman SE. Azaribine, homocystinemia and thrombosis. Arch Dermatol 1977; 113:1301.

Serfontein WJ, Ubbink JB, DeVilliers LS, Rapley CH, Becker PJ. Plasma pyridoxal-5-phosphate as risk index for coronary artery disease. Atherosclerosis 1985; 55:357.

Serfontein WJ, Ubbink JB, DeVilliers LS, Becker PJ. Depressed plasma pyridoxal-5-phosphate levels in tobacco-smoking men. Atherosclerosis 1986; 59:341.

Slavik M, Hyanek J, Elis J, Homolka J. Typical hyperaminoaciduria after high doses of 6-azauridine triacetate. Biochem Pharmacol 1969; 18:1782.

Slavik M, Smith KJ, Blanc O. Decrease of serum pyridoxal phosphate levels and homocystinemia after administration of 6-azauridine triacetate and their prevention by administration of pyridoxine. Biochem Pharmacol 1982; 22:2349.

Smolin LA, Crenshaw TD, Kurtycz D, Benevenga NJ. Homocyst(e)ine accumulation in pigs fed diets deficient in vitamin B_6: Relationship to atherosclerosis. J Nutr 1983; 113:2022.

Solberg LA, Strong JP. Risk factors and atherosclerotic lesions. A review of autopsy studies. Arteriosclerosis 1983; 3:187.

Stabler SP, Marcell PD, Podell ER, Allen RH, Savage DG, Lindenbaum J. Elevation of total homocysteine in the serum of patients with cobalamin or folate deficiency detected by capillary gas chromatography-mass spectrometry. J Clin Invest 1988; 81:466.

Subar AF, Block G, James LD. Folate intake and food sources in the U.S. population. Am J Clin Nutr 1989; 50:508.

Suzman M. Effect of pyridoxine and low animal protein diet in coronary artery disease. Circ., Suppl. IV 1973; 254, Abst. 987.

Swift M, Morrell D. Cardiovascular risk in homocystinuria family members. Am J Hum Genet 1982; 34:1016.

Swift ME, Shultz TD. Relationship of vitamins B_6 and B_{12} to homocysteine levels: Risk for coronary heart disease. Nutr Rep Int 1986; 34:1.

Tiller JR, Schilling RSF, Morris JN. Occupational toxic factor in mortality from coronary heart disease. Br Med J 1968; 4:407.

Vermaak WJH, Barnard HC, Potgeiter GM, Du T, Theron H. Vitamin B_6 and coronary artery disease. Epidemiological observations and case studies. Atherosclerosis 1987; 55:357.

Wilcken DEL, Wilcken B. The pathogenesis of coronary artery disease. A possible role for methionine metabolism. J Clin Invest 1976; 57:1079.

Wilcken DEL, Gupta VJ. Cysteine-homocysteine mixed disulfide: Differing plasma concentrations in normal men and women. Clin Sci 1979a; 57:211.

Wilcken DEL, Gupta VJ. Sulphur containing amino acids in chronic renal failure with particular reference to homocysteine and cysteine-homocysteine mixed disulphide. Eur J Clin Invest 1979b; 9:301.

Wilcken DEL, Gupta VJ, Betts AK. Homocysteine in the plasma of renal transplant recipients: Effects of cofactors for methionine metabolism. Clin Sci 1981; 61:743.

Wilcken DEL, Reddy GSR, Gupta VJ. Homocysteinemia, ischemic heart disease and the carrier state for homocystinuria. Metabolism 1983; 32:363.

Wilcken DEL, Dudman NPB, Tyrell PA. Homocystinuria due to cystathionine β-synthase deficiency: The effects of betaine treatment in pyridoxine responsive patients. Metabolism 1985; 34:1115.

Wilcken DEL, Dudman NPB, Tyrell PA, Robertson MR. Folic acid lowers elevated plasma homocysteine in chronic renal insufficiency: Possible implications for prevention of vascular disease. Metabolism 1988; 37:697.

CARCINOGENESIS

5

Vegetables, Fruits, and Carotenoids and the Risk of Cancer

Regina G. Ziegler

Environmental Epidemiology Branch, Epidemiology and Biostatistics Program, Division of Cancer Etiology, National Cancer Institute, National Institutes of Health, Bethesda, Maryland

Amy F. Subar

Applied Research Branch, Surveillance Program, Division of Cancer Prevention and Control, National Cancer Institute, National Institutes of Health, Bethesda, Maryland

Carotenoids are naturally occurring pigmented compounds, usually yellow to red in color, that are abundant in plants and are introduced into animal tissues through dietary intake. To date approximately 600 distinct carotenoids have been identified, approximately 10% of which are considered to be "provitamin A" because they can be metabolically converted to vitamin A in humans (Olson, 1989). Beta-carotene is the most abundant of the provitamin A carotenoids in the U.S. food supply. In addition to their role as vitamin A precursors, carotenoids also have antioxidant and immunological properties which may be important in cancer etiology and prevention (reviewed in Bendich and Olson, 1989).

POSSIBLE ROLES IN CANCER PREVENTION

Several mechanisms have been proposed whereby carotenoids may directly play a role in cancer prevention. The most widely discussed is their antioxidant potential. Highly reactive free radicals and singlet oxygen can damage cell membranes and genetic material. Carotenoids may prevent oxidative degradation, which has been proposed as a step in the development of malignancy (reviewed in Burton, 1989). It should be noted, however, that antioxidant properties are shared by other dietary constituents, such as vitamins C and E. In addition, an immunological role has been proposed for carotenoids. There is preliminary evidence that carotenoids may enhance the immune response responsible for killing cancer cells, possibly by protecting macrophages, natural killer cells, and cytotoxic T cells from oxidation (reviewed in Bendich, 1989).

STRUCTURE

Most of the naturally occurring carotenoids possess 40 carbon atoms. More than 600 have been identified, not including cis-trans and optically active isomers (Britton and Goodwin, 1982). Most of the carotenoids in food or human blood are hydrocarbon carotenoids, such as beta-carotene, alpha-carotene, and lyco-pene, or C^{40} xanthophylls, such as cryptoxanthin, lutein, and zeaxanthin (Straub, 1987). Figure 1 presents the chemical structures of the carotenoids abundant in food and in animal tissues.

MEASURING THE CAROTENOID CONTENT OF FOODS

Originally carotenoids were considered important in nutrition because of their vitamin A activity. Only in the last 15 years has there been significant interest in evaluating carotenoids for roles unrelated to their conversion to vitamin A. Thus, food composition tables in the U.S. present vitamin A and not carotenoid values for individual foods (USDA, 1976–1987). Vitamin A activity in these tables was first expressed in international units (IU); in 1967, the FAO/WHO Expert Group recommended that retinol equivalents (RE) be used (FAO/WHO Expert Group, 1967). REs take into consideration the inefficient utilization of dietary carotenoids as vitamin A relative to dietary retinol (Committee on Dietary Allowances, 1980). Both poor absorption of carotenoids and limited metabolic conversion to vitamin A are involved. Table 1 lists the estimated vitamin A activity of selected retinoids and carotenoids using all-*trans*-retinol as the standard (Beecher and Khachik, 1984). It is obvious that using the vitamin A activity in REs as the sole index of the total carotenoid content of foods leads to an un-derestimate of the carotenoids actually present, since most carotenoids have no provitamin A activity.

As interest increased regarding the precise carotenoid content of foods, in-vestigators made reasonable assumptions about the vitamin A values listed in food composition tables. The vitamin A activity assigned to fruits and vegetables was assumed to be entirely from provitamin A carotenoids. Formulas were derived to calculate carotenoid content, based on the poor utilization of various carotenoids as vitamin A: 1 RE of vitamin A = 6 μg beta-carotene or 12 μg of other provitamin A carotenoids = 1 μg retinol. Such calculations were reasonable for estimating beta-carotene, the most abundant provitamin A carotenoid in foods, but were less appropriate for other provitamin A carotenoids and ignored the carotenoids without vitamin A activity (Beecher and Khachik, 1984).

Very few food composition tables currently provide carotenoid values directly

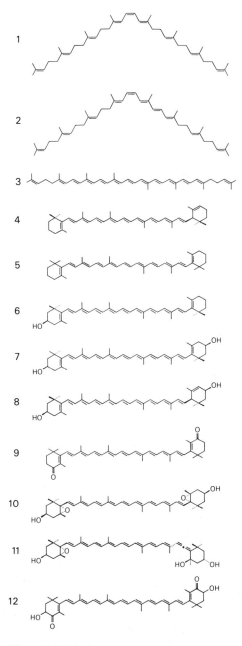

Figure 1 Polyenes and carotenoids in foods that may also be found in animal tissues. 1, phytoene; 2, phytofluene; 3, lycopene; 4, alpha-carotene; 5, beta-carotene; 6, beta-cryptoxanthin; 7, zeaxanthin; 8, lutein; 9, canthaxanthin; 10, violaxanthin; 11, neoxanthin; 12, astaxanthin. (From Bendich and Olson, 1989.)

Table 1   Vitamin A Activity of Various Naturally Occurring Retinoids and Carotenoids

Retinoid or carotenoid	Vitamin A activity
Retinoids	
All-*trans*-retinol	100
11-*cis*-retinol	75
13-*cis*-retinol	85
Carotenoids	
All-*trans*-beta-carotene	17
9-*cis*-beta-carotene	6
All-*trans*-beta-carotene	8–9
Lycopene	0
Beta-cryptoxanthin	8–10
Lutein	0
3-keto-β-carotene	9
Beta-carotene-5,6-epoxide	3–4
Beta-apo-8′-carotenal	12
Beta-apo-10′-carotenal	0

Source: From Beecher and Khachik, 1984.

(Beecher and Khachik, 1984). The U.S. Department of Agriculture's Revised Handbook 8 (USDA, 1976–1987) presents vitamin A data for vegetables and fruits based on the Association of Official Analytic Chemists methods (Horwitz, 1980). The AOAC methods only separate major classes of compounds, such as hydrocarbon carotenoids and xanthophylls, and do not separate individual carotenoids. State-of-the-art analyses of the carotenoid content of foods are now being performed by USDA in conjunction with the National Cancer Institute using high-performance liquid chromatography (HPLC). Such procedures are able to quickly separate and quantitate alpha- and beta-carotene, lycopene, and some individual xanthophylls, such as lutein and beta-cryptoxanthin (Beecher and Khachik, 1989).

As updated carotenoid values become available, they are published in the scientific literature and used to update the vitamin A values in USDA Revised Handbook 8. Footnotes indicate when the vitamin A values are based on HPLC methods (Beecher and Khachik, 1984). Most investigators, however, have not had the opportunity to utilize updated carotenoid data in evaluating the carotenoid content of the diet and in investigating the role of beta-carotene, other individual carotenoids, and carotenoids in general in the etiology of cancer.

In a recent study (Micozzi et al., 1990) which analyzed by HPLC the carotenoid content of selected foods, fresh green leafy vegetables were found to be moderately high in beta-carotene and very high in xanthophylls, especially lutein. Fresh yellow-orange vegetables, such as carrots, acorn squash, and sweet potato, contained primarily alpha- and beta-carotene. Tomatoes were rich in lycopene, a hydrocarbon carotenoid without provitamin A activity.

The above study and others summarized by Beecher and Khachik (1989) show that cooking vegetables results in a large decrease in total xanthophylls (25–68%) and a smaller decrease in total hydrocarbon carotenoids (3–12%). The actual loss depends on the vegetable and the length and type of cooking. In addition, the geographic area in which produce is grown affects its carotenoid content (Beecher and Khachik, 1989).

MAJOR SOURCES OF CAROTENOIDS IN THE U.S. DIET

Table 2 identifies the leading sources of vitamin A in the U.S. diet, based on frequency of food consumption data from the 1987 National Health Interview

Table 2 Food Sources of Vitamin A and Beta-Carotene in the U.S. Population: The 1987 National Health Interview Survey

Food(s)	% Contribution to total daily vitamin A intake	Cumulative % of vitamin A	Cumulative % of provitamin A[a]
Carrots	28.0	28.0	43.7
Liver	11.1	39.1	—
Sweet potato	9.2	48.3	58.1
Ready-to-eat cereals	7.8	56.1	—
Milk (fluid)	6.7	62.8	—
Spinach	5.5	68.3	66.7
Beef stew	5.0	73.3	74.5
Vegetable soup	3.7	77.0	80.3
Cheese (hard)	3.0	80.0	—
Margarine	2.9	82.9	—
Collards	2.8	85.7	84.7
Broccoli	2.6	88.3	88.8
Salad	2.0	90.3	91.9
Eggs	1.8	92.1	—
Cantaloupe	1.7	93.8	94.6
Ice cream	1.3	95.1	—
Spaghetti (incl. sauce and cheese)	1.2	96.3	96.0
Butter	1.1	97.4	—
Orange juice	1.0	98.4	97.6
Mayonnaise	0.7	99.1	—

[a] Derived from values for vitamin A by excluding all animal sources. The data reflect current vitamin A values from USDA Revised Handbook 8 (USDA, 1976–1987) updated by analytical data for tomatoes. Data do *not* represent total carotenoid content.

Survey (NHIS). The 1987 NHIS is a large, representative survey of the non-institutionalized U.S. adult population aged 19–99 years. The data in Table 2 reflect not only the concentration of vitamin A in individual foods but also their frequency of consumption and usual portion size. For example, liver, which is infrequently consumed by Americans, is the second leading source of vitamin A in the U.S. diet because of its high vitamin density. The primary sources of provitamin A carotenoids were derived from the vitamin A data in Table 2 by excluding animal sources of vitamin A. A limited number of vegetables—carrots, sweet potatoes, spinach, beef stew containing carrots, vegetable soup, collards/greens, broccoli, and green salad—provide nearly 92% of the provitamin A carotenoid content of the U.S. diet. The data also indicate that fruits in general are poor sources of beta-carotene. However, vegetables (and some fruits) which are high in carotenoids which are not converted to vitamin A, such as lycopene-rich tomatoes, do not appear on this list though they may be significant sources of total carotenoids. This table illustrates the difficulty in estimating carotenoid values from vitamin A data. It should be noted that carotenoids have also been found in small amounts in dairy products, eggs, shellfish, and poultry (Dimitrov, 1986).

ABSORPTION, TRANSPORT, AND LOCALIZATION

Dietary carotenoids are absorbed directly through the intestine; some are incorporated into chylomicra, appearing in the blood via the lymph (Bendich and Olson, 1989). The typical efficiency of absorption of carotenoids is assumed to be about one-third that of vitamin A (all-*trans*-retinol), based on the calculated absorption of beta-carotene. Research suggests that absorption of beta-carotene may be reduced by in vivo structural changes such as double-bond isomerization, ring opening, and oxidation (Beecher and Khachik, 1984). Carotenoids, which are fat-soluble, are transported in the blood primarily by low-density lipoproteins and, to a lesser extent, by high- and very-low-density lipoproteins (Parker, 1989). Most of the carotenoids distributed in human tissue are localized in adipose tissue (80–85%), followed by liver (8–12%) and muscle (2–3%). In addition, high concentrations of carotenoids are found in the corpus luteum and adrenal glands. Of the total body pool of carotenoids, serum contains approximately 1% (Bendich and Olson, 1989). Depending on an individual's vitamin A status, protein status, and metabolic characteristics, a significant amount of the provitamin A carotenoids are converted to retinal by the intestinal mucosa and to a lesser extent by the liver and other organs. Based on data for beta-carotene, the efficiency of conversion is assumed to be approximately 50%. The two possible pathways of conversion are central and eccentric cleavage. The retinal formed can then be reduced to retinol for use in vitamin A functions (Bendich and Olson, 1989).

CAROTENOIDS IN HUMAN SERUM

The individual carotenoids in human serum are also being measured by HPLC at present. Five to 10 distinct carotenoids have been identified in serum from U.S. subjects. Beta-carotene, alpha-carotene, cryptoxanthin, lycopene, and lutein are the major components with lycopene occurring at the highest concentrations (Parker, 1989). It is important to note that the levels of beta-carotene and retinol in the blood are not highly correlated. Serum beta-carotene is believed to reflect relatively recent diet while serum vitamin A appears to be maintained within a narrow range in well-nourished populations.

RELATIONSHIP BETWEEN DIETARY INTAKE
AND BLOOD LEVELS

A recent study involving 30 men showed that for seven major plasma carotenoids, individuals maintain relatively constant carotenoid profiles. Fasting serum levels seemed to reflect relatively long-term dietary patterns and not occasional large intakes of carotenoid-rich foods (Brown et al., 1989a). The study showed that maximum plasma concentrations of beta-carotene occurred 24–48 hr after a dose of pure beta-carotene or beta-carotene in carrots, and that plasma responses were highly variable among subjects. A three- to fourfold difference in plasma levels was noted between the lowest and highest responders. However, concentrations were consistently about 20% higher when pure beta-carotene, rather than an equivalent dose of beta-carotene in carrots, was administered. An equivalent intake of broccoli or tomato juice did not change the levels of plasma carotenoids. Another feeding study of 61 men and women also indicated that there is wide interindividual variation in fasting plasma beta-carotene levels following beta-carotene doses (Dimitrov et al., 1988). Individuals on high-fat diets showed significantly greater increases than those on low-fat diets. While the two feeding studies discussed above relied primarily on fasting blood samples, another small study showed that a test meal high in calories (790 kcal) and fat (45% of calories), and moderate in vitamin A (40–50% of the Recommended Dietary Allowance) and carotenoids (20% of the average daily intake), did not alter seven major plasma carotenoids during the 4 hr after the meal (Brown et al., 1989b). This suggests that subjects may not need to be fasting to obtain useful blood carotenoid values.

Several epidemiological studies have shown limited associations between dietary carotenoid intake, as measured by food frequency questionnaires, and plasma carotenoid levels ($r = 0.21$–0.29) (Willett et al., 1983; Russell-Briefel et al., 1985; Roidt et al., 1988). In addition, factors other than dietary intake were shown to affect plasma carotenoid levels. Women exhibited significantly higher levels than men in two studies (Willett et al., 1983; Nierenberg et al., 1989).

Cigarette smoking (Russell-Briefel et al., 1985; Roidt et al., 1988), alcohol intake (Russell-Briefel et al., 1985; Roidt et al., 1988; Nierenberg et al., 1989), and body mass index (Willett et al., 1983; Roidt et al., 1988; Nierenberg et al., 1989) were all found to be negatively correlated with plasma carotenoid values, while plasma cholesterol was found to be positively correlated (Willett et al., 1983; Russell-Briefel et al., 1985; Roidt et al., 1988).

CAROTENOIDS, VITAMIN A, AND CANCER

Early cancer research focused on the possible protective effects of vitamin A and the chemically similar retinoids because of the traditional importance of vitamin A in normal differentiation and the efficacy of retinoids in limiting carcinogenesis in animal experiments. However, when epidemiological studies suggested that vegetables and fruits might reduce the risk of cancer, attention also turned to the carotenoids concentrated in these foods. Beta-carotene was emphasized since it is the most abundant of the carotenoids that can be metabolized to vitamin A by humans. But as evidence accumulated that beta-carotene need not be converted to vitamin A before it modulates carcinogenesis, other carotenoids began to be considered. Fortunately, carotenoids and vitamin A can be independently evaluated in epidemiological studies using either dietary intake or blood nutrient levels. This chapter reviews the evidence from human studies that beta-carotene and other carotenoids are directly involved in cancer prevention.

EPIDEMIOLOGICAL APPROACHES

To evaluate the evidence first prospective and then a limited number of retrospective studies will be considered. In a prospective study dietary information and/or blood samples are collected from a healthy group of people, and the cohort followed over time. When a sufficient number of cancer diagnoses or deaths have occurred, the data collected earlier are compared for the cases and either all the noncases in the cohort or controls selected from the cohort and matched to the cancer cases. In a retrospective study patients with a particular cancer are identified and comparable controls selected. Then information about usual diet prior to signs and symptoms of disease, blood samples, or both are collected and compared for the cases and controls. In prospective studies the exposure, whether low dietary intake or low blood nutrient levels, can be ascertained prior to clinical disease. However, only the common cancers occur in sufficiently large numbers to be evaluated in these studies; and it is often difficult to stabilize blood nutrients during the waiting period while cancers accrue. With retrospective studies it is relatively easy to identify large numbers of cases and to focus on the less common cancers. The interview can assess in depth many potential risk factors for a specific cancer without trying to cover the pertinent risk factors for all cancers.

While there is a possibility for bias when cancer patients recall usual dietary patterns, no clear evidence of bias exists in a number of well-conducted studies. However, selecting an appropriate time for blood collection so that nutrient levels will not be influenced by disease or treatment is often impossible in a retrospective study.

In this chapter the results of the epidemiological studies are evaluated by examining whether there is an association between carotenoids and cancer, its direction, and its statistical significance, and whether there is a graded response to increasing exposure and the statistical significance of the trend. Associations and trends can be biologically meaningful without being statistically significant; studies with small numbers may lack the power to attain statistical significance.

PROSPECTIVE STUDIES OF CAROTENOID INTAKE AND CANCER

Six prospective studies have examined the relationship between carotenoid intake and cancer (Hirayama, 1979, 1985; Shekelle et al., 1981; Kvale et al., 1983; Colditz et al., 1985; Wang and Hammond, 1985; Paganini-Hill et al., 1987) (Table 3). The earliest was published a little over 10 years ago (Hirayama, 1979). Three monitored cancer incidence (Shekelle et al., 1981; Kvale et al., 1983; Paganini-Hill et al., 1987) and three monitored cancer mortality (Hirayama, 1985; Colditz et al., 1985; Wang and Hammond, 1985). Only one study asked about most of the major carotenoid sources in the diet and formed a quantitative index of carotenoid intake using food composition tables (Paganini-Hill et al., 1987). A second study did develop an approximate carotenoid index but had to rely on summaries of diet histories rather than the original data (Shekelle et al., 1981). The other four studies used the frequency of consumption of a limited number of vegetables and fruits, not all of which were especially high in carotenoids (Kvale et al., 1983; Hirayama, 1985; Colditz et al., 1985; Wang and Hammond, 1985).

In three of the four studies that examined all cancers combined, risk was inversely related to vegetable and fruit or carotenoid intake (Hirayama, 1985; Colditz et al., 1985; Paganini-Hill et al., 1987). The two studies that analyzed men and women separately noted the inverse relationship with all cancer in both sexes (Hirayama, 1985; Paganini-Hill et al., 1987). Lung was the site most frequently involved. Decreased risk with increased intake was seen in four of the five studies that evaluated lung cancer (Shekelle et al., 1981; Kvale et al., 1983; Hirayama, 1985; Wang and Hammond, 1985), even though the single study that developed a quantitative measure of carotenoid intake found no association with lung cancer (Paganini-Hill et al., 1987). Cancer at several other sites [stomach (Hirayama, 1985), cervix (Hirayama, 1985), head and neck (Shekelle et al., 1981), breast (Paganini-Hill et al., 1987), and bladder (Paganini-Hill

Table 3 Prospective Studies of Dietary Carotenoids and Cancer

Authors, date	Study population	Exposure evaluated	Cancer site	No. of cases[a]	Evidence of association[b]
Hirayama, 1979, 1985	Japan Men, women	Green-yellow vegetables	All cancer	14,740	tr, neg (M,F)
			Stomach	5,247	tr, neg (M,F)
			Lung	1,917	tr, neg (M only)
			Cervix	589	+, neg
Shekelle, 1981	Western Electric Co. employees, Chicago, IL	Carotenoids in vegetables, fruits, and soups	All cancer	208	—
			Nonmelanoma skin	36	—
	Men		Lung	33	+, tr, neg
			Prostate	29	—
			Colon	29	—
			Rectum	20	—
			Bladder	19	—
			Epidermoid head, neck	14	(+), neg
Kvale, 1983	Norway Men	Vegetables (excl. potatoes) Fruits, berries	Lung	70	(+), neg
Colditz, 1985	Elderly MA residents Men, women	Six vegetables and fruits	All cancer	42	+, tr, neg

Reference	Cohort	Dietary factor	Cancer site	No. of cases[a]	Results[b]
Wang, 1985	Volunteers from 25 U.S. states (American Cancer Society cohort) Men	Fruits and fruit juices Green salad	Lung	671	tr(?), neg tr(?), neg
Paganini-Hill, 1987	Residents of CA retirement community (Leisure World) Men, women	Carotenoids	All cancer	638	(tr), neg (M) +(?), neg (F)
			Breast	123	(+), neg (F)
			Colon	110	—
			Prostate	92	—
			Bladder	58	(tr), neg (M) tr, neg (F)
			Lung	55	—

[a] Refers to the number of cancer cases used to evaluate a relationship with carotenoids. This number may be less than the cancer incidence or mortality within the cohort because of missing information on diet and potential confounders.

[b] A + indicates a statistically significant association, e.g., a significant difference in dietary intake between cases and noncases/controls or a significant difference in cancer rates between subgroups of the cohort stratified by dietary intake; (+) indicates an apparent association that is not statistically significant; + (?) indicates an apparent association that was not tested for statistical significance. Tr indicates a statistically significant test for trend in cancer rates or rate ratios with changes in dietary intake; (tr) indicates an apparent trend that is not statistically significant; neg implies a decreased risk of cancer with increased intake.

et al., 1987)] was reported to be reduced with increased intake of vegetables and fruits or carotenoids in a single study. However, two studies failed to find a protective effect for colon cancer (Shekelle et al., 1981; Paganini-Hill et al., 1987); two failed to find one for prostate cancer (Shekelle et al., 1981; Paganini-Hill et al., 1987); and one of two studies failed to find a protective effect for bladder cancer (Shekelle et al., 1981; Paganini-Hill et al., 1987). Only two of these studies systematically evaluated cancer at different sites (Shekelle et al., 1981; Paganini-Hill et al., 1987). In addition, the less common cancers would not yet have occurred in sufficient numbers in these cohorts to be analyzed.

Taken together, these six prospective studies of diet and cancer strongly suggest that high levels of vegetable and fruit consumption are associated with a reduced risk of lung cancer and possibly other cancers. The causal agent is more difficult to identify. Only one study systematically investigated the relationship of all the major nutrients to risk of lung cancer (Shekelle et al., 1981). Carotenoid intake alone was significantly associated with reduced risk. Vitamin C, which like carotenoids is found primarily in vegetables and fruits, was not implicated in the two studies that evaluated it (Shekelle et al., 1981; Kvale et al., 1983). No decrease in risk of lung cancer with high retinol (preformed vitamin A) consumption was noted in two studies (Shekelle et al., 1981; Paganini-Hill et al., 1987) although results of a third study did suggest such a relationship (Kvale et al., 1983). Finding a reduction in risk with consumption of carotenoids but not retinol suggests that the active carotenoids do not first have to be metabolized into vitamin A to be protective.

The maximum follow-up time in these prospective studies ranged from 5 years (Colditz et al., 1985; Paganini-Hill et al., 1987) to 11–12 years (Kvale et al., 1983; Wang and Hammond, 1985) to 17–19 years (Shekelle et al., 1981; Hirayama, 1985). In the longer duration studies, it seems likely that current diet assessed at onset of follow-up did not reflect preclinical disease. One of the studies with extended follow-up did examine the influence of time between dietary interview and diagnosis of lung cancer on the strength of the carotenoid association and found no effect (Shekelle et al., 1981).

In general, these studies did not demonstrate in their published reports that smoking was adequately controlled. Intake of vegetables and fruits and carotenoids is decreased among smokers (Stryker et al., 1988; Subar et al., 1990). In a recent study the carotenoid intake of male smokers was reported to be 80–90% that of male nonsmokers; the comparable range for females was 70–80% (Stryker et al., 1988). Thus uncontrolled confounding by smoking might generate an apparent protective effect for diet in studies of lung cancer and other smoking-related cancers, such as head and neck, bladder, and cervix. Most of the studies adjusted for smoking intensity. Only one study adjusted for duration of smoking (Shekelle et al., 1981), which is a stronger predictor of lung cancer risk than intensity

(Doll and Peto, 1978). Also, some of these studies were limited in their ability to control for confounding because of small numbers of cancers.

PROSPECTIVE STUDIES OF BLOOD CAROTENOID LEVELS AND CANCER

Prospective epidemiological studies have considered not only vegetable and fruit and carotenoid intake but also carotenoid levels in serum or plasma prior to the onset of cancer. These six studies are presented in Table 4 (Willett et al., 1984; Stahelin et al., 1984, 1991; Nomura et al., 1985; Menkes et al., 1986; Schober et al., 1987; Wald et al., 1988b; Burney et al., 1989; Helzlsouer et al., 1989; Connett et al., 1989). In the 5 years since the earliest of these studies was published, the approach has become more sophisticated. Originally total carotenoids were assayed spectrophotometrically (Willett et al., 1984); then HPLC was used to separate and measure beta-carotene. Recently, blood levels of other individual carotenoids, such as lycopene and lutein, have also been determined (Burney et al., 1989; Helzlsouer et al., 1989; Comstock et al., 1991).

In five of these prospective studies controls matched to the individuals who developed cancer were selected from the cohort so that a limited number of the stored blood samples would need to be thawed (Willett et al., 1984; Nomura et al., 1985; Menkes et al., 1986; Schober et al., 1987; Wald et al., 1988b; Burney et al., 1989; Helzlsouer et al., 1989; Connett et al., 1989). The sixth study measured beta-carotene in each participant's blood immediately after it was collected (Stahelin et al., 1991). Four of the studies used cancer incidence (Willett et al., 1984; Nomura et al., 1985; Menkes et al., 1986; Schober et al., 1987; Wald et al., 1988b; Burney et al., 1989; Helzlsouer et al., 1989); two, cancer mortality (Stahelin et al., 1991; Connett et al., 1989).

All of the studies systematically tested for associations with each of the common cancers in their populations. In all five studies that measured beta-carotene, risk of lung cancer was reduced among subjects with high blood beta-carotene levels (Nomura et al., 1985; Menkes et al., 1986, Wald et al., 1988b; Connett et al., 1989; Stahelin et al., 1991). The inverse associations were statistically significant in four of these studies (Nomura et al., 1985; Menkes et al., 1986; Wald et al., 1988b; Stahelin et al., 1991) and trends were apparent in all five. Although total carotenoid levels were not related to lung cancer risk in one study (Willett et al., 1984), in another study total carotenoid levels demonstrated a stronger inverse association with lung cancer than beta-carotene levels (Connett et al., 1989). In all three studies that examined stomach cancer, risk was reduced with high beta-carotene levels (Nomura et al., 1985; Wald et al., 1988b; Stahelin et al., 1991) although the relationship was not as pronounced as for lung cancer. For colon cancer inverse associations with beta-carotene were observed

Table 4 Prospective Studies of Serum or Plasma Carotenoids and Cancer

Authors, date	Study population	Exposure evaluated	Cancer site	No. of cases, controls[a]	Evidence of association[b]
Willett, 1984	14 centers in U.S. hypertension study (HDFP) Men, women	Total carotenoids	All cancer	111,210	—
			Lung	17,28	—
			Breast	14,31	—
			Leukemia, lymphoma	11,23	+, pos
			Gastrointestinal	11,22	—
			Prostate	11,21	—
Stahelin, 1984, 1991	Chemical co. employees, Basel, Sw Men	Beta-carotene	Lung	68	+, tr(?), neg
			Stomach	20	+, neg
			Colon	17	—
			Other cancers	99	—
Nomura, 1985	Japanese in heart disease study, Oahu, HI Men	Beta-carotene	Colon	81,302	(+), neg
			Lung	74,302	+, tr, neg
			Stomach	70,302	(+), neg
			Rectum	32,302	—
			Bladder	27,302	—
Menkes, 1986		Beta-carotene	Lung	99,196	+, tr, neg
Schober, 1987	Washington County, MD	Beta-carotene	Colon	72,143	—
Burney, 1989	Men, women	Total carotenoids Beta-carotene Lycopene	Pancreas	22,44	+, tr, neg
Helzlsouer, 1989		Beta-carotene Lycopene	Bladder	35,70	(+), (tr), neg

Study	Cohort	Nutrient	Cancer site	No. of cases[a]	Result[b]
Wald, 1988b	Users of BUPA medical center, London, UK. Men	Beta-carotene	All cancer	271,533	+, tr, neg
			Skin	56,107	—
			Lung	50,99	+, tr, neg
			Colorectal	30,59	(+), neg
			Central nervous system	17,34	(+), neg
			Bladder	15,29	(+), neg
			Stomach	13,26	+(?), neg
			Other	90,179	—
Connett, 1989	22 centers in U.S. heart disease study (MRFIT) Men	Total carotenoids	All cancer	156,311	—
		Beta-carotene			—
		Total carotenoids	Lung cancer	66,131	+, tr, neg
		Beta-carotene			(+), (tr), neg
		Total carotenoids	Gastrointestinal	28,56	—
		Beta-carotene			—
		Total carotenoids	Colon	14,28	—
		Beta-carotene			—

[a] Refers to the number of cases and matched controls selected from the cohort that were used to evaluate a relationship with blood carotenoid levels or to the number of cases alone if the entire cohort was utilized in analysis.

[b] A + indicates a statistically significant association, e.g., a significant difference in blood nutrient levels between cases and controls or a significant difference in relative risks between subgroups of the study population stratified by blood nutrient levels; (+) indicates an apparent association that is not statistically significant; + (?) indicates an apparent association that was not tested for statistical significance. Tr indicates a statistically significant test for trend in relative risks with changes in blood nutrient levels; (tr) indicates an apparent trend that is not statistically significant; tr(?) indicates an apparent trend that was not tested for statistical significance. Pos implies an increased risk of cancer with increased nutrient levels; neg implies a decreased risk of cancer with increased nutrient levels.

in only two of five investigations (Nomura et al., 1985; Wald et al., 1988b); for bladder cancer, in one of three investigations (Wald et al., 1988b).

The apparent reduction in risk of pancreas and bladder cancer with high serum lycopene levels (Burney et al., 1989; Helzlsouer et al., 1989) is provocative but needs to be replicated by further research. The absence of parallel effects for beta-carotene suggests that high lycopene levels measure something more specific than frequent consumption of vegetables and fruits and that not all antioxidant carotenoids may be equally effective in vivo.

In general, the specificity of the beta-carotene associations noted in these prospective studies of blood nutrient levels and cancer has not been adequately explored. Blood levels of other carotenoids and other constituents of vegetables and fruits, such as vitamin C and folacin, have not been systematically evaluated. For example, only the study that assayed for micronutrients immediately after blood collection was able to measure vitamin C because of its lability in stored serum and plasma. Vitamin C was significantly reduced in those men who subsequently developed stomach cancer but unaltered in those who developed lung cancer (Stahelin et al., 1991). Techniques are now available to stabilize the vitamin C in blood for long-term storage (Margolis et al, 1990) and need to be considered in future cohort studies. Vitamins A and E were the only nutrients routinely assayed along with beta-carotene. Among the six studies strong or consistent associations for vitamin A similar to those seen for beta-carotene were not seen, suggesting that beta-carotene need not first be converted to vitamin A to be active. Inverse associations with blood vitamin E levels were noted in three of the six studies (Willett et al., 1984; Stahelin et al., 1984; Menkes et al., 1986) but may have resulted from inverse associations of blood lipoprotein levels with risk of cancer.

Except for one study with five years of follow-up (Willett et al., 1984), the maximum follow-up time in these cohorts ranged from 8 to 12 years. However, median times between blood collection and cancer diagnosis or death are likely to be much shorter and, in general, were not presented. Among the five studies that examined the impact of elapsed time between blood collection and lung cancer (Stahelin et al., 1984; Nomura et al., 1985; Menkes et al., 1986; Wald et al., 1988b; Connett et al., 1989), four were able to demonstrate that lowered blood beta-carotene levels in the subjects who eventually developed lung cancer were not likely to be a result of preclinical disease (Stahelin et al., 1984; Nomura et al., 1985; Menkes et al., 1986; Wald et al., 1988b) even though data from three studies suggest that beta-carotene levels are reduced in the years immediately preceding lung cancer diagnosis (Wald et al., 1988b) or death (Stahelin et al, 1984; Connett et al., 1989). It is interesting to note that in the London BUPA cohort serum levels of beta-carotene, vitamin A, and vitamin E were all reduced in those men who subsequently developed lung cancer but the low levels of vitamin A and vitamin E were restricted to those men who were diagnosed within a few years after blood collection and thus were attributed to metabolic consequences of cancer (Wald et al., 1986, 1987). Only the reduced beta-carotene levels were thought to be etiologically important (Wald et al., 1988b).

Degradation of carotenoids during extended storage of blood samples is a worrisome problem. At present the precise stability of individual carotenoids under different storage conditions is not known although several groups, including the U.S. National Institute for Standards and Technology and the U.S. Centers for Disease Control, are conducting relevant experiments. The scope of the problem is illustrated by one cohort study where 83% of the serum samples had undetectable levels of beta-carotene after storage at $-23°$ to $-40°C$ for 12–19 years (Friedman et al., 1986). In another study which stored samples at $-50°$ to $-70°C$, 15% of the specimens had no beta-carotene (<2 $\mu g/dl$) after 8–10 years (Connett et al., 1989). A third study reported a gradual decline of approximately 5% per year in beta-carotene levels in serum stored at $-40°C$ for up to 10 years (Wald et al., 1988b). Not even storage at $-70°C$ has been proved totally reliable (Nomura et al, 1985; Menkes et al., 1986). If degradation of carotenoids leads to a less precise measurement of exposure, then the power of a study to detect associations is diminished. However, to compensate to the extent possible, most of these prospective studies matched controls to cases by length of storage (Willett et al., 1984; Menkes et al., 1986; Schober et al., 1987; Wald et al., 1988b; Connett et al., 1989) and/or standardized for storage interval in analysis (Willett et al., 1984).

A recent study of carotenoid stability indicates that plasma samples frozen immediately after plasma separation were no different from those maintained at room temperature in the dark for 24 hr (Craft et al., 1988). Six individual carotenoids (lutein/zeanthin, precryptoxanthin, cryptoxanthin, lycopene, alpha-carotene, and beta-carotene) were stable in plasma stored at $-70°C$ for 28 months or at $-20°C$ for 5 months. However, after 15 months carotenoids maintained at $-20°C$ were significantly decreased. Such results suggest that the validity of data based on blood samples stored for long periods at temperatures greater than $-70°C$ may be questionable.

Of more concern than the ability of carotenoid degradation to obscure relationships is its potential to generate associations that do not exist. Such bias can occur if the carotenoids in the blood collected from cases and controls degrade at different rates. This situation probably occurred in a prospective study conducted in Guernsey, England (Wald et al., 1984). Plasma beta-carotene levels were lower among the 39 women who developed cancer during 7–14 years of follow-up than among the 78 matched controls, and a trend was apparent. But further investigation indicated that beta-carotene had degraded markedly during storage at $-20°C$ and was likely to have been more rapidly destroyed in blood samples from the cases because of repeated freezing and thawing (Wald et al., 1988a).

In these prospective studies of blood carotenoid levels and cancer, as in the studies of dietary carotenoids, control of smoking is critical because plasma beta-carotene and total carotenoids have been shown to be reduced among smokers relative to nonsmokers (Russell-Briefel et al., 1985; Stryker et al., 1988; Nierenberg et al., 1989), and plasma beta-carotene is inversely correlated with frequency of smoking (Stryker et al., 1988). One reason is that smokers consume fewer vegetables, fruits, and carotenoids; but in addition, beta-carotene levels may rise less sharply with increasing carotenoid intake in smokers. In a recent study, men and women who smoked one pack a day had on the average 72 and 79%, respectively, of the plasma beta-carotene levels of nonsmokers with similar carotenoid intake (Stryker et al., 1988). The possibility exists that beta-carotene in the blood may quench free radicals in cigarette smoke. Thus adjusting beta-carotene effects for smoking may lead to an underestimate of the protective effect of beta-carotene. Nonetheless, control of smoking is still necessary for a conservative estimate of the relationship between blood carotenoid levels and risk of any smoking-related cancer.

Dietary intake and blood nutrient levels are imperfect but complementary ways of evaluating carotenoids. High dietary intake of carotenoids may simply reflect high intake of vegetables and fruits and their constituents, such as vitamin C, folate, dietary fiber, and indoles. High levels of beta-carotene in serum or plasma may reflect high dietary intake of carotenoids, vegetables, and fruits or other dietary and genetic factors that influence the low-density lipoprotein fraction which transports beta-carotene in blood. The concordance of the studies of dietary carotenoids and blood beta-carotene levels—both measures are associated with a reduced risk of lung cancer—suggests that beta-carotene may be the protective factor. This is the simplest explanation although a role for other carotenoids or other constituents of vegetables and fruits is consistent with the findings.

In comparing prospective studies of the influence of dietary carotenoids and blood beta-carotene levels, the latter are often considered more valid because a well-characterized chemical species is being measured. However, conclusions based on the former have more immediate public health relevance since recommendations about reducing cancer risk must be expressed in practical terms of dietary intake.

RETROSPECTIVE STUDIES OF CAROTENOID INTAKE AND LUNG CANCER

In addition to the prospective studies reviewed, a number of retrospective studies of carotenoids and specific cancers have been conducted. Lung has been the site studied most intensively because of the prevalence of this cancer and the increasing evidence from epidemiological studies that diet may be involved in its etiology. The 11 retrospective studies of carotenoid intake and lung cancer are summarized in Table 5 (MacLennan et al., 1977; Hinds et al., 1984; Ziegler et al., 1984, 1986; Samet et al., 1985; Wu et al., 1985; Pisani et al., 1986; Byers et al., 1987; Bond et al., 1987; Pastorino et al., 1987; Fontham et al., 1988; Marchand et al., 1989). Retrospective studies of blood carotenoid levels and lung cancer are not included. The severity of this particular cancer and its treatment suggests that appetite and metabolism would be altered after diagnosis and complicate the interpretation of blood nutrient levels.

All 11 studies of diet and lung cancer showed decreased risk with increased intake of carotenoids and/or vegetable and fruit subgroups. In all the studies either the inverse associations or the tests for trend were statistically significant. In nine of the studies indices of carotenoid intake were developed (Hinds et al., 1984; Ziegler et al., 1984, 1986; Samet et al., 1985; Wu et al., 1985; Byers et al., 1987; Bond et al., 1987; Pastorino et al., 1987; Fontham et al., 1988; Marchand et al., 1989) by including most of the carotenoid-rich vegetables and fruits in the dietary interview, and weighting the frequencies of consumption according to carotenoid content from food composition tables.

Two of these studies attempted to determine whether beta-carotene or other carotenoids or another constituent of vegetables and fruits was primarily responsible for the protective effect. In one study the frequencies of consumption of dark green and dark yellow-orange vegetables were compared with a carotenoid index, and more pronounced decreases in lung cancer risk were associated with the two food group measures (Ziegler et al., 1986). Two explanations were presented: (1) beta-carotene was protective; and these two food groups, rich in beta-carotene, were better measures of its intake than an approximate index of the hydrocarbon carotenoids; or alternatively (2) the protective agent might be another constituent of these vegetable subgroups, and not necessarily a carotenoid. In another study total vegetable intake was more strongly associated with reduced risk of lung cancer than estimates of the intake of beta-carotene or of the other carotenoids with vitamin A activity (Marchand et al., 1989). In addition, tomatoes, which are rich in lycopene; dark green vegetables, rich in lutein; and cruciferous vegetables, rich in indoles, seemed about as protective as carrots, which are rich in beta-carotene. These observations suggested that constituents of vegetables other than beta-carotene might be important in the prevention of lung cancer. Further research regarding individual carotenoid content of foods will enable estimation of the intake of the specific carotenoids and will thus facilitate studies to identify the actual protective factor(s).

In general, in these retrospective studies of diet and lung cancer other factors concentrated in vegetables and fruits have been rarely investigated. Inverse associations with vitamin C were noted in four studies (Hinds et al., 1984; Byers et al., 1987; Fontham et al., 1988; Marchand et al., 1989) and with dietary fiber in two studies (Byers et al., 1987; Marchand et al., 1989); but in every situation but one (Fontham et al., 1988) the associations were weaker than with carotenoids.

Table 5 Retrospective Studies of Dietary Carotenoids and Lung Cancer

Authors, date	Study population	Exposure evaluated	Cases, controls Type of controls		Evidence of association[a]
MacLennan, 1977	Singapore Chinese Men, women	8 vegetables (6 green leafy vegs.)		233, 300 Hospital	+, neg
Hinds, 1984	Oahu, HI Multiethnic Men, women	Carotenoids	M: F:	261, 444 103, 183 Population	+, tr(?), neg tr(?), pos
Ziegler, 1984, 1986	New Jersey Men	Carotenoids Dark green vegs. Dark yellow-orange vegs.		763, 900 Population	(tr), neg tr, neg tr, neg
Samet, 1985	New Mexico Men, women	Carotenoids		447, 759 Population	+, (tr), neg
Wu, 1985	Los Angeles, CA Women	Carotenoids		220, 440 Neighborhood	+, tr(?), neg
Pisani, 1986	Lombardy, Italy Men, women	Carrots Leafy green vegetables		417, 849 Hospital	tr, neg tr, neg
Byers, 1987	Upstate New York Men, women	Carotenoids	M: F:	296, 587 154, 315 Neighborhood	+, tr, neg —
Bond, 1987	Chemical co. employees, Texas Men	Carotenoids		734[b] Cohort[c]	+, tr(?), neg

Pastorino, 1987	Milan, Italy Women	47, 159 Hospital	Carotenoids	+, neg
Fontham, 1988	Southern Louisiana Men, women	1253, 1274 Hospital	Carotenoids	(+), (tr), neg
			Vegetables	(+), (tr), neg
			Fruits	+, tr, neg
Marchand, 1989	Oahu, HI Multiethnic Men, women	M: 230, 597	Beta-carotene	+, tr, neg
			Other provitamin A carotenoids	+(?), tr, neg
			Vegetables	+, tr, neg
			Fruits	—
		W: 102, 268 Population	Beta-carotene	+, tr, neg
			Other provitamin A carotenoids	+(?), tr, neg
			Vegetables	+, tr, neg
			Fruits	—

[a] A + indicates a statistically significant association, e.g., a significant difference in dietary intake between cases and controls or a significant difference in relative risks between subgroups of the study population stratified by dietary intake; (+) indicates an apparent association that is not statistically significant; +(?) indicates an apparent association that was not tested for statistical significance. Tr indicates a statistically significant test for trend in relative risks with changes in dietary intake; (tr) indicates an apparent trend that is not statistically significant; tr(?) indicates an apparent trend that was not tested for statistical significance. Pos implies an increased risk of cancer with increased intake; neg implies a decreased risk of cancer with increased intake.

[b] Represents the combined number of cases and controls participating in the study. Separate numbers of cases and controls were not given.

[c] Controls matched to the cases were selected from the cohort.

Retinol intake was considered in nine studies (Hinds et al., 1984; Ziegler et al., 1984, 1986; Samet et al., 1985; Wu et al., 1985; Bond et al., 1987; Byers et al., 1987; Pastorino et al., 1987; Fontham et al., 1988; Marchand et al., 1989) and seemed unrelated to lung cancer risk in all but one (Fontham et al., 1988).

In many of these retrospective studies, as in the prospective studies described earlier, it is not clear that the carotenoid–lung cancer associations were adequately adjusted for smoking. Emphasis was placed on adjusting for smoking intensity although duration of smoking may have been a more potent confounder.

Six of the studies used general population (Hinds et al., 1984; Ziegler et al., 1984, 1986; Samet et al., 1985; Marchand et al., 1989) or neighborhood (Wu et al., 1985; Byers et al., 1987) controls rather than hospital controls. This approach eliminates the possibility that the dietary patterns that predispose toward many chronic diseases, such as heart disease, stroke, and diabetes, and characterize many hospitalized individuals of the same age as cancer patients may generate the dietary differences between cancer cases and controls observed in a study.

Even though all 11 of these retrospective studies indicate that intake of vegetables, fruits, and carotenoids may significantly reduce the risk of lung cancer, the more detailed findings are not as consistent. All seven of the studies conducted in men detected a decreased risk of lung cancer with high carotenoid intake (Hinds et al., 1984; Ziegler et al., 1984, 1986; Samet et al., 1985; Byers et al., 1987; Bond et al., 1987; Fontham et al., 1988; Marchand et al., 1989). Four studies observed the same relationship in women (Samet et al., 1985; Wu et al., 1985; Pastorino et al., 1987; Marchand et al., 1989); three did not (Hinds et al., 1983; Byers et al., 1987; Fontham et al., 1988). One study included whites and Hispanics and found the protective effect of dietary carotenoids restricted to whites (Samet et al., 1985), while another study with both white and black subjects found protection by dietary carotenoids in both races (Fontham et al., 1988). Two studies reported that protection was primarily among smokers who had stopped smoking (Samet et al., 1985; Byers et al., 1987), but a third found it predominantly among current smokers (Ziegler et al., 1986). A fourth study noted protective effects in both current and ex-smokers (Fontham et al., 1988); a fifth reported different patterns for men and women (Marchand et al., 1989).

One consistent finding of these case-control studies is that protection by carotenoids is not restricted to squamous cell lung cancer. Of the six studies that investigated histological specificity, all found inverse associations of carotenoid intake with lung adenocarcinoma (Wu et al., 1985; Pisani et al., 1986) or small-cell lung cancer (Fontham et al., 1988) or both (Ziegler et al., 1984; Byers et al., 1987; Marchand et al., 1989), although the associations seemed strongest with squamous cell disease. This result suggests that carotenoids might modulate carcinogenesis in sites other than just those involving squamous epithelium.

Vitamin A plays an important role in the normal differentiation of squamous epithelium. Failure to observe a similar histological specificity for carotenoids weakens the argument (De Vet, 1989) that beta-carotene functions through a mechanism involving cleavage into retinol in peripheral tissues.

When the six studies that used a carotenoid index and population or neighborhood controls are considered, the smoking-adjusted relative risks of lung cancer among those in the lowest quartile or tertile of carotenoid intake, compared to those in the highest quartile or tertile, ranged from 1.3 to 2.7 (Hinds et al., 1984; Ziegler et al., 1984, 1986; Samet et al., 1985; Wu et al., 1985; Byers et al., 1987; Marchand et al., 1989). Nonetheless, these relative risks suggest that the levels of vegetable and fruit consumption characteristic of about 30% of a typical community may be sufficient for a noticeable reduction (22–63%) in lung cancer risk. What needs to be more carefully examined is the range of carotenoid intake over which an effect is observed. It is important to determine whether vegetables, fruits, and carotenoids seem to reduce lung cancer risk only among individuals with nutritionally inadequate diets or whether increased carotenoid intake beyond that normally consumed might benefit well-nourished individuals.

RETROSPECTIVE STUDIES OF CAROTENOID INTAKE AND OTHER CANCERS

For cancers other than lung cancer, too few retrospective studies of the role of diet have been conducted or the results are too inconsistent to definitely implicate carotenoids. Those cancers for which there is suggestive evidence from retrospective studies that vegetables, fruits, and carotenoids are protective include mouth, pharynx, larynx, esophagus, stomach, colon, rectum, bladder, and cervix.

It needs to be emphasized that for these other sites evidence of reduced risk with high vegetable and fruit intake does not necessarily imply that the dietary etiology is the same as that observed with lung cancer. For example, we conducted a population-based case-control study of esophageal cancer among black men in Washington, D.C., the U.S. metropolitan area with the highest esophageal cancer mortality rates for nonwhite males (Ziegler et al., 1981). Heavy alcohol intake was the dominant risk factor. However, even after controlling for alcohol, low vegetable and fruit consumption was significantly associated with an increased risk of esophageal cancer. Also associated with increased risk were low dairy product and egg consumption and low fresh or frozen meat and fish consumption (Table 6). Low intake of vitamin C, riboflavin, and vitamin A, as well as of carotenoids, were also all associated with elevated risk. These results suggested that generally poor nutrition, characterized by inadequate intake of the basic food groups, was the dominant dietary risk factor. Multiple micronutrient deficiencies might be involved. This explanation is consistent with the geographic pattern of

Table 6 Adjusted[a] Relative Risks of Esophageal Cancer in Washington, D.C. Black Males by Food Group and Micronutrient Intake[b]

Food group or micronutrient	Level of consumption			
	Highest tertile	Middle tertile	Lowest tertile	*p* for trend
Meat and fish	1.0	1.3	1.2	0.39
Fresh or frozen meat and fish	1.0	1.6	2.2	0.01
Processed meat and fish	1.0	0.9	0.9	0.34
Dairy products and eggs	1.0	1.7	1.9	0.02
Vegetables and fruits	1.0	1.7	2.0	0.02
Vegetables	1.0	1.5	1.6	0.07
Fruits	1.0	2.4	2.0	0.05
Complex carbohydrates	1.0	1.1	1.2	0.24
Vitamin A	1.0	1.5	1.5	0.10
Carotenoids	1.0	1.3	1.3	0.17
Vitamin C	1.0	1.2	1.8	0.03
Thiamin	1.0	1.2	1.2	0.34
Riboflavin	1.0	1.0	1.7	0.05

[a] Adjusted for ethanol consumption. Smoking was not a risk factor in this study.
[b] Includes 120 cases and 250 controls.
Source: Adapted from Ziegler et al., 1981.

this cancer. Internationally it is endemic in regions with limited diets and impoverished agriculture; within a country it seems associated with low socioeconomic status.

Cervical cancer is another cancer that has been linked with carotenoids, vegetables, and fruits. It is primarily a squamous cell epithelial tumor like lung cancer. It is associated with low socioeconomic status and thus possibly with poor nutrition. Several epidemiological studies have suggested that carotenoids, vitamin C, or folacin might be protective (Ziegler et al., 1990). However, in a recent community-based case-control study of invasive cervical cancer conducted in five areas of the United States, no increased risk was noted with low intake of carotenoids, vegetables, fruits, or the vegetable subgroups rich in beta-carotene (Table 7) (Ziegler et al., 1990). The range of carotenoid intake in the study was estimated to be three- to fourfold and typical of low socioeconomic groups in the United States. Although the results of this study need to be confirmed, they suggest that carotenoids may not protect against all epithelial tumors.

To summarize, low intake of vegetables, fruits, and carotenoids is consistently associated with an increased risk of lung cancer in both prospective and retro-

Table 7 Adjusted[a] Relative Risks of Invasive Squamous Cell Cervical Cancer in U.S. White Women by Carotenoid and Food Group Intake[b]

Nutrient or food group	Level of consumption				
	Highest quartile	Quartile 3	Quartile 2	Lowest quartile	*p* for trend
Carotenoids	1.0	0.67	0.85	1.19	0.18
Vegetables and fruits	1.0	0.64	0.96	1.11	0.34
Fruits	1.0	1.00	0.93	1.35	0.26
Vegetables	1.0	0.92	1.16	1.16	0.43
Dark green vegetables	1.0	0.98	1.33	1.00	0.69
Dark yellow-orange vegetables	1.0	0.89	1.14	1.22	0.32

[a] Adjusted for number of sexual partners, age at first intercourse, number of cigarettes/day, duration of oral contraceptive use, history of nonspecific genital infection, years since last Pap smear, age at diagnosis, and study center.
[b] Includes 271 cases and 502 controls.
Source: Adapted from Ziegler et al., 1990.

spective studies. In addition, low levels of beta-carotene in blood are consistently associated with the subsequent development of lung cancer. The simplest explanation is that beta-carotene is protective. Since retinol is not related in a similar manner to lung cancer risk, beta-carotene appears to function through a mechanism that does not require its conversion to vitamin A. However, the importance of other carotenoids and other constituents of vegetables and fruits has not been adequately explored.

Both prospective and retrospective studies suggest that vegetable and fruit intake may reduce the risk of certain other cancers. Because of fewer studies and less consistency among studies, however, the epidemiological evidence is at present less persuasive than for lung cancer.

CLINICAL TRIALS INVOLVING BETA-CAROTENE

A number of clinical trials of the efficacy of beta-carotene in cancer prevention are underway. Chemoprevention clinical trials at the National Cancer Institute emphasize the administration of compounds with known antioxidant properties, such as beta-carotene, vitamin E, vitamin C, and selenium. Only a few clinical trials are currently underway which involve dietary modification designed to increase carotenoid or vegetable and fruit consumption. However, several clinical trials are being initiated that attempt to show the effects of decreased fat and increased fiber consumption. The people in these trials who adhere to a low-fat, high-fiber diet are likely to increase their vegetable and fruit consumption as well as their intake of carotenoids, vitamin C, folacin, and other micronutrients.

SIGNIFICANCE OF FINDINGS AND IMPLICATIONS

Epidemiological studies suggest that increased vegetable and fruit consumption may reduce cancer risk. There is no evidence at present that a *moderate* increase in vegetable and fruit intake has adverse health effects. In fact, on any given day, only 83% and 59% of American adults consume at least one serving of a vegetable or fruit, respectively (Patterson and Block, 1988). While there is legitimate concern regarding the pesticide content of produce, the benefits of consuming vegetables and fruits appear to outweigh the possible risks. Furthermore, through the substitution of vegetables and fruits for other foods in an individual's diet, additional beneficial changes are likely to occur, including increased micronutrient intake; decreased calorie, fat, and sugar intake; and reduced weight. Although clinical trials to evaluate vegetable and fruit consumption directly have not been completed, it seems prudent to recommend increased intake, based on the likely benefit and unlikely risk. Thus the National Cancer Institute, the National Academy of Sciences, and the U.S. Department of Agriculture all suggest increasing vegetable and fruit consumption.

Also important is consumption of a variety of vegetables and fruits. Given the present state of knowledge, increasing only those vegetables and fruits rich in beta-carotene cannot be definitively recommended. Although beta-carotene is a plausible protective agent, other carotenoids, other micronutrients such as vitamin C or folacin, and other plant constituents such as dietary fiber or indoles may also play a role.

While beta-carotene supplements and multiple-vitamin supplements at doses comparable to the Recommended Dietary Allowances are not known to cause adverse health effects, they are not an acceptable substitute for increased vegetable and fruit intake since the protective factor(s) in vegetables and fruits has not been identified. Even if clinical trials clearly implicate beta-carotene as beneficial, vegetables and fruits could still contain additional crucial substances.

The National Cancer Institute currently suggests increasing vegetable and fruit intake to five servings a day. The recommendation is not based on epidemiological studies of cancer or overall morbidity and mortality. Instead it is derived from data describing U.S. dietary patterns and reflects what seems achievable by Americans on a Western diet and what provides adequate intake of important micronutrients. More research to clarify the health benefits of various levels of intake of vegetables and fruit would facilitate determining future guidelines. In the interim, diets oriented toward including five servings of vegetables and fruit a day are nutrient-dense and may reduce cancer risk.

REFERENCES

Beecher GR, Khachik F. Evaluation of vitamin A and carotenoid data in food composition tables. J Natl Cancer Inst 1984; 73:1397–1404.

Beecher GR, Khachik F. Analysis of micronutrients in food. In: Moon TE, Micozzi MS, eds. Nutrition and cancer. New York, Marcel Dekker, 1989, 103–158.

Bendich A. Carotenoids and the immune response. J Nutr 1985; 119:112–115.

Bendich A, Olson JA. Biological actions of carotenoids. FASEB J 1989; 3:1927–1932.

Bond GG, Thompson FE, Cook RR. Dietary vitamin A and lung cancer: results of a case-control study among chemical workers. Nutr Cancer 1987; 9:109–121.

Britton G, Goodwin TW. Carotenoid chemistry and biochemistry. Elmsford, NY: Pergamon Press, 1982.

Brown ED, Micozzi MS, Craft NE, Bieri JG, Beecher G, Edwards BK, Rose A, Taylor PR, Smith JC, Jr. Plasma carotenoids in normal men after a single ingestion of vegetables or purified β-carotene. Am J Clin Nutr 1989a; 49:1258–1265.

Brown ED, Rose A, Craft N, Seidel KE, Smith JC, Jr. Concentrations of carotenoids, retinol, and tocopherol in plasma in response to ingestion of a meal. Clin Chem 1989b; 35:310–312.

Burney PGJ, Comstock GW, Morris JS. Serologic precursors of cancer: Serum micronutrients and the subsequent risk of pancreatic cancer. Am J Clin Nutr 1989; 49:895–900.

Burton GW. Antioxidant action of carotenoids. J Nutr 1989; 119:109–111.

Byers TE, Graham S, Haughey BP, Marshall JR, Swanson MK. Diet and lung cancer risk: Findings from the Western New York Diet Study. Am J Epidemiol 1987; 125:351–363.

Colditz GA, Branch LG, Lipnick RJ, Willett WC, Rosner B, Posner BM, Hennekens CH. Increased green and yellow vegetable intake and lowered cancer deaths in an elderly population. Am J Clin Nutr 1985; 41:32–36.

Committee on Dietary Allowances, Food and Nutrition Board. *Recommended Dietary Allowances*, 9th rev. ed. Washington, DC: National Academy of Sciences, 1980.

Comstock GW, Helzlsouer KJ, Bush TL. Prediagnostic serum levels of carotenoids and vitamin E as related to subsequent cancer in Washington County, Maryland, Am J Clin Nutr 1991; 53:2603–2645.

Connett JE, Kuller LH, Kjelsberg MO, Polk BF, Collins G, Rider A, Hulley SB. Relationship between carotenoids and cancer: The Multiple Risk Factor Intervention Trial (MRFIT) Study. Cancer 1989; 64:126–134.

Craft NE, Brown ED, Smith JC, Jr. Effects of storage and handling conditions on concentrations of individual carotenoids, retinol, and tocopherol in plasma. Clin Chem 1988; 34:44–48.

De Vet HCW. The puzzling role of vitamin A in cancer prevention. Anticancer Res 1989; 9:145–152.

Dimitrov NV. Beta-carotene: Biological properties and applications. A year in nutritional medicine. New Canaan, 1986, 167–202.

Dimitrov NV, Meyer C, Ullrey DE, Chenoweth W, Michelakis A, Malone W, Boone C, Fink G. Bioavailability of β-carotene in humans. Am J Clin Nutr 1988; 48:298–304.

Doll R, Peto R. Cigarette smoking and bronchial carcinoma: Dose and time relationships among regular smokers and lifelong nonsmokers. J Epidemiol Commun Hlth 1978; 32:303–313.

Fontham ETH, Pickle LW, Haenszel W, Correa P, Lin Y, Falk RT. Dietary vitamins A and C and lung cancer risk in Louisiana. Cancer 1988; 62:2267–2273.

Food and Agriculture Organization/World Health Organization Expert Group. Requirements of vitamin A, thiamine, riboflavin and niacin. FAO Rep Series, No. 41. Rome: FAO, 1967.

Friedman GD, Blaner WS, Goodman DS, Vogelman JH, Brind JL, Hoover R, Fireman BH, Orentreich N. Serum retinol and retinol-binding protein levels do not predict subsequent lung cancer. Am J Epidemiol 1986; 123:781–789.

Helzlsouer KJ, Comstock GW, Morris JS. Selenium, lycopene, a-tocopherol, β-carotene, retinol, and subsequent bladder cancer. Cancer Res 1989; 49:6144–6148.

Hinds MW, Kolonel LN, Hankin JH, Lee J. Dietary vitamin A, carotene, vitamin C and risk of lung cancer in Hawaii. Am J Epidemiol 1984; 119:227–237.

Hirayama T. Diet and cancer. Nutr Cancer 1979; 1:67–81.

Hirayama T. A large scale cohort study on cancer risks with special reference to the risk reducing effects of green-yellow vegetable consumption. Int Symp Princess Takamatsu Cancer Res Fund 1985; 16:41–53.

Horwitz W. Official Methods of Analysis of the Association of Analytic Chemists. Washington, DC: AOAC, 1980, 230–231, 734–740.

Kvale G, Bjelke E, Gart JJ. Dietary habits and lung cancer risk. Int J Cancer 1983; 31:397–405.

MacLennan R, DaCosta J, Day NE, Law CH, Nq YK, Shanmugaratnam K. Risk factors for lung cancer in Singapore Chinese, a population with high female incidence rates. Int J Cancer 1977; 20:854–860.

Marchand LL, Yoshizawa CN, Kolonel LN, Hankin JH, Goodman MT. Vegetable consumption and lung cancer risk: A population-based case-control study in Hawaii. J Natl Cancer Inst 1989; 81:1158–1164.

Margolis SA, Paule RC, Ziegler RG. The differential measurement of ascorbic and dehydroascorbic acid in sera preserved in dithiothreitol or metaphosphoric acid. Clin Chem, 1990; 36:1750–1755.

Menkes MS, Comstock GW, Vuilleumier JP, Helsing KJ, Rider AA, Brookmeyer R. Serum β-carotene, vitamins A and E, selenium, and the risk of lung cancer. N Engl J Med. 1986; 315:1250–1254.

Micozzi MS, Beecher GR, Taylor PR, Khachik F. Carotenoid analyses of selected raw and cooked foods associated with a lower risk for cancer. J Natl Cancer Inst 1990; 82:282–285.

Nierenberg DW, Stukel TA, Baron JA, Dain BJ, Greenberg ER. Determinants of plasma levels of beta-carotene and retinol. Am J Epidemiol 1989; 130:511–521.

Nomura AMY, Stemmerman GN, Heilbrun LK, Salkeld RM, Vuilleumier JP. Serum vitamin levels and the risk of cancer of specific sites in men of Japanese ancestry in Hawaii. Cancer Res 1985; 45:2369–2372.

Olson JA. Provitamin A function of carotenoids: The conversion of β-carotene into vitamin A. J Nutr 1989; 119:105–108.

Paganini-Hill A, Chao A, Ross RK, Henderson BE. Vitamin A, β-carotene, and the risk of cancer: A prospective study. J. Natl Cancer Inst 1987; 79:443–448.

Parker RS. Carotenoids in human blood and tissues. J Nutr 1989; 119:101–104.

Patterson BH, Block G. Food choices and the cancer guidelines. Am J Public Hlth 1988; 78:282–286.

Pastorino U, Pisani P, Berrino F, Andreoli C, Barbieri A, Costa A, Mazzoleni C, Gramegna G, Marubini E. Vitamin A and female lung cancer: A case-control study on plasma and diet. Nutr Cancer 1987; 10:171–179.

Pisani P, Berrino F, Macaluso M, Pastorino U, Crosignani P, Baldasseroni A. Carrots, green vegetables, and lung cancer: A case-control study. Int J Epidemiol 1986; 15:463–468.

Roidt L, White E, Goodman GE, Wahl PW, Omen GS, Rollins B, Karkeck JM. Association of food frequency questionnaire estimates of vitamin A intake with serum vitamin A levels. Am J Epidemiol 1988; 128:645–654.

Russell-Briefel R, Bates MW, Kuller LH. The relationship of plasma carotenoids to health and biochemical factors in middle-aged men. Am J Epidemiol 1985; 122:741–749.

Samet JM, Skipper BJ, Humble CG, Pathak DR. Lung cancer risk and vitamin A consumption in New Mexico. Ann Rev Respir Dis 1985; 131:198–202.

Schober SE, Comstock GW, Helsing KJ, Salkeld RM, Morris JS, Rider AA, Brookmeyer R. Serologic precursors of cancer I. Prediagnostic serum nutrients and colon cancer risk. Am J Epidemiol 1987; 126:1033–1041.

Shekelle RB, Lepper M, Liu S, Maliza C. Raynor WJ, Jr, Rossof AH. Dietary vitamin A and risk of cancer in the Western Electric Study. Lancet 1981; 2:1185–1190.

Stacewicz-Sapuntzakis M, Bowen PE, Kikendall JW, Burgess M. Simultaneous determination of serum retinol and various carotenoids: Their distribution in middle-aged men and women. J Micronutr Anal 1987; 3:27–45.

Stahelin HB, Rosel F, Buess E, Brubacher G. Cancer, vitamins, and plasma lipids: Prospective Basle study. J Natl Cancer Inst 1984; 73:1463–1468.

Stahelin HB, Gey KF, Eichholzer M, Ludin E. β-carotene and cancer prevention: The Basle study. Am J Clin Nutr 1991; 53:265S–269S.

Straub O. Key to carotenoids. Boston: Birkhauser Verlag, 1987.

Stryker WS, Kaplan LA, Stein EA, Stampfer MJ, Sober A, Willett WC. The relation of diet, cigarette smoking, and alcohol consumption to plasma β-carotene and α-tocopheral levels. Am J Epidemiol 1988; 127:283–296.

Subar AF, Harlan LC, Mattson ME. Food and nutrient intake differences between smokers and non-smokers in the U.S. Am J Public Hlth 1990; 80:1323–1329.

United States Department of Agriculture. Composition of foods: Raw, processed, prepared. USDA Agriculture Handbook No. 8, Revised sections 8–1 through 8–16. Washington, DC, 1976–1987.

Wald NJ, Boreham J, Hayward JL, and Bulbrook RD. Plasma retinol, β-carotene, and vitamin E in relation to the future risk of breast cancer. Br J Cancer 1984; 49:321–324.

Wald N, Boreham J, Bailey A. Serum retinol and subsequent risk of cancer. Br J Cancer 1986; 54:957–961.

Wald NJ, Thompson SG, Densem JW, Boreham J, Bailey A. Serum vitamin E and subsequent risk of cancer. Br J Cancer 1987; 56:69–72.

Wald NJ, Nicolaides-Bouman A, Hudson GW. Plasma retinol, β-carotene, and vitamin E levels in relation to the future risk of breast cancer (letter). Br J Cancer 1988a; 57:235.

Wald NJ, Thompson SG, Densem JW, Boreham J, Bailey A. Serum β-carotene and subsequent risk of cancer: Results from the BUPA study. Br J Cancer 1988b; 57:428–433.

Wang L, Hammond EC. Lung cancer, fruit, green salad, and vitamin pills. Chin Med J 1985; 98:206–210.

Willett WC, Stampfer MJ, Underwood BA, Speizer FE, Rosner B, Hennekens CH. Validation of a dietary questionnaire with plasma carotenoid and α-tocopherol levels. Am J Clin Nutr 1983; 38:631–639.

Willett WC, Polk BF, Underwood BA, Stampfer MJ, Pressel S, Rosner B, Taylor JO, Schneider K, Hames CG. Relation of serum vitamins A and E and carotenoids to the risk of cancer. N Engl J Med 1984; 310:430–434.

Wu AH, Henderson BE, Pike MC, Yu MC. Smoking and other risk factors for women. J Natl Cancer Inst 1985; 74:747–751.

Ziegler RG, Morris LE, Blot WJ, Pottern LM. Hoover R, Fraumeni JF, Jr. Esophageal cancer among black men in Washington, D.C. II. Role of nutrition. J Natl Cancer Inst 1981; 67:1199–1206.

Ziegler RG, Mason TJ, Stemhagen A, Hoover R, Schoenberg JB, Gridley G, Virgo PW, Altman R, Fraumeni JF, Jr. Dietary carotene and vitamin A and risk of lung cancer among whites in New Jersey. J Natl Cancer Inst 1984; 73:1429–1435.

Ziegler RG, Mason TJ, Stemhagen A, Hoover R, Schoenberg JB, Gridley G, Virgo PW, Fraumeni JF, Jr. Carotenoid intake, vegetables, and the risk of lung cancer among white men in New Jersey. Am J Epidemiol 1986; 123:1080–1093.

Ziegler RG, Brinton LA, Hamman RF, Lehman HF, Levine RS, Mallin K, Norman SA, Rosenthal JF, Trumble AC, Hoover RN. Diet and the risk of invasive cervical cancer among white women in the United States. Am J Epidemiol 1990; 132:432–445.

6

Intervention Trials with Beta-Carotene in Precancerous Conditions of the Upper Aerodigestive Tract

Harinder Garewal

University of Arizona Cancer Center and
Veterans Affairs Medical Center
Tucson, Arizona

Glenn J. Shamdas

University of Arizona Cancer Center
Tucson, Arizona

INTRODUCTION

Vitamin A plays an essential role in the normal differentiation of epithelial tissues (Hicks, 1983). Certain carotenoids, a group of some 300 different compounds that are the red, orange, and yellow pigments in plants, can serve as precursors for vitamin A (retinol) and have antioxidant and anticarcinogenic properties of their own. Beta-carotene is biologically one of the most important carotenoids, since it can be converted in mammalian tissues to vitamin A. In the developing world, carotenoids serve as the dietary source for approximately 80–90% of vitamin A as compared with only about 50% in the United States. Carotenoids that are not converted to vitamin A circulate with fats and are deposited in many tissues throughout the body. These deposited carotenoids probably have a direct protective role in tissues which may be responsible for the majority of anticarcinogenic activity.

Epidemiological Studies

Epidemiological studies have provided evidence for an association between low intake of carotenoid-containing foods, i.e., vegetables and fruits, and a higher risk of many cancers including those of the upper aerodigestive tract (Bjelke, 1975; Hirajama, 1979; Peto et al., 1981; Nomura et al., 1982; Winn et al., 1984; Greenwald et al., 1986). This is reviewed in more detail in an accompanying chapter in this book. These studies are particularly suggestive of such an association for lung cancer and cancer of the oral cavity.

Laboratory and Animal Studies

Carotenoids, particularly beta-carotene, have been shown to have antimutagenic activity in bacterial systems. Similarly, in many tissue culture systems, beta-carotene has a profound inhibitory effect on transformation induced by chemicals and radiation (Som et al., 1984; Bertram et al., 1988). Beta-carotene can block genotoxic damage induced in Chinese hamster ovary cells by tumor promoters such as extract of areca nut, which is an integral part of betel quid, that is linked to oral cancer causation (Stich and Dunn, 1986).

The precise mechanism(s) of action of retinoids and carotenoids in cancer inhibition have not yet been determined. They produce salutary effects on cellular differentiation, immunological function, and interaction of cells with growth factors, such as epidermal growth factor, all of which may be important in their cancer-inhibiting activities.

Of particular relevance to the prevention of cancer of the upper aerodigestive tract is the ability of these compounds to produce profound inhibition of the formation of precancerous and cancerous lesions in the hamster cheek pouch model in which lesions are induced by applying the carcinogen 7,12-dimethyl-benz(a)anthracene (DMBA) (Shklar et al., 1980a,b; Burge-Bottenbley and Shklar, 1983; Schwartz et al., 1986). The hamster cheek pouch does not normally develop spontaneous tumors and offers a more reliable growth and microscopic system for the study of tumor prevention than models based on the use of transplanted tumors. One of its major advantages is that a characteristic sequence of tumor development occurs which is very similar to that seen in natural human oral cancer, i.e., the development first of precancerous lesions followed by epidermoid cancer within a consistent time sequence. This model has been used to screen potential chemopreventive agents by testing their ability to inhibit DMBA-induced tumors. Beta-carotene, either locally applied or administered systemically, causes significant inhibition of tumor formation in this model (Schwartz et al., 1986). In fact, in this model system, beta-carotene can actually induce regression of established tumors when directly injected into the lesion. Vitamin E has also been shown to be very active in this system (Shklar, 1982; Odukoya et al., 1984).

These observations on the anticarcinogenic activity of carotenoids have led to attempts at clinically testing their efficacy in the inhibition of human cancer. As discussed below, the reversal of precancerous lesions is one of the most useful clinical approaches available for screening agents for this purpose. In this chapter, we will summarize recent trials using beta-carotene, used either alone or in combination with other agents, for the suppression of preneoplasia.

IMPORTANCE OF INTERVENTION TRIALS IN PRECANCEROUS LESIONS

It is now generally accepted that cancer develops through a series of sequential changes involving initiation, promotion, and progression to malignancy (Fig. 1). Most of the early steps in this pathway occur at the subcellular level and are not reflected as phenotypically identifiable lesions. Premalignant lesions are the first clinically identifiable lesions along this pathway that "mark" a mucosa as having been affected by carcinogens. Therefore, the search for treatments that can cause reversal or suppression of premalignancy constitutes an important strategy for the inhibition of carcinogenesis, i.e., prevention of cancer.

CANCER OF THE ORAL CAVITY

Squamous cell oral cancer is a common neoplasm with an incidence that varies from region to region throughout the world. Some of the highest rates occur in developing countries, particularly India, Sri Lanka, South Vietnam, Papua in New Guinea, the Philippines, Hong Kong, Taiwan, and parts of Brazil, where up to 25% of all cancers are found in the oral cavity (Dunham, 1968; Baden, 1978). In Europe, France has the highest incidence of oral pharyngeal cancer which is approximately twice that seen in the United States (U.S. Dept. of State, 1982). In the U.S., oral cancer accounted for approximately 30,000 new cancer cases in 1988 resulting in about 9000 deaths (Silverberg and Lubera, 1988). This variation in incidence is related to exposure to known etiological agents. Strong

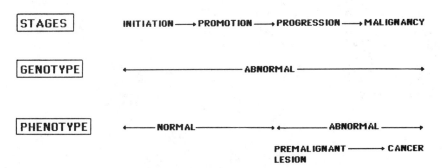

Figure 1 Carcinogenesis occurs via a series of stages resulting in the transformation of a normal cell to a malignant one. The earliest stages probably result in genetic damage and are not clinically recognizable as phenotypic abnormalities. As illustrated, pre-malignant lesions represent the earliest clinically recognizable change indicating that a tissue has been affected by carcinogenesis; hence their importance to cancer prevention trials.

support exists for exogenous factors such as tobacco and alcohol use as being major causative agents (U.S. Dept. Health and Human Services, 1982). In developing countries tobacco and betel nut chewing is a widespread custom, particularly in the Orient, and is responsible for most of these malignancies (Muir and Kirk, 1960). Clearly, efforts at prevention of this disease must focus on the reduction or elimination of these noxious habits. Additionally, however, in view of the known link to carcinogenic exposure, the concept of using compounds that might inhibit the carcinogenesis pathway is particularly relevant to this disease.

Oral Premalignant Lesions

Oral cavity premalignant lesions are generally classified as leukoplakia or erythroplakia. Leukoplakia is defined as a whitish patch that cannot be removed by scraping and cannot be classified clinically or microscopically as any other disease entity (Fig. 2). Biopsy usually shows hyperkeratosis with varying degrees of dysplasia. Erythroplakia is a lesion that has a reddish, velvety appearance. These lesions are considered premalignant based on the following lines of evidence: (1) Oral cancers are very often histologically and clinically associated

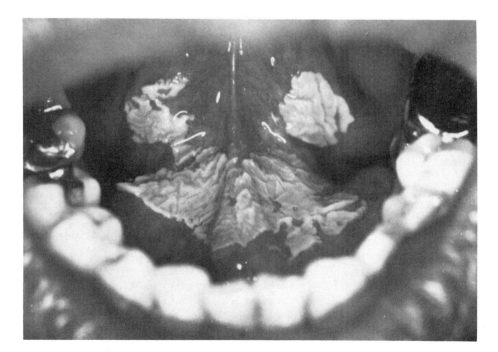

Figure 2 Oral leukoplakia. White lesion on floor of the mouth and lower surface of the tongue.

with leukoplakic changes elsewhere in the oral cavity. (2) Epidemiological studies show that almost all new cases of oral cancer in regions of the world with endemically high incidence of head and neck cancer arise in patients with previous evidence of premalignant change. (3) Prospective follow-up of leukoplakia patients has revealed a significant incidence of transformation to malignancy. The malignant transformation rate in leukoplakia depends on the characteristics of the lesion, the most important of which is the presence or absence of dysplasia. Rates of <1% to >15% have been reported, depending mainly on the degree of dysplasia and duration of follow-up. Presently, the standard treatment of this lesion depends on the index of suspicion for malignant transformation and consists primarily of surgical excision and/or cryosurgery. Clearly these modalities are not suitable for all lesions, particularly the larger ones. Furthermore, these lesions may merely be markers for an overall defect in the oral mucosa, i.e., "field cancerization," induced by carcinogens. If this is indeed the case, local treatment, e.g., excision of the visible lesions only, will not decrease cancer risk elsewhere. Because of easy accessibility to examination and follow-up, oral leukoplakia is an excellent lesion in which to evaluate agents by efficacy in reversing premalignant changes.

Clinical Trials in Leukoplakia (Table 1)

Retinoids

Several clinical trials have been conducted demonstrating the efficacy of various retinoids, both natural and synthetic, in reversing leukoplakia. In one study, 13-*cis*-retinoic acid (13-cRA, isotretinoin), *trans*-retinoic acid (tretinoin), or an aromatic retinoid (etretinate) was used to treat 75 patients with leukoplakia (Koch, 1978). Patients were given approximately 70 mg daily of one of these agents for 8 weeks. The overall response rate (complete and partial) was 87% for 13-cRA, 59% for tretinoin, and 91% for etretinate. The treatment was associated with considerable toxicity. Relapses occurred in over 50% of patients after therapy was discontinued, most often within 1–2 months of treatment cessation. A second study performed by the same group involving 45 patients compared etretinate given orally to oral etretinate plus topical etretinate paste for 6 weeks. A high response rate was again observed in both groups (Koch, 1981).

An 82% response rate was reported in 11 patients treated with 13-cRA lozenges (Shah et al., 1983). Similar results were reported with oral 13-cRA (Hong et al., 1986). The dose used was 1–2 mg/kg/day given for 3 months. Relapses again were frequent after cessation of treatment.

Beta-Carotene

Stich and colleagues have conducted a series of studies demonstrating that beta-carotene alone or in combination with vitamin A can decrease the incidence of

Table 1 Retinoid/Carotenoid Trials in Oral Leukoplakia

Investigator	Agent	CR (%)	PR (%)	OR (%)	Number of patients	Country
Koch (1978)[a]	a. *trans*-Retinoic acid	NS	NS	59	27	Germany
	b. 13-cRA	NS	NS	87	24	
	c. Etretinate	NS	NS	91	24	
Shah et al. (1983)	13-cRA (lozenges)	27	55	82	11	USA
Hong et al. (1986)	13-cRA	8	59	67	24	USA
Stich et al. (1988b)[b]	a. BC	15	NS	NS	27	India
	b. BC + Vit A	27	NS	NS	51	
Stich et al. (1988a)	Vit A	57	NS	NS	21	India
Garewal et al. (1989)	BC	8	63	71	24	USA

[a] Response criteria not fully defined.
[b] Only complete remission rate reported.
NS = not stated; CR = complete response; PR = partial response; OR = overall response; BC = beta-carotene.

micronucleated cells in exfoliated oral mucosal cells from populations at high risk for oral cancer (Stich et al., 1988b). Increased frequency of micronucleated cells probably reflects genotoxic damage produced by carcinogens. Stich et al. also performed trials in leukoplakia patients using vitamin A alone or in combination with beta-carotene conducted mainly in India (Stich et al., 1988b). It should be emphasized that this study population differs from that of other trials in that the lesion is primarily related to chewing of betel nuts in this region of the world. In one study, treatment consisted of beta-carotene (180 mg/week), group 1, or beta-carotene plus vitamin A (100,000 IU/week), group 2, or placebo, group 3, given twice weekly for 6 months. After 6 months of treatment, 15% of patients in group 1, 27% in group 2, compared with only 3% in group 3 had complete remissions of their disease. In addition, the frequency of micronucleated cells was significantly reduced in groups 1 and 2 compared with group 3. The appearance of new leukoplakias was also strongly inhibited in the treatment groups. In a more recent trial using 200,000 IU of vitamin A alone per week for 6 months, Stich et al. reported a 57% response rate with suppression of new lesions (Stich et al., 1988a). Cessation of treatment was associated with recurrence of lesions. These studies suggest that continued treatment with beta-carotene and/ or low doses of vitamin A might be effective in preventing recurrence.

We have recently completed a trial of beta-carotene alone in oral leukoplakia (Garewal et al., 1990). All patients were given 30 mg of beta-carotene daily for 3–6 months. A response rate of 71% was noted in 24 evaluable patients. Of great importance was the fact that no significant toxicity was observed throughout the duration of this trial. No patient had to discontinue or reduce drug dosage because of side effects. Since beta-carotene has been shown to produce changes in the cellular immune system in animal and in in vitro studies, we took the opportunity of this clinical trial to test whether similar changes were produced in humans in vivo. A significant increase in the number of cells expressing a natural killer (NK) cell marker (Leu 11) was observed in 16 patients who had measurements done at baseline and after 2 months of beta-carotene therapy. The percentage (mean $\pm$ standard deviation) of peripheral blood mononuclear cells expressing this NK cell marker increased from 4.1 $\pm$ 1.5 at baseline to 28.8 $\pm$ 6.5 at 2 months ($p < 0.05$). A larger trial to confirm these results as well as test the role of continued beta-carotene therapy to prevent relapse was recently initiated at our institution.

RESPIRATORY TRACT PREMALIGNANT LESIONS

When there is continuous injury caused by carcinogens, the columnar cells of the normal respiratory epithelium are replaced by metaplastic stratified squamous epithelium. This change is called bronchial squamous metaplasia, a precursor of lung cancer.

Vitamin A deficiency leads to the development of bronchial squamous metaplasia (Saccomanno et al., 1974), and administration of vitamin A or its analogs has been shown to reverse these changes (Harris et al., 1973; Nettesheim et al., 1979). These observations have generated several studies to determine the effect of retinoids in patients with a high risk of developing lung cancer.

Saccomanno et al. (1982) reported the use of 13-cRA (1–2.5 mg/kg/day) in 21 patients with abnormal sputum cytology but no evidence of invasive carcinoma. In follow-up sputum cytology performed at 2-week intervals, the retinoid did not alter the cytological diagnosis in any patient. Unfortunately, in light of the long latency period for the development of cancer after metaplastic change, the short treatment period (4–40 weeks) precludes definitive conclusions.

In 1982, Mathe et al. (Gouveia et al., 1982; Mathe et al., 1982) reported their experience with oral etretinate (25 mg/day for 6 months) in 52 cigarette smokers with bronchial metaplasia. Bronchoscopy and extensive rebiopsy of previously involved sites were performed after 6 months of treatment. Reductions in the percentage of sections showing metaplasia occurred in 76% of 30 evaluable patients. Complete resolution of metaplastic changes was noted in 3% of those patients who had also stopped smoking. In a subsequent study of 40 heavy smokers with a high degree of bronchial metaplasia in their biopsies, the same authors showed a significant response using the same dosage of oral etretinate (Misset et al., 1986). When a second bronchoscopy was performed on 36 evaluable patients, the index of metaplasia decreased significantly from 34% to 26%. As in the earlier study, 11% of the patients who had stopped smoking during therapy demonstrated complete resolutions of their bronchial metaplasia. These results suggest that retinoids may play an active role in reversing the preneoplastic process.

Several studies with beta-carotene are presently in progress. A large-scale, collaborative trial conducted by the National Cancer Institute and the National Public Health Institute of Finland is currently studying the efficacy of beta-carotene and vitamin E in decreasing lung cancer incidence in a population of 28,000 cigarette smokers (Albanes et al., 1986). This randomized, double-blind, 6-year intervention study was started in 1984 and evaluates four different treatment groups: placebo, beta-carotene, vitamin E, and beta-carotene in combination with vitamin E.

The combination of beta-carotene with vitamin A is also being tested in populations at high risk for lung cancer and mesothelioma due to occupational exposure to asbestos. Tin miners from Yunnan province in southern China have a high incidence of lung cancer because of heavy smoking and previous exposure to radiation and asbestos. Treatment arms consist of beta-carotene, vitamin A, vitamin E, and selenium.

The Seattle lung cancer chemoprevention trial is using beta-carotene in combination with retinol (Goodman and Ommen, 1990). This trial was initiated in 1983 as a pilot chemoprevention trial in high-risk groups: cigarette smokers, age 50–67 with a 20-pack-a-year or greater history of smoking, and asbestos workers, age 45–74, with chest X-ray and/or work history evidence of significant exposure. These trials have presently achieved their recruitment targets, demonstrating high adherence with study medications, and have found no increase of potentially relevant toxicity symptoms and signs in participants receiving active agents vs. placebo. The two populations have now been combined and the trial has been expanded to test the hypothesis that a combination of retinol with beta-carotene will decrease the incidence of lung cancer in these two high-risk groups.

Another trial utilizing asbestos-exposed individuals combines beta-carotene with retinol and is being conducted in Tyler, Texas. End points in several of these studies include evaluation of reversal of metaplastic changes in addition to decrease in incidence of cancer. The results of these well-designed studies should be of considerable importance.

LARYNGEAL PAPILLOMATOSIS

Laryngeal papillomatosis is a proliferation of polypoid lesions on the vocal cords, which may precede squamous cell carcinoma. Retinoids have been administered because of their antiproliferative activity against transforming epithelial tissues and the lack of any other nontoxic, effective treatment (Bichler and Daxenbichler, 1982).

In a study conducted at the University of Arizona, five patients with recurrent progressive laryngeal papillomatosis were treated with 13-cRA 1–2 mg/kg/day (Alberts et al., 1986a). Two patients achieved complete regression of their laryngeal lesions, one for 24 months and the other for 36 and a third patient had a partial response lasting 12 months. The two other patients showed no improvement while on retinoids and no additional benefit occurred in these nonresponders when doses were increased. Bichler had similar results employing etretinate (1 mg/kg/day) in 42 patients with laryngeal papillomatosis who manifested moderate to severe dysplastic changes (Bichler, 1983); a complete response was achieved in 67% of these patients and a partial response in 26%.

These results demonstrate that retinoids have activity in laryngeal papillomatosis. No studies with carotenoids have been reported in this disease. Such trials would be of interest to test whether similar response rates can be achieved with the less toxic carotenoids, such as beta-carotene, that cannot be metabolized to the retinoids used in the above trials, i.e., 13-cRA or etretinate.

ESOPHAGEAL LESIONS

The National Cancer Institute and the Cancer Institute of the Chinese Academy of Medical Sciences are conducting two randomized, double-blind, 5-year intervention trials in esophageal cancer in a rural area of China (Linxian). This particular region of China has a very high incidence of esophageal cancer. Treatment arms consist of vitamin A, beta-carotene, zinc, riboflavin, niacin, vitamin C, molybdenum, selenium, and vitamin E in eight separate intervention groups (Li et al., 1986). This study will determine the impact of supplementation with vitamins and minerals on the incidence of esophageal cancer. A second study, the dysplasia trial, will evaluate the effect of these vitamins and minerals, including beta-carotene, on a high-risk population with severe esophageal dysplasia, a premalignant lesion associated with esophageal cancer. In this lesion, profound cellular atypia is observed in the squamous epithelial lining of the lumen of the esophagus. All the study participants undergo sampling of the esophageal mucosa to confirm dysplasia. Patients with dysplasia who do not have cancer are included in the trial. Participants will be evaluated for disease progression or regression. Pilot phases of these studies have been completed and have shown that patient recruitment and compliance were feasible.

OTHER LESIONS

Several other sites are the targets of clinical trials with beta-carotene, either alone or in combination with other agents. Among these are skin, colon, and cervical lesions.

A related area of current interest is the prevention of second primary tumors in patients cured of their initial cancer. This is of particular importance to upper aerodigestive tract cancers where the incidence of second primaries is high. For instance, patients with squamous cell head and neck cancer have an increased incidence of second primary tumors, either synchronous or metachronous, of the upper aerodigestive tract (Muir and Kirk, 1960; Shapshay et al., 1980; McGuirt et al., 1982; Karp et al., 1985). In fact, patients with early lesions have a high cure rate of their primary tumor, but may succumb to a second malignancy. Approximately 10–40% of such patients will develop second primary tumors, a rate that is related to continued exposure to carcinogens. This is considered to be the result of a diffuse mucosal abnormality, often referred to as "field cancerization," resulting from carcinogen exposure (Slaughter et al., 1953). This patient population, with its high cancer risk and high rate of premalignant lesions, represents an excellent target for chemopreventive agents. Trials incorporating beta-carotene in an effort to reduce this increased risk are currently in the planning stages.

SUITABILITY OF AGENTS FOR CHEMOPREVENTION

Prevention and treatment are two different goals in the control of cancer. Potential chemopreventive agents must have properties that are not required for drugs used in advanced cancer. Chemopreventive agents must be essentially nontoxic to promote widespread use. The use of vitamins and related compounds is a definite advantage since it allows consideration of supplementation by dietary adjustments. Finally, the cost of the agent should not be prohibitive.

With the above considerations in mind, it is evident that the toxicity of the most frequently used retinoids, such as 13-cRA, would preclude widespread use for cancer prevention. For example, at the doses used in the leukoplakia studies, these drugs very often produce dermatological, hepatic, and other side effects. In addition, their teratogenicity is a significant problem. Similar considerations apply to high doses of vitamin A. Beta-carotene, on the other hand, fulfills all the criteria for a suitable chemopreventive agent in that it is nontoxic (Bendich, 1988), inexpensive, and a naturally occurring nutrient. Early trials have suggested that beta-carotene might have activity in reversing oral preneoplastic lesions and perhaps inhibiting the occurrence of new ones. Therefore, beta-carotene may emerge as an important agent in head and neck cancer prevention.

As indicated earlier, relapse rates after discontinuation of treatment are high, perhaps because of continued exposure to carcinogens or variations in individual susceptibility. Therefore, the role of maintenance therapy with beta-carotene in preventing lesion occurrence and recurrence needs to be studied. Because of the toxicity of the retinoids such maintenance studies are not practical with these agents but are quite feasible with the nontoxic beta-carotene. Therefore, even under conditions where beta-carotene is proven to be ineffective or less effective

Table 2 Cancer Prevention Trials Using Beta-Carotene

Investigator, location	Cancer	Study group	Other agents
1. Hennekens, Boston	All	Physicians	Aspirin
2. NCI, Finland	Lung	Smokers	Vitamin E
3. Goodman, Seattle	Lung	Smokers	Retinol
4. Kuller, Pittsburgh	Lung	Smokers	—
5. Ommen, Seattle	Lung	Asbestos	Retinol
6. McLarty, Tyler, Texas	Lung	Asbestos	Retinol
7. NCI, China	Lung	Tin miners	Retinol, selenium
8. Greenberg Hannover	Colon	Polyps	—
9. Bowen, Chicago	Colon	Polyps	—
10. NCI, China	Esophagus	Dysplasia	Multivitamins, minerals
11. NCI, China	Esophagus	General population	Multivitamins, minerals
12. Luande, Tanzania	Skin	Albino	—
13. Greenberg, Hannover	Skin	Previous skin cancer	—
14. Safal, New York	Skin	Previous skin cancer	Vitamins C, E
15. Garewal, Tucson	Oral	Leukoplakia	—

in treatment of the primary lesion than the more toxic retinoids, its role in maintenance of a response may be valuable. Table 2 provides a list of chemoprevention clinical trials presently being conducted with the support of the National Cancer Institute that use beta-carotene alone or in combination with other agents.

RECOMMENDATIONS

Premalignant lesions of the upper aerodigestive tract offer excellent target lesions for screening potential chemopreventive agents for ''reversing'' or inhibiting the progression of carcinogenesis in a clinical setting. Early results of trials with beta-carotene, alone or in combination with other agents, have been very promising, particularly in lesions of the oral cavity. Results of ongoing trials of other disease sites should be available in the next several years. If these agents are indeed shown to be capable of suppressing premalignant lesions at multiple sites, then a strong case could be made for recommending an increase in their intake as an approach to the prevention of cancer.

ACKNOWLEDGMENT

This work was supported in part by USPHS grant CA-27502. HSG is a recipient of an American Cancer Society Career Development Award.

REFERENCES

Albanes D, Virtamo J, Rautalahti M, Pikkarainen J, Taylor PR, Greenwald P, Heinonen OP. Pilot study: The U.S. Finland lung cancer prevention trial. J Nutr Growth Cancer 1986; 3:207–214.

Alberts DS, Coulthard SW, Meyskens FL. Regression of aggressive laryngeal papillomatosis with 13-cis-retinoic acid (Accutane). J Biol Response Mod 1986a; 5:124–128.

Alberts DS, Coulthard SW, Meyskens FL. Regression of bronchial epidermoid metaplasia in heavy smokers with etretinate. Cancer Detect Prev 1986b; 9:157–160.

Baden E. Tabac et cancers de la region oropharyngee et des broaches. Donees actuelles. Rev. Med. Julouse 1978; 14:549–560.

Bendich A. The safety of beta-carotene. Nutr Cancer 1988; 11:207–214.

Bertram JS, Peng A, Rundhang JE. Carotenoids have intrinsic cancer preventive action. FASEB J 1988; 2:A1413.

Bichler E. The role of aromatic retinoid in treatment of laryngeal keratinizing disorders and dysplasias. In: Proceedings of the 13th international congress of chemotherapy, Vienna: 201–229.

Bichler E, Daxenbichler G. Retinoic acid-binding protein in human squamous cell carcinomas of the ORL region. Cancer 1982; 49:619–621.

Bjelke E. Dietary vitamin A and human lung cancer (1975). Int J Cancer 1975; 15:561–565.

Burge-Bottenbley A, Shklar G. Retardation of experimental oral cancer development by retinyl acetate. Nutr Cancer 1983; 5:121–129.

Dunham LJ. A geographic study of a relationship between oral cancer and plants. Cancer Res 1968; 28:2369–2371.

Garewal HS, Meyskens FL, Killen D, Reeves D, Kiersh TA, Elletson H, Strosberg A, King D, Steinbronn K. Response of oral leukoplakia to beta-carotene. J Clin Oncol 1990: 8:1715–1720.

Goodman GE, Ommen GS. Seattle lung cancer chemoprevention trial. Proc Am Soc Clin Oncol 1990: 9 (abstract).

Gouveia J, Mathe G, Hercend T, Gros F, Lemaigre G, Santelli G, Homasson JP, Gaillard JP, Angebault M, Bonniot JP, Lededente A, Marsac T, Panot R, Preket S. Degree of bronchial metaplasia in heavy smokers and its regression after treatment with a retinoid. Lancet 1982; 1:710–712.

Greenwald P, Sondik E, Lynch BS. Diet and chemoprevention in NCI's research strategy to achieve national cancer control objectives. Ann Rev Public Health 1986; 7:267–291.

Harris CC, Silverman T, Smith JM, Jackson F, Boren HG. Proliferation of tracheal epithelial cells in normal and vitamin A deficient Syrian golden hamster. J Natl Cancer Inst 1973; 51:1059–1062.

Hicks RM. The scientific basis for regarding vitamin A and its analogs as anticarcinogenic agents. Proc Nutr Soc 1983; 42:83–93.

Hirajama T. Diet and cancer. Nutr Cancer 1979; 1:67–81.

Hong WK, Endicott J, Itri LM, Doos W, Batsakis JG, Bell R, Fofonoff S, Byers R, Atkinson EN, Vaughan C, Toth BB, Kramer A, Dimery IW, Skipper P, Strong S. 13-Cis retinoic acid in the treatment of oral leukoplakia. N Engl J Med 1986; 315:1501–1505.

Karp DD, Guralnik E, Guidice LA. Multiple primary cancers: A prevalent and increasing problem. Proc Am Soc Clin Oncol 1985; 4:13.

Koch HF. Biochemical treatment of precancerous oral lesions: The effectiveness of various analogues of retinoic acid. J Maxillofac Surg 1978; 6:59–63.

Koch HF. Effect of retinoids on precancerous lesions of oral mucosa. In Orfanos CE, Braun-Falco O, Farber EM, Grupper CL, Polano MK, Schuppli R (eds): Retinoids: Advances in basic research and therapy, Berlin: Springer-Verlag, 1981: 307–312.

Li J-Y, Taylor PR, Li G-Y, Blot WJ, Yu Y, Ezshow AG, Sun YH, Yang CS, Yang Q, Tangrea JA, Zheng SF, Greenwald P, Cahill J. Intervention studies in Linxian, China: An update. J Nutr Growth Cancer 1986; 3:192–206.

Mathe G, Gouveia J, Hercend T, et al. Correlation between precancerous bronchial metaplasia and cigarette consumption, the preliminary results of retinoid treatment. Cancer Detect Prev 1982; 5:461–466.

McGuirt WF, Mathews B, Kaufman JA. Multiple simultaneous tumors in patients with head and neck cancer. Cancer 1982; 50:1195–1199.

Misset JL, Mathe G, Santelli G, Gouveia J, Homasson JP, Sudre MC, Gaget H. Regression of bronchial epidermoid metaplasia in heavy smokers with etretinate. Cancer Detect Prev 1986; 9:157–160.

Muir CS, Kirk R. Betel, tobacco and cancer of the mouth. Br J Cancer 1960; 14:597–608.

Nettesheim P, Synder C, Kim JCS. Vitamin A and the susceptibility of respiratory tract tissues to carcinogenic insult. Environ Health Persp 1979; 29:89–93.

Nomura A, Yamakawa H, Ishidate T, Kamiyama S, Musvda H, Stemmermann GN, Heilburn LW, Hankin JH. Intestinal metaplasia in Japan: Association with diet. J Natl Cancer Inst 1982; 68:401–405.

Odukoyo O, Hawach F, Shklar G. Retardation of experimental oral cancer by topical vitamin E. Nutr Cancer 1984; 6:98–104.

Peto R, Doll R, Buckley JD, Sparr MB. Can dietary beta-carotene materially reduce human cancer rates? Nature 1981; 2910:201–208.

Saccomanno G, Archer VE, Auerbach O, Saunders RP, Brennan LM. Development of carcinoma of the lung as reflected in exfoliated cells. Cancer 1974; 33:256–270.

Saccomanno G, Moran PG, Schmidt RD, Hartshorn DF, Brian DA, Dreher WH, Sowada BJ. Effects of 13-cis retinoids on premalignant and malignant cells of lung origin. Acta Cytol 1982; 26:78–85.

Schwartz J, Suda D, Light G. Beta-carotene is associated with the regression of hamster buccal pouch carcinoma and induction of tumor necrosis factor in macrophages. Biochem Biophys Res Commun 1986; 136:1130–1135.

Shah JP, Strong EW, DeCosse JJ, Itri L, Sellers P. Effect of retinoids on oral leukoplakia. Am J Surg 1983; 146:466–470.

Shapshay S, Hong WK, Fried M, Sismums A, Vaughn CW, Strong S. Simultaneous carcinomas of the esophagus and upper aerodigestive tract. Otolaryngol Head Neck Surg 1980; 88:373–377.

Shklar G, Marefat P, Kornhauser A, Trickler DP, Wallace KD. Retinoid inhibition of lingual carcinogenesis. Oral Surg 1980a; 49:325–332.

Shklar G, Schwartz J, Grau D, Tuckler DP, Wallace KD. Inhibition of hamster buccal pouch carcinogenesis by 13-cis retinoic acid. Oral Surg 1980b; 50:45–52.

Shklar G. Oral mucosal in hamsters: Inhibition by vitamin E. J Natl Cancer Inst 1982; 68:791–797.

Silverberg E, Lubera J. Cancer Statistics. Ca 1988; 38:5–22.

Slaughter DP, Southwick HW, Smejkal W. Field cancerization in oral stratified squamous epithelium, clinical implications of multicentric origin. Cancer 1983; 5:963–968.

Som S, Chatterjee M, Bannerjee MR. Beta-carotene inhibition of 7,12-dimethylbenz(a)anthracene-induced transformation of murine mammary cells in vitro. Carcinogenesis 1984; 5:937–940.

Stich HF, Dunn BP. Relationship between cellular levels of beta-carotenes and sensitivity to genotoxic agents. Int J Cancer 1986; 38:713–717.

Stich HF, Hornby AP, Mathew B, Sankaranarayanan R, Nair MK. Response of oral leukoplakias to the administration of vitamin A. Cancer Lett 1988a; 40:93–101.

Stich HF, Rosin MP, Hornby AP, Mathew B, Sankaranarayanan R, Nair MN. Remission of oral leukoplakias and micronuclei in tobacco/betel quid chewers treated with beta-carotene plus vitamin A. Int J Cancer 1988b; 42:195–199.

U.S. Department of Health and Human Services. The health consequences of smoking and cancer: A report of the Surgeon General, 1982, 82–5017.

U.S. Department of State. U.S. national report on aging for the United Nations World Assembly on Aging, 1982, 12–17.

Winn DM, Ziegler RG, Pickle LW, Gudley G, Blott WJ, Hoover RN. Diet in the etiology of oral and pharyngeal cancer among women from the southern U.S. Cancer Res 1984; 44:1216–1222.

7

Epidemiological Studies of Vitamin E and Cancer Risk

Paul Knekt

Social Insurance Institution
Helsinki, Finland

INTRODUCTION

Cancer is a major public health problem. There is evidence that about 80–90% of all incident cancers are determined by potentially controllable external factors (Doll and Peto, 1981). It has been postulated that dietary factors may account for about one-third of all deaths from cancer. However, there is still a lack of definitive evidence about which dietary characteristics most influence cancer risk. From the public health point of view, it would be of special significance to identify preventive agents in the diet. Accumulating evidence suggests that vitamin E is a nutrient which may reduce the incidence of various cancers.

It has been suggested that vitamin E has anticancer effects as a lipid antioxidant and free radical scavenger (Tappel, 1980; Ames, 1983). Vitamin E may trap chain reactions started by oxygen radicals of endogenous or exogenous origin (e.g., produced as byproducts of normal metabolism or after infections, or caused by nitroso compounds or by radiation), thus protecting cells from lipid peroxidation (Ames, 1983). According to the antioxidant hypothesis, vitamin E may also trap secondarily propagated radicals from the chain reaction of polyunsaturated fatty acids peroxidation and exogenous radicals caused by environmental agents, e.g., carcinogens, mutagens and drugs (Gey, 1986). Selenium has antioxidant properties through its role as an integral component in the enzyme glutathione peroxidase and through other mechanisms (Helzlsouer, 1983). It has been suggested that vitamin E may interact with selenium because vitamin E may reduce the oxidative damage seen in selenium deficiency (Hoekstra, 1975; Combs and Scott, 1977; Diplock, 1978).

The effect of vitamin E on carcinogenesis has been investigated in a number of animal experiments. They, as well as in vitro studies, have shown that vitamin E can block the formation of carcinogenic nitrosamines (Mergens, 1982; Chen et al., 1988). The mechanisms by which vitamin E opposes other carcinogens are not clearly understood. It has been demonstrated that vitamin E inhibits other chemical carcinogenesis as well as the growth of transplanted and spontaneous tumor cells (Birt, 1986; Mirvish, 1986; Shamberger, 1986; Chen et al., 1988; Knekt, 1988a). However, different studies have yielded somewhat conflicting results. Most of the studies have concentrated on mammary gland, colon, oral, and skin carcinogenesis. In animal models, vitamin E has been shown to inhibit oral carcinogenesis and to inhibit or have no effect on mammary gland carcinogenesis. Vitamin E has also been reported to inhibit or to enhance skin carcinogenesis and to inhibit, to have no effect on, or to enhance colon carcinogenesis. Single studies have reported an inhibitory effect on vitamin E on ear duct and forestomach carcinogenesis but no effect on urinary bladder and contradictory results on liver carcinogenesis (Birt, 1986; Chen et al., 1988; Knekt, 1988a). The effect of vitamin E has been reported to depend on the level of dietary selenium and fat. It may also depend on other factors such as the amount of vitamin E administered, method of administration, carcinogen used, dosage of the carcinogen, route of administration, and species of animals used.

Although some part of the animal studies support the hypothesis that vitamin E has an anticancer effect, these findings cannot be directly applied to human cancer. The purpose of this chapter is to present some of the evidence regarding the effect of vitamin E on human cancer.

BACKGROUND

Vitamin E is the group name for eight fat-soluble naturally occurring chemical formations, four tocopherols and four tocotrienols, together with synthetic compounds having varying degrees of biological activity. The most active of these compounds is alpha-tocopherol (Tomassi and Silano, 1986). Alpha-tocopherol and vitamin E are used as synonyms in this chapter. Vitamin E is naturally present in plant lipids and there is apparently a strong proportionality between tocopherol and the linoleic acid content of most fats and oils (Hove and Harris, 1951). The primary sources of vitamin E are vegetable oils, especially sunflower, cottonseed, and safflower (Bakemeier, 1988). Vitamin E is also found in a wide variety of foods. In the average diet its main sources are vegetable oils and margarine, cereals, and vegetables (Food and Nutrition Board, 1980; Piironen, 1986; Bakemeier, 1988).

Recently recommended dietary allowances (RDA) of vitamin E are 10 mg alpha-tocopherol equivalents (15 IU) in adult males, and 8 mg alpha-tocopherol equivalents (12 IU) in adult females per day (Food and Nutrition Board, 1980). This is likely to be met by the tocopherols occurring naturally in well-balanced diets of 1500–3000 kcal. Thus, nutritional deficiency of the vitamin is rare in the developed world. Estimates of the daily average intake of naturally occurring alpha-tocopherols in the American diet range, for example, from 5 to 20 mg (Tomassi and Silano, 1986). According to the antioxidant hypothesis, high polyunsaturated fatty acid intake or selenium deficiency might increase the requirement of vitamin E. Vitamin E is the least toxic of the fat-soluble vitamins, and doses of up to 1200 IU/day have been used without causing any apparent harm (Farrell and Bieri, 1975; Council on Scientific Affairs, 1987; Bendich and Machlin, 1988). Thus it has been suggested that the minimum daily intake of vitamin E should be higher than the present RDA (Gey et al., 1987). The intake should, however, be related to the empirical evidence of a possible protective effect against cancer.

Most epidemiological studies on the relationship between vitamin E and human cancer were made during the last decade. Four different study designs have been used: ecological studies; cross-sectional (case control) studies; longitudinal (cohort) studies; and clinical trials. Only a few ecological studies have been carried out so far. The majority of the studies at the individual level are cross-sectional or longitudinal, thus presenting indirect evidence of a possible protective effect of vitamin E intake against cancer occurrence. These studies have been based on the dietary intake or blood level of vitamin E. The longitudinal studies have been of the nested case control type. Clinical intervention trials, providing more definitive answers to the question of whether supplementary vitamin E will reduce cancer risk, have been started but the results will not be available for several years.

ECOLOGICAL STUDIES

The diet of populations with a high incidence of stomach cancer may have low levels of vitamin E and other micronutrients (Weisburger et al., 1980). Deficiency in vitamin E intake was accentuated in areas with high risk of gastric cancer in Colombia (Correa et al., 1983), but intercountry comparisons linking per capita intake of vitamin E to gastric cancer mortality demonstrate a relatively weak association (Howson et al., 1986). In one study, lower serum vitamin E levels were found in an area in northern China where the risk of esophageal cancer is higher than that reported for normal U.S. adults (Yang et al., 1984). Another study showed a progressive decline in serum vitamin E levels in populations living in areas of increasing risk of esophageal cancer (van Helden et al., 1987). Thus, several ecological studies have reported an inverse association between vitamin E intake and the risk of different cancers of the gastrointestinal tract.

Although the results are suggestive, the fact that adjustments for the intake of other micronutrients and other confounding factors have not been made in these studies limit the possibilities of drawing reliable conclusions about relationships between vitamin E intake and cancer occurrence.

DIETARY STUDIES

In most cohort and case control studies on diet and cancer, consumption of vegetables has been found to be inversely related to the risk of several different cancers (e.g., cancers of the lung, stomach, and colon) (Peto et al., 1981; Hennekens, 1986; Surgeon General, 1988). It has generally been postulated that these associations are mainly due to carotenoids. However, another explanation for these findings may be that the vitamin E found in many vegetables inhibits the development of cancer. With respect to establishing the role of vitamin E, a major problem in interpreting the results of these studies is that the studies have apparently not distinguished between the possible effects of vitamin E and other factors. The evidence that the association between intake of vegetables and cancer risk is due to their vitamin E content is thus weak.

The few cross-sectional studies focusing on the association between calculated intake of vitamin E and the risk of cancer generally do not reveal a protective effect of vitamin E. In a case control study based on 246 stomach cancer cases and an equal number of matched population controls, there was no difference between cases and controls in the average daily consumption of vitamin E or alpha-tocopherol calculated from quantitative diet history questionnaire data (Risch et al., 1985). The intake of some vegetables was, however, inversely associated with the risk of stomach cancer, suggesting that some other correlate of vegetable intake is the protective factor. Graham et al. (1988) found no association between the level of ingestion of vitamin E and the risk of colon cancer in a study regarding the current diet of 428 colon cancer cases and 428 matched controls. Byers et al. (1987) compared the vitamin E intake of 450 lung cancer patients and 902 controls in a population-based case control study. The intake of vitamin E was estimated by detailed interviews using a modified food frequency method. A nonsignificant inverse gradient between the intake of vitamin E and the risk of lung cancer was observed among men. For women there was no association. In a small study of nine lung cancer cases and nine matched controls it was assessed with a 28-day dietary history interview (Lopez-S and LeGardeur, 1982) that the intake of vitamin E 1 year prior to diagnosis was possibly inversely associated with the incidence of lung cancer. On the basis of a semiquantitative frequency questionnaire, Stryker et al. (1988) reported lower vitamin E intake among 204 malignant melanoma cases than among 248 controls. Use of supplements and consumption of several food sources of vitamin E, however, were not associated with a reduced risk of melanoma. A study of 290 breast cancer cases and 307 hospital-based controls did not reveal any differences between the vitamin E intake of cases and controls based on semiquantitative dietary history interviews (Gerber et al., 1988). In another study (Toniolo et al., 1989), no significant difference in usual vitamin E intake estimated on the basis of a dietary history questionnaire was observed between 250 breast cancer cases and 499 controls chosen as a stratified random sample from the general population.

The result of case control studies may be biased because knowledge of cancer may lead cancer patients to describe their past diet somewhat differently from the way they would have done had they been healthy controls. This drawback is, however, not present in longitudinal studies. A longitudinal nested case control study of 29 thyroid cancer cases and 87 matched controls did not disclose any difference in the present regular vitamin E intake between the two groups (Glattre et al., 1989).

There are some limitations in the use of the dietary vitamin E data which have to be considered when interpreting the lack of association between vitamin E intake and cancer risk: (1) Vitamin E is present in a variety of commonly consumed foods, and it is thus difficult to identify population groups with substantially different levels of intake. It is also possible that the general adequacy of human diets in vitamin E precludes a study of any association between a deficiency state and cancer risk. (2) There are some factors that may cause random variations in estimates of vitamin E intake, thus masking any true association with cancer risk. It is difficult to quantify the consumption of some of the main sources of vitamin E (e.g., vegetable oils). The estimates of individual dietary intake of vitamin E obtained using food history recall are not necessarily a valid representation of the intake prior to the onset of cancer. (3) Studies have used food rather than pure vitamins. Exact identification of vitamin E has been difficult because of the lack of adequate food consumption tables for that micronutrient. (4) Different tissues may vary in their vitamin E requirement; thus the rate of cancer occurrence may differ due to vitamin E status.

SERUM STUDIES

Cross-Sectional (Case Control) Studies

All the vitamin E present in the human body derives from the diet. There is no single storage organ for vitamin E, but the liver, adipose tissue, and muscle contain most of the body's tocopherol (Bieri et al., 1983). Although only a small amount of the total body tocopherol is found in the blood, serum vitamin E levels are directly related to dietary and supplemental intake of the vitamin (Davies et al., 1969; Willett et al., 1983b,c; Knekt et al., 1988c). It has been suggested that serum vitamin E levels tend to reflect intake of the nutrient over a longer period (Machlin, 1980). The serum tocopherol level can thus be used as a proxy

Table 1 Summary of Case Control Studies of the Relationship Between Serum/Plasma
Vitamin E/Alpha-Tocopherol Level of Cancer Risk

Ref.	Site of cancer	No. of cases	Direction of association		
			Inverse	No	Positive
Atukorala et al. (1979)	Lung	26		X	
Lopez-S et al. (1982)	Lung	29	X		
Miyamoto et al. (1987)	Lung	37	X		
Krishnamurthy et al. (1986)	Oral	30	X		
Stryker et al. (1988)	Melanoma	204	X		
Rougereau et al. (1987)	GI, lower	190	X		
	GI, other	570	X		
	Hormonal	197			X
	Lung	71	X		
	Nervous system	40	X		
Hayes et al. (1988)	Prostate	134	X		
Gerber et al. (1988)	Breast	314			X
Heinonen et al. (1987)	Gynecological	88		X	
Heinonen et al. (1985)	Ovary	11			X
Romppanen et al. (1985)	Vulva	6		X	

measure of vitamin E intake in studies relating nutritional vitamin E intake to cancer incidence.

The results of the few cross-sectional studies on the association between the blood vitamin E level and different cancers are somewhat contradictory, showing both inverse association, no association, and positive association (Table 1). Atukorala et al. (1979) found no differences in serum vitamin E levels between newly diagnosed lung cancer patients and patients of similar age with nonmalignant diseases. Lopez-S and LeGardeur (1982) reported significantly lower serum vitamin E levels among persons with primary lung carcinoma than among matched hospitalized controls, and Miyamoto et al. (1987) found significantly lower serum vitamin E levels in lung cancer patients than in controls. In the same study, healthy family members of lung cancer patients also had lower vitamin E levels than controls, although they had higher levels than the cancer cases, suggesting that familial factors, dietary or metabolic, may influence serum vitamin E levels. In a comparative study of serum alpha-tocopherol from 30 oral cancer cases and 30 age-matched healthy controls, alpha-tocopherol levels were observed to be lower among cancer patients than among controls (Krishnamurthy and Jaya, 1986). Stryker et al. (1988) found nonsignificantly lower plasma alpha-tocopherol levels among 204 patients with malignant melanoma than among 248 controls. In a study of 1068 cancer patients and 880 healthy controls, Rougereau et al. (1987) noted a significantly lower blood vitamin E level among several cancer sites (e.g., gastrointestinal, lung, and nervous system) than among controls. The only exception was the combined group of hormone-related cancers (i.e., prostate, breast, uterus, and ovary), which presented a nonsignificant positive association. Gerber et al. (1988) found significantly higher mean plasma vitamin E levels in breast cancer cases than in controls after adjustment for the levels of triglycerides and cholesterol in a hospital-based study based on 319 cases and 344 controls. Despite the higher plasma level among cancer cases there was no difference in vitamin E intake between cases and controls. This finding suggests that the high plasma vitamin E level may be a consequence and not a cause of tumor development. Ninety-four patients with prostate cancer had significantly lower concentrations of serum alpha-tocopherol than hospital controls (Hayes et al., 1988). No differences in serum levels of vitamin E were observed between 88 gynecological cancer cases combined (i.e., vulvar, cervical, endometrial, and ovarian carcinogenesis) and 31 healthy controls (Heinonen et al., 1987). Two Finnish studies based on small numbers of subjects found no differences between patients with cancers of the female reproductive organs (i.e., vulvar and ovarian) and patients without carcinoma (Heinonen et al, 1985; Romppanen et al., 1985).

The cross-sectional studies have presented an inverse association with respect to some sites of cancer (e.g., cancers of the lung, oral cavity, gastrointestinal tract, nervous system, and skin) but not all (e.g., cancer of female reproductive organs). The results of these studies should, however, be interpreted with caution, partly because it is impossible to know whether the low level of serum vitamin E preceded the cancer or vice versa, and partly because of uncontrolled confounding factors.

Longitudinal (Cohort) Studies

Basic Associations

The association between the serum vitamin E level and the subsequent cancer risk has been examined in 14 longitudinal studies, all of the nested case control type within the main study. In 13 of the studies, vitamin E determinations were based on stored frozen serum or plasma samples collected at the baseline examination and thawed for analysis at the end of follow-up. Only one study used fresh plasma samples analyzed at the baseline (Stähelin et al., 1984). The study population, number of cases and controls, number of years of follow-up, site of cancer, matching variables, mean level of vitamin E among controls, and mean case control difference in the vitamin E levels of the different studies are presented in Table 2. The number of cancer cases in the studies varied from 25 to 453.

Eleven of the studies reported lower serum vitamin E levels in subjects who developed cancer than in controls (Table 2). Most of the studies were based on

Table 2 Summary[a] of Longitudinal Studies of Relationship Between Plasma/Serum Vitamin E/Alpha-Tocopherol Levels and Cancer Risk

Study (ref.)	Study subjects			Sex	Age at entry (years)	No. of years of follow-up	Site of cancer	Matching variables	Storage temperature (°C)	Control mean vitamin E (mg/liter)	Mean case-control difference (mg/liter)	Stated statistical significance
	Population at risk	No. of cases	No. of controls									
Basel study, Stähelin et al. (1984)	4,224	115	308	Male	26–71	7–9	All, 3 sites	Age, sex	Fresh	16.2	−0.9	ns
Guernsey study, Wald et al. (1984)	5,004	39	78	Female	28–75	7–14	Breast	Age, gynecological variables, breast disease	−20	6.0	−1.3	$p < 0.025$
Hypertension Detection and Follow-up Program, Willett et al. (1984)	4,480	111	210	Both	30–69	5	All, 5 sites	Age, sex, race, time of blood collection	−70	12.6	−1.0	ns
Honolulu Heart Program, Nomura et al. (1985)	6,860	284	302	Male	52–71	10	5 sites	Randomly selected controls	−75	12.3	0.0	ns
Eastern Finland Heart Survey, Salonen et al. (1985)	12,155	51	51	Both	30–64	4	All, 2 sites	Age, sex, smoking	−20	5.0	−0.1	ns
Washington County Study, Menkes et al. (1986)	25,802	99	196	Both	25–64	8	Lung	Age, sex, race, smoking, time of blood collection	−73	11.9	−1.4	$p < 0.001$

Study												
Washington County Study, Schober et al. (1987)	25,802	72	143	Both	25–64	9	Colon	Age, sex, race, smoking, time of blood collection	−73	12.7	−1.0	$p = 0.10$
Zoetermeer study, Kok et al. (1987)	10,532	69	138	Both	5–99	6–9	All, lung	Age, sex, smoking	−20	8.5	−1.3	$p < 0.005$
London study, Wald et al. (1987)	22,000	271	533	Male	35–64	2–9	All, 6 sites	Age, smoking, duration of storage of the serum sample	−40	10.3	−0.2	ns
Malmö study, Fex et al. (1987)	10,000	25	50	Male	46–48	3–8	All	Restricted sex, age, population group	−20	3.0	−0.3	ns
Social Insurance Institution Study, Knekt (1988b)	15,093	313	578	Female	15–99	7–10	All, 4 sites	Age, sex, time of blood collection	−20	10.4	−0.4	$p < 0.05$
Social Insurance Institution Study, Knekt et al. (1988a)	21,172	453	841	Male	15–99	7–10	All, 9 sites	Age, sex, time of blood collection	−20	8.3	−0.3	$p < 0.05$
Guernsey study, Russell et al. (1988)	5,086	30	288	Female	26–88	8	Breast	Age, menopausal status, time of blood collection	−20	6.2	+0.3	ns
Washington County Study, Burney et al. (1989)	25,620	22	44	Both	40–89	12	Pancreas	Age, sex, race, hours since last meal	−70	11.8	+1.1	ns

[a] Update of Table 2 in Knekt (1988a).

relatively small numbers of cases, and only five of them reported statistically significant differences between cases and controls in the total sample (Wald et al., 1984; Menkes et al., 1986; Kok et al., 1987; Knekt, 1988b; Knekt et al., 1988a). In one study a significant difference was observed in a subpopulation of nonsmoking men in eastern Finland (Salonen et al., 1985); in another study in a population of healthy employees studied as a cohort study including all subjects rather than matched controls (Gey et al., 1987); and in one study only during the first year of follow-up (Wald et al., 1987). Overall, the studies show 3% lower mean vitamin E levels among cases than among controls, which was a significant difference.

A gradient, suggesting an increased cancer risk associated with a decreasing serum level of vitamin E, was reported (Wald et al., 1984; Menkes et al., 1986; Kok et al., 1987; Knekt et al., 1988a). However, most pronounced in some studies was an elevated cancer risk at the lowest levels of serum vitamin E (Wald et al., 1984; Knekt 1988b).

Effect Modification

Although the results of longitudinal studies on the association between serum vitamin E and cancer are somewhat conflicting, it is possible that vitamin E does provide protection against cancer. This may be concealed in population studies: exposure to factors inducing cancer may vary in different populations and living conditions. There may, for example, be differences in the diet (e.g., consumption of saturated and unsaturated fats and nitrates), alcohol consumption, reproductive behavior, and smoking habits. In addition, vitamin E may provide protection only against some specific exposures inducing cancer, and thus only under certain circumstances. So far the associations between serum vitamin E and cancer risk in different subgroups of populations have been studied rarely, probably because rather few cancer cases are available in the majority of those studies.

In one study, the association between the vitamin E level and cancer risk was studied within categories of body mass index and serum cholesterol (Knekt, 1988a). There was a significant association with respect to all sites of cancer among subjects of normal weight, but not among obese persons. Overnutrition resulting in obesity may thus override the possible protective effect of vitamin E. It has been suggested that diets high in polyunsaturated fat lower serum cholesterol levels (Grundy, 1979). It is also known that alpha-tocopherol is an antioxidant stabilizing unsaturated lipids against autooxidation (Bieri et al., 1983). These suggestions are in agreement with the findings among women (Knekt, 1988b) that vitamin E provides protection against cancer at low levels of serum cholesterol. No interaction between serum vitamins A and E has been reported (Schober et al., 1987; Knekt et al., 1988a).

The results concerning the proposed biochemical interaction (Hoekstra, 1975; Tappel, 1980) between selenium and vitamin E in the protection against peroxidative cell damage are contradictory. In one study (Salonen et al., 1985), subjects with both low serum selenium and low serum alpha-tocopherol levels had a significantly elevated risk of all cancers combined, and in two other studies a nonsignificantly elevated risk (Willett et al., 1983a; Knekt et al., 1988a). However, the inverse association between serum alpha-tocopherol and cancers unrelated to smoking seemed to be strongest among men with a low level of serum selenium (Knekt, 1988a). There was also a strong inverse association between serum alpha-tocopherol and the incidence of hormone-related cancers combined, and especially for breast cancer among women with low levels of serum selenium (Knekt, 1988b). On the other hand, a study on colon cancer (Schober et al., 1987), a study on pancreatic cancer (Burney et al., 1989), and a study on five individual cancers (the bladder, colon, lung, rectum, and stomach) and all these five cancers combined (Nomura et al., 1985) found no such interaction. In one study, persons with both high selenium levels and vitamin E in the lowest tertile appeared to have an increased risk of lung cancer (Menkes et al., 1986).

In some studies (Salonen et al., 1985; Wald et al., 1987; Knekt et al., 1988a), the inverse association between serum vitamin E and all sites of cancer was mainly concentrated among nonsmoking men. Reliable studies of this effect among women have not been made because of the small number of smokers. The major part of cancer in nonsmokers is necessarily caused by factors other than tobacco smoke. Thus, the possible protective effects of vitamin E may mainly be related to some of these other carcinogens, and possibly to small amounts of carcinogens derived from tobacco smoke by passive smoking (Repace, 1984). These findings may also be due to differences in nutrient intake between smokers and nonsmokers. Because of social class differences and possibly because of health behavior clustering, nonsmoking men may, for example, consume a diet richer in polyunsaturated fatty acids and thus the vitamin E/cancer mechanism functions more specifically.

Site-Specific Cancers

The effect of vitamin E may differ with regard to cancers of different anatomical sites since the risk factors may differ. Several investigators have examined the relationship between serum vitamin E level and cancers of specific sites. However, with a few exceptions, the number of cancer cases has been small. Lung cancer has been examined in eight studies, and the number of cases in the different studies varies from 15 to 144. Smoking is the dominant risk factor for lung cancer and, accordingly, no significant association with vitamin E status was generally observed. Stähelin et al. (1984), Kok et al. (1987), Wald et al. (1987), and Knekt et al. (1988a) found nonsignificantly lower mean vitamin E levels among cases. Likewise, Salonen et al. (1985) found no substantial difference between cases and controls. Willett et al. (1984) and Nomura et al. (1985) reported nonsignificantly higher vitamin E levels among lung cancer cases than among controls. The hypothesis that large amounts of some substance in tobacco smoke may inhibit the effect of vitamin E was supported by the finding of the study by Knekt et al. (1988a) that an inverse association exists among nonsmokers but not among smokers between serum vitamin E and cancers which are regarded as smoking-related. On the other hand, Menkes et al. (1986) demonstrated a protective effect of vitamin E against lung cancer. It is thus possible that the interaction between smoking and serum alpha-tocopherol may also vary between different populations.

Several studies have reported the association between serum vitamin E level and subsequent cancer occurrence of different organs of the gastrointestinal tract; the number of cancer cases varies for different sites of gastrointestinal cancers from 11 to 81 (Table 3). With one exception for colorectal cancer among men (Knekt et al., 1988a), all studies performed on cancers of the colon, rectum, or colon and rectum combined (Stähelin et al., 1984; Nomura et al., 1985; Schober et al., 1987; Wald et al., 1987; Knekt et al., 1988b) reported a nonsignificantly lower mean level of serum vitamin E among cases than among controls. In studies based on a limited number of gastrointestinal cancers combined, Willett et al. (1984) found a nonsignificant inverse association, and Salonen et al. (1985)

Table 3 Summary[a] of Longitudinal Studies of Relationship Between Plasma/Serum Vitamin E/Alpha-Tocopherol Levels and Risk of Gastrointestinal Cancers

Ref.	Site of cancer	No. of cases	Mean case control difference (%)
Stähelin et al. (1984)	Stomach	19	0
	Colorectal	14	-13
Willett et al. (1984)	Gastrointestinal	11	-12
Salonen et al. (1985)	Gastrointestinal	18	?
Nomura et al. (1985)	Stomach	70	-1
	Colon	81	-1
	Rectum	32	-6
Wald et al. (1987)	Stomach	13	$+5$
	Colorectal	30	-4
Schober et al. (1987)	Colon	72	-8
Knekt et al. (1988a)	Stomach	48	-7
	Colorectal	21	$+9$
Knekt et al. (1988b)	Upper gastrointestinal tract	35	-6
	Colorectal	37	-9

[a] Update of Table 3 in Knekt (1988a).

reported no association. The results on stomach cancer are contradictory. Nomura et al. (1985) and Knekt et al. (1988a,b) found a nonsignificant inverse association, and Wald et al. (1987) reported a nonsignificant positive association. Stähelin et al. (1984) found no association in one study population using a nested case control design and Gey et al. (1987) reported a significant inverse association in the same study population using a cohort design.

Thus several of the studies on serum alpha-tocopherol and the risk of gastrointestinal cancers are consistent with the hypothesis of the protective effect of vitamin E against those cancers. This effect may be due to the fact that intake of vitamin E may inhibit the formation of nitrosamines and also provide protection against tissue damage resulting from intake of polyunsaturated fats, both of which have been suggested as etiological agents for gastrointestinal cancer (Risch et al., 1985). The discrepancy in the results is possibly due to the fact that other risk factors (e.g., saturated fats and alcohol) (Committee on Diet, Nutrition, and Cancer, 1982) may confound the association.

Five studies have reported on hormone-related cancers, i.e., cancers of the breast, endometrium, or ovary among women and cancer of the prostate among men (Wald et al., 1984; Willett et al., 1984; Knekt, 1988b; Knekt et al., 1988a; Russell et al., 1988). The number of cancer cases varied between 11 and 67 for different sites. Alpha-tocopherol levels were not notably associated with incidence of these cancers, suggesting that hormonal exposure in some instances overrides the possible protective effect of vitamin E. A significant inverse association has been reported between serum vitamin E and breast cancer in a prospective study (Wald et al., 1984), but another study based on the same population has failed to confirm the finding (Russell et al., 1988). An elevated risk of breast cancer and hormone-related cancers was reported among persons with a low serum selenium level (Knekt, 1988b). A nonsignificant inverse association was observed (Knekt, 1988b) with respect to cancer of the cervix uteri, which is not hormonally related but is chiefly related to the number of sexual partners (Doll and Peto, 1981).

An inverse association between serum alpha-tocopherol and the risk of cancer of the pancreas was reported among men in one study (Knekt et al., 1988a) and a strongly protective effect of low vitamin E level in another (Burney et al., 1989). Two studies reported a nonsignificant positive (Nomura et al., 1985; Wald et al., 1987) and one study an inverse (Knekt et al., 1988a) association with respect to bladder cancer. No significant associations were reported with respect to leukemias and lymphomas (Willett et al., 1984; Knekt, 1988a) and the nervous system (Wald et al., 1987; Knekt, 1988a). A nonsignificant inverse association with basal cell carcinoma (Knekt et al., 1988a) and with skin cancer (Wald et al., 1987) was reported. Because almost all these studies are based on small numbers of cases, no definite conclusions can be drawn for these sites. The main evidence available of a possible association between vitamin E and cancer risk among humans comes from the epidemiological longitudinal studies based on serum vitamin levels. Straightforward conclusions of a possible protective effect of vitamin E cannot, however, be drawn from these studies. Several alternative hypotheses may explain the associations observed. These hypotheses are discussed as follows.

Confounding Factors

The association between the serum vitamin E level and cancer risk may be a direct effect of dietary or serum vitamin E or it may be due to confounding by other factors associated with vitamin E. The possible confounding by sex, age, and time of blood collection were used as matching variables in several studies (Table 2). Generally, adjustment for smoking and other potential confounding factors resulted in only minor changes in the associations (Menkes et al., 1986; Kok et al., 1987; Knekt, 1988b; Knekt et al., 1988a). Despite the control of several confounding factors in the different studies, the possibility remains that the observed associations between alpha-tocopherol and cancer risk are not causal, but due to some other correlates of serum alpha-tocopherol or vitamin E intake.

It is also possible that people whose diets are rich in vitamins may have more healthy habits than other people. The intake of vitamin E may also coincide with the intake of some other substances that are responsible for the observed protective effect. For example, consumption of vegetables is known to be inversely associated with the risk of several cancers (Howson et al., 1986; Surgeon General, 1988) and, besides vitamin E, vegetables contain several other micronutrients and nonnutritional compounds which may inhibit carcinogenesis. The confounding caused by simultaneous intake of other micronutrients or other possible anticarcinogens has not generally been taken into account in studies on serum alpha-tocopherol and cancer. The only exception is the study by Stähelin et al. (1984), which reported the association with citrus fruit intake (vitamin C). Possible adjustment would not have altered the results of that study.

The association between serum retinol, beta-carotene, and selenium and the risk of subsequent cancer has been investigated in several longitudinal studies (Knekt, 1988a). The results support the hypothesis of an inverse association between these micronutrients and the occurrence of cancer. It is also well known that the serum level of alpha-tocopherol is positively associated with serum levels of beta-carotene and selenium (Willett et al., 1983c; Russell-Briefel et al., 1985; Knekt et al., 1988c). It is thus possible that the alpha-tocopherol/cancer association may be secondary to the association between serum beta-carotene or selenium and cancer. However, in several studies the adjustments for serum beta-carotene, retinol, and selenium have not materially altered the association between alpha-tocopherol and cancer (Kok et al., 1987; Menkes et al., 1986; Schober et al., 1987; Knekt, 1988b; Knekt et al., 1988a), thus suggesting an independent association between the serum alpha-tocopherol level and cancer risk.

Serum cholesterol is a potential confounder of the association between serum vitamin E and the risk of cancer. Vitamin E is transported in the lipoproteins (Davies et al., 1969; Takahashi et al., 1977) and it is thus highly correlated with serum cholesterol (Davies et al., 1969; Willett et al., 1984; Menkes et al., 1986; Knekt et al., 1988a). Several studies report an inverse association between serum cholesterol level and the risk of cancer (Sidney and Farquhar, 1983; McMichael et al., 1984). One of the many possible explanations is that a low level of serum cholesterol is a cause of cancer and that the serum vitamin E/cancer association is secondary to the serum cholesterol/cancer association. There is still a great deal of doubt surrounding this contention. In several of the studies on the association between serum vitamin E and the occurrence of cancer, adjustment has been made for serum cholesterol level. Willett et al. (1984) and Wald et al. (1987) reported that adjustment for lipid values reduced the difference. Adjustment for serum cholesterol did not alter the association in other studies (Nomura et al., 1985; Schober et al., 1987; Knekt, 1988b; Knekt et al., 1988a). One study reported a significant independent association for both the serum cholesterol and the serum alpha-tocopherol level (Knekt, 1988a). Another study did not adjust for serum lipid values (Wald et al., 1984) and in yet another (Menkes et al., 1986) it is unclear whether the results were adjusted for serum lipids. In summary, it is possible that the vitamin E/cancer association is not fully secondary to the serum cholesterol/cancer association.

Preclinical Disease

Although measurements of vitamin E in prediagnostic serum in the longitudinal studies reduce the likelihood that vitamin E levels in cases are affected by cancer, it is still possible that a depressed level of serum vitamin E is a consequence of preclinical cancer at the baseline study when the blood samples were collected. The inverse association between serum vitamin E level and the risk of cancer has been reported as being restricted to the first year of follow-up, indicating that the association may be due to preclinical cancer (Wald et al., 1987). However, other evidence suggests that preclinical cancer is probably not the only explanation for the inverse association; inverse associations have also been found after exclusion of the cancer cases occurring during the first years of follow-up (Wald et al., 1984; Kok et al., 1987; Knekt et al., 1988a). No trends with time have been detected when the serum vitamin E levels of cases and of matched controls have been compared for different time periods (Menkes et al., 1986; Schober et al., 1987). Exclusion of persons at the lower end of the scale of several variables (e.g., hematocrit, body mass index, and cholesterol) did not notably alter the associations (Knekt et al., 1988a). Thus, the inverse association between vitamin E level and cancer occurrence cannot be fully explained by preclinical cancer.

Validity Aspects

Several factors may impair the usefulness of single stored serum vitamin E as a measure of vitamin E intake. There is evidence that the level of serum alpha-tocopherol, and thus the intake of vitamin E, is influenced by changing living conditions, e.g., sociodemographic factors such as region, occupation, social class, and marital status, and on factors related to health behavior such as smoking, supplementation, and obesity (Russell-Briefel et al., 1985; Comstock et al., 1988; Knekt et al., 1988c). Thus, a single sample for each person may not be sufficient to reflect serum levels or dietary intake of vitamin E over a lengthy period of time (Tangney et al., 1987), and the possible associations observed between serum vitamin E and cancer occurrence may be concealed (Freudenheim and Marshall, 1988). On the other hand, the results of one study (Knekt, 1988a), showing a relatively high intraindividual repeatability over a period of several years, suggest that the level of alpha-tocopherol in the serum changes slowly and that consequently a single measurement should give a useful gauge of the general levels in serum and, perhaps, also of the general vitamin E intake.

The serum level of vitamin E may change without any changes taking place in the dietary intake of vitamin E (Urbach et al., 1952). Changes in the intake of fats and cholesterol and other circumstances influencing the level of serum lipoproteins also alter the serum vitamin E level (Horwitt et al., 1972). Another potential confounding factor when serum vitamin E is used as a measure of long-term dietary intake of vitamin E is the occasional use of vitamin E supplements (Davies et al., 1969; Willett et al., 1983c; Comstock et al., 1988).

The association between the serum vitamin E level and cancer risk may be affected by random or systematic variations in the serum vitamin E determinations. The reported repeatability of the measurements within individual days and from day to day reported has, however, been rather good (Willett et al., 1984; Salonen et al., 1985; Menkes et al., 1986; Knekt, 1988a). Any random errors in the serum vitamin E levels may weaken the observed vitamin E–cancer relationship. Because the serum samples of each cancer case and its matched controls were handled similarly and analyzed in random order in several studies (Willett et al., 1984; Menkes et al., 1986; Schober et al., 1987; Knekt, 1988b; Knekt et al., 1988a; Burney et al., 1989), any effects of systematic variation in the laboratory analyses will not have affected the case control comparisons within the sets.

Little is known about the effects of blood sample storage conditions on alpha-tocopherol levels. It has been suggested that storage at about $-70°C$ degrades the alpha-tocopherol levels only slightly (Willett et al., 1984; Nomura et al., 1985; Menkes et al., 1986). Some degradation has occurred when samples have been stored at $-20°C$ (Wald et al., 1984; Salonen et al., 1985), an effect that increases with time (Wald et al., 1984, 1987).

Three of the studies based on serum samples stored at $-20°C$ have reported a significant inverse association between serum vitamin E level and cancer risk (Wald et al., 1984; Knekt, 1988b; Knekt et al., 1988a). This finding may be artefactual in the event that vitamin E degradation has occurred and done so to a greater extent in the samples from the cases than in those from the controls.

A reassay of serum samples from the study by Wald et al. (1984) 5 years after the samples were assayed showed a roughly 50% degradation of the mean alpha-tocopherol level (Wald et al., 1988). In the earlier study no records were kept of the number of times the sample had been withdrawn from storage, but it is possible that the serum samples from the cancer cases were thawed more often than those from the controls (Russell et al., 1988). Thus, the inverse association found may be due to degradation (Wald et al., 1988). This conclusion is supported by the fact that Russell et al. (1988) found no significant difference between the serum vitamin E level of cases and controls in their study of different women drawn from the same population but presenting no degradation (Russell et al., 1988).

Although the samples were stored at $-20°C$ for over 10 years prior to analysis in the studies by Knekt (1988b) and Knekt et al. (1988a), they had not been thawed and refrozen or exposed to ambient light during this period. Accordingly, several observations suggested relatively minor degradation in vitamin E levels in the samples during storage (Knekt, 1988a): (1) The mean level of alpha-tocopherol was not much lower than that reported in studies based on fresh serum samples (Atukorala et al., 1979; Willett et al., 1984; Gey, 1986) and was comparable to the level of samples stored frozen at various temperatures and for different durations (Willett et al., 1984; Menkes et al., 1986; Kok et al, 1987: Wald et al., 1987). (2) There were only small differences in intraindividual reliability coefficients of serum alpha-tocopherol between samples stored for 2 years and for over 10 years. (3) The mean levels of serum alpha-tocopherol were no lower in persons examined at the beginning of the follow-up than in those studied later. (4) The known relationship between alpha-tocopherol and other variables was confirmed by the data. The study was designed to eliminate any possible bias due to loss during storage (Knekt, 1988a). In particular, the serum samples from cases and controls were handled identically during storage, and the duration of storage was used as a matching factor. Thus, it seems reasonable to conclude that the loss of alpha-tocopherol during storage did not bias the findings.

CLINICAL TRIALS

Although the hypothesis that adequate vitamin E intake reduces the risk of cancer is partly supported by animal experiments, in vitro studies, and human case control and follow-up studies, the evidence that vitamin E provides direct protection against cancer is still inconclusive. To provide reliable evidence there is a need for large-scale randomized and placebo-controlled trials studying whether intake of vitamin E supplements will reduce future cancer risk.

The first small-scale studies on the effect of vitamin E supplementation in patients with mammary dysplasia indicated an improvement in clinical signs, suggesting that the risk of breast cancer may be reduced by vitamin E supplementation (London et al., 1985a; Chen et al., 1988). However, these findings have not been confirmed by later well-designed, double-blind, randomized, placebo-controlled trials. A trial on 128 women with confirmed mammary dysplasia did not demonstrate any difference in mammary dysplasia between a group treated with alpha-tocopherol and a control group during a relatively short follow-up period (London et al., 1985b). Another trial on 73 patients reported no beneficial effect of vitamin E on clinically palpable benigh breast findings (Ernster et al., 1985). One trial on 200 patients, which studied the prevention of recurrence of colorectal polyps, revealed only a small reduction in the rate of polyp recurrence associated with vitamins C and E supplementation (McKeown-Eyssen et al., 1988).

Generalization of the findings from chemopreventive trials needs large-scale studies. A number of such randomized, placebo-controlled trials testing whether the intake of vitamin E and other micronutrient supplements (e.g., beta-carotene, vitamin A, vitamin C, selenium) can lower cancer incidence are currently under way (Hennekens, 1986; Bertram et al., 1987; Cullen, 1988; Surgeon General, 1988). The trials are directed at prevention of cancers of different sites and to subjects in various categories of cancer risk. In studies focusing on the prevention of colon cancer the target study group consists of individuals with familial polyposis in one study, of individuals with adenomatous polyps in another, and of volunteers in a third. In two studies on the prevention of lung cancer the populations under study include male smokers and tin miners. The target study group in a study on the prevention of skin cancer consists of persons with prior basal cell carcinomas. In a multifactorial trial focusing on all sites of cancer the population under study includes nurses and dentists. The follow-ups of these trials have been too short to allow any result to be presented yet.

SUMMARY

It has been suggested that vitamin E has anticarcinogenic properties because of its role as a lipid antioxidant and free radical scavenger, and as a blocker of nitrosation. Although the results of several animal studies have shown that vitamin E inhibits cancer at various sites (e.g., the mouth, skin, and mammary gland) in some circumstances (e.g., depending on dietary selenium and fat), the findings cannot be directly applied to human cancer.

The role of vitamin E intake in the etiology of cancer has not been widely studied epidemiologically in humans, and the results are conflicting. In several studies on diet and cancer, consumption of vegetables, which are a source of vitamin E, has been found to be inversely related to the risk of lung and other cancers. However, in these studies the possibility cannot be excluded that the associations are mainly due to other substances (such as carotene) in the vegetables. The results of the few studies specifically on vitamin E intake and cancer risk disclose only weak associations with respect to lung cancer and do not generally support the hypothesis of a protective effect, possibly due to methodological issues.

The results of the few cross-sectional studies on the blood vitamin E level and cancer have shown inverse associations, especially with respect to lung cancer. Because of methodological issues, firm conclusions cannot be drawn from these results. Most longitudinal studies on the blood vitamin E level and cancer occurrence have reported slightly lower mean levels of serum vitamin E among cancer cases than among controls. The number of cancer cases in most studies has been relatively small, and therefore information about associations for different sites of cancer or in subgroups of populations is relatively scarce. The strength of the association seems, however, to vary among populations and subgroups of populations as well as among different sites of cancer. The association is strongest for gastrointestinal cancers. The strength of the association may also depend on smoking status and the levels of serum selenium and serum cholesterol. Although the association does not generally seem to be due to preclinical cancer or different confounding factors such as serum cholesterol, selenium, or vitamin A, it is still possible that the associations are due to some other substances present in the sources of vitamin E. It is conceivable that the associations observed in the cross-sectional and longitudinal studies are not causal. To obtain a reliable answer to the issue of a causal connection between vitamin E intake and the occurrence of cancer, randomized intervention trials are needed. In light of the potential chemopreventive actions of vitamin E and the safety of this nutrient, it is being given in ongoing intervention trials. It will, however, take several years before the results of these trials are available.

Some of the findings from human studies agree with the hypothesis that a sufficient intake of vitamin E provides protection against cancer. The possible preventive effect may interact with other causes of cancer. Thus there are probably cancers whose incidence does not depend on the vitamin E intake. However, the question as to whether an increase in vitamin E intake reduces the incidence of cancer has not been answered. To establish the possible anticarcinogenic effect of vitamin E and to estimate its magnitude in humans, data are needed from ongoing intervention trials on human populations and results from large-scale observational studies in various circumstances. Until these convincingly demonstrate that ample intake of vitamin E inhibits cancer in humans, vitamin E supplements should not be recommended for this purpose.

REFERENCES

Ames BN. Dietary carcinogens and anticarcinogens. Science 1983; 221:1256–1264.

Atukorala S, Basu TK, Dickerson JWT, Donaldson D, Sakula A. Vitamin A, zinc and lung cancer. Br J Cancer 1979; 40:927–931.

Bakemeier AH. The potential role of vitamins A, C, and E and selenium in cancer prevention. Oncology Nursing Forum 1988; 15:785–791.

Bendich A, Machlin LJ. Safety of oral intake of vitamin E. Am J Clin Nutr 1988; 48:612–619.

Bertram JS, Kolonel LN, Meyskens FL Jr. Rationale and strategies for chemoprevention of cancer in humans. Cancer Res 1987; 47:3012–3031.

Bieri JG, Corash L, Hubbard VS. Medical uses of vitamin E. N Engl J Med 1983; 308:1063–1071.

Birt DF. Update on the effects of vitamins A, C, and E and selenium on carcinogenesis. Proc Soc Exp Biol Med 1986; 183:311–320.

Burney PGJ, Comstock GV, Morris JS. Serologic precursors of cancer: Serum micronutrients and the subsequent risk of pancreatic cancer. Am J Clin Nutr 1989; 49:895–900.

Byers TE, Graham S, Haughey BP, Marshall JR, Swanson MK. Diet and lung cancer risk: Findings from the Western New York Diet Study. Am J Epidemiol 1987; 125:351–363.

Chen LH, Boissonneault GA, Glauert HP. Vitamin C, vitamin E and cancer. (Review.) Anticancer Research 1988; 8:739–748.

Combs GF Jr, Scott ML. Nutritional interrelationships of vitamin E and selenium. BioScience 1977; 27:467–473.

Committee on Diet, Nutrition, and Cancer. Assembly of Life Sciences. National Research Council. Diet, nutrition and cancer. Washington, DC: National Academy Press, 1982.

Comstock GW, Menkes MS, Schober SE, Vuilleumier J-P, Helsing KJ. Serum levels of retinol, beta-carotene, and alpha-tocopherol in older adults. Am J Epidemiol 1988; 127:114–123.

Correa P, Cuello C. Fajardo LF, Haenszel W, Bolanos O, Ramirez de B. Diet and gastric cancer: Nutrition survey in a high-risk area. J Natl Cancer Inst 1983; 70:673–678.

Council on Scientific Affairs. Vitamin preparations as dietary supplements and as therapeutic agents. J Am Med Assoc 1987; 257:1929–1936.

Cullen JW. The National Cancer Institute's intervention trials. Cancer 1988; 62:1851–1864.

Davies T, Kelleher J, Losowsky MS. Interrelation of serum lipoprotein and tocopherol levels. Clin Chim Acta 1969; 24:431–436.

Diplock AT. The biological function of vitamin E and the nature of the interaction of the vitamin with selenium. World Rev Nutr Diet 1978; 31:178–183.

Doll R, Peto R. The causes of cancer: Quantitative estimates of avoidable risks of cancer in the United States today. J Natl Cancer Inst 1981; 66:1192–1308.

Ernster VL, Goodson WH, Hunt TK, Petrakis NL, Sickles EA, Miike R. Vitamin E and benign breast "disease": A double-blind, randomized clinical trial. Surgery 1985; 97:490–494.

Farrell PM, Bieri JG. Megavitamin E supplementation in man. Am J Clin Nutr 1975; 28:1381–1386.

Fex G, Pettersson B, Åkesson B. Low plasma selenium as a risk factor for cancer death in middle-aged men. Nutr Cancer 1987; 10:221–229.

Food and Nutrition Board, National Research Council. Recommended dietary allowances, 9th ed. Washington, DC: National Academy of Sciences, 1980.

Freudenheim JL, Marshall JR. The problem of profound mismeasurement and the power of epidemiological studies of diet and cancer. Nutr Cancer 1988; 11:243–250.

Gerber M, Cavallo F, Marubini E, Richardson S, Barbieri A, Capitelli E, Costa A, Crastes de Paulet A, Crastes de Paulet P, Decarli A, Pastorino U, Pujol H. Liposoluble vitamins and lipid parameters in breast cancer. A joint study in northern Italy and southern France. Int J Cancer 1988; 42:489–494.

Gey KF. On the antioxidant hypothesis with regard to arteriosclerosis. Bibl Nutr Dieta 1986; 37:53–91.

Gey KF, Brubacher GB, Stähelin HB. Plasma levels of antioxidant vitamins in relation to ischemic heart disease and cancer. Am J Clin Nutr 1987; 45:1368–1377.

Glattre E, Thomassen Y, Thoresen SO, Haldorsen T, Lund-Larsen PG, Theodorsen L. Prediagnostic serum selenium in a case-control study of thyroid cancer. Int J Epidemiol 1989; 18:45–49.

Graham S, Marshall J, Haughey B, Mittelman A, Swanson M, Zielezny M, Byers T, Wilkinson G, West D. Dietary epidemiology of cancer of the colon in western New York. Am J Epidemiol 1988; 128:490–503.

Grundy SM. Dietary fats and sterols. In: Levy RI, Rifkind BM, Dennis BH, Ernst N, eds. Nutrition, lipids, and coronary heart disease. New York: Raven Press, 1979, pp. 89–118.

Hayes RB. Bogdanovicz JFAT, Schroeder FH, Bruijn de A, Raatgever JW, Maas van der PJ, Oishi K, Yoshida O. Serum retinol and prostate cancer. Cancer 1988; 62:2021–2026.

Heinonen PK, Koskinen T, Tuimala R. Serum levels of vitamins A and E in women with ovarian cancer. Arch Gynecol 1985; 237:37–40.

Heinonen PK, Kuoppala T, Koskinen T, Punnonen R. Serum vitamins A and E and carotene in patients with gynecologic cancer. Arch Gynecol Obstet 1987; 241:151–156.

Helden van PD, Beyers AD, Bester AJ, Jaskiewicz K. Esophageal cancer: Vitamin and lipotrope deficiencies in an at-risk South African population. Nutr Cancer 1987; 10:247–255.

Helzlsouer KJ. Selenium and cancer prevention. Semin Oncol 1983; 10:305–310.

Hennekens CH. Vitamin A analogues in cancer chemoprevention. In: DeVita VT Jr, Hellman S, Rosenberg SA, eds. Important advances in oncology. Philadelphia: Lippincott, 1986, pp. 23–35.

Hoekstra WG. Biochemical function of selenium and its relation to vitamin E. Fed Proc 1975; 34:2083–2089.

Horwitt MK, Harvey CC, Dahm CH Jr, Searcy MT. Relationship between tocopherol and serum lipid levels for determination of nutritional adequacy. Ann NY Acad Sci 1972; 203:223–236.

Hove EL, Harris PL. Note on the linoleic acid-tocopherol relationship in fats and oils. J Am Oil Chem Soc 1951; 28:405.

Howson CP, Hiyama T, Wynder EL. The decline in gastric cancer: Epidemiology of an unplanned triumph. Epidemiol Rev 1986; 8:1–27.

Knekt P. Serum alpha-tocopherol and the risk of cancer. Helsinki: Publications of the Social Insurance Institution, Finland, ML:83, 1988a, 1–148.

Knekt P. Serum vitamin E level and risk of female cancers. Int J Epidemiol 1988b; 17:281–286.

Knekt P, Aromaa A, Maatela J, Aaran R-K, Nikkari T, Hakama M, Hakulinen T, Peto R, Saxén E. Teppo L. Serum vitamin E and risk of cancer among Finnish men during a 10-year follow-up. Am J Epidemiol 1988a; 127:28–41.

Knekt P, Aromaa A, Maatela J, Alfthan G, Aaran R-K, Teppo L, Hakama M. Serum vitamin E, serum selenium and risk of gastrointestinal cancer. Int J Cancer 1988b; 42:846–850.

Knekt P. Seppänen R, Aaran R-K. Determinants of serum alpha-tocopherol in Finnish adults. Prev Med 1988c; 17:725–735.

Kok FJ, van Duijn CM, Hofman A, Vermeeren R, de Bruijn AM, Valkenburg HA. Micronutrients and the risk of lung cancer. N Engl J Med 1987; 316:1416.

Krishnamurthy S, Jaya S. Serum alpha-tocopherol, lipo-peroxides, and ceruloplasmin and red cell glutathione and antioxidant enzymes in patients of oral cancer. Ind J Cancer 1986; 23:36–42.

London RS, Murphy L, Kitlowski KE. Hypothesis: Breast cancer prevention by supplemental vitamin E. J Am Coll Nutr 1985a; 4:559–564.

London RS, Sundram GS, Murphy L, Manimekalai S, Reynolds M, Goldstein PJ. The effect of vitamin E on mammary dysplasia: A double-blind study. Obstet Gynecol 1985b; 65:104–106.

Lopez-S A, LeGardeur BY. Vitamins A, C, and E in relation to lung cancer incidence. (Abstract.) Am J Clin Nutr 1982; 35:851.

Machlin LJ, ed. Vitamin E: A comprehensive treatise. New York: Marcel Dekker, 1980.

McKeown-Eyssen G, Holloway C, Jazmaji V, Bright-See E, Dion P, Bruce WR. A randomized trial of vitamins C and E in the prevention of recurrence of colorectal polyps. Cancer Res 1988; 48:4701–4705.

McMichael AJ, Jensen OM, Parkin DM, Zaridze DG. Dietary and endogenous cholesterol and human cancer. Epidemiol Rev 1984; 6:192–216.

Menkes MS, Comstock GW, Vuilleumier JP, Helsing KJ, Rider AA, Brookmeyer R. Serum beta-carotene, vitamins A and E, selenium, and the risk of lung cancer. N Engl J Med 1986; 315:1250–1254.

Mergens WJ. Efficacy of vitamin E to prevent nitrosamine formation. Ann NY Acad Sci 1982; 393:61–69.

Mirvish SS. Effects of vitamins C and E on N-nitroso compound formation, carcinogenesis, and cancer. Cancer 1986; 58 (suppl):1842–1850.

Miyamoto H, Araya Y, Ito M, Isobe H, Dosaka H, Shimizu T, Kishi F, Yamamoto I, Honma H, Kawakami Y. Serum selenium and vitamin E concentrations in families of lung cancer patients. Cancer 1987; 60:1159–1162.

Nomura AMY, Stemmermann GN, Heilbrun LK, Salkeld RM, Vuilleumier JP. Serum vitamin levels and the risk of cancer of specific sites in men of Japanese ancestry in Hawaii. Cancer Res 1985; 45:2369–2372.

Peto R, Doll R, Buckley JD, Sporn MB. Can dietary beta-carotene materially reduce human cancer rates? Nature 1981; 290:201–208.

Piironen V. Tokoferolit ja tokotrienolit elintarvikkeissa ja keskimääräisessä suomalaisessa ruokavaliossa. (Väitöskirja.) (English summary: Tocopherols and tocotrienols in foods and in the average Finnish diet.) (Dissertation.) Helsinki: Helsingin yliopisto, Elintarvikekemian ja teknologian laitoksen EKT-sarja 726, 1986.

Repace JL. Consistency of research data on passive smoking and lung cancer. Lancet 1984; 1:156.

Risch HA, Jain M, Choi NW, Fodor JG, Pfeiffer CJ, Howe GR, Harrison LW, Craib KJ, Miller AB. Dietary factors and the incidence of cancer of the stomach. Am J Epidemiol 1985; 122:947–959.

Romppanen U, Tiumala R, Punnonen R, Koskinen T. Serum vitamin A and E levels in patients with lichen sclerosus and carcinoma of the vulva: Effect of oral etretinate treatment. Ann Chir Gynaecol 1985; 74 (suppl 197):27–29.

Rougereau A, Person O, Rougereau G. Fat soluble vitamins and cancer localization associated to an abnormal ketone derivative of D3 vitamin: Carcinomedin. Int J Vit Nutr Res 1987; 57:367–373.

Russell-Briefel R, Bates MW, Kuller LH. The relationship of plasma carotenoids to health and biochemical factors in middle-aged men. Am J Epidemiol 1985; 122:741–749.

Russell MJ, Thomas BS, Bulbrook RD. A prospective study of the relationship between serum vitamins A and E and risk of breast cancer. Br J Cancer 1988; 57:213–215.

Salonen JT, Salonen R, Lappeteläinen R, Mäenpää PH, Alfthan G, Puska P. Risk of cancer in relation to serum concentrations of selenium and vitamins A and E: Matched case-control analysis of prospective data. Br Med J 1985; 290:417–420.

Schober SE, Comstock GW, Helsing KJ, Salkeld RM, Morris JS, Rider AA, Brookmeyer R. Serologic precursors of cancer. I. Prediagnostic serum nutrients and colon cancer risk. Am J Epidemiol 1987; 126:1033–1041.

Shamberger RJ. Chemoprevention of cancer. In: Reddy BS, Cohen LA, eds. Diet, nutrition and cancer: A critical evaluation. Vol. 2. Boca Raton, FL: CRC, 1986, pp. 43–62.

Sidney S, Farquhar JW. Cholesterol, cancer, and public health policy. Am J Med 1983; 75:494–508.

Stryker WS, Stampfer MJ, Stein EV, Kaplan L, Louis TA, Sober A, Willett WC. Diet, plasma levels of beta-carotene and alpha-tocopherol and risk of malignant melanoma. (Abstract.) Am J Epidemiol 1988; 128:889–890.

Stähelin HB, Rösel F, Buess E, Brubacher G. Cancer, vitamins, and plasma lipids: Prospective Basel Study. J Natl Cancer Inst 1984; 73:1463–1468.

Surgeon General's report on nutrition and health. Washington, DC: U.S. Department of Health and Human Services. DHHS (PHS) Publication No. 88-50210, 1988.

Takahashi Y, Uruno K, Kimura S. Vitamin E binding proteins in human serum. J Nutr Sci Vitaminol 1977; 23:201–209.

Tangney CC, Shekelle RB, Raynor W, Gale M, Betz EP. Intra- and interindividual variation in measurements of beta-carotene, retinol, and tocopherols in diet and plasma. Am J Clin Nutr 1987; 45:764–769.

Tappel AL. Vitamin E and selenium protection from in vivo lipid peroxidation. Ann NY Acad Sci 1980; 355:18–29.

Tomassi G, Silano V. An assessment of the safety of tocopherols as food additives. Food Chem Toxic 1986; 24:1051–1061.

Toniolo P, Riboli E, Protta F, Charrel M, Cappa APM. Calorie-providing nutrients and risk of breast cancer. J Natl Cancer Inst 1989; 81:278–286.

Urbach C, Hickman K, Harris PL. Effect of individual vitamins A, C, E, and carotene administered at high levels on their concentration in the blood. Exp Med Surg 1952; 10:7–20.

Wald NJ, Boreham J, Hayward JL, Bulbrook RD. Plasma retinol, beta-carotene and vitamin E levels in relation to the future risk of breast cancer. Br J Cancer 1984; 49:321–324.

Wald NJ, Thompson SG, Densem JW, Boreham J, Bailey A. Serum vitamin E and subsequent risk of cancer. Br J Cancer 1987; 56:69–72.

Wald NJ, Nicolaides-Bouman A, Hudson GA. Plasma retinol, beta-carotene and vitamin E levels in relation to the future risk of breast cancer. Br J Cancer 1988; 57:235.

Weisburger JH, Reddy BS, Hill P. Cohen LA, Wynder EL, Spingarn NE. Nutrition and cancer: On the mechanisms bearing on causes of cancer of the colon, breast, prostate, and stomach. Bull NY Acad Med 1980; 56:673–696.

Willett WC, Polk BF, Morris JS, Stampfer MJ, Pressel S, Rosner B, Taylor JO, Schneider K, Hames CG. Prediagnostic serum selenium and risk of cancer. Lancet 1983a; 2:130–134.

Willett WC, Stampfer MJ, Underwood BA, Speitzer FE, Rosner B, Hennekens CH. Validation of a dietary questionnaire with plasma carotenoid and alpha-tocopherol levels. Am J Clin Nutr 1983b; 38:631–639.

Willett WC, Stampfer MJ, Underwood BA, Taylor JO, Hennekens CH. Vitamins A, E, and carotene: Effects of supplementation on their plasma levels. Am J Clin Nutr 1983c; 38:559–566.

Willett WC, Polk BF, Underwood BA, Stampfer MJ, Pressel S, Rosner B, Taylor JO, Schneider K, Hames CG. Relation of serum vitamins A and E and carotenoids to the risk of cancer. N Engl J Med 1984; 310:430–434.

Yang CS, Sun Y, Yang QU, Miller KW, Li G, Zheng S-F, Ershow AG, Blot WJ, Li J. Vitamin A and other deficiencies in Linxian, a high esophageal cancer incidence area in northern China. J Natl Cancer Inst 1984; 73:1449–1453.

8

Folate Deficiency and Cancer

C. E. Butterworth, Jr.

University of Alabama at Birmingham
Birmingham, Alabama

INTRODUCTION

Background

The folate family of compounds has played a prominent role in the study of carcinogenesis and in the treatment of cancer for more than 40 years. A milestone in the history of folic acid research occurred in 1945 when Angier et al., announced the successful synthesis of folic acid, thus confirming its chemical structure to be pteroylglutamic acid (PGA). This achievement not only made it possible to obtain pure material of known chemical structure for reference work and nutritional studies, it also opened the way for the synthesis of new analogs and derivatives. Prior to 1945 investigators had been dependent on purified extracts from various biological sources including liver, yeast, spinach leaves, and bacterial fermentation products. Folic acid received its name in 1941 after it had been extracted in concentrated form from spinach leaves (Latin *folium*, leaf) (Mitchell et al., 1941). Synthetic PGA identified the common component of these extracts and explained their nutritional properties in various assay systems. During the years immediately following the synthesis of PGA, i.e., the "monoglutamyl" form of folic acid, it became possible to synthesize certain "polyglutamyl" or "conjugated" forms of folate as well as the biological antagonists aminopterin and methotrexate (Farber et al., 1947, 1948). It also became possible to synthesize citrovorum factor ("leucovorin"), which helped establish the vital role of 5 formyltetrahydropteroylglutamate in the transport of single-carbon units (Sauberlich and Baumann, 1948). In later years this product came into use in a successful treatment regimen known as "leucovorin rescue" following high doses of folate antagonists for cancer chemotherapy (Gilman et al., 1985).

Undoubtedly, the crucial role of folate in the biosynthesis of nucleotides necessary for cell division, nucleic acid metabolism, and genetic expression has made it an ideal subject for wide-ranging clinical and laboratory investigations. Probably no other single vitamin has been the subject of such intense scrutiny. In some respects it is paradoxical that the successful use of folic acid antagonists in leukemia and certain forms of cancer has tended to obscure the role of folate in normal nutrition, including any potential ability to minimize risks of cancer initiation. This chapter reviews certain old and new evidence which suggests that folate deficiency may be associated with an increased risk of cancer and that optimal intakes may have a protective effect.

Anticancer Effects of Fermentation *L. casei* Factor

One of the earliest references linking folate to cancer appeared in 1944 and carries the intriguing title: "Folic Acid: A Tumor Growth Inhibitor" (Leuchtenberger et al., 1944). Actually, this report was based on investigations using fermentation *L. casei* factor, produced by a strain of *Corynebacterium*, since the chemical synthesis of PGA had not yet been achieved. It was later learned that the "fermentation *L. casei* factor" is pteroyltriglutamate, i.e., folic acid with two additional glutamic acid units in γ-peptide linkage. In the first of this series of three brief reports, Leuchtenberger et al. (1944) reported striking inhibition of growth of sarcoma 180 transplants in mice treated with intravenous injections of "fermentation *L. casei* factor." Subsequently, it was shown (Leuchtenberger et al., 1945; Lewisohn et al., 1946) that intravenous injections of this material led to the complete disappearance of tumors in 38 of 89 mice (43%) with biopsy-proven spontaneous breast cancer. Treated animals lived longer than controls and showed no signs of toxicity. The occurrence of new tumors was markedly diminished in the treated mice. Evidence was also presented that the anticancer effect was associated with the triglutamyl form of the vitamin since injections of liver *L. casei* factor were ineffectual. Indeed, evidence suggested that high doses of the liver *L. casei* factor produced more rapid growth of tumors, but the results were considered inconclusive. It is now known that liver *L. casei* factor is in the monoglutamyl form. It seems remarkable in retrospect that the line of investigation started by this group was never independently confirmed or refuted. Nevertheless, these three reports stand in evidence that supraphysiological doses of folate directly interfere with growth of certain tumors, or that the triglutamate form, which does not normally circulate, may interfere in some way with vitamin turnover and balance. Another possible explanation is that the injections strengthen a flagging repair mechanism that is already in existence. In any case these results stimulated interest in the polyglutamyl (or conjugated) forms of folate and led to the synthesis of these compounds by SubbaRow and his associates (Farber et al., 1947).

Studies of Synthetic Conjugated Forms of Folate

In 1947 Farber et al. (1947) described the results of a clinical study of two folic acid "conjugates": pteroyl-α-diglutamate (diopterin) and pteroylglutamyl-γ-glutamyl-γ-glutamate (teropterin). These compounds were given parenterally in high doses to 90 adults with various forms of advanced cancer. The diglutamate form, diopterin, was given in doses as high as 300 mg/day orally for an unspecified period, the average duration of treatment being 5 weeks. Pteroyltriglutamate was given intravenously in a total dose of 12,740 mg to one patient over a period of 6 weeks. Another received the same material, presumably orally, for a total dose of 19,000 mg. In both instances there was no evidence of toxicity (Farber et al., 1947). It should be noted that each agent tested is capable of being converted to folic acid by enzymes present in normal human tissue. Although reduction in the size of tumors occurred "frequently enough to warrant further experimental studies (Farber et al., 1947), this line of investigation was abandoned when overshadowed by subsequent events.

Anticancer Effects of Folic Acid Antagonists

In 1948 Farber and colleagues reported the occurrence of dramatic temporary remissions in the course of acute childhood leukemia following therapy with the newly designed folic acid analog, aminopterin (4-aminopteroylglutamic acid). It is fair to say that this report and the discovery of other folic acid antagonists such as methotrexate revolutionized the treatment of childhood leukemia, and of other forms of cancer, over the course of many subsequent years. In this report reference was made to "an acceleration phenomenon" in the leukemic process associated with the use of folic acid conjugates (teropterin and diopterin). Unfortunately, the evidence for such a phenomenon is largely anecdotal; there is virtually no scientific documentation of it in peer-reviewed journal articles. Indeed, the studies reported in 1947 give no hint that the treatment of cancer in adults with high doses of folate caused any acceleration of the disease (Farber et al., 1947). Nevertheless, the tacit belief seems to have developed that folic acid intake should be restricted as a matter of principle in all forms of cancer and leukemia. Physicians apparently became fearful that giving folate might predispose to cancer or exacerbate existing cases. Research on nutritionally active folic acid compounds such as the polyglutamates came to a standstill, while efforts were concentrated on developing new folate antagonists and therapeutic regimens. A growing body of evidence now indicates that inadequate dietary intake of folate may be associated with an increased risk or prevalence of certain forms of cancer. Moreover, some studies suggest that adequate or high folate intake may be associated with lower risks for cancer of the cervix (Brock et al., 1988; Butterworth et al., 1991), lung (Heimburger et al., 1988), colon (Lashner et al., 1989), and esophagus (Jaskiewicz et al., 1988). In other words, optimal intake of folate may be a protective or preventive measure. There is no convincing evidence that adequate dietary intake or even ordinary supplements of folate contribute to the primary occurrence of cancer.

COCARCINOGENIC EFFECTS OF FOLATE DEFICIENCY AND FOLATE ANTAGONISTS

Knowledge that has evolved since the discovery of aminopterin now provides a rational metabolic basis by which folate deficiency might contribute to the etiology of some forms of cancer. When Farber and his colleagues (1948) were studying acute leukemia in children in 1948 the origins of the disease were largely unknown and considered a mystery. Although the viral nature of avian leukosis, the Rous sarcoma, and breast cancer in mice had been clearly demonstrated, the role of viruses as a cause of human leukemia was regarded as theoretical for at least another 10 years. Reviewing the subject in 1959, Schwarz and Schoolman noted that "studies have been gradually supporting evidence for the virus theory of the etiology of leukemia." A major advance had occurred in 1957 when Friend reported the induction of leukemia in mice by cell-free extracts from human patients.

As a result of progress in virology and molecular biology, research emphasis has gradually shifted away from the empirical use of cytotoxic therapeutic agents, such as aminopterin, toward the study of basic mechanisms including chemical carcinogenesis and the expression of viral oncogenes. Eto and Krumdieck (1986) reviewed the literature concerning relationships of vitamin B_{12} and folate deficiencies to cancer. They cite a significant body of evidence that deficiency of either vitamin enhances the activity of various chemical carcinogens although neither deficiency is carcinogenic by itself. The cocarcinogenic effect of nutrient deficiency can be demonstrated either by dietary deprivation or by the use of vitamin antagonists. It is of considerable importance that Barich et al. (1986) demonstrated that the folate antagonist methotrexate can have a dual effect; it can act as a cocarcinogen as well as an antitumor agent. Not only is it possible for nutrient deficiency to favor the initiation of cancer by exogenous carcinogens, it is also possible to demonstrate that deficiency can alter the regulation of expression of naturally occurring oncogenes. For example, Hsieh et al. (1989) reported that diets deficient in folate, vitamin B_{12}, and other methyl donors lead to striking increases in the expression of endogenous oncogenes and retrovirus-like sequences in mouse liver.

Branda et al. (1988) described an interesting effect of folate deficiency on a major determinant of cancer lethality: the propensity to form metastases. Cells from a cultured line of murine B_{16} melanoma (F10 strain) were grown in either folate-deficient or folate-sufficient media. It was demonstrated that deficient cells had increased numbers of DNA strand breaks, increased volume, and abnormal deoxyuridine suppression tests. The folate-deficient cells consistently initiated more pulmonary metastases when injected into host mice than did control cells. Thus, folate deficiency may have an important bearing on the metastatic potential of tumor cells, and conceivably even on local spread and survival. Therefore it is evident that folate status has an effect on cancer ecology that is not limited to tumor initiation.

ROLE OF FOLATE IN MAINTENANCE OF CHROMOSOME STRUCTURE AND FUNCTION

Chromosome Breaks; Folate-Sensitive Fragile Sites; Translocation Effects

It has been demonstrated that folic acid deficiency leads to chromosome breaks at specific heritable fragile sites (Sutherland, 1979) as well as at other locations (Yunis and Soreng, 1984). Many folate-sensitive breaks occur at positions known to be associated with translocations seen in cancer. It is believed that such translocations disrupt patterns of regulation by adjacent segments of genetic information in Burkitt's lymphoma as well as in cases of acute myeloblastic leukemia and chronic myeloid leukemia (Rowley, 1982).

Rowley (1989) discussed the consequences of the well-studied translocations from chromosome 9 to 22 which forms the Philadelphia chromosome and which is believed to be responsible for human chronic myeloid leukemia. As a result of this translocation a latent protooncogene, Abelson (*ABL*) from chromosome 9, hybridizes with the gene at the breakpoint cluster region (*BCR*) of chromosome 22. The fused gene is expressed as a large chimeric protein product with features of both the Abelson virus and the *BCR* gene.

It is important to emphasize that once a translocation has occurred, folate coenzymes remain essential to the survival and function of the cell. Indeed, the newly constituted cell may have a folate requirement that is greater or metabolically different from the parent cell line. In this way a folate antagonist could have a more selective impact on the mutant cell line than on the original one.

DNA Methylation; Histone Binding

In addition to the role of folate in the biosynthesis of structural components of DNA such as purines and thymidine, considerable interest now centers on broader relationships of folate to chromatin structure, DNA methylation, and histone binding. The organization of chromosomes was reviewed by Castro (1987), along with a discussion of the effects of nutrient deficiencies in the causation of chromosomal breaks and exchanges. A major tool employed in the study of chromosomal organization has been the assessment of sensitivity to micrococcal nuclease digestion. Since segments of DNA bound to histone, or coiled around the nucleosome core, are inaccessible to the enzyme, the length of DNA fragments released after digestion is a reflection of binding. Actively transcribing segments of DNA have an altered conformation and are more susceptible to nuclease digestion than bulk DNA (Weintraub and Groudine, 1976). Razin and Riggs (1980) discussed the evidence that DNA methylation, particularly of cytosine units, is a key element in the regulation of gene function. It was also shown that DNA is consistently undermethylated in malignant and premalignant cells of the colon (Goelz et al., 1985).

It is relevant to the present discussion to note that in eukaryotes approximately 165 base pairs (bp) of DNA are coiled around an octameric histone core to form a nucleosome, the fundamental packaging unit of condensed DNA. One nucleosome is attached to another by a variable stretch of "linker" DNA consisting of 20–60 bp. A separate histone, H-1, is attached to DNA at its point of entry into and exit from the coil, forming a bridge between strands of linker DNA (Fig. 1). Castro (1983) showed that the internucleosomal repeat length of DNA in rat liver extracts is decreased by a high-carbohydrate, fat-free ("lipogenic") diet. The term *lipogenic* ordinarily implies a diet lacking in folate, vitamin B_{12}, and certain methyl donors which leads to the development of a fatty liver. However, in the cited studies a fixed allowance of vitamins, including folate and vitamin

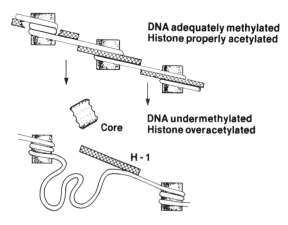

DNA adequately methylated
Histone properly acetylated

Core

DNA undermethylated
Histone overacetylated

H-1

Figure 1 Scheme showing the organization of nucleosomes with approximately two and one-half turns of DNA coiled about the octameric histone core. Histone H-1 is believed to stabilize the coil, but its binding to linker DNA is diminished when butyrate inhibits deacetylation. Folate-derived methyl groups exposed along the major grove of DNA are believed to guide the attachment of the coil to the core (see text). (From Butterworth, 1985. Used with permission.)

B_{12}, was supplied, during manipulation of other calorie sources (Castro and Sevall, 1980). Thus the term lipogenic is used in a slightly different context here; it cannot be stated with certainty whether or not a relative deficiency of lipotropic factors existed. However, the authors postulated that the fat-free feeding program is lipogenic because it induces nuclear transcription and synthesis of enzymes necessary to convert carbohydrate to fat. Presumably the uncoiled DNA is more accessible to micrococcal nuclease digestion, yielding more of the shorter fragments which contain approximately 210 base pairs. Although the basic mechanism is not established, the importance of this dietary effect is the similarity to chromosome changes associated with hypomethylation and steroid hormone action which also affect nuclear transcription. Thus there may well be an interaction between lipogenic diets and folate status.

Krumdieck (1983) advanced the novel hypothesis that the spacing of methyl groups exposed along the major groove of DNA constitutes a type of binary code to direct and regulate the binding of DNA to histones. The protruding methyl groups of thymine and methylcytosine can be visualized as "recognition points" or space-occupying knobs. Incorporation of uracil into DNA, which occurs during deficiency of folate and other methyl donors (Goulian et al., 1980), would result in improper recognition sites. While uracil (in the form of dUMP) is capable of replacing thymidylate in the base-pairing process, it lacks a methyl group and presumably does not facilitate the binding of histone to DNA. In times of folate deficiency, cells are arrested in the S phase of the mitotic cycle, tend to be enlarged (megaloblastic), and display an immature pattern of nuclear chromatin. In summary, it is believed that a lack of methyl groups along the major groove of DNA interferes with histone binding and results in transcription of otherwise suppressed genetic sequences. A further consequence would be exposure of DNA to attack by endogenous nucleases, thereby increasing the risk of chromosome breaks and incorporation of viral genomes.

Histone Acetylation

Another important determinant of DNA binding to histones is the reversible acetylation of lysine residues. The ability to reversibly acetylate histones appears to be essential for completion of the cell division cycle, for DNA replication and genetic expression. Megee et al. (1990) studied structure-function relationships through the creation of directed point mutations in the H-4 histone of yeast which structurally resembles mammalian histone. Four lysine residues strategically located at positions 5, 8, 12, and 16 appear to be essential for normal chromosome function. Substitution of arginine or asparagine at all four positions is lethal, while partial substitution causes impaired growth, formation of enlarged cells, and slow progression through the division cycle. These morphological effects in yeast are reminiscent of the megaloblastic changes associated with folate deficiency in other organisms. There is evidence that acetyl groups bound to histone are subject to rapid turnover and that the process of deacetylation is inhibited by butyrate. A detailed review of butyrate effects was presented by Kruh (1982). Since butyrate favors acetylation of histones (H-4 and others), this appears to be another mechanism for bringing about dissociation of DNA from the histone binding sites and activation of gene expression. It is of interest that exposure of erythroleukemia cells in tissue culture to sodium butyrate induces hemoglobin synthesis (Ohlsson-Wilhelm et al., 1984). The regulation of genetic expression thus appears to be affected by either the extent of DNA methylation or the extent of histone acetylation, or both. In either case the dissociated DNA would be exposed to the risk of having a viral gene inserted at a breakpoint, or undergoing a translocation.

Steroid Hormone Effects

The process of gene expression is complicated further by the action of steroid hormones, which are believed to act by removing histone attachments at specific binding sites in target tissue DNA. Pater et al. (1988) reported that a specific set of nucleotide sequences confers responsiveness to glucocorticoids and progesterone, promoting colony formation in cultured rat kidney cells carrying genes for the human papillomavirus type 16 and the *ras* oncogene. In other work, Hsieh et al. (1989) demonstrated in mice that methyl-deficient diets cause profound increases in the hepatic synthesis of certain gene products, including a 16-fold increase in RNA expressing the *C-myc* oncogene. Taken together, these studies suggest that when a target tissue such as the cervix is folate-deficient, it would have enhanced vulnerability to sex hormone stimulation and the expression of viral oncogenes.

CLINICAL STUDIES

Inborn Errors of Folate Metabolism; Hematological Disorders

In 1978 Branda et al., described a family in which 32 individuals had severe hematological disease including anemia, pancytopenia, and leukemia. Among four generations 17 of the 32 family members died of their disease and several others were reported to have chromosomal abnormalities, particularly hypodiploidy. One member of the family, the proband, had severe aplastic anemia with megaloblastic features and was found to have impaired uptake of folate by stimulated lymphocytes and bone marrow cells. There was marked improvement in his aplasia following treatment with high doses of folic acid. Five other family members were found to have a similar defect in cellular uptake of folate. In spite of improvement in anemia the proband developed lymphedema of the lower extremities and died several years later with chylous pleural effusion and ascites

(Arthur et al., 1983). Although these manifestations are common with thoracic duct obstruction due to lymphoma, it is not known whether or not a lymphoma was present. The proband's children were subsequently found to have evidence of impaired folate homeostasis, altered patterns of sister chromatid exchange, and low mitotic indices. However, no clear relationships could be established between the observed cytogenetic abnormalities and the high incidence of hematological disease among family members.

Cancer of the Upper Aerodigestive Tract and Esophagus

Schantz et al. (1989) recently described studies in 23 young adults (less than 40 years of age) who had squamous cell carcinomas (SCC) of the upper aerodigestive tract (nasopharynx, oral cavity, pharynx, and larynx). Cytogenetic studies revealed an increased number of chromatid breaks per cell in lymphocyte cultures exposed to bleomycin from SCC cases than from controls or subjects with non-SCC tumors. The authors suggest that the occurrence of SCC in this population depends not only on exposure to a responsible carcinogen, but potentially on an inherent genetic sensitivity. The chromosome sensitivity was most apparent in non-tobacco users and in patients less than 30 year old. It is not known if folate metabolism or nutritional status was a factor, but the possibility merits consideration in view of folate's role in chromosome repair.

The incidence of esophageal cancer in developed countries has been linked to excessive use of alcohol and tobacco, although some high-incidence areas exist, such as in northern Iran, in which the use of tobacco and alcohol is restricted or prohibited (Ghadirian, 1987). As a result, low socioeconomic status and poor nutrition have been implicated as major risk factors in a number of epidemiological studies. As noted below, both alcohol and tobacco smoke may inactivate or suppress the function of folic acid and vitamin B_{12} in the tissues exposed to them. In this way the use of alcohol and tobacco could exaggerate marginal deficiency of these vitamins by direct contact in the upper aerodigestive tract. In a study of esophageal cancer among black males in Washington, D.C., Zeigler et al. (1981) observed that the least nourished third of the population had twice the risk of cancer mortality as the best nourished. No specific micronutrient deficiency could be identified. There was no independent association of risk with the use of tobacco or alcohol, and the major predictor was poor general nutrition.

In the republic of Transkei, southern Africa, squamous cell carcinoma of the esophagus is the most common form of cancer, yet epidemiological studies do not indicate a close correlation with patterns of alcohol and tobacco usage (Jaskiewicz et al., 1988). Instead, evidence is accumulating to support an association with low socioeconomic status and inadequate dietary intake of several key nutrients caused by poor agricultural conditions. In a recent survey of 1000 cytological specimens obtained by brush biopsy of the esophagus from subjects in low-, intermediate-, and high-incidence areas, morphological features similar to those seen with folate deficiency in the cervix were observed (Jaskiewicz et al., 1987). Published photographs of esophageal cells not only resemble those of the cervix with regard to folate deficiency and dysplasia but also display features suggestive of koilocytosis as seen with papillomavirus infection (Jaskiewicz et al., 1987). Morphological features compatible with folic acid deficiency were present in all population groups but were most common in the high-risk area where they were present in 22.8% of adults. Nutritional status assessment by biochemical analyses in this population revealed significantly lower red blood cell folate values among eight subjects with dysplastic and cancer cells than in 18 controls ($p = 0.05$) (van Helden et al., 1987). This is one of only a few studies presenting direct assay results of folate in connection with cancer epidemiology. There was also evidence of multiple nutrient deficiencies (vitamins A, E, B_{12}, and red blood cell folate) which was more pronounced in the high-incidence area than in the intermediate- and low-incidence districts. The red blood cell folate value (ng/ml, mean $\pm$ SD) in the high-incidence district was 222 ± 51 ($n = 17$) while the corresponding value in the low-incidence district was 307 ± 99 ($n = 14$; $p < 0.005$) (van Helden et al., 1987). Red blood cell folate is considered a reliable indicator of nutritional status since it reflects long-term folate intake, whereas serum folate reflects the recent level of consumption. It was also observed that DNA from tumors of the esophagus was hypomethylated in four subjects when compared with DNA extracted from the normal part of the esophagus in the same patient (van Helden et al., 1987).

Collectively these studies provide strong support for the view that nutritional deficiency predisposes to the development of esophageal cancer in this geographic region. Folate deficiency appears to be a crucial factor, along with deficiency of other lipotropic nutrients including vitamin B_{12}, and methyl donors such as choline and methionine.

Bronchial Squamous Metaplasia with Atypia (Dysplasia)

It is widely believed that atypical bronchial squamous metaplasia is an intermediate step in the transition from normal to malignant bronchial epithelium in smokers (Robbins and Kumar, 1987). As in the cervix, malignant changes tend to occur in areas of metaplasia and are accompanied by nuclear immaturity, irregular nuclear borders, and altered patterns of cytoplasmic differentiation. In view of the direct exposure of the bronchial mucosa to high concentrations of noxious substances contained in tobacco smoke, Krumdieck postulated that localized vitamin deficiency could mediate chemical carcinogenesis (Heimburger et al., 1988). Tobacco smoke is known to contain cyanates, isocyanates, nitrites, and nitrous oxide along with many other potentially reactive compounds. It has been demonstrated that cyanate is capable of inactivating tetrahydrofolate, while butyl nitrite is capable of inactivating both folate and vitamin B_{12} (Francis et al., 1977; Khaled et al., 1986). It was reasoned that high doses of folate and vitamin B_{12} given systemically might offset the localized, point-of-contact inactivation of these nutrients. In a randomized, double-blind intervention trial it was observed that daily oral supplements of 10 mg of folic acid plus 0.5 mg of hydroxocobalamin were associated with significant improvement in sputum cytology (Heimburger et al., 1988). Hydroxocobalamin was chosen because of its ability to scavenge cyanide compounds through conversion to cyanocobalamin. It is not possible to conclude from this study which nutrient exerted the favorable effect. The authors were careful to point out that the experimental program should not be construed as a means to prevent lung cancer in individuals who continue to smoke. Nevertheless the findings focus attention on basic mechanisms involving folate and vitamin B_{12} during intermediate stages of oncogenesis. Further study is needed to determine optimal levels of intake of these nutrients for individuals exposed to noxious agents whether through voluntary inhalation, or occupational or environmental exposure.

Cancer of the Colon

Lashner et al. (1989) have evaluated the effect of folate supplementation on the incidence of dysplasia or cancer in a case control study of 99 subjects with chronic ulcerative colitis (CUC). Because of the known high incidence of colon carcinoma in association with CUC, it is standard medical practice to follow patients closely and to obtain at least one biopsy from each 10 cm of colon during an annual colonoscopy. All subjects were free of dyplasia and cancer at the beginning of the study but had had pancolitis for at least 7 years at the time evaluation was made. A 62% lower incidence of dysplasia or cancer was observed among subjects who were receiving a daily folate supplement either in the form of a multivitamin product or a 1-mg daily prescription. The outcome fell just short of statistical significance in spite of the magnitude of the difference. However, the effect of folate supplementation did not change with adjustment and could not be attributed entirely to bias or confounding. The authors recommend folate supplementation for patients with chronic ulcerative colitis as a possible chemopreventive measure for cancer pending the outcome of larger case control studies.

Cervical Dysplasia and Cancer

Muir (1990) has commented that cancer of the cervix is by far the commonest cancer in women in the developing world, with an incidence of some 370,000 new cases each year. He notes that nearly every chromosome carries at least one protooncogene, many of which occur at specific sites and are associated consistently with certain forms of cancer. Most tumors can be characterized by mutations which either activate an oncogene or inactivate tumor suppressor genes.

Thus the "spacing" effect of a viral gene insertion, or a chromosome translocation at a folate-sensitive fragile site, could have disastrous effects on the regulation of cell proliferation.

The possibility of a link between folic acid metabolism and cancer of the cervix was brought into focus by a report of Whitehead et al. (1973). These investigators described the occurrence of megaloblastic features in cervical epithelial cells from women who were using oral contraceptive steroid hormones. Despite the fact that clinical signs of deficiency were lacking, and serum values for folate and vitamin B_{12} were normal, the abnormal cytological manifestations disappeared within 3 weeks of supplementation with 10 mg of folic acid orally each day. Citing evidence that folate is required for expression of estrogenic effects in target organs of experimental animals, the authors postulated that folate deficiency had occurred at the end-organ level due to hormonal stimulation. This introduced the important concept of localized vitamin deficiency. Although this paper did not describe cytological manifestations in terms conventionally related to dysplasia, there is evidence that megaloblastic features are "deceptively similar" to those observed in early cervical cancer (Koss, 1979).

Earlier, Lloyd and Garry (1963) had described a patient with pernicious anemia in whom the cervical biopsy was suspected of showing cancer, yet the abnormal cells disappeared after vitamin B_{12} was given as treatment for the primary disorder. It has been reported that oral supplementation with 10-mg daily doses of folate over a period of 3 months resulted in general improvement in cytological manifestations, and in less severe biopsy readings in cases of cervical dysplasia than in a similar group of control subjects receiving a placebo (Butterworth et al., 1982). This study suggested that a localized folate deficiency in the cervix is sometimes indistinguishable from early cancer and may be an integral part of the premalignant process. It was pointed out that localized folate deficiency could interfere with DNA synthesis, repair, and methylation, or alter susceptibility to oncogenic viruses or chemical carcinogens. At the time of this report it was the prevailing view that most cases of cervical dysplasia tended to grow progressively worse and that remissions were rare. Current evidence suggests that perhaps half of the cases of early dysplasia may revert to normal spontaneously.

Brock et al. (1988) reported dietary intake studies and measurements of certain plasma nutrients in 117 Australian women with in situ cervical cancer compared with 196 controls. The average daily nutrient intake for the previous year was estimated by a food frequency questionnaire. There appeared to be a protective effect on cancer risk associated with upper quartiles of intake of carotene, vitamin C, and folate. However, the protective trend was not significant when the results were corrected for other risk factors. Biochemical assessment of nutritional status regarding folate was not performed. Higher intake levels of fruit juices were associated with a protective effect, even after adjustment for other variables, but the specific nutrient responsible could not be identified. Fruit juices are generally considered to be good sources of all three of the protective nutrients, namely, carotene, vitamin C, and folate.

A recently reported epidemiological study presents evidence that young women of childbearing age whose red blood cell folate concentration is in the upper tertile have significantly reduced risk of having cervical dysplasia in association with human papillomavirus (HPV) type 16 (Butterworth et al., 1991). The study was conducted over a 5-year period and involved a total of 294 women with dysplasia and 170 normal controls. It was observed that the influence of four well-recognized risk factors (cigarette smoking, oral contraceptive use, parity, and HPV infection) was significantly less among women with red blood cell folate concentrations in the upper tertile ($\geq$290 ng/ml) than among those in the middle tertile (180–289) or lower tertile ($\leq$180). Among women with a positive test for HPV-16 the ratio of cases to controls (rate ratio) was 1.2, 5.3, and 3.3 in the upper, middle, and lower tertiles, respectively, of red cell folate concentration. Apparently there is a protective effect associated with the presence of higher tissue folate levels as reflected in the higher red cell folate values in this population. It seems remarkable that the risk of HPV-16-associated cervical dysplasia was nearly five times as great among women in the middle tertile of red cell folate concentration, while the risk was slightly lower but still significantly great among those in the lowest tertile. This pattern might be explained by the failure of HPV genome insertion due to the occurrence of chromosome breaks which are not repaired with very low tissue levels of folate. The results imply that perhaps two-thirds of this low-income population, most of whom use oral contraceptives, would benefit from an intake of folic acid that would place them in the upper tertile. Further studies are needed to determine optimal levels of folate intake to afford maximal protection.

FOLATE DEFICIENCY AND SUSCEPTIBILITY TO HUMAN PAPILLOMAVIRUS (HPV) AND OTHER ONCOGENIC VIRUSES

Since the reports of zur Hausen in 1977 and of Meisels and Morin in 1981, it has become increasingly apparent that human papillomaviruses (HPV) are primary factors in the causation of many cases of squamous cell carcinoma of the cervix. Of more than 60 known strains of HPV, types 16 and 18 are most commonly associated with dysplastic lesions. Some evidence suggests that the virus may exist in asymptomatic carriers (Macnab et al., 1986), presumably in the cytoplasm, while in affected individuals the viral genome is incorporated into the host chromosome (Dürst et al., 1985). Reference has already been made to the increased expression of the Moloney murine leukemia virus in extracts of liver from folate-deficient mice (Hsieh et al., 1989).

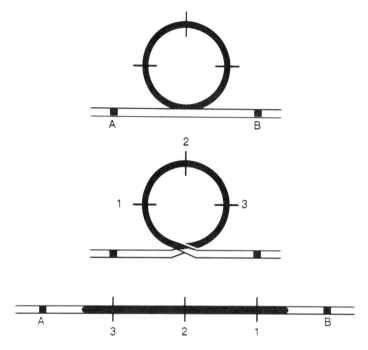

Figure 2 Diagram illustrating hypothetical situation by which a circular viral genome, e.g., from a polyoma virus, may be incorporated into a linear strand of host DNA. Simultaneous breaks along homologous strands are repaired by cross-ways rejoining as in crossing over. Note that potential interactions between genes at point A and point B would be altered by the new spatial arrangement. (Redrawn from Watson, 1970.)

It was postulated many years ago that the genome of the polyoma virus, which, like HPV, is a circular DNA molecule, might gain access to the host genome by a process resembling "crossing over" (Watson, 1970). In this situation homologous segments of the two molecules could become aligned in such a way that a simultaneous break might be repaired by joining the end of one molecule to the end of the other (see Fig. 2). The result would be insertion of a linear stretch of viral DNA into the host genome. There is evidence that the HPV genome exists as a supercoiled circular molecule like that of the polyoma virus DNA (Vinograd et al., 1965). Mechanisms which favor incorporation of the viral genome are not well understood but certainly would be affected by factors involved in DNA synthesis and repair. Nutritional folate status is obviously a candidate for scrutiny in view of its established role in this area and its connection with fragile sites.

Popescu et al. (1987) observed that in an established line of cultured cells derived from cervical carcinoma the DNA genome of HPV-18 is integrated at a single site on chromosome 12. Direct in situ DNA hybridization suggested that a heritable folate-sensitive fragile site at the same location may facilitate integration of the viral gene. This key observation emphasizes the potential importance of folate deficiency in exposing a heritable fragile site to the risk of insertion of viral DNA sequences. Chromosome 12 also contains the Ki-*ras* 2 oncogene, but the linkage is not close. Further details are presented in a review by Wettstein (1990).

The propensity for folate deficiency to cause chromosome breaks both at hereditary and constitutive fragile sites suggests that an inadequate supply of folate could favor the opportunistic insertion of a viral genome. It seems clear that a delicate balance must be maintained between optimal and suboptimal nutrient status since folate would be required for survival of the cell and for viral replication after incorporation. Thus it would be desirable if an optimal folate status could be maintained at all times in order to minimize the risks for incorporation of a viral genome.

SUMMARY

A growing body of evidence indicates that folic acid deficiency favors the onset of malignant transformation of cells by several possible mechanisms. Although suppression of folate function through the use of folate antagonists has been shown to have beneficial effects *after* the onset of some forms of cancer, it is now apparent that either nutritional deprivation or antagonism may increase the potential for neoplastic changes in otherwise normal cells, *before* cancer is established. Unconfirmed reports have described striking beneficial effects of intravenous injections of triglutamyl folate in two types of cancer in experimental animals. Several broad lines of investigation have been concerned with cancer initiation by altered regulation of genetic expression including both endogenous and exogenous oncogenes. Folate appears to be an important factor in regulating the supply of methyl groups for DNA methylation, which in turn is a major determinant of histone binding, chromosome structure, and gene transcription. Folate also plays a crucial role in the prevention of chromosome breaks at heritable and constitutive fragile sites. Chromosome breaks are essential elements in two of the most important concepts concerning oncogenesis: first, that translocations disrupt internal regulatory mechanisms based on control of endogenous oncogenes by adjacent genomic segments; and second, that chromosome breaks permit incorporation of viral oncogenes into the host genome.

Clinical intervention trials as well as epidemiological studies have shown an association between low-folate status and increased risk of dysplasia or cancer of the cervix, colon, bronchus, and esophagus. Other evidence suggests that folate status modifies responsiveness of target tissue to steroid hormone stimulation. This relationship could have clinical relevance in understanding localized nutrient deficiency and prevention of hormone-dependent malignancies. Recent developments indicate that genetic regulation is affected by histone acetylation as well as by DNA methylation. Future investigations will be needed to explore the new interface of interaction between one-carbon and two-carbon metabolism at the level of the chromosome.

REFERENCES

Angier RB, Boothe JH, Hutchings BL, et al. Synthesis of a compound identical with the L. casei factor isolated from liver. Science 1945; 102:227.

Arthur DC, Danzl TJ, Branda RF. Cytogenetic studies of a family with a hereditary defect of cellular folate uptake and high incidence of hematologic disease. In: Butterworth CE, Jr., Hutchinson ML, eds. Nutritional factors in the induction and maintenance of malignancy. New York: Academic Press, 1983.

Barich LL, Schwarz J, Barich D. Oral methotrexate in mice: A co-carcinogenic as well as an anti-tumor agent to methylcholanthrene-induced cutaneous tumors. J. Invest Dermatol 1986; 39:615–619.

Branda RF, Moldow CF, MacArthur JR, Wintrobe MM, Anthony BK, Jacob HS. Folate-induced remission in aplastic anemia with familial defect of cellular folate uptake. N Engl J Med 1978; 298:469–75.

Branda RF, McCormack JJ, Perlmutter CA, Mathews LA, Robison SH. Effects of folate deficiency on the metastatic potential of murine melanoma cells. Cancer Res 1988; 48:4529–4534.

Brock KE, Berry G, Mock PA, MacLennan R, Truswell AS, Brinton LA. Nutrients in diet and plasma and risk of in situ cervical cancer. J Natl Cancer Inst 1988; 80:580–585.

Butterworth CE, Jr. Vitamin deficiency and cancer. Med Oncol Tumor Pharmacother 1985; 2:165–174.

Butterworth CE Jr, Hatch KD, Gore H, Mueller H, Krumdieck CL. Improvement in cervical dysplasia associated with folic acid therapy in users of oral contraceptives. Am J Clin Nutr 1982; 35:73–82.

Butterworth CE, Jr. Hatch KD, Macaluso M, et al. Folate deficiency and cervical dysplasia (submitted for publication, 1991).

Castro CE. Nucleosomal repeat length in rat liver nuclei is decreased by a high carbohydrate, fat-free diet. J Nutr 1983; 113:557–565.

Castro CE. Nutrient effects on DNA and chromatin structure. Ann Rev Nutr 1987; 7:407–421.

Castro CE, Sevall JS. Alteration of higher order structure of rat liver chromatin by dietary composition. J Nutr 1980; 110:105–116.

Dürst M, Kleinheinz A, Hotz M, Gissmann L. The physical state of human papillomavirus type 16 DNA in benign and malignant genital tumors. J Gen Virol 1985; 66:1515–1522.

Eto I, Krumdieck CL. Role of vitamin B-12 and folate deficiencies in carcinogenesis. Adv Exp Med and Biol 1986; 206:313–330.

Farber S, Cutler EC, Hawkins JW, Harrison JH, Pierce EC 2nd, Lenz GG. The action of pteroylglutamic conjugates on man. Science 1947; 106:619–621.

Farber S, Diamond LK, Mercer RD, Sylvester RF Jr, Wolff JA. Temporary remissions in acute leukemia in children produced by folic acid antagonist, 4-aminopteroyl-glutamic acid (aminopterin). N Engl J Med 1948; 238:787–793.

Francis KT, Thompson RW, Krumdieck CL. Reaction of tetrahydrofolic acid with cyanate from urea solutions: Formation of an inactive folate derivative. Am J Clin Nutr 1977; 30:2028–2032.

Friend C. Cell-free transmission in adult Swiss mice of a disease having the character of a leukemia. J Exp Med 1957; 105:307–318.

Ghadirian P. Food habits of the people of the Caspian Littoral of Iran in relation to esophageal cancer. Nutr Cancer 1987; 9:147–57.

Gilman AG, Goodman LS, Rall TW, Murad F (eds). The pharmacological basis of therapeutics, 7th ed. New York: Macmillan, 1985, 1266.

Goelz SE, Vogelstein B, Hamilton SR, Feinberg AP. Hypomethylation of DNA from benign and malignant human colon neoplasms. Science 1985; 228:187–190.

Goulian M, Bleile B, Tseng BY. Methotrexate-induced misincorporation of uracil in DNA. Proc Natl Acad Sci USA 1980; 77:1956–1960.

Heimburger DC, Alexander CB, Birch R, Butterworth CE Jr, Bailey WC, Krumdieck CL. Improvement in bronchial squamous metaplasia in smokers treated with folate and vitamin B_{12}. Report of a preliminary randomized double-blind intervention trial. JAMA 1988; 259:1525–1530.

Hsieh LL, Wainfan E, Hoshina S, Dizik M, Weinstein IB. Altered expression of retrovirus-like sequences and cellular oncogenes in mice fed methyl-deficient diets. Cancer Res 1989; 49:3795–3799.

Jaskiewicz K, Venter FS, Marasas WF. Cytopathology of the esophagus in Transkei. J Natl Cancer Inst 1987; 79:961–967.

Jaskiewicz, K, Marasas WFO, Lazarus C, Beyers AD, van Helden PD. Association of esophageal cytological abnormalities with vitamin and lipotrope deficiencies in populations at risk of esophageal cancer. Anticancer Res 1988; 8:711–715.

Khaled MA, Watkins CL, Krumdieck CL. Inactivation of B_{12} and folate coenzymes by butyl nitrite as observed by NMR: Implications on one-carbon transfer mechanism. Biochem Biophys Res Commun 1986; 135:201–207.

Koss LG. Diagnostic cytology and its histopathologic bases, 3rd ed. Philadelphia: J.B. Lippincott, 1979.

Kruh J. Effects of sodium butyrate, a new pharmacological agent, on cells in culture. Mol Cell Biochem 1982; 42:65–82.

Krumdieck CL. Role of folate deficiency in carcinogenesis. In: Butterworth CE, Jr., Hutchinson ML, eds. Nutritional factors in the induction and maintenance of malignancy. New York: Academic Press, 1983, 225–245.

Lashner BA, Heidenreich PA, Su GL, Kane SV, Hanauer SB. Effect of folate supplementation on the incidence of dysplasia and cancer in chronic ulcerative colitis. A case-control study, Gastroenterology 1989; 97:255–259.

Leuchtenberger C, Lewisohn R, Laszlo D, Leuchtenberger R. "Folic acid": A tumor growth inhibitor. Proc Soc Exp Biol Med 1944; 55:204–205.

Leuchtenberger R, Leuchtenberger C, Laszlo D, Lewisohn R. The influence of "folic acid" on spontaneous breast cancers in mice. Science 1945; 101:46.

Lewisohn R, Leuchtenberger C, Leuchtenberger R, Keresztesy JC. The influence of liver L. casei factor on spontaneous breast cancer in mice. Science 1946; 104:436–437.

Lloyd HED, Garry J. Atypical cells in vaginal smears in pernicious anemia. Am J Obstet Gynecol 1963; 85:408–412.

Macnab JCM, Walkinshaw SA, Cordiner JW, Clements JB. Human papillomavirus in clinically and histologically normal tissue of patients with genital cancer. N Engl J Med 1986; 315:1052–1058.

Megee PC, Morgan BA, Mittman BA, Smith MM. Genetic analysis of histone H4: Essential role of lysines subject to reversible acetylation. Science 1980; 247:841–845.

Meisels A, Morin C. Human papillomavirus and cancer of the uterine cervix. Gynecol Oncol 1981; 12:S111–S123.

Mitchell HK, Snell EE, Williams RJ. The concentration of "folic acid." J Am Chem Soc 1941; 63:2284.

Muir CS. Epidemiology, basic science, and the prevention of cancer: Implications for the future. Cancer Res 1990; 50:6441–6448.

Ohlsson-Wilhelm BM, Farley BA, Kosciolek B, La Bella S, Rowley PT. K562 Human erythroleukemia cell variants resistant to growth inhibition by butyrate have deficient histone acetylation. Am J Hum Genet 1984; 36:1225–1238.

Pater MM, Hughes GA, Hyslop DE, Nakshatri H, Pater A. Glucocorticoid-dependent oncogenic transformation by type 16 but not type 11 human papilloma virus DNA. Nature 1988; 335:832–835.

Popescu NC, Amsbaugh SC, DiPaolo JA. Human papillomavirus type 18 DNA is integrated at a single chromosome site in cervical carcinoma cell line SW756. J Virol 1987; 61:1682–1685.

Razin A, Riggs AD. DNA methylation and gene function. Science 1980; 210:604–610.

Robbins SL, Kumar V. Basic Pathology, 4th ed. Philadelphia: W. B. Saunders, 1987, 185.

Rowley JD. Identification of the constant chromosome regions involved in human hematologic malignant disease. Science 1982; 216:749–751.

Rowley JD. The Philadelphia chromosome translocation: A paradigm for understanding leukemia. In: Fortner JG, Rhoads JE, eds. Accomplishments in cancer research. Philadelphia: J.B. Lippincott, 1989, 105–116.

Sauberlich HE, Baumann CA. A factor required for the growth of Leuconostoc citrovorum. J Biol Chem 1948; 176:165–173.

Schantz SP, Hsu TC, Ainslie N, Moser RP. Young adults with head and neck cancer express increased susceptibility to mutagen-induced chromosome damage. JAMA 1989; 262:3313–3315.

Schwartz SO, Schoolman HM. The etiology of leukemia: The status of the virus as causative agent—A review. Blood 1959; 14:279–294.

Sutherland GR. Heritable fragile sites on human chromosomes. I. Factors affecting expression in lymphocyte culture. Am J Hum Genet 1979; 31:125–135.

van Helden PD, Beyers AD, Bester AJ, Jaskiewicz K. Esophageal cancer: Vitamin and lipotrope deficiencies in an at-risk South African population. Nutr Cancer 1987; 10:247–255.

Vinograd J, Lebowitz J, Radloff R, Watson R, Laipis P. The twisted circular form of polyoma viral DNA. Biochemistry 1965; 53:1104–1111.

Watson JD. Molecular biology of the gene, 2nd ed. Menlo Park: W.A. Benjamin, 1970.

Weintraub H, Groudine M. Chromosomal subunits in active genes have an altered conformation. Science 1976; 193:848–856.

Wettstein FO. State of viral DNA and gene expression in benign vs malignant tumors. In: Pfister H, ed. Papillomaviruses and human cancer. Boca Raton: CRC Press, 1990, 155–79.

Whitehead N, Reyner F, Lindenbaum J. Megaloblastic changes in the cervical epithelium. Association with oral contraceptive therapy and reversal with folic acid. JAMA 1973; 226:1421–1424.

Yunis JJ, Soreng AL. Constitutive fragile sites and cancer. Science 1984; 226:1199–1204.

Ziegler RG, Morris LE, Blot WJ, Pottern LM, Hoover R, Fraumeni JF. Esophageal cancer among black men in Washington D.C. II. Role of nutrition. J Natl Cancer Inst 1981; 67:1199–1206.

zur Hausen H. Human papillomaviruses and their possible role in squamous cell carcinomas. Curr Top Microbiol Immunol 1977; 78:1–30.

NEUROLOGICAL FUNCTIONS

9

Relationship of Vitamin B$_6$, Vitamin B$_{12}$, and Folate to Neurological and Neuropsychiatric Disorders

Howerde E. Sauberlich

University of Alabama at Birmingham
Birmingham, Alabama

Considerable attention has been given to the metabolic roles of vitamin B$_6$, vitamin B$_{12}$, and folate. More recently, the importance of these vitamins in neurological diseases has been recognized. This chapter will consider interactions of vitamin B$_6$, vitamin B$_{12}$, and folate in neurological disorders.

VITAMIN B$_6$ (PYRIDOXINE)

General Considerations

Vitamin B$_6$ was established in 1934 as a nutritional factor required to prevent rat acrodynia (György, 1934, 1935, 1971; Sauberlich, 1981). The isolated vitamin was called pyridoxine and is the common commercial and pharmaceutical form of vitamin B$_6$. The vitamin occurs in nature in three forms: pyridoxine, pyridoxal, and pyridoxamine. All three forms exist as phosphorylated derivatives, with pyridoxal-5'-phosphate functioning as the coenzyme form of vitamin B$_6$. However, the various forms of the vitamin are readily converted in the body into pyridoxal phosphate by the action of pyridoxal kinase. The predominent form of vitamin B$_6$ in human plasma is pyridoxal phosphate (Coburn and Mahuren, 1983). Pyridoxal phosphate functions as a coenzyme in a large number and variety of enzyme actions concerned almost entirely with protein and amino acid metabolism (Sauberlich and Canham, 1980; Sauberlich, 1985). Examples are its roles in the formation of serotonin from 5-OH-tryptophan, transamination reactions, biosynthesis of delta-aminolevulinic acid (a precursor essential for hemoglobin formation), and in the conversion of homocysteine to cystathionine and its further conversion to cysteine.

Vitamin B_6 deficiency in experimental animals, such as the pig, results in peripheral nervous system changes that include degeneration of the peripheral nerves, spinal roots, posterior root ganglia, and sensory ganglia (Follis and Wintrobe, 1945; Swank and Adams, 1948). The changes resemble those observed with vitamin B_{12} deficiency. However, the changes respond to vitamin B_6 administration, but not to vitamin B_{12}.

Clinically, vitamin B_6 deficiency in the human is manifested often as central nervous system changes and with the occurrence of abnormal electroencephalograms (Coursin, 1964; Sauberlich, 1964, 1981). Seborrheic dermatitis and eczema may occur in the regions of the mouth, nose, and ears. Cheilosis, glossitis, and angular stomatitis may be present. Hyperirritability and convulsive seizures may occur with children. Hypochromic, microcytic anemia is only rarely observed in children or adults (Coursin, 1964; Harris and Horrigan, 1964). A subclinical deficiency of vitamin B_6 is often detected by an increased excretion of xanthurenic acid due to altered metabolism of tryptophan (Sauberlich et al., 1972).

Genetic Defects

An overt clinical deficiency of vitamin B_6 appears to be relatively rare. Most often a deficiency is associated with a genetic defect that results in a vitamin B_6 dependency syndrome. These conditions can usually be controlled with the use of therapeutic doses of vitamin B_6.

Most vitamin B_6 syndromes, or vitamin B_6-related inborn errors of metabolism, fall into the following categories: (1) xanthurenic aciduria due to a defect in tryptophan metabolism as a result of reduced kynureninase activity; (2) homocystinuria due to reduced gamma-cystathionase or cystathionine-beta-synthase activity; (3) convulsions due to reduced brain glutamic acid decarboxylase activity; and (4) anemia due to reduced delta-aminolevulinic acid synthase activity (Ebadi, 1978; Sturman, 1978, 1981; Sauberlich, 1981; Merrill and Henderson, 1987). Fortuantely, these syndromes usually respond to continuous high daily doses of pyridoxine (Scriver, 1973; Rosenberg, 1976; Grieco, 1977; Bankier et al., 1983; Crowell and Roach, 1983; Krishnamoorthy, 1983; Stephenson and Byrne, 1983; Fowler, 1985; Merrill and Henderson, 1987).

Mental retardation and psychiatric manifestations are often accompanied by accumulation of homocysteine in plasma as the first indication of a cystationine-beta-synthase deficiency. The deficiency in the enzyme appears to be caused by more than one type of gene mutation (Fowler, 1985). Consequently, many but not all cases of the enzyme deficiency are responsive to pyridoxine supplements (Abbott et al., 1987; Ferraris et al., 1988; Ueland and Refsum, 1989).

Pyridoxine-dependent seizures due to an increased requirement of the vitamin within the central nervous system require prompt diagnosis and treatment in order to prevent irreversible neurological damage (Bankier et al., 1983; Crowell and Roach, 1983; Krishnamoorthy, 1983; Stephenson and Byrne, 1983).

Vitamin B_6 Deficiency and Neuropathy

Alcoholism

Alcoholic patients may exhibit peripheral neuropathy, convulsions, and sideroblastic anemia. Alcohol has a systemic effect on the maintenance of blood pyridoxal phosphate levels (Li, 1978; Li and Lumeng, 1985) and can interfere in the utilization of iron for heme synthesis. Biochemical evidence of a vitamin B_6 deficiency has been observed in 20–30% of alcoholic patients.

Nervous System Disorders

In early studies with the rat, vitamin B_6 deficiency resulted in epileptiform convulsions. Subsequent investigations have shown that in vitamin B_6 deficiency, a marked reduction occurs in the level of gamma-aminobutyric acid (GABA) in the brain (Roberts et al., 1964; Ebadi, 1978). GABA is an established inhibitory neurotransmitter that is formed from glutamic acid by the pyridoxal phosphate-dependent glutamic acid decarboxylase enzyme. Moreover, other neurotransmitters, including serotonin, dopamine, and norepinephrine as well as histamine and taurine, are produced by pyridoxal phosphate-dependent enzymes (Coburn, 1985; Dakshinamurti et al., 1985). Vitamin B_6 deficiency results in peripheral nervous system changes in experimental animals. Although the neurological condition resembles that observed in a vitamin B_{12} deficiency, it responds only to vitamin B_6 supplementation.

Autistic Children

The benefit of vitamin B_6 supplements, usually in conjunction with magnesium, has been studied in autistic children. Some autistic children have been reported to show clinical improvement during double-blind trials of short-term treatment with a combination of vitamin B_6 and magnesium (Rimland et al., 1978; Barthelemy et al., 1981; Martineau et al., 1988a,b). However, to appropriately assess the efficacy of this treatment will require long-term, well-designed, and placebo-controlled studies with large numbers of autistic children (Martineau et al., 1988a,b).

Carpal Tunnel Syndrome

Carpal tunnel syndrome is a common peripheral neuropathy often associated with hypoesthesia, paresthesia, and pain in the hand (Kopell and Goodgold, 1968; Phalen, 1970; Amadio, 1985). Surgical treatment is sometimes required to relieve the compression of the median nerve at the wrist (Smith et al., 1984; Amadio,

1985, 1987). However, a number of reports have suggested that pyridoxine supplements may be of benefit in some patients (Bernstein, 1990; Ellis et al., 1981, 1982; Ellis, 1987; Kasdan and Janes, 1987). Ellis and colleagues explored extensively the use of pyridoxine supplements in the treatment of carpal tunnel syndrome (Ellis, 1987; Ellis and Preston, 1985; Ellis et al., 1976, 1979, 1981, 1982; Folkers et al., 1978; Shizukuishi et al., 1980). The treatment usually involved the daily use of 50 to 300 mg of pyridoxine (Ellis, 1987; Ellis and Folkers, 1990; Folkers and Ellis, 1990). Since many of the reports were based on studies that lacked a satisfactory scientific design, the treatment with pyridoxine has been met with skepticism (Smith et al., 1984; Scheyer and Hass, 1985; Amadio, 1987; Kasdan and James, 1987). Nevertheless some studies showed a beneficial effect from pyridoxine, while in others it was without benefit (McCann and Davis, 1979; Beyers et al., 1984; Smith et al., 1984; D'Souza, 1985; Guzman et al., 1989).

Kasdan and Janes (1987) reviewed 994 patients with a diagnosis of carpal tunnel syndrome. Of the diagnosed cases, 27% received surgical treatment with success in approximately 97% of patients. In 494 patients treated with pyridoxine at a dosage of 100 mg twice daily, 68% had satisfactory improvement. The investigators suggested that the use of vitamin B_6 may be helpful in many cases of carpal tunnel syndrome.

Although D'Souza (1985) obtained complete remission of the carpal tunnel syndrome in 16 of 19 patients with daily pyridoxine supplements of 100–200 mg for up to 6 months, Scheyer and Haas (1985) failed to observe any benefit from comparable pyridoxine treatment in 13 patients. From a recent study of 12 patients with carpal tunnel syndrome, Guzman et al. (1989) concluded that pyridoxine supplementation may serve as an adjuvant treatment of carpal tunnel syndrome patients undergoing surgery.

The therapeutic effectiveness of pyridoxine supplementation in the treatment of patients with carpal tunnel syndrome remains controversial. Perhaps only selected patients may benefit from the supplements (Amadio, 1985). Beyers et al. (1984) categorized their patients with symptoms suggestive of carpal tunnel syndrome into four groups based on standardized electrodiagnostic criteria: (a) carpal tunnel syndrome, (b) peripheral neuropathy, (c) peripheral neuropathy and carpal tunnel syndrome, and (d) none. As a result, they suggested that the positive response observed in patients with carpal tunnel syndrome receiving pyridoxine supplements may be related to an unrecognized peripheral neuropathy. The etiology of carpal tunnel syndrome appears uncertain, but it is known to occur frequently in association with abnormal metabolism such as diabetes mellitus, alcoholism, pregnancy, obesity, and hypothyroidism (Taylor, 1971). Consequently, divergence in response to pyridoxine supplementation may relate to diverse factors that may have induced the syndrome in the patient studied.

Drugs and Vitamin B$_6$ Metabolism

Oral Contraceptive Agents

Nearly 25 years ago it was observed that women using oral contraceptive agents (OCA) excreted elevated amounts of xanthurenic acid in the urine following a test load of L-tryptophan. Pyridoxine supplements of 25 mg/day corrected the abnormal excretion (Rose, 1978a,b; Bermond, 1982; Miller, 1985). The abnormal tryptophan metabolism associated with using OCA is probably the result of direct inhibition of kynureninase by estrogen. In the rat, the four- to five-fold excess of apokynureninase in the liver can be activated by pyridoxine supplements (Bender, 1982; Bender et al., 1982). Thus, the normalization of tryptophan metabolism by pyridoxine supplements is due to an increase in kynureninase activity which thereby overcomes the inhibition. In some instances women on OCA complain of nervousness, depression, irritability, or headaches (Baumblatt and Winston, 1970; Adams et al., 1973). Usually the condition is improved or corrected with daily supplements of 10–25 mg of pyridoxine (Adams et al., 1973; Rose, 1978a; Bermond, 1982). Oral contraceptive agents may lower plasma pyridoxal phosphate levels and alter tryptophan metabolism, but whether the requirement for vitamin B$_6$ is truly increased remains unclear (Baumblatt and Winston, 1970; Luhby et al., 1971; Rose et al., 1972; Leklem et al., 1975; Shane and Contractor, 1975; Miller et al., 1978; Rose, 1978a). Rose (1978a) concluded that the available evidence does not justify the routine supplementation of dietary vitamin B$_6$ intake with pyridoxine in OCA users.

Antibiotics, Anticonvulsants, and Other Antimetabolites

Isoniazid, like other hydrazides, forms a hydrazone with vitamin B$_6$ to cause the vitamin to be inactive or inhibited (Bauernfeind and Miller, 1978; Brown et al., 1984a; Bhagavan, 1985; Pellock et al., 1985; Ueland and Refsum, 1989). Consequently, prolonged use of isoniazid to treat tuberculosis can induce signs of vitamin B$_6$ deficiency, including peripheral neuritis and a pellagra-like dermatitis. Administration of 15–50 mg of vitamin B$_6$ daily in combination with the isoniazid will cure or prevent the condition without affecting the beneficial effects of the chemotherapeutic agent. Other medications, such as hydralazine, penicillamine, cyloserine, corticosteroids, and anticonvulsants, may also antagonize vitamin B$_6$ and increase the daily requirement of the vitamin from 2 mg to intakes of 60–120 mg (Bauernfeind and Miller, 1978; Ebadi, 1978; Bhagavan, 1985).

Celiac Disease

In general, celiac disease, which is due to a sensitivity to the gliadin fraction of wheat gluten, is associated with an impaired absorption of folate and iron and, to a lesser degree, an impaired absorption of vitamin B$_{12}$ (Hoffbrand, 1974; Chanarin, 1980b). Consequently, the patients usually have low plasma and eryth-

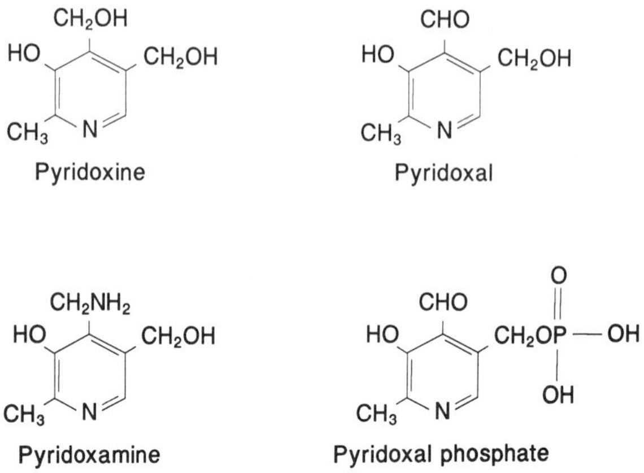

Figure 1   Structures of several forms of vitamin B_6.

rocyte folate levels. In addition, about 25% may have reduced serum vitamin B_{12} levels. The condition is usually treated with use of a gluten-free diet and supplements of folate. Iron and vitamin B_{12} supplements may also be necessary.

Adults with celiac disease often show signs of mental depression. A Swedish study of 12 celiac patients treated with daily oral doses of 80 mg of pyridoxine for 6 months observed significant improvement in the signs of depression (Hallert et al., 1983). Folate supplementation for 1 year was without improvement in mood. The benefits of pyridoxine therapy in these patients, if substantiated, could be of clinical importance because of the debilitating effects of the mental depression of celiac disease.

Toxicity of Vitamin B_6

Since little vitamin B_6 is stored in the body (25–30 mg), an excess intake of the vitamin is excreted unaltered or as its metabolite, 4-pyridoxic acid. Consequently, excess intakes of the vitamin are usually removed readily from the body without any evidence of toxicity. For instance, the treatment of patients with genetic defects in vitamin B_6 metabolism, premenstrual syndrome, and certain types of mental disorders often involves the use of daily supplements of 100–300 mg of vitamin B_6 for extended periods without apparent side effects (Scriver, 1973; Rosenberg, 1976; Abraham and Hargrove, 1980; O'Brien, 1982; Coburn et al., 1983; Rudman and Williams, 1983; Pauling, 1984; Gunn, 1985; London et al. 1985; Smallwood et al., 1986; Bendich and Cohen, 1990; Bernstein, 1990). Even higher doses of 600–3000 mg per day of pyridoxine have been administered to autistic, schizophrenic, and hyperkinetic children (Pauling et al., 1973; Rimland et al., 1978; Brenner, 1982). Side effects were not reported.

However, prolonged high intakes of the vitamin have been reported to result in toxic effects (Berger and Schaumburg, 1984; Davidson, 1984; Dalton, 1985; Parry and Bredesen, 1985; Podell, 1985; Friedman et al., 1986; Waterstron and Gilligan, 1987). For example, in a preliminary report of an uncontrolled study, a vitamin B_6 dependency, resulting in abnormal electroencephalograms and convulsion, was observed in three of eight normal adult men who ingested daily supplements of 200 mg of pyridoxine for over a month (Canham et al., 1963). More recent studies suggest that the administration of 500 mg of pyridoxine or even less per day over a prolonged period may result in sensory nerve damage (Schaumburg et al., 1983; Parry and Bredesen, 1985; Cohen and Bendich, 1986; Dalton and Dalton, 1987; Bendich and Cohen, 1990). Discontinuance of the pyridoxine supplementation appeared to reverse the neurological changes, although this may require a period of several weeks or longer (Podell, 1985; Cohen and Bendich, 1986; Friedman et al., 1986; Dalton and Dalton, 1987). It is interesting that either a deficiency of vitamin B_6 or an excess of the vitamin may induce adverse neurological changes.

VITAMIN B_{12} (COBALAMIN)

General Considerations

An anemia was described in 1822 that became known as Addisonian pernicious anemia (Castle, 1961). It was not until 1926 that a dietary factor was associated with this megaloblastic anemia (Minot and Murphy, 1926). Subsequently, it was found that a gastric intrinsic factor was essential for the absorption of the dietary (or extrinsic) factor (Castle, 1953). In 1948 a crystalline red substance was isolated by Rickes et al. (1948) and termed vitamin B_{12}. A similar report was made shortly thereafter by British investigators (Smith and Parker, 1948). Only microgram quantities of the vitamin were required to produce a positive hematological response in patients suffering with pernicious anemia.

Vitamin B_{12} is a relatively stable compound with a complex structural formula that consists of a corrin nucleus linked through aminopropanol to a nucleotide containing dimethylbenzimidazole. An atom of cobalt is present in the corrin ring system that is also attached to the dimethylbenzimidazole group. Compounds with this structure are called cobalamins. Several congeners of vitamin B_{12} exist (Chanarin, 1980a). The commercial form of vitamin B_{12} has cyanide attached to the cobalt atom. Although little cyanocobalamin exists in nature, this is a stable form of the vitamin. The active coenzyme forms of vitamin B_{12} are 5-deoxyadenosylcobalamin and methylcobalamin. Vitamin B_{12} is present in the liver predominantly as 5-deoxyadenosylcobalamin (65–75%) with the remainder consisting of hydroxocobalamin (20–30%) and methylcobalamin (1–5%). In blood the predominant form is methylcobalamin (Linnell, 1975).

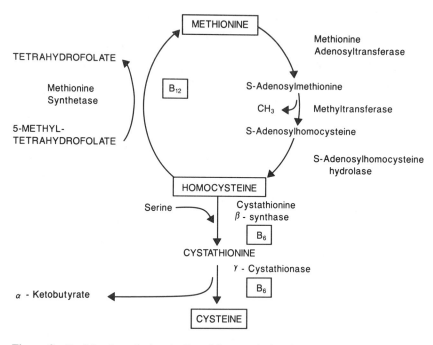

Figure 2   Participation of vitamin B_{12}, folate, and vitamin B_6 in the metabolism of methionine and homocysteine.

The 5-deoxyadenosylcobalamin form of vitamin B_{12} serves as a cofactor for the mitchondrial mutase enzyme that catalyzes the isomerization of methylmalonyl coenzyme A to succinyl coenzyme A. The metabolism of odd-chain-length fatty acids is dependent on this reaction. The methylcobalamin form is essential for the activation of methionine synthase (methyltransferase) that participates in the removal of the methyl group from folate in the homocysteine-methionine trans-methylation reaction. Consequently, a vitamin B_{12} deficiency results in folate being "trapped" as methyltetrahydrofolate (Chanarin, 1980a; Chanarin et al., 1985; Herbert, 1987; Herbert and Colman, 1988).

Although vitamin B_{12} is essential for the normal maturation of erythrocytes and for the normal functioning of all cells, increased attention has recently been given to its role in the nervous system. In the human, vitamin B_{12} deficiency causes a degeneration of peripheral nerves, portions of the posterior and lateral column of the spinal cord, and probably changes in the brain (Hillman, 1985; Herbert and Colman, 1988). Not all subjects with megaloblastic anemia due to vitamin B_{12} deficiency exhibit evidence of neuropathy. Conversely, vitamin B_{12} deficiency may also result in neurological changes without changes in the blood

(Lindenbaum et al., 1988). However, prolonged vitamin B_{12} deficiency produces irreversible damage to the nervous system, apparently as a result of inadequate myelin synthesis. It should be noted that because of their close metabolic inter-relationship, a deficiency of either vitamin B_{12} or folate can result in a morpho-logically identical macrocytic anemia, megaloblastic bone marrow changes, and hypersegmented polymorphonuclear neutrophils (Chanarin, 1980a; Chanarin et al., 1985; Herbert, 1987; Herbert and Colman, 1988).

Genetic Defects

In rare instances, hereditary disorders of vitamin B_{12} metabolism may result in neurological dysfunctions (Carmel et al., 1988b; Cooper and Rosenblatt, 1987). Therapy with hydroxycobalamin provided a favorable neurological response and usually a dramatic reduction in the excretion of methylmalonic acid associated with the condition (Shinnar and Singer, 1984; Mamlok et al., 1986; Mitchell et al., 1986). Prompt recognition and early treatment of the vitamin B_{12} disorder are essential.

Vitamin B_{12} Deficiency and Neuropathy

General

A vitamin B_{12} deficiency neuropathy may develop in patients as a result of intestinal malabsorption rather than classical pernicious anemia (Dastur et al., 1975). The neurological features of vitamin B_{12} deficiency either from malab-sorption or pernicious anemia are identical (Victor and Adams, 1983; McCombe and McLeod, 1984). The neurological features indicate spinal cord compression, characterized by symmetrical posterolateral degeneration in the spinal cord, usu-ally accompanied by peripheral sensory neuropathy (Martin, 1988). Histological observations indicate primary demyelinating changes (Dastur et al., 1975; Victor and Adams, 1983).

By the late 1950s, serum vitamin B_{12} levels were recognized as a valuable clinical test. Serum levels of vitamin B_{12} could be used to diagnose vitamin B_{12} deficiency in pernicious anemia as well as dietary deficiency of the vitamin before anemia developed. Serum vitamin B_{12} levels in the range of 75–112 pmol/liter (100–150 ng/liter) are indicative of early vitamin B_{12} deficiency, although anemia and macrocytosis may be absent (Strachan and Henderson, 1965).

A number of reports indicate that the usual criteria for diagnosing vitamin B_{12} deficiency and pernicious anemia are not sufficiently sensitive. In the extensive study of Lindenbaum and associates (1988), 28% (40 patients) of the 141 con-secutive patients with neuropsychiatric abnormalities due to vitamin B_{12} deficiency had no macrocytosis or anemia. Serum vitamin B_{12} levels were frequently in the low normal range. Sixteen patients had levels between 75 and 150 pmol/liter (100 and 200 ng/liter). The patients commonly suffered from paresthesia of the

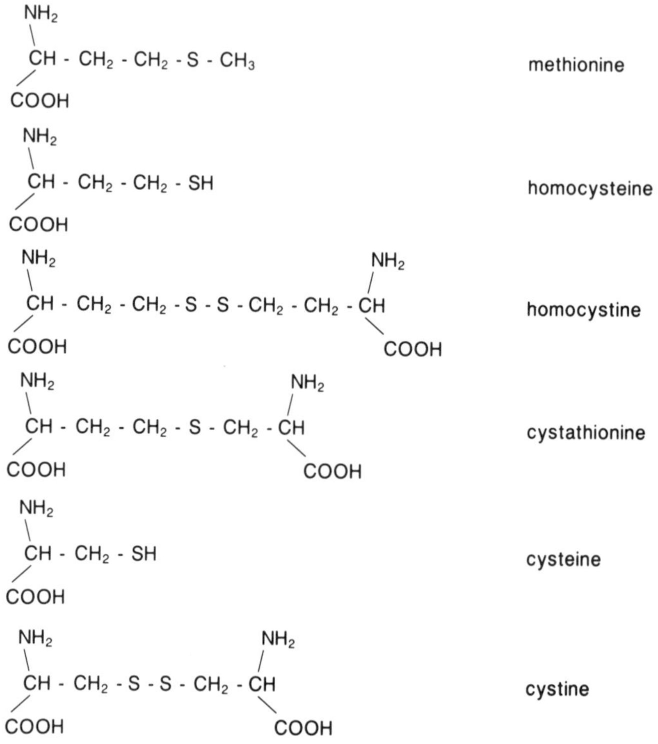

$$NH_2$$
$$\text{CH - CH}_2\text{ - CH}_2\text{ - S - CH}_3 \qquad\qquad\qquad \text{methionine}$$
$$COOH$$

$$NH_2$$
$$\text{CH - CH}_2\text{ - CH}_2\text{ - SH} \qquad\qquad\qquad\qquad \text{homocysteine}$$
$$COOH$$

$$NH_2 \qquad\qquad\qquad\qquad\qquad\qquad NH_2$$
$$\text{CH - CH}_2\text{ - CH}_2\text{ - S - S - CH}_2\text{ - CH}_2\text{ - CH} \qquad \text{homocystine}$$
$$COOH \qquad\qquad\qquad\qquad\qquad COOH$$

$$NH_2 \qquad\qquad\qquad\qquad NH_2$$
$$\text{CH - CH}_2\text{ - CH}_2\text{ - S - CH}_2\text{ - CH} \qquad\qquad \text{cystathionine}$$
$$COOH \qquad\qquad\qquad\qquad COOH$$

$$NH_2$$
$$\text{CH - CH}_2\text{ - SH} \qquad\qquad\qquad\qquad\qquad \text{cysteine}$$
$$COOH$$

$$NH_2 \qquad\qquad\qquad\qquad NH_2$$
$$\text{CH - CH}_2\text{ - S - S - CH}_2\text{ - CH} \qquad\qquad\qquad \text{cystine}$$
$$COOH \qquad\qquad\qquad\qquad COOH$$

Figure 3 Structures of methionine metabolites.

extremities, ataxia, memory loss, and weakness of the limbs as well as cerebral symptoms and changes in mood and personality, Of significance was the elevated serum level of total homocysteine and methylmalonic acid in 36 of 37 patients measured. All of the patients responded to vitamin B_{12} therapy. The responses included a marked reduction in the serum levels of methylmalonic acid and of total homocysteine, and improvement in neuropsychiatric abnormalities and hematological findings. The investigators concluded that neuropsychiatric disorders due to vitamin B_{12} deficiency may occur frequently in the absence of anemia or an elevated mean red cell volume (Lindenbaum et al., 1988). These findings suggest that measurement of serum levels of total homocysteine and methylmalonic acid both before and after cobalamin treatment would be useful in the diagnosis of such patients.

Megaloblastic anmeia is commonly considered an early manifestation of vitamin B_{12} deficiency, while neurological symptoms have generally been considered to be late manifestations of a deficiency of the vitamin (Victor and Lear,

1956; Babior and Bunn, 1987). Neurological disorders in the absence of anemia have been described for vitamin B_{12}-deficient patients but such cases have been considered to be exceptional or unusual (Babior and Bunn, 1987). Strachan and Henderson (1965) described psychiatric syndromes due to vitamin B_{12} deficiency in patients with normal bone marrow and normal hematological parameters. It is now recognized that chronic deficiency of vitamin B_{12} can lead to neurological abnormalities, mania, and dementia with associated degeneration of the spinal cord as well as brain damage (Goggans, 1984; Gross et al., 1986; Jones et al., 1987; Karnaze and Carmel, 1987; Beck, 1988; Hector and Burton, 1988; Lindenbaum et al., 1988; Martin, 1988; Steiner et al., 1988). The exact relationship of vitamin B_{12} deficiency to neurological abnormalities remains unknown (Carmel et al., 1988a,b; Steiner et al., 1988).

Nitrous Oxide

The use of nitrous oxide as an anesthetic was reported to induce a neurological dysfunction in two adult women (Schilling, 1986). Further evaluation revealed that the subjects had an acute subclinical vitamin B_{12} deficiency. Other studies in humans and animals demonstrated that nitrous oxide acutely and severely interferes with vitamin B_{12} metabolism (Deacon et al., 1978; Blanco and Peters, 1983; Chanarin et al., 1985; Banerjee and Matthews, 1990).

Vegans

Vegan diets from which animal proteins are rigidly removed have seen increased use. These diets are often deficient in vitamin B_{12} and, hence, pose a risk of producing a deficiency, particularly in pregnant and lactating women. Higginbottom and associates (1978) described vitamin B_{12} deficiency in a 6-month-old infant who had been exclusively breast-fed by a strict vegetarian mother. Severe manifestations of central nervous system involvement were observed. The infant was described as hypothermic, in a deep coma, flaccid, and completely unresponsive. As a consequence of the severe vitamin B_{12} deficiency, the infant suffered from methylmalonic aciduria, homocystinuria, and a moderate cystathionuria. A dramatic response occurred in vitamin B_{12} therapy. The infant was discharged after 14 days. Such observations reiterate the importance of vitamin B_{12} supplementation in strict vegetarians and, in particular, vegan women who breast-feed their infants.

Vitamin B_{12} and Psychiatric Disease

General

An association between vitamin B_{12} deficiency and psychiatric disease was first observed by Addison in 1868 who noted that the "mind occasionally wanders" in pernicious anemia patients (Roos and Willanger, 1977; Moss et al., 1987).

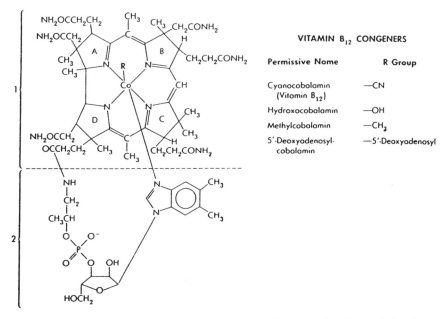

VITAMIN B$_{12}$ CONGENERS

Permissive Name	R Group
Cyanocobalamin (Vitamin B$_{12}$)	—CN
Hydroxocobalamin	—OH
Methylcobalamin	—CH$_3$
5'-Deoxyadenosyl-cobalamin	—5'-Deoxyadenosyl

Figure 4   Structures of vitamin B$_{12}$ and congeners. [Reproduced with permission from *Goodman and Gilman's Pharmacological Basis of Therapeutics*, 7th ed., edited by Alfred Goodman Gilman, Louis S. Goodman, Theodore W. Rall, and Ferid Murad, Macmillan, New York, 1985.]

Subsequently, numerous reports have noted psychiatric and behavioral problems concomitant with vitamin B$_{12}$ deficiency (Samson et al., 1952; Holmes, 1956; Weiner and Hope, 1959; Smith, 1960; Shulman, 1967a; Zucker et al., 1981; Cole and Prchal, 1984; Petrie and Ban, 1985; Hector and Burton, 1988; Levitt and Jaffe, 1989). Although this mental dysfunction may occur at any age, it is noted more frequently in elderly patients (Crantz, 1985; Moss et al., 1987; Green, 1989). Since the psychiatric symptoms may precede hematological and neurological changes of vitamin B$_{12}$ deficiency by moths or even years, an early diagnosis of pernicious anemia or deficiency of the vitamin may be missed (Strachan and Henderson, 1965; Lindenbaum et al., 1988). If the vitamin B$_{12}$ deficiency is recognized before irreversible neurological damage has occurred, vitamin B$_{12}$ therapy may effectively reverse the symptoms (Krein et al., 1984; Hillman, 1985; Herbert and Colman, 1988).

Alzheimer-Type Dementia

Low serum vitamin B$_{12}$ concentrations occur more frequently in patients with Alzheimer-type dementia than in nondemented patients or in patients with other types of dementia (Cole and Prchal, 1984). This observation is of interest since vitamin B_{12} deficiency is recognized to induce memory loss, confusion, and neurological damage (Samson et al., 1952; Homes, 1956; Weiner and Hope, 1959; Smith, 1960; Strachan and Henderson, 1965; Shulman, 1967a).

Other investigators also reported a high incidence of low serum vitamin B_{12} concentrations in elderly patients with organic psychosyndromes, dementia, or confusional states (Droller and Dossett, 1959; Dawson and Donald, 1966). However, in several studies no association was observed between low serum vitamin B_{12} and confusion or memory state among elderly patients (Cape and Shinton, 1961; Elwood et al, 1971). Most patients with Alzheimer-type dementia fail to respond to vitamin B_{12} therapy (Shulman, 1967b; Hughes et al., 1970; Kral et al., 1970), suggesting that irreversible changes may have occurred as a result of prolonged low serum vitamin B_{12} concentrations (Coyle et al., 1983). Whether a direct causal relationship exists between Alzheimer-type dementia and low serum vitamin B_{12} concentrations is unclear.

FOLATE (FOLIC ACID, FOLACIN)

General Considerations

The anemia due to a deficiency of either folate or vitamin B_{12} has the common morphological features of megaloblastic erythropoiesis. In 1926, Addisonian pernicious anemia was recognized as a condition associated with diet. However, the subsequent efforts of Wills (1933) demonstrated that another dietary factor, now known as folate, was associated with the megaloblastic anemia of pregnant women. The yellow vitamin was isolated from spinach in 1941 (Mitchell et al., 1941). Folic acid is the commercially synthesized form of the vitamin. Folate occurs in animals and plants in the form of numerous derivatives, particularly as polyglutamates. The predominant form of folate in human plasma is 5-methyltetrahydrofolate. Folate derivatives participate in various reactions that involve the transfer of single carbon units. As such, the vitamin participates in thymidine and purine biosynthesis, formate metabolism, formation of methionine from homocysteine, choline synthesis, and glycine formation from serine. The formation of thymidylate, essential for deoxyribonucleic acid synthesis and cell division, is dependent on the presence of both folate and vitamin B_{12}. Consequently, a deficiency of either will result in a megaloblastic anemia.

In addition to megaloblastic anemia, folate deficiency may result in several clinical symptoms. They include tiredness, weakness, pallor, sleeplessness, forgetfulness, periods of euphoria, and sometimes glossitis and anorexia. Although folate deficiency has not been considered to produce neurological complications (Herbert, 1972; Anderson and Talbot, 1981; Herbert and Colman, 1988), this consideration appears to be in question (Martin, 1988). Folate deficiency is relatively common as indicated from nutrition surveys (Subar et al., 1989, Sauberlich, 1990). Low blood folate levels have been observed in young women and the elderly (Grinblat, 1985; Marcus & Freedman, 1985). In addition to low dietary intakes, folate deficiency may result from excessive alcohol consumption, pregnancy, and certain medications, especially oral contraceptive agents (Rose et al., 1984; Roe, 1985; Kanazawa & Herbert, 1986; Subar et al., 1989; Sauberlich, 1990).

Genetic Defects Involving Folate

Occasionally, patients with inborn errors of folate metabolism are observed with neurological disorders and psychotic problems (Luhby et al., 1961; Santiago-Borrero et al., 1973; Freeman et al., 1975). Some patients responded partially to treatment with large amounts of folic acid (Luhby et al., 1961; Santiago-Borrero et al., 1973; Freeman et al., 1975; Botez et al., 1976). Several patients have been reported with a complete inability to absorb any form of folate from the gastrointestinal tract (Luhby et al, 1961; Santiago-Borrero et al., 1973). These patients were mentally retarded, had seizures and other neurological manifestations, and had severe megaloblastic anemia. The anemia responded only to large doses of folate administered by injection. Thus, an increasing body of evidence supports the concept that folate deficiency per se can affect the nervous system and give rise to neurological signs and symptoms.

A child has been described who had congenital folate malabsorption (Corbeel et al., 1985). The child had convulsions, diarrhea, anemia, and the appearance of mental retardation. The authors concluded from their investigations that folate deficiency was caused by a defect in folate transport across both the intestine and the blood-brain barrier. The convulsions were dramatically controlled with a therapeutic trial of methionine, folate, and vitamin B_{12}. Additional inborn errors of metabolism that involve folate have been summarized by Chanarin (1980b) and Davis (1986).

Patients with 5,10-methylenetetrahydrofolate reductase deficiency may have demyelination in the brain and subacute combined degeneration of the spinal cord (Clayton et al., 1986; Hyland et al., 1988). This enzyme catalyzes the synthesis of the methyl donor, 5-methyltetrahydrofolate, which is the main form of plasma and tissue folate. Consequently, patients with this enzyme deficiency have reduce concentrations of folate in plasma, erythrocytes, and spinal cord (Rowe, 1983; Hyland et al., 1988). The patients also may have elevated concentrations of homocyst(e)ine in their blood and urine, along with reduced concentrations of methionine in plasma and reduced concentrations of S-adenosyl-methionine and of the neurotransmitter amine metabolites in cerebral spinal fluid (Erbe, 1979; Harpey et al., 1983; Rowe, 1983; Wendel and Bremer, 1984; Clayton et al., 1986; Hyland et al., 1988; Kang et al., 1988). The mechanism of demyelination found in these patients is unknown, but may be associated with impaired *S*-adenosylmethionine metabolism (Hyland et al., 1988). *S*-Adenosyl-methionine serves in several important methylation reactions in the brain and has antidepressant effects (Reynolds et al., 1984). The use of *S*-adenosylmethionine resulted in significant improvement in severely depressed patients (Bottiglieri et al., 1988; Carney et al., 1988; Janicak et al., 1988; Potkin et al., 1988; Rosenbaum et al., 1988; Tolbert, 1988).

Patients with hereditary deficiency of 5, 10-methylenetetrahydrofolate reductase require prompt therapy with folic acid or folinic acid (N^5-formyltetrahydro-folate; citrovorum factor; leucovorin); some cases may require, in addition, supplements of vitamin B_6, vitamin B_{12}, methionine, or betaine to prevent neurological deterioration (Harpey et al., 1981; Wendel and Bremer, 1984). Children with homocystinuria and a suspected deficiency of 5,10-methylenete-trahydrofolate reductase activity have been reported to have periodic rages and seizures (Murphy et al., 1985). Therapy with folic acid provided a dramatic improvement in patients.

Fragile X Syndrome

Folate has been reported to be effective in the treatment of patients with fragile X syndrome (Lejeune, 1981, 1982; Harpey, 1982; Brown et al., 1984b; Erbe, 1984; Erbe and Wang, 1989; Simensen and Rogers, 1989). This inherited disorder is second only to Down syndrome among the genetic causes of mental retardation (Simensen and Rogers, 1989). One in 2610 males and one in 4221 females have been reported to be afflicted by the fragile X syndrome (Turner et al., 1986). Intellectual functioning is more severely affected in the male than in the female heterozygote. Although early treatment of the child with folate may be of some benefit (Simensen and Rogers, 1989), long-term studies are needed to adequately assess the effectiveness of therapy.

Folate Deficiency and Neuropathy

Although less frequent, folate deficiency may produce neurological changes identical to that of vitamin B_{12} deficiency (Grant et al., 1965; Pincus et al., 1972; Marcus and Freedman, 1985; Grinblat, 1985; Davis, 1986). Neurological signs and symptoms that could be associated with folate deficiency have now received considerable attention (Hansen et al., 1964; Fleming and Dada, 1966; Fehling et al., 1974; Manzoor and Runcie, 1976; Reynolds, 1976; Botez et al., 1979; Grinblat, 1985; Marcus and Freedman, 1985; Abou-Saleh and Coppen, 1986; Martin, 1988). Folate deficiency has been associated with a high incidence of forgetfulness and irritability, sometimes with hostility and paranoid behavior (Vatassery and Maletta, 1983; Herbert and Colman, 1988). In an experiment conducted on himself, Herbert described, after 4 months on a folate-deficient diet, mental changes that included forgetfulness, irritability, and insomnia (Herbert, 1962). Folate supplementation promptly reversed the mental changes. An association of dementia in patients with low serum folate concentrations was reported by Reynolds et al. (1973). However, Shulman (1972) did not observe any correlation between psychiatric illness and folate status. Increased alertness and drive, along with behavioral changes, have been reported in epileptic patients administered folate (Neubauer, 1970; Chi'en et al., 1975). Many drugs used to treat epilepsy are antifolates. Some patients with neurological disease have shown improvement in peripheral neuropathy when folate was administered (Grant et al., 1965; Reynolds, 1976). An association was reported between folate deficiency and dementia, particularly in the elderly (Sneath et al., 1973; Grinblat, 1985; Marcus and Freedman, 1985; Martin, 1988; Green, 1989; Levitt and Jaffe, 1989). Some patients with neurological disease have normal serum vitamin B_{12} levels but respond to folate therapy (Carney and Sheffield, 1970; Botez et al., 1976; 1978; Manzoor and Runcie, 1976).

Folate deficiency is commonly observed in patients with depressive illness and other psychiatric disturbances. Therapeutic trials have demonstrated significant improvement with the administration of 10 mg of folate per day (Abou-Saleh and Coppen, 1986). Botez et al. (1984) studied 49 patients with low serum and cerebrospinal fluid folate levels. The patients showed major neurological symptoms or exhibited depression and minor neurological signs. Supplementation of the patients with 10 mg/day of folate for 7–11 months resulted in significant improvement in their intellectual functioning.

On rare occasions, folate deficiency may result in subacute combined degeneration of the spinal cord. Such patients suffer from hematological, neurological, and psychiatric manifestations (Lever et al., 1986). Treatment with 5-methyltetrahydrofolate provided striking improvement in the manifestations of the deficiency. 5-Methyltetrahydrofolate represents the folate form that is transported into the central nervous system (Spector and Lorenzo, 1975).

Nervous tissue contains relatively high concentrations of folate. Its function is uncertain but it is assumed to be associated with synaptic events. Evidence exists to support this view. Folate deficiency in epileptic patients induced by drug therapy may lead to neuropsychiatric complications and peripheral neuropathy (Reynolds, 1976). Other reports describe an association between folate deficiency and peripheral neuropathy, organic brain syndromes, pyramidal tract damage, and dementia (Grant et al., 1965; Jensen and Olesen, 1969; Reynolds et al., 1973; Manzoor and Runcie, 1976; Enk et al., 1980).

Gimsing et al. (1989) studied the function of vitamin B_{12} and folate in chronic alcoholic men with peripheral neuropathy and encephalopathy. The 46 male patients studied had no hematological signs of folate or vitamin B_{12} deficiency. Erythrocyte folate and plasma vitamin B_{12} concentrations were all normal, while only 8% had low plasma folate concentrations. However, one-half of the patients had a functional deficiency of folate as determined by the deoxyuridine suppression test and by the formiminoglutamic acid excretion test. Based on the results of the functional tests, the investigators considered folate deficiency as a contributing factor in the development of neuropathy in chronic alcoholics, but not in the development of alcoholic encephalopathy. However, it is recognized that the neuropathy in the chronic alcoholic is of multifactorial origin (Davis, 1986). Kanazawa and Herbert (1986) have also observed a high incidence of an abnormal deoxyuridine suppression test in alcoholics at the time of hospital admission.

Drugs and Folate Metabolism

Because of the antifolate action of anticonvulsants, such as diphenylhydantoin, primidone, and phenobarbitone, prolonged use of the agents may result in a folate-deficient status (Reynolds, 1968, 1975; Chanarin, 1980b; Hiilesmaa et al., 1983; Hendel et al., 1984; Edeh and Toone, 1985; Lambie and Johnson, 1985; Marcus and Freedman, 1985; Reynolds and Trimble, 1985; Davis, 1986; Danskey et al., 1987; Deb et al., 1987; Goggin et al., 1987). This may be reflected in megaloblastic anemia (Flexner and Hartman, 1960) and in reduced folate levels in serum and cerebrospinal fluid (Dastur and Dave, 1987). Folate treatment has been used to correct the megaloblastic anemia that may occur in some patients on anticonvulsants (Martindale, 1982). Although folate levels in the cerebrospinal fluid are normally two to three times the serum levels, a specific role for folate in cerebral metabolism remains undefined (Dreyfus and Geel, 1981). Occasionally subjects on anticonvulsants have neuropsychiatric symptoms, neuropathy, or myelopathy (Edeh and Toone, 1985; Lambie and Johnson, 1985). Although the mechanism of action is uncertain, the drugs appear to impair folate absorption and tissue transport, or inhibit folate coenzyme formation (Hendel et al., 1984; Lambie and Johnson, 1985; Reynolds and Trimble, 1985).

It has been recognized for some time that the use of certain oral contraceptive agents may result in folate and/or vitamin B_{12} deficiency (Shojania et al., 1968, 1971; Sojania, 1971; Davis, 1986). Only rarely do megaloblastic abnormalities occur (Paton, 1969; Streiff, 1970; Toghill and Smith, 1971; Wood et al., 1972). Recently, a patient was described who had used oral contraceptives for 4 years and developed peripheral polyneuropathy and megaloblastic anemia (Kornberg et al., 1989). A folate deficiency appeared to be the primary problem. The significance and mechanism of action of oral contraceptive agents on folate metabolism remains unclear.

Toxicity of Vitamin B_{12} and Folate

Folate and vitamin B_{12} appear to be nontoxic even with intakes that exceed the Recommended Dietary Allowances (1989) by several hundred times (Butterworth and Tamura, 1989). However, exceedingly high concentrations of folate can have

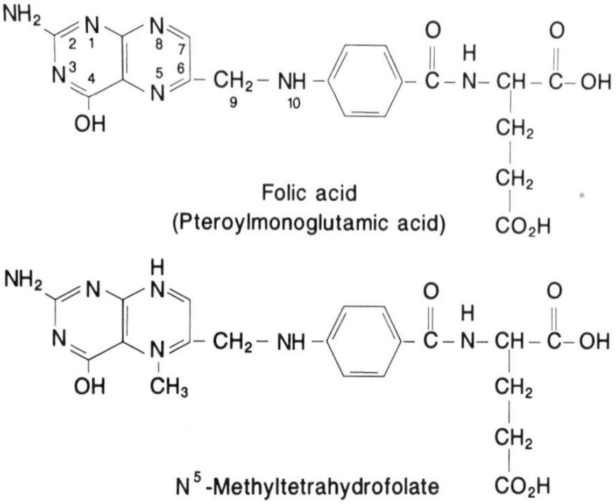

Figure 5 Structures of folic acid and N^5-methyltetrahydro-folate.

convulsant effects (Colman and Herbert, 1979). Such were observed in an epileptic patient administered 14.4 mg of folic acid by rapid intravenous infusion (Chi'en et al., 1975). However, oral doses of up to 1000 mg/day of folic acid for 5 months were tolerated with no side effects in adolescents (Brown et al., 1984b; Zettner et al., 1981).

SUMMARY

Although folate is closely related to vitamin B_{12} nutritionally and biochemically, its potential role in normal mental function is largely unknown at present. However, vitamin B_{12} deficiency must be seriously considered as a causative factor in neurological damage and dementia. In addition, vitamin B_6 deficiency can result in central nervous system changes, with the occurrence of abnormal electroencephalograms and convulsive seizures. Although the changes resemble those observed with vitamin B_{12} deficiency, vitamin B_6 appears to function largely in an independent manner in the central nervous system. Genetic defects may result in dependency syndromes of vitamin B_6, vitamin B_{12}, or folate. With early recognition, these conditions can usually be controlled with therapeutic doses of the involved vitamin.

The abnormal tryptophan metabolism and neurological manifestations observed in some women on OCA usually respond to pyridoxine supplements. However, routine supplementation with pyridoxine in OCA users is not recommended. Various other medications such as isoniazid, penicillamine, cycloserine, and anticonvulsants may antagonize vitamin B_6 and increase the daily requirement of the vitamin. Supplements of vitamin B_6 have been reported to benefit patients with carpal tunnel syndrome, celiac disease, or autism. These observations require further study to establish their clinical importance. Caution should be noted in that prolonged daily administration of 500 mg pyridoxine and above may result in sensory nerve damage. The neurological changes appear to reverse with discontinuance of the vitamin supplements.

A vitamin B_{12} deficiency may result in neurological changes without the development of macrocytic anemia. Vitamin B_{12} levels in the serum may be within the acceptable range. However, these patients usually have elevated serum levels of methylmalonic acid and of total homocysteine. Vitamin B_{12} therapy results in an improvement of the neurological disorders and a lowering of the serum methylmalonic acid and homocysteine levels. Early recognition of a vitamin B_{12} deficiency is essential if irreversible neurological damage is to be prevented.

Because of their close metabolic interrelationship, a deficiency of either vitamin B_{12} or folate will result in morphologically identical macrocytic anemia and megaloblastic bone marrow changes. However, folate deficiency appears to produce neurological changes less frequently than vitamin B_{12} deficiency. Occasionally subjects on anticonvulsants have neuropsychiatric symptoms, neuropathy, or myelopathy, which respond to folate treatment.

The extent to which dietary changes and supplements of vitamin B_6, vitamin B_{12}, or folate can ameliorate the symptoms and signs of neurological dysfunctions requires further exploration.

NOTE ADDED IN PROOF

Since the above chapter was prepared two relevant publications have appeared. Surtees et al. observed diminished concentration of methyl-group carriers in the cerebrospinal fluid (CSF) of six children with congenital human immunodeficiency virus (HIV) infection and neurological disease. The concentration of neopterin in CSF was elevated in each of the five subjects tested. The findings suggested that defective methylation may be related to the neurological damage cause by HIV infection.

Godfrey et al. observed borderline or low levels of red blood cell folate in 41 subjects (33% of 121) with major depression or schizophrenia. In a controlled trial, oral supplements of 15 mg daily of methyl folate resulted in significant improvement in clinical and social recovery over a period of 3 months. The findings support evidence that impaired methylation reactions in the central nervous system may be related to some forms of mental illness.

ACKNOWLEDGMENT

This work was supported in part by USPHS/NIH Grant 5PO1-CA28103.

REFERENCES

Abbott MH, Folstein, SE, Abbey H, Pyeritz RR. Psychiatric manifestations of homocystinuria due to cystathionine β-synthase deficiency: Prevalence, natural history, and relationships to neurologic impairment and vitamin B_6-responsiveness. Am J Med Genet 1987; 26:959–969.

Abou-Saleh MT, Coppen A. The biology of folate in depression: Implications for nutritional hypotheses of the psychoses. Psychiat Res 1986; 20:91–101.

Abraham GG, Hargrove JT. Effect of vitamin B_6 on premenstrual symptomatology in women with premenstrual tension syndrome: A double-blind crossover study. Infertility 1980; 3:155–165.

Adams PW, Rose DP, Folkard J, Wynn V, Seed M, Strong R. Effect of pyridoxine hydrochloride (vitamin B_6) upon depression associated with oral contraception. Lancet 1973; 1:897–904.

Amadio PC. Pyridoxine as an adjunct in the treatment of carpal tunnel syndrome. J Hand Surg 1985; 10A:237–241.

Amadio PC. Carpal tunnel syndrome, pyridoxine, and the work place. J Hand Surg 1987; 12A:875–880.

Anderson SA, Talbot JM. A review of folate intake, methodology, and status. Bethesda: Life Sciences Research Office, FASEB, 1981.

Babior BM, Bunn HF. Megaloblastic anemia. In: Braunwald E, Isselbacher KJ, Petersdorf RG, Wilson JD, Martin JB, Fauci AS, eds. Harrison's principles of internal medicine, 11th ed. New York: McGraw-Hill, 1987, 1498–1504.

Banerjee RV, Matthews RG. Cobalamin-dependent methionine synthase. FASEB J. 1990; 4:1450–1459.

Bankier A, Turner M, Hopkins IJ. Pyridoxine dependent seizures: A wider clinical spectrum. Arch Dis Child 1983; 58:415–418.

Barthelemy C, Garreau B, Leddt I, Ernouf D, Muh JB, Lelord G. Behavioral and biological effects of oral magnesium, vitamin B_6 and combined magnesium-vitamin B_6 administration in autistic children. Magnesium Bull 1981; 2:150–153.

Bauernfeind JC, Miller ON. Vitamin B_6: Nutritional and pharmaceutical usage, stability, bioavailability, antagonists, and safety. In Human vitamin B_6 requirements. Proceedings of a Workshop, June 11–12, 1976, Letterman Army Institute of Research, Presidio of San Francisco, Calif. A report of the Committee on Dietary Allowances, Food and Nutrition Board, National Academy of Sciences, Washington, DC, 1978, 78–110.

Baumblatt MJ, Winston F. Pyridoxine and the pill. Lancet 1970; 1:832.

Beck WS. Cobalamin and the nervous system. N Engl J Med 1988; 318:1752–1754.

Bender DA. The tryptophan load test for vitamin B_6 status is inappropriate for women receiving oestrogens. Proc Nutr Soc 1982; 41:120A.

Bender DA, Tagoe CE, Vale JA. Effects of oestrogen administration on vitamin B_6 and tryptophan metabolism in the rat. Br J Nutr 1982; 47:609–614.

Bendich A, Cohen M. Vitamin B_6 safety issues. Ann NY Acad Sci 1990; 585:321–330.

Berger A, Schaumburg HH. More on neuropathy from pyridoxine use. N Engl J Med 1984; 311:986–987.

Bermond P. Therapy of side effects of oral contraceptive agents with vitamin B_6. Acta Vitaminol Enzymol 1982; 4:45–54.

Bernstein AL. Vitamin B_6 in clinical neurology. Ann NY Acad Sci 1990; 585:250–260.

Beyers CM, DeLisa JA, Frankel DL, Kraft GH. Pyridoxine metabolism in carpal tunnel syndrome with and without peripheral neuropathy. Arch Phys Med Rehabil 1984; 65:712–716.

Bhagavan HN. Interaction between vitamin B_6 and drugs. In: Reynolds RD, Leklem JE, eds. Vitamin B_6: Its role in health and disease. New York: Alan R. Liss, 401–415.

Blanco G, Peters HA. Myeloneuropathy and macrocytosis associated with nitrous oxide abuse. Arch Neurol 1983; 40:416–418.

Botez MI, Cadotte M, Beaulieu R, Pichette LP, Pison C. Neurologic disorders responsive to folic acid therapy. Can Med Assoc J 1976; 115:217–223.

Botez MI, Peyronnard JM, Bachevalier J, Charron L. Polyneuropathy and folate deficiency. Arch Neurol 1978; 35:581–584.

Botez MI, Peyronnard JM, Berube LB, Labrecque R. Relapsing neuropathy, cerebral atrophy and folate deficiency. Appl Neurophysiol 1979; 42:171–183.

Boetz MI, Botez T, Maag U. The Wechsler subtests in mild organic brain damage associated with folate deficiency. Psychol Med 1984; 14:431–437.

Bottiglieri T, Chary TK, Laundry M, Carney MWP, Godfrey P, Toone KB, Reynolds EH. Transmethylation in depression. Ala J Med Sci 1988; 25:296–301.

Brenner A. The effects of megadose selected B-complex vitamins on children with hyperkinesis: Controlled studies with long-term follow-up. J Learn Disabil 1982; 15:258–264.

Brown A, Mallett M, Fiser D, Arnold WC. Acute isoniazid intoxication: Reversal of CNS symptoms with large doses of pyridoxine. Pediatr Pharmacol 1984a; 4:199–202.

Brown WT, Jenkins EC, Freidman E, Brooks J, Cohen IL, Duncan C, Hill AL, Malik MN, Morris V, Wolf E, Wisniewski K, French JH. Folic acid therapy in the fragile X syndrome. Am J Med Genet 1984b; 17:289–297.

Butterworth CE, Jr, Tamura T. Folic acid safety and toxicity: A brief review. Am J Clin Nutr 1989; 50:353–358.

Canham JE, Nunes WT, Eberlin EW. Electroencephalographic and central nervous system manifestations of B_6 deficiency and induced B_6 dependency in normal human adults. Proceedings of the Sixth International Congress of Nutrition, Edinburgh, August 9–15, 1963. Edinburgh: E&S Livingstone, Ltd., 1963, 537.

Cape RD, Shinton NK. Serum vitamin B_{12} concentration in the elderly. Gerontol Clin 1961; 3:163–172.

Carmel R, Karnaze DS, Weiner JM. Neurologic abnormalities in cobalamin deficiency are associated with higher cobalamin "analogue" values than are hematologic abnormalities. J Lab Clin Med 1988a; 111:57–62.

Carmel R, Watkins D, Goodman SI, Rosenblatt DS. Hereditary defect of cobalamin metabolism (cbl G mutation) presenting as a neurologic disorder in adulthood. N Engl J Med 1988b; 318:1738–1741.

Carney MWP, Sheffield BF. Associations of subnormal serum foalte and vitamin B_{12} and effects of replacement therapy. J Nerv Ment Dis 1970; 150:404–412.

Carney MWP, Chary TKN, Bottiglieri T, Reynolds EH. Switch and S-adenosylmethionine. Ala J Med Sci 1988; 25:316–319.

Castle WB. Development of knowledge concerning the gastric intrinsic factor and its relation to pernicious anemia. N Engl J Med 1953; 249:603–614.

Castle WB. A century of curiosity about pernicious anemia. Trans Am Clin Climatol Assoc 1961; 73:54–80.

Chanarin I. The cobalamins (vitamin B_{12}). In Barker BM, Bender DA, eds. Vitamins in medicine, 4th ed., Vol. 1, London: Heinemann Medical, Ltd., 1980a, 173–246.

Chanarin I. The folates. In: Barker BM, Bender DA, eds. vitamins in medicine, 4th ed., Vol. 1. London: Heinemann Medical, Ltd., 1980b, 247–314.

Chanarin I, Deacon R, Lumb M, Muir M, Perry J. Cobalamin-folate interrelations: A critical review. Blood 1985; 66:479–489.

Chi'en LT, Krumdieck CL, Scott CW, Jr, Butterworth CE, Jr. Harmful effect of megadoses of vitamins: Electroencephalogram abnormalities and seizures induced by intravenous folate in drug-treated epileptics. Am J Clin Nutr 1975; 28:51–58.

Clayton PT, Smith I, Harding B, Hyland K, Leonard JV, Leeming RJ. Subacute combined degeneration of the spinal cord, dementia and parkinsonism due to an inborn error of folate metabolism. J Neurol Neurosurg Psychiat 1986; 49:920–927.

Coburn SP. Metabolic and clinical studies of vitamin B_6 in mental disorders. In: Reynolds RD, Leklem JE, eds. Vitamin B_6: Its role in health and disease. New York: Alan R. Liss, 1985, 123–159.

Coburn SP, Mahuren JD. A versatile cation-exchange procedure for measuring the seven major forms of vitamin B_6 in biological samples. Anal Biochem 1983; 129:310.

Coburn SP, Schaltenbrand WE, Mahuren JD, Clausman RJ, Townsend D. Effect of megavitamin treatment on mental performance and plasma vitamin B_6 concentrations in mentally retarded young adults. Am J Clin Nutr 1983; 38:352–355.

Cohen M, Bendich A. Safety of pyridoxine: A review of human and animal studies. Toxicol Lett 1986; 34:129–139.

Cole MG, Prchal JF. Low serum vitamin B_{12} in Alzheimer-type dementia. Age and Ageing 1984; 13:101–105.

Colman N, Herbert V. In: Kumar S, ed. Biochemistry of brain. Oxford: Pergamon Press, 1979, 127–142.

Cooper BA, Rosenblatt DS. Inherited defects of vitamin B_{12} metabolism. Ann Rev Nutr 1987; 7:291–320.

Corbeel L, Van den Berghe G, Jaeken J, Van Tornout J, Eeckels R. Congenital folate malabsorption. Eur J Pediatr 1985; 143:284–290.

Coursin DB. Vitamin B_6 metabolism in infants and children. Vit Hormones 1964; 22:755–786.

Coyle J, Price D, DeLong M. Alzheimer's disease: A disorder of cortical cholinergic innervation, Science 1983; 219:1184–1190.

Crantz JG. Vitamin B_{12} deficiency in the elderly. Clin Geriatr Med 1985; 1:701–710.

Crowell GF, Roach ES. Pyridoxine-dependent seizures. Am Fam Physician 1983; 27:183–187.

Dakshinamurti K, Paulose CS, Siow YL. Neurobiology of pyridoxine. In: Reynolds RD, Leklem JE, eds. Vitamin B_6: Its role in health and disease. New York: Alan R. Liss, 1985, 99–121.

Dalton K. Pyridoxine overdose in premenstrual syndrome. Lancet 1985; 1:1168–1169.

Dalton K, Dalton MJT. Characteristics of pyridoxine overdose neuropathy syndrome. Acta Neurol Scan 1987; 76:8–11.

Dansky LV, Andermann E, Rosenblatt D, Sherwin AL, Andermann F. Anticonvulsants, folate levels, and pregnancy outcome: A prospective study. Ann Neurol 1987; 21:176–182.

Dastur DK, Dave UP. Effect of prolonged anticonvulsant medication in epileptic patients: Serum lipids, vitamins B_6, B_{12}, and folic acid, proteins, and fine structure of liver. Epilepsia 1987; 28:147–159.

Dastur DK, Santhadevi N, Quadros EV, Gagrat BM, Wadia NH, Desai MM, Singhal BS, Bharucha EP. Interrelationships between the B-vitamins in B_{12}-deficiency neuromyelopathy. A possible malabsorption-malnutrition syndrome. Am J Clin Nutr 1975; 28:1255–1270.

Davidson RA. Complications of megavitamin therapy. South Med J 1984; 77:200–203.

Davis RE. Clinical chemistry of folic acid. Adv Clin Chem 1986; 25:233–294.

Dawson AA, Donald D. The serum vitamin B_{12} in the elderly. Gerontol Clin 1966; 8:220–225.

Deacon R, Lumb M, Perry J, Chanarin I, Minty B, Halsey MJ, Nunn JF. Selective inactivation of vitamin B_{12} in rats by nitrous oxide. Lancet 1978; 2:1023–1024.

Deb S, Cowie VA, Richens A. Folate metabolism and problem behavior in mentally handicapped epileptics. J Ment Def Res 1987; 31:163–168.

Dreyfus PM, Geel SE. Vitamin and nutritional deficiencies. In: Siegel GL, Albers RW, Agranoff BW, Katzman R, eds. Basic neurochemistry. Boston: Little, Brown, 1981; 661–679.

Droller H, Dossett J. Vitamin B_{12} levels in senile dementia and confusional states. Geriatrics 1959; 14:367–373.

D'Souza M. Carpal tunnel syndrome: Clinical or neurophysiological diagnosis? Lancet 1985; 1:1104.

Ebadi M. Vitamin B_6 and biogenic amines in brain metabolism. In Human vitamin B_6 requirements. Proceedings of a workshop of the Food and Nutrition Board, National Research Council, National Academy of Sciences, Washington, D.C. 1978; 129–161.

Edeh J, Toone BK. Antiepileptic therapy, folate deficiency, and psychiatric morbidity: A general practice survey. Epilepsia 1985; 26:434–440.

Ellis JM. Treatment of carpal tunnel syndrome with vitamin B_6. South Med J 1987; 80:882–884.

Ellis JM, Folkers K. Clinical aspects of treatment of carpal tunnel syndrome with vitamin B_6. Ann NY Acad Sci 1990; 585:302–320.

Ellis J, Preston H. Free of pain: Vitamin B_6 deficiency U.S.A. The cause of soft tissue rheumatism. Revised edition, Dallas; Southwest Publ. Co., 1985.

Ellis JM, Kishi T, Azuma J, Folkers K. Vitamin B_6 deficiency in patients with a clinical syndrome including the carpal tunnel defect. Biochemical and clinical response to therapy with pyridoxine. Res Commun Chem Pathol Pharmacol 1976; 13:743–756.

Ellis J, Folkers K, Watanabe T, Kaji M, Saji S, Caldwell J, Temple C, Wood F. Clinical results of a cross-over treatment with pyridoxine and placebo of the carpal tunnel syndrome. Am J Clin Nutr 1979; 32:2040–2046.

Ellis J, Folkers K, Levy M, Takemura K, Shizukuishi S, Ulrish R, Harrison P. Therapy with vitamin B_6 with and without surgery for treatment of patients having the idiopathic carpal tunnel syndromes. Res Commun Chem Pathol Pharmacol 1981; 33:331–344.

Ellis J, Folkers K, Levy M, Shizukuishi S, Lewandowski J, Nishii S, Shubert H, Ulrich R. Response of vitamin B_6 deficiency and the carpal tunnel syndrome to pyridoxine. Proc Natl Acad Sci USA 1982; 79:7494–7498.

Elwood P, Shinton N, Wilson C, Sweetnam W, Frazer A. Haemoglobin, vitamin B_{12}, and folate levels in the elderly. Br J Haematol 1971; 21:557–563.

Enk C, Hougaard K, Hippe E. Reversible dementia and neuropathy associated with folate deficiency 16 years after partial gastrectomy. Scand J Haematol 1980; 25:63–66.

Erbe RW. Genetic defects of folate metabolism, Adv Hum Genet 1979; 9:293–354.

Erbe RW. Folic acid therapy in the fragile X syndrome. Editorial comment. Am J Med Genet 1989; 17:299–301.

Erbe RW, Wang J-C. Folate metabolism in humans. Am J Med Genet 1984; 17:277–287.

Fehling C, Jagerstad M, Lindstrand K, Elmquist D. Folate deficiency and neurological disease. Arch Neurol 1974; 30:263–265.

Ferraris S, Bonetti G, Biasetti S, Bracco G, Ponzone A. Folates and homocystinuria. Case report. J Inher Metab Dis 1988; 11:310–311.

Fleming AF, Dada TO. Folic acid and neurological disease. Lancet 1966; i:97.

Flexner JM, Hartman RC. Megaloblastic anaemia associated with anticonvulsant drugs. Am J Med 1960; 28:386–396.

Folkers K, Ellis J. Successful therapy with vitamin B_6 and vitamin B_2 of carpal tunnel syndrome and need for determination of the RDAs for vitamin B_6 and B_2 for disease states. Ann NY Acad Sciences 1990; 585:292–301.

Folkers K, Ellis J, Watanable T, Saji S, Kaji M. Biochemical evidence for a deficiency of vitamin B_6 in the carpal tunnel syndrome based on a cross-over clinical study. Proc Natl Acad Sci USA 1978; 75:3410–3412.

Follis RH, Wintrobe MM. A comparison of the effects of pyridoxine and pantothenic acid deficiencies on the nervous tissues of swine. J Exp Med 1945; 81:539–551.

Fowler B. Recent advances in the mechanism of pyridoxine-responsive disorders. J Inher Metab Dis 1985; 8:76–83.

Freeman JM, Finkelstein JD, Mudd SH. Folate: Responsive homocystinuria and schizophrenia. N Engl J Med 1975; 292:491–496.

Friedman MA, Resnick JS, and Baer RL. Subepidermal vesicular dermatosis and sensory peripheral neuropathy caused by pyridoxine abuse. J Am Acad Dermatol 1986; 14:915–917.

Gimsing P, Melgaard B, Andersen K, Vilstrup H, Hippe E. Vitamin B_{12} and folate function in chronic alcoholic men with peripheral neuropathy and encephalopathy. J Nutr 1989; 119:416–424.

Godfrey PSA, Toone BK, Carney MWP, et al. Enhancement of recovery from psychiatric illness by methylfolate. Lancet 1990; 336:392–395.

Goggans FC. A case of mania secondary to vitamin B_{12} deficiency. Am J Psychiatr 1984; 141:300–301.

Goggin T, Gough H, Bissessar A, Crowley M, Baker M, Callaghan N. A comparative study of the relative effects of anticonvulsants drugs and dietary folate on the red cell folate status of patients with epilepsy. Quart J Med 1987: 65:911–919.

Grant HC, Hoffbrand AV, Wells DG. Folate deficiency and neurologic disease. Lancet 1965; 2:763–767.

Green R. The role of folate and vitamin B_{12} in neurotransmitter metabolism and degenerative neurological changes associated with aging: Proceedings of a workshop. J Nutr 1989; 119:841–842.

Grieco AJ. Homocystinuria: Pathogenetic mechanisms. Am J Med Sci 1977; 273:120–132.

Grinblat J. Folate status in the aged. Clin Geriatr Med 1985; 1:711–728.

Gross JS, Weintraub NT, Neufeld RR, Libow LS. Pernicious anemia in the demented patient without anemia or macrocytosis. J Am Geriat Soc 1986; 34:612–614.

Gunn ADG. Vitamin B_6 and the premenstrual syndrome (PMS). Int J Vit Nutr Res., Suppl 27, 1985; 213–224.

Guzman FJL, Gonzalez-Bietrago JM, de Arriba F, Mateos F, Moyano JC, Lopez-Alburquerque T. Carpal tunnel syndrome and vitamin B_6. Klin Wochenschr 1989; 67:38–41.

György P. Vitamin B_2 and the pellagra-like dermatitis in rats. Nature 1934; 133:498.

György P. Vitamin B_2 complex. I. Differentiation of lactoflavin and ''rat antipellagra'' factor. Biochem J 1935; 29:741.

György P. Developments leading to the metabolic role of vitamin B_6. Am J Clin Nutr 1971; 24:1250.

Hallert C, Åström J, Walan A. Reversal of psychopathology in adult coeliac disease with the aid of pyridoxine (vitamin B_6). Scand J Gastroenterol 1983; 18:299–304.

Hansen HA, Nordqvist P, Sourander P. Megaloblastic anemia and neurologic disturbances combined with folic acid deficiency. Acta Med Scand 1964; 176:243–251.

Harpey JP. Treatment of fragile X. Pediatrics 1982; 69:670.

Harpey JP, Rosenblatt DS, Cooper BA, LeMöel G, Roy C, Lafourcade J. Homocystinuria caused by 5, 10-methylenetetrahydrofolate reductase deficiency: A case in an infant responding to methionine, folinic acid, pyridoxine, and vitamin B_{12} therapy. J Pediatr 1981; 98:275–279.

Harpey JP, LeMöel G, Zittoun J. Follow-up in a child with 5,10-methylenetetrahydrofolate reductase deficiency. J Pediatr 1983; 103:1007.

Harris JW, Horrigan DL. Pyridoxine-responsive anemia: Prototype and variations on the theme. Vit Hormones 1964; 22:721–753.

Hector M, Burton JR. What are the psychiatric manifestations of vitamin B_{12} deficiency? J Am Geriatr Soc 1988; 36:1105–1112.

Hendel J, Dam M, Gram L, Winkel P, Jorgensen I. The effects of carbamazepine and valproate on folate metabolism in man. Acta Neurol Scand 1984; 69:226–231.

Herbert V. Experimental folate deficiency. Trans Assoc Am Physicians 1962; 75:307–320.

Herbert V. Folate deficiency. J Am Med Assoc 1972; 222:834 (letter to the editor).

Herbert V. The 1986 Herman award lecture. Nutrition science as a continually unfolding story: The folate and vitamin B-12 paradigm. Am J Clin Nutr 1987; 46:387–402.

Herbert VC, Colman N. Folic acid and vitamin B_{12}. In: Shils ME, Young VR, eds. Modern nutrition in health and disease, Philadelphia: Lea and Febiger, 1988, 388–416.

Higginbottom MC, Sweetman L, Nyhan WL. A syndrome of methylmalonic aciduria, homocystinuria, megaloblastic anemia and neurologic abnormalities in a vitamin B_{12}-deficient breast-fed infant of a strict vegetarian. N Engl J Med 1978; 299:317–323.

Hiilesmaa VK, Teramo K, Granström M-L, Bardy AH. Serum folate concentrations during pregnancy in women with epilepsy: Relation to antiepileptic drug concentrations, number of seizures, and fetal outcome. Br Med J 1983; 287:577–579.

Hillman RS. Vitamin B_{12}, folic acid, and the treatment of megaloblastic anemias. In: Gilman LJ, Goodman LS, Rall TW, Murad F, eds. Goodman and Gilman's pharmacological basis of therapeutics, 7th ed. New York: Macmillan, 1985, 1323–1337.

Hoffbrand AV. Anaemia in adult coeliac disease. Clin Gastroenterol 1974; 3:71–89.

Holmes J. Cerebral manifestations of vitamin B_{12} deficiency. Br Med J 1956; 1394–1403.

Hughes D, Elwood P, Shinton N, Wrighton R. Clinical trial of the effect of vitamin B_{12} levels in the elderly subjects with low serum B_{12} levels, Br Med J 1970; 2:458–460.

Hyland K, Smith I, Bottiglieri T, Perry J, Wendel U, Clayton PT, Leonard JV. Demyelination and decreased S-adenosylmethionine in 5,10-methylene tetrahydrofolate reductase deficiency. Neurology 1988; 38:459–462.

Janicak PG, Lipinski J, Davis JM, Comaty JE, Waternaux C, Cohen B, Altman E, Sharma RP. S-Adenosylmethionine in depression. A literature review and preliminary report. Ala J Med Sci 1988; 25:306–313.

Jensen ON, Olesen OV. Folic acid concentrations in psychiatric patients. Acta Psychiat Scan 1969; 45:289–294.

Jones SJ, Yu YL, Rudge P, Kriss A, Gilois C, Hirani N, Nijhawan R, Norman P, Will R. Central and peripheral SEP defects in neurologically symptomatic and asymptomatic subjects with low vitamin B_{12} levels. J Neurol Sci 1987; 82:55–65.

Kanazawa S, Herbert V. Detection of folate deficiency in alcoholism using the peripheral blood lymphocyte deoxyuridine suppression test. J Nutr Sci Vitaminol 1986; 32:251–257.

Kang S-S, Wong PWK, Zhou J, Sora J, Lessick M, Ruggie N, Grcevich G. Thermolabile methlyentetrahydrofolate reductase in patients with coronary artery disease. Metabolism 1988; 37:611–613.

Karnaze DS, Carmel R. Low serum cobalamin levels in primary degenerative dementia. Do some patients harbor atypical cobalamin deficiency states? Arch Intern Med 1987; 147:429–431.

Kasdan ML, Janes C. Carpal tunnel syndrome and vitamin B_6. Plastic Reconstruct Surg 1987; 79:456–459.

Kopell HP, Goodgold J. Clinical and electrodiagnostic features of carpal tunnel syndrome. Arch Phys Med 1968; 49:371–375.

Kornberg A, Segal R, Theitler J, Yona R, Kaufman S. Folic acid deficiency, megaloblastic anemia and peripheral polyneuropathy due to oral contraceptives. Isr J Med Sci 1989; 25:142–145.

Kral V, Solyom L, Enesco H, Ledwidge B. Relationships of vitamin B12 and folic acid to memory function. Biol Psychiat 1970; 2:19–26.

Krein BM, Troncoso J, Kahn SB, Mancall EL. Irreversible neurologic degeneration secondary to vitamin B_{12} deficiency without anemia: Report of a case. J AOA 1984; 84:348–350.

Krishnamoorthy KS. Pyridoxine-dependency seizure: report of a rare presentation. Ann Neurol 1983; 13:103–104.

Lambie DG, Johnson RH. Durgs and folate metabolism. Drugs 1985; 30:145–155.

Lejeune J. Metabolisme des monocarbones et syndrome de 'X fragile. Bull Acad Natl Med 1981; 165:1197–1206.

Lejeune J. Is the fragile X syndrome amenable to treatment? Lancet 1982; 1:100 (letter).

Leklem JE, Brown RR, Rose DP, Linkswiler HM. Vitamin B$_6$ requirements of women using oral contraceptives. Am J Clin Nutr 1975; 28:535–541.

Lever EG, Elwes RDC, Williams A, Reynolds EH. Subacute combined degeneration of the cord due to folate deficiency: Response to methyl folate treatment. J Neurol Neurosurg Psychiat 1986; 49:1203–1207.

Levitt AJ, Jaffe RT. Folate, B$_{12}$, and life course of depressive illness. Biol Psychiat 1989; 25:867–872.

Li TK. Factors influencing vitamin B$_6$ requirements in alcoholism. In Human vitamin B$_6$ requirements. Washington, DC, 1978, National Academy of Sciences, 210–225.

Li T-K, Lumeng L. Vitamin B$_6$ metabolism in alcoholism and alcoholic liver disease. In: Reynolds RD, Leklem JE, eds. Vitamin B$_6$: Its role in health and disease. New York: Alan R. Liss, 1985, 257–269.

Lindenbaum J, Healton EB, Savage DG, Brust JCM, Garrett TJ, Podell ER, Marcell PD, Stabler SP, Allen RH. Neuropsychiatric disorders caused by cobalamin deficiency in the absence of anemia or macrocytosis. N Engl J Med 1988; 318:1720–1728.

Linnell J. The fate of cobalamins in vivo. In: Babior BM, ed. Cobalamin: Biochemistry and pathophysiology. New York: John Wiley and Sons, 1975, 287–333.

London RS, Murphy L, Kitlowski KE. Treatment of premenstrual syndrome with vitamin B$_6$: physicians attitudes and perceptions. In: Reynolds RE, Leklem JE, eds. Vitamin B$_6$: Its role in health and disease. New York: Alan R. Liss, 1985, 468–477.

Luhby AL, Eagle FJ, Roth E, Cooperman JM. Relapsing megaloblastic anemia in an infant due to a specific defect in gastrointestinal absorption of folic acid. Am J Dis Child 1961; 102:482–483.

Luhby AL, Brin M, Gordon M, Davis P, Murphy M, Spiegel H. Vitamin B$_6$ metabolism in users of oral contraceptive agents. I. Abnormal urinary xanthurenic acid excretion and its correction by pyridoxine. Am J Clin Nutr 1971; 24:684–693.

Mamlok RJ, Isenberg JN, Rassin DK, Norcross K, Tallan HH. A cobalamin metabolic defect with homocystinuria, methylmalonic aciduria and macrocytic anemia. Neuropediatrics 1986; 17:94–99.

Manzoor M, Runcie J. Folate responsive neuropathy: Report of ten cases. Br Med J 1976; 1:1176–1178.

Marcus DL, Freedman ML. Folic acid deficiency in the elderly. J Am Geriatr Soc 1985; 33:552–558.

Martin DC. B$_{12}$ and folate deficiency dementia. Clin Geriatr Med 1988; 4:841–852.

Martindale J. Phenytoin and some other anticonvulsants. in: Reynolds RR, ed. The extrapharmacopoeia. London: Pharmaceutical Press, 1982, 1235.

Martineau J, Barthelemy C, Cheliakine C, Lelord G. Brief report: An open middle-term stiudy of combined vitamin B$_6$-magnesium in a subgroup of autistic children selected on their sensitivity to this treatment. J Autism Dev Dis 1988a; 18:435–447.

Martineau J, Barthelemy C, Roux S, Lelord G. The effects of combined pyridoxine plus magnesium administration on the conditioned evoked potentials in children with autistic behavior. In: Reynolds RR, Leklem JE, eds. Clinical and physiological applications of vitamin B$_6$. New York: Alan R. Liss, 1988b, 357–362.

McCann VJ, Davis RE. Carpal tunnel syndrome, diabetes and pyridoxal. Aust. NZ J Med 1978; 8:638–640.

McCombe PA, McLeod JG. The peripheral neuropathy of vitamin B_{12} deficiency. J Neurol Sci 1984; 66:117–126.

Merrill AH, Jr, and Henderson JM. Diseases associated with defects in vitamin B_6 metabolism or utilization. Ann Rev Nutr 1987; 7:137–156.

Miller LT. Oral contraceptives and vitamin B_6 metabolism. In Vitamin B_6: Its role in health and disease. Reynolds RD, Leklem JE, eds. New York: Alan R. Liss, 1985, 243–255.

Miller LT, Dow MJ, Kokkeler SC. Methionine metabolism and vitamin B_6 status in women using oral contraceptives. Am J Clin Nutr 1978; 31:619–625.

Minot GR, Murphy WP. Treatment of pernicious anemia by a special diet. J Am Med Assoc 1926; 87:470–476.

Mitchell GA, Watkins D, Melancon SB, Rosenblatt, DS Geoffroy G, Orquin J, Hormsy MB, Dallaire L. Clinical heterogeneity in cobalamin C variant of combined homocystinuria and methylmalonic aciduria. J Pediatr 1986; 108:410–415.

Mitchell HK, Snell EE, Williams RJ. Concentration of "folic acid." J Am Chem Soc 1941; 63:2284.

Moss R, D'Amico S, Maletta G. Mental dysfunction as a sign of organic illness in the elderly. Geriatrics 1987; 42:35–42.

Murphy JV, Thome LM, Michals K, Matalon R. Folic acid responsive rages, seizures and homocystinuria. J Inher Metab Dis 1985; 2:109–110.

Neubauer C. Mental deterioration in epilepsy due to folate deficiency. Br Med J 1970; 2:759–761.

O'Brien PMS. The premenstrual syndrome: A review of the present status of therapy. Drugs 1982; 24:140–151.

Parry GJ, Bredesen DE. Sensory neuropathy with low-dose pyridoxine. Neurology 1985; 35:1466–1468.

Paton A. Oral contraceptives and folate deficiency. Lancet 1969; 1:418.

Pauling L. Sensory neuropathy from pyridoxine use. N Engl J Med 1984; 310:197.

Pauling L, Robinson AB, Oxley SS, Bergeson M, Harris D, Kerry P, Blephen J, Keaveny IT. Results of a loading test of ascorbic acid, niacinamide, and pyridoxine in schizophrenic subjects and controls. In: Hawkins D, Pauling L, eds. Orthomolecular psychiatry: Treatment of schizophrenia. San Francisco: W. H. Freeman, 1973, 18–34.

Pellock JM, Howell J, Kendig EL, Baker H. Pyridoxine deficiency in children treated with isoniazid. Chest 1985; 5:658–661.

Petrie WM, Ban TA. Vitamins in psychiatry: Do they have a role? Drugs 1985; 30:58–65.

Phalen GS. Reflections on 21 years' experience with carpal tunnel syndrome. J Am Med Assoc 1970; 212:1365–1367.

Pincus JA, Reynolds EH, Glaser GH. Subacute combined system degeneration of folate deficiency. J Am Med Assoc 1972; 221:496–497.

Podell RN. Nutritional supplementation with megadoses of vitamin B_6. Postgrad Med 1985; 77:113–116.

Potkin SG, Bell K, Plan L, Bunney WE, Jr. Rapid antidepressant response with Same. A double-blind study. Ala J Med Sci 1988; 25:313–316.

Recommended Dietary Allowances. Food and Nutrition Board, National Research Council, National Academy of Sciences, Washington, DC, 10th ed., 1989.

Reynolds EH. Mental effects of anticonvulsants and folic acid metabolism. Brain 1968; 91:197–214.

Reynolds EH. Chronic antiepileptic toxicity: A review. Epilepsia 1975; 16:319–352.

Reynolds EH. Neurological aspects of folate and vitamin B_{12} metabolism. Clin Haematol 1976; 5:661–696.

Reynolds EH, Trimble MR. Adverse neuropsychiatric effects of anticonvulsant drugs. Drugs 1985; 29:570–581.

Reynolds EH, Rothfeld P, Pincus JH. Neurological disease associated with folate deficiency. Br Med J 1973; 2:398–400.

Reynolds EH, Carney MWP, Toone BK. Methylation and mood. Lancet 1984; 2:196–198.

Rickes EL, Brink NG, Koniuszy FR, Wood TR, Folkers K. Crystalline vitamin B_{12}. Science 1948; 107:396–397.

Rimland B, Callaway E, Dreyfus P. The effect of high doses of vitamin B_6 on autistic children: A double-blind crossover study. Am J Psychiat 1978; 135:472–475.

Roberts E, Wein J, Simonsen DG. Gamma-aminobutyric acid (gamma ABA), vitamin B_6, and neuronal function–A speculative synthesis. Vit Hormones 1964; 22:503–559.

Roe DA. Drug effects on nutrient absorption, transport, and metabolism. Drug-Nutrient Interact 1985; 4:117–135.

Roos D, Willanger R. Various degrees of dementia in a selected group of gastrectomized patients with low serum B_{12}. Acta Neurol Scand 1977; 55:377–384

Rose DP. Oral contraceptives and vitamin B_6. In Human vitamin B_6 requirements. Proceedings of a workshop of the Food and Nutrition Board, National Research Council, National Academy of Sciences, Washington, DC, 1978a, 193–201.

Rose DP. The interactions between vitamin B_6 and hormones. Vit Hormones 1978b; 36:53–99.

Rose DP, Strong R, Adams PW, Harding PE. Experimental vitamin B_6 deficiency and the effect of oestrogen-containing oral contraceptives on the tryptophan metabolism and vitamin B_6. Clin Sci 1972; 42:465–477.

Rose RC, Hoyumpa AM, Jr, Allen RH, Middleton HM, III, Henderson LM, Rosenberg IH. Transport and metabolism of water-soluble vitamins in intestine and kidney. Fed Proc 1984; 43:2423–2429.

Rosenbaum JF, Maurizio F, Falk WE, Pollack M.H., Cohen LS, Cohen BM, Zubenko GS. An open-label pilot study of oral-S-adenosylmethionine in major depression. Ala J Med Sci 1988; 25:301—306.

Rosenberg LE. Vitamin responsive inherited metabolic disorders. Adv Hum Genet 1976; 6:1–74.

Rowe PB. Inherited disorders of folate metabolism. In: Stanbury JB, Wyngaarden JB, Fredrickson DC, Goldstein JL, Brown MS, eds. The metabolic basis of inherited disease. New York: McGraw-Hill, 1983, 498–521.

Rudman D, Williams PJ. Megadose vitamins: Use and misuse. N Engl J Med 1983; 309:488–490.

Samson D, Scott S, Christian R, Engel G. Cerebral metabolic disturbance and delirium in pernicious anemia. Arch Intern Med 1952; 90:4.

Santiago-Borrero PJ, Santini R, Jr, Perez-Santiago E, Maldonado N, Millan S, Coll-

Camaley G. Congenital isolated defects of folic acid absorption. J Pediatr 1973; 82:450–455.

Sauberlich HE. Human requirements for vitamin B_6. Vit Hormones 1964; 22:807–823.

Sauberlich HE. Vitamin B_6 status assessment: Past and present. In: Leklen JE, Reynolds RD, eds. Methods in vitamin B_6 nutrition. New York: Plenum Press, 1981, 203–239.

Sauberlich HE. Interaction of vitamin B_6 with other nutrients. In: Reynolds RD, Leklen JE, eds. Vitamin B_6: Its role in health and disease. New York: Alan R. Liss, 1985, 193–217.

Sauberlich, HE. Evaluation of folate nutrition of population groups. In: Folic acid metabolism in health and disease. New York: Wiley-Liss, 1990, 211–235.

Sauberlich HE, Canham JE. Vitamin B_6. In: Goodhart RS, Shils ME, eds. Modern nutrition in health and disease, 6th ed. Philadelphia: Lea and Febiger, 1980, 209–216.

Sauberlich HE, Canham JE, Baker EM, Raica N, Jr, Herman YF. Biochemical assessment of the nutritional status of vitamin B_6 in the human. Am J Clin Nutr 1972; 25:629–742.

Schaumburg H, Kaplan J, Windebank A, Vick N, Rasmus S, Pleasure D, Brown M. Sensory neuropathy from pyridoxine abuse: A new megavitamin syndrome, N Engl J Med 1983; 309:445–448.

Scheyer RD, Hass DC. Pyridoxine in carpal tunnel syndrome. Lancet 1985; 2:42.

Schilling RF. Is nitrous oxide a dangerous anesthetic for vitamin B_{12}-deficient subjects? J Am Med Assoc 1986; 255:1605–1606.

Scriver CR. Vitamin-responsive inborn errors of metabolism. Metabolism 1973; 22:1319–1344.

Shane B, Contractor SF. Assessment of vitamin B_6 status. Studies on pregnant women and oral contraceptive users. Am J Clin Nutr 1975; 28:739–747.

Shinnar S, Singer HS. Cobalamin C mutation (methylmalonic aciduria and homocystinuria) in adolescence. N Engl J Med 1984; 311:451–454.

Shizukuishi S, Nishii S, Ellis J, Folkers K. The carpal tunnel syndrome as a probable primary deficiency of vitamin B_6 rather than a deficiency of a dependency state. Biochem Biophys Res Commun 1980; 95:1126–1130.

Shojania AM. Effect of oral contraceptives on vitamin B_{12} metabolism. Lancet 1971; 1:932.

Shojania AM, Hornady GJ, Barnes PH. Oral contraceptives and serum-folate levels. Lancet 1968; 1:1376–1377.

Shojania AM, Hornady GJ, Barnes PH. The effect of oral contraceptives on folate metabolism. Am J Obstet Gynecol 1971; 111:782–791.

Shulman R. Psychiatric aspects of pernicious anaemia: A prospective controlled investigation. Br Med J 1967a; 266–270.

Shulman R. Vitamin B_{12} deficiency and psychiatric illness. Br J Psychiat 1967b; 113:252–256.

Shulman R. The present status of vitamin B_{12} and folic acid deficiency in psychiatric illness. Can Psychiatr Assoc 1972; 17:205–216.

Simensen RJ, Rogers RC. Fragile-X syndrome. Am Fam Physician 1989; 39:185–193.

Smallwood J, Ah-Kye D, Taylor I. Vitamin B_6 in the treatment of pre-menstrual mastalgia. Br J Clin Prac 1986; 40:532–533.

Smith A. Megaloblastic madness. Br Med J 1960; 1840–1845.

Smith EL, Parker LFJ. Purification of antipernicious anaemia factor. Biochem J 1948; 43:viii–ix.

Smith GP, Rudge PJ, Peters TJ. Biochemical studies of pyridoxal and pyridoxal phosphate status and therapeutic trial of pyridoxine in patients with carpal tunnel syndrome. Ann Neurol 1984; 15:104–107.

Sneath P, Chanarin I, Hodkinson HM, McPherson CK, Reynolds EH. Folate status in a geriatric population and its relation to dementia. Age and Ageing 1973; 2:177–182.

Spector R, Lorenzo AV. Folate transport in the central nervous system. Am J Physiol 1975; 229:777–782.

Steiner I, Kidron D, Soffer D, Wirguin I, Abramsky O. Sensory peripheral neuropathy of vitamin B_{12} deficiency: A primary demyelinating disease. J Neurol 1988; 235:163–164.

Stephenson JBP, Byrne KE. Pyridoxine responsive epilepsy: Expanded pyridoxine dependency: Arch Dis Child 1983; 58:1034–1036.

Strachan RW, Henderson JG. Psychiatric syndromes due to avitaminosis B_{12} with normal blood and bone marrow. Quart J Med 1965; 34:303–317.

Streiff RR. Folate deficiency and oral contraceptives. J Am Med Assoc 1970; 214:105–108.

Sturman JA. Vitamin B_6 and the metabolism of sulfur amino acids. In: Human vitamin B_6 requirements. Proceedings of a Workshop, June 11–12, 1976, Letterman Army Institute of Research, Presidio of San Francisco, California. A report of the Committee on Dietary Allowances, Food and Nutrition Board, National Academy of Sciences, Washington, DC, 1978, 37–60.

Sturman JA. Vitamin B_6 and sufur amino acid metabolism. In: Leklem JE, Reynolds RD, eds. Methods in vitamin B_6 nutrition. New YorK: Plenum Press, 1981, 341–371.

Subar AF, Block G, James LD. Folic acid intake and food sources in the U.S. population. Am J Clin Nutr 1989; 50:508–516.

Surtees R, Hyland K, Smith I. Central-nervous-system methyl-group metabolism in children, with neurological complications of HIV infection. Lancet 1990; 335:619–621.

Swank RL, Adams RD. Pyridoxine and pantothenic acid deficiency in swine. J Neuropathol Exp Neurol 1948; 7:274–286.

Taylor N. Carpal tunnel syndrome. Am J Phys Med 1971; 50:192–213.

Toghill PJ, Smith PG. Folate deficiency and the pill. Br Med 1971; 1:608–609.

Tolbert LC. MAT kinetics in affective disorders and schizophrenia. Ala J Med Sci 1988; 25:291–296.

Turner G, Robinson H, Laing S, Purvis-Smith S. Preventive screening for the fragil X syndrome. N Engl J Med 1986; 315:607–609.

Ueland PM, Refsum H. Plasma homocysteine, a risk, factor for vascular disease: Plasma levels in health, disease, and drug therapy (review article). J Lab Clin Med 1989; 44:473–501.

Vatassery GT, Maletta GJ. Relationship between nutrition and dementia in the elderly. Psychiat Med 1983; 1:429–443.

Victor M, Adams RD. Deficiency diseases of the nervous system. In: Petersdorf RG, Adams RD, Braumwald E, Isselbacher KJ, Martin JB, Wilson JD, eds. Harrison's principles of internal medicine, 10th ed. New York: McGraw-Hill, 1983, 2112–2118.

Victor M, Lear AA. Subacute combined degeneration of the spinal cord: Current concepts of the disease process: value of serum vitamin B_{12} determinations in clarifying some of the common clinical problems. Am J Med 1956; 20:896–911.

Waterstrom JA, Gilligan BS. Pyridoxine neuropathy. Med J Aust 1987; 146:640–642.

Weiner J, Hope J. Cerebral manifestations of vitamin B_{12} deficiency. J Am Med Assoc 1959; 170:1038–1041.

Wendel U, Bremer HJ. Betaine in the treatment of homocystinuria due to 5,10-methylenetetrahydrofolate reductase deficiency. Eur J Pediatr 1984; 142:147–150.

Wills L. Nature of the haemopoietic factor in marmite. Lancet 1933; 1:1283–1286.

Wood JK, Goldstone AH, Allan NC. Folic acid and the pill. Scand J Haematol 1972; 9:539–544.

Zettner A, Boss GR, Seegmiller JE. A long-term study of the absorption of large oral doses of folic acid. Ann Clin Lab Sci 1981; 11:516–524.

Zucker DK, Livingston RL, Nakra R, Clayton PJ. B_{12} deficiency and psychiatric disorders: Case report and literature review. Biol Psychiat 1981; 16:197–205.

10

Vitamin and Mineral Intake and Cognitive Functioning

David Benton

University College
Swansea, Wales, United Kingdom

INTRODUCTION

It will appear unlikely to many nutritionists that the majority of those living in the West will benefit from the taking of vitamins and mineral supplements. The argument goes that as the diet supplies sufficient protein and calories, then the necessary micronutrients come associated with the protein and calories. A minority viewpoint is that some individuals will benefit from vitamin and mineral supplements for one of two reasons. First, the diet may be such that a subclinical deficiency results; second, in particular individuals there may be a genetically determined need for a high intake.

An examination of the literature produces some evidence to justify further examination of the view that some diets are deficient in minerals and vitamins. For example, Greenwood and Richardson (1979), when they reviewed the literature dealing with the adequacy of the diets of adolescents, concluded that "specific nutrient deficiencies have been identified in a significant proportion of the adolescent population. They included iron, calcium, vitamin A, vitamin C. . . ." Sandstead et al. (1971) studied the nutritional status of preschool children from economically depressed areas: biochemical assays gave grounds for concern about the adequacy of diet in the case of vitamin A in 96% of subjects; the figure for iron was 35%, for folic acid 17%, and for thiamine 13%. These and similar data suggest the possibility that subclinical deficiencies of vitamins and minerals exist in sections of the population.

Individuals with a genetically determined higher need for certain vitamins present a second group that will benefit from supplementation. Williams (1956) pointed out that there may be a 2000% variation in individual vitamin requirements, and formulated the concept of a geneotrophic disease in which, because of genetic factors, the afflicted individual requires a larger intake of one or more specific nutrients.

Psychological measures have infrequently been used to study the adequacy of diet. Cognitive tasks reflect the summated activity of billions of neurons and countless biochemical pathways and their associated enzymes. It may well be that relatively small dietary deficiencies, which are dismissed as causing only minor changes to the activity of a single enzyme, will along with many other similar minor effects have a measurable and potentially important cumulative influence on cerebral functioning. It can be argued that if subclinical deficiencies exist then a disruption of cognitive functioning will be one of the first indications. This chapter therefore reviews the studies that have related vitamin and mineral supplementation to psychological functioning.

VITAMIN AND MINERALS SUPPLEMENTATION OF CHILDREN

Boggs et al. (1965) selected nine preschool children, of low intelligence on a Headstart program, and found that the taking of vitamin/mineral supplements in a double-blind crossover study significantly improved both the teachers' ($p <$ 0.0001) and parents' ratings of their behavior ($p < 0.04$). The increase in intelligence scores approached significance. The extent to which these findings reflect a carefully selected sample is unclear.

Schoenthaler (1987) studied young offenders, guilty of serious crimes, in two penal institutions. He used a 7-day dietary diary to distinguish those who were well nourished (43%) from those with deficient intakes (57%) of minerals and vitamins. A multivitamin and mineral supplement was given for 3 months to all offenders, irrespective of the quality of their diet: it was argued that those with a poor diet would respond, while the well nourished would not. In one institution a mood scale was administered and it was found that, when compared with those eating an adequate diet, the taking of a supplement was associated with improved mood in those with a poor diet ($p < 0.05$).

More recently, interest in the impact of mineral and vitamin supplements on cognitive functioning was stimulated by the report that their administration was associated with increased nonverbal intelligence in 12-year-old British school children (Benton and Roberts, 1988). In this study, using a double-blind procedure, 60 children were randomly given either a supplement containing a wide range of vitamins and minerals, or a placebo. Figure 1 illustrates the findings. The scores on the Calvert nonverbal test of those taking the supplement increased

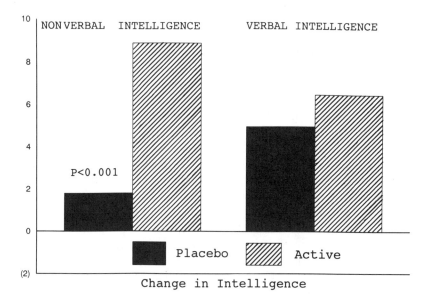

Figure 1 Impact of vitamin/mineral supplementation on the intelligence of British schoolchildren. Twelve-year-old schoolchildren took either a placebo or multivitamin/mineral supplement. Data presented are changes in scores on verbal and nonverbal intelligence tests taken before and after taking the supplement for 8 months. The taking of the active supplement significantly improved scores on the nonverbal test.

markedly; on average they were nine IQ points more than those receiving placebo ($p < 0.001$).

At the same time, Schoenthaler et al (1991) were studying a group of 15-year-old adolescent offenders in juvenile treatment facilities in Oklahoma. In a double-blind placebo study the 40 offenders, who received a multimineral/vitamin supplement for 13 weeks, committed significantly fewer violent and other antisocial acts ($p < 0.009$). Any adverse behavior was logged by staff, unaware of the type of tablet taken. Cameras were used to ensure continuous surveillance. In fact the improvement in behavior occurred rapidly, within a matter of days. A subgroup also took the Wechsler Intelligence Scale for Children (WISCR); the taking of the supplement was associated with a significant six-point increase in intelligence, whereas the scores of those taking the placebo declined by one point ($p < 0.05$). The authors commented that the statistically significant increase seemed to be due primarily to large rises in the scores of about a quarter of the subjects who had received the active tablet.

The Benton and Roberts (1988) study stimulated several attempts to replicate the findings. Although some of the resulting data are negative, a consistent picture may be emerging. Nelson et al. (1990) examined 227 children, aged 7–12 years, who took a vitamin/mineral supplement for 4 weeks. This double-blind placebo study found no evidence that supplementation induced changes in intelligence scores. The Nelson et al. study can not be seen as a replication study as it differs from the original in many ways; the tests, the composition of the tablets, and the time for which they were taken were all different.

In contrast, Crombie et al. (1990) went to great trouble to replicate the Benton and Roberts (1988) design using the same tests and tablets. In this double-blind study Crombie et al. (1990) studied 86 children from one school and found a small, but nonsignificant, advantage of 2.4 points on the Calvert nonverbal test for those taking the supplement as opposed to the placebo. As a similar trend was not apparent with other tests, their concluding statement was that "although the possibility of a weak effect of supplementation on the Calvert non-verbal test cannot be ruled out, overall our study does not support the hypothesis that vitamin and mineral supplementation leads to improved performance in non-verbal tests of reasoning." This conclusion may turn out to be prophetic as there is reason to believe that supplementation affects not the ability to reason but rather the ability to sustain attention.

Under double-blind conditions, Benton and Buts (1990) gave 167 Belgian schoolchildren either a supplement or a placebo for 5 months. Based on a 15-day dietary diary the intake of 11 minerals and vitamins was calculated. In 45% of the individuals the calculated intake of one or more nutrients was less than 50% of the U.S. Recommended Dietary Allowance on six or more occasions. These individuals were classified in the group consuming a poor diet. Although in terms of the macronutrients the two diets were broadly similar, for five vitamins and five minerals the intake of boys on the poorer diet was significantly less.

Figure 2 shows that the boys who were eating the poorer diet scored significantly better on the Calvert nonverbal test following vitamin/mineral supplementation for 5 months ($p < 0.02$). A similar finding resulted when boys were divided into those attending schools for the more academically gifted and those attending technical/manual schools. The less academic boys who received a supplement scored significantly better on the nonverbal test than those who received a placebo ($p < 0.02$), although this was not true for girls. It may be that the impact of nutrition subtly interacts with background and the immediate environment.

Most of the studies so far described have examined children in their early teenage years. Benton and Cook (1991) argued that if these children had diets deficient in minerals and vitamins, then younger children may also be a high-risk group for similar dietary deficiencies. When parents were asked about food consumption patterns of their 6-year-old children they often described their children as having a poor appetite and food fads. Forty-three children of 6 years of age were given four subtests of the British Ability Scale that could be combined to give an intelligence score. In a double-blind study the tests were given before

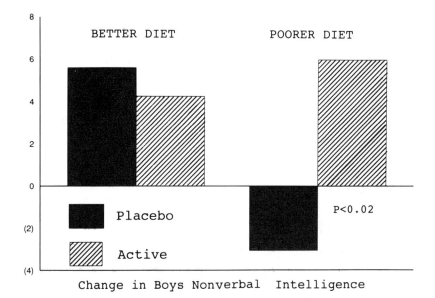

Figure 2 Impact of vitamin/mineral supplementation on the nonverbal intelligence of Belgian schoolchildren consuming different diets. One hundred and three thirteen-year-old Belgian boys recorded their diets for 15 days and the daily consumption of 11 vitamins and minerals was calculated from food tables. The sample was divided into two groups; one that tended to have a higher (65%), and the other a lower (35%), intake of minerals and vitamins. The figure reports changes in non-verbal intelligence that resulted from the taking of a vitamin/mineral supplement for 5 months. In those with a poorer diet the supplement significantly improved nonverbal intelligence.

and after taking either a vitamin/mineral supplement or a placebo for 6 or 8 weeks. Figure 3 illustrates the results. The scores of the children receiving the active tables increased by 7.6 points whereas the scores of those receiving the placebo decreased by 1.7 points ($p < 0.001$). To the psychologist administering the tests the difference appeared to be one of concentration and attitude. Those who proved to be on the placebo when the code was broken had a tendency to take a quick look at the problem and say that they did not know the answer. Those who proved to be on the active tablet tended to think about a problem for a period of time during which they sometimes came up with a correct answer.

The suggestion that a subclinical deficiency of vitamins exists in a section of the population is supported by a study by Heseker et al. (1990). They screened 1228 subjects aged 17–29 for low levels of blood vitamins and selected 197 who received supplements or a placebo for 8 weeks under a double-blind procedure.

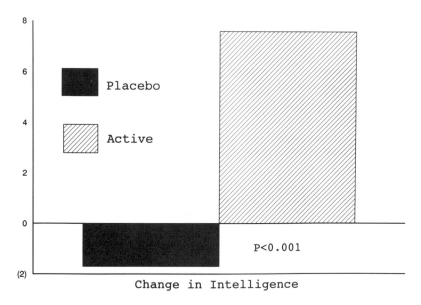

Figure 3   Impact of vitamin/mineral supplementation on the intelligence of 6-year-old children. The intelligence of 47 six-year-old children was measured before and after taking either a placebo or vitamin/mineral supplement for 6 or 8 weeks. The scores of those taking the active tablet increased and those taking the placebo decreased.

The taking of the supplement was associated with improvement on several indices of mood. The results of this study are interesting in that they show that psychological parameters are capable of measuring differences between those who receive adequate and borderline (less than fifth percentile) nutrition.

EVALUATION OF STUDIES OF THE IMPACT OF THE SUPPLEMENTATION OF CHILDREN

This chapter discusses nine studies, of which seven reported positive findings. This consistency should not be taken to imply that all, or even most, children respond. However, this consistency suggests that there is a phenomenon worthy of further study (Table 1). Any apparent inconsistency in this area can be explained by the assumption that there is a subgroup of children who benefit from supplementation. The evidence from Crombie et al. (1990), Nelson et al. (1990), and Benton and Buts (1990) is that most children do not respond. The subgroup of boys who responded in the Benton and Buts (1990) study had a significantly lower intake of calcium, iron, magnesium, zinc, phosphorus, and vitamins A, B_1, B_2, B_6, and nicotinic acid than the boys who failed to respond. The diets of

Table 1 Summary of Studies on the Effects of Dietary Supplementation on Tests of Verbal and Nonverbal Intelligence

Investigators	Subjects	Age	*n*	Test	Response
1. Boggs et al. (1965)	Preschool (Headstart)	<6	9	IQ	+
2. Schoenthaler (1987)	Young criminals, U.S. prisons	?	57	Mood	+
3. Benton and Roberts (1988)	British school-children	12	60	Calvert	+
4. Schoenthaler et al, (1991)	Juvenile offenders, Oklahoma	15	40	Wechsler	+
5. Crombie et al. (1990)	British school-children	11?	86	Calvert	N.S.
6. Benton and Buts (1990)	Belgian school-children	13	167	Calvert	+
7. Heseker et al. (1990)	German university students and others	17–29	197	Psycho-motor; mood	+
8. Nelson et al. (1990)	British school-children	7–12	227	IQ	N.S.
9. Benton and Cook (1991)	British school-children	6–7	43	IQ	+

the boys in both the Nelson et al. (1990) and Crombie et al. (1990) studies were significantly better than that eaten by the Belgian boys who responded to supplementation (Benton and Buts, 1990). So far three studies have described a subsample with a poor diet that responded to supplementation (Schoenthaler, 1987, 1991; Benton and Buts, 1990). Other studies reporting beneficial responses have chosen their sample either on the basis of dietary problems (Benton and Cook, 1990, unpublished) or social disadvantage such that nutritional deficiencies may have existed (Boggs et al., 1965).

The findings in Figs. 2 and 3 suggest a mechanism by which supplementation may influence scores on intelligence tests. In all these studies intelligence tests are taken twice, before and after consuming tablets for a period of time. There is a reasonable expectation that the scores on intelligence tests are going to be higher the second time they are taken, simply because the test is familiar. The surprising finding is that when the supplement caused an improvement, the placebo was associated with a worse performance than usually observed when taking a test for a second time (Benton and Roberts, 1988; Benton and Buts, 1990; Benton and Cook, 1991). A possible, if not likely, explanation is that children with a poor diet are poorly motivated or have difficulty sustaining attention. Having taken the test before they know it is difficult, maybe perceive it as boring, and simply do not try very hard. The Calvert nonverbal test, which was used in both Fig. 1 and 2, takes 40 min and subjectively appears to require the child to work rapidly; more than any other test it requires that the child sustain attention for a prolonged period. The fact that the girls in Fig. 2 did not respond to supplementation may reflect sex differences in the attitude of girls toward school work, although this explanation needs to be experimentally examined.

A more general comment is that future work would benefit from the use of more sensitive psychological measures: a remarkable aspect of the findings in this area is that such a global measure as intelligence has been found to be influenced by vitamin/mineral supplements. The use of measures such as reaction times, or tests of the ability to sustain attention, may be instructive as they are more likely to reflect subtle changes in cognitive functioning.

CONCLUSIONS CONCERNING THE IMPACT OF SUPPLEMENTATION ON INTELLIGENCE

Any suggestion that vitamin and mineral supplementation improves the intelligence of children is bound to be viewed skeptically. However, the data suggest hypotheses that should be studied.

1. The majority of children do not respond to vitamin/mineral supplementation with increased performance on intelligence tests.
2. A subgroup of children with a diet low in vitamins and minerals are apathetic and/or have a poor ability to sustain attention.
3. Vitamin and mineral supplements do not improve performance, but rather prevent the adverse effects of a poor diet.
4. The effects of consuming a poor diet will subtly interact with the attitudes and expectations of the individual, the nature of the task, and the social setting in which it is performed.

The finding, in 7 of the 9 studies described, that vitamin/mineral supplements changed either the behavior or the intelligence of children suggests the hypothesis that some children in Western industrialized societies are consuming diets marginally deficient in vitamins and minerals (see Table 1). This view so radically conflicts with the conventional assumption that the intake of mineral and vitamins is adequate in the majority of the population that a substantial body of data will be required before this assumption is commonly accepted.

THIAMINE SUPPLEMENTATION OF CHILDREN

Harrell (1946) examined 120 children who lived together on a farm used as an orphanage. They ate the same diet, which, following analysis at Columbia University, was estimated to supply 1 mg of thiamine a day. The World Health Organization (WHO) Recommended Daily Allowance for children aged 10–12 is 1 mg/day for boys and 0.9 mg/day for girls, so a priori the diet would have been thought to supply an adequate amount of thiamine. Under a double-blind procedure the children took either a placebo or 2 mg thiamine on a daily basis.

A range of tests were taken before and after taking the tablets for a year. There were remarkable improvements in those taking the thiamine rather than the placebo; they were significantly taller, had better eyesight, quicker reaction times, and scored better on tests of memory and intelligence.

NUTRITIONAL SUPPLEMENTS AND MENTALLY HANDICAPPED CHILDREN

For 4 months, using a double-blind procedure, 16 mentally retarded children (IQ 17–70) were given a supplement that contained eight minerals and 11 vitamins (Harrell et al., 1981). The IQs of those receiving the supplement increased significantly when compared with those receiving the placebo ($p < 0.05$). In a second but not double-blind stage, those who had previously received the placebo received the supplement and IQs increased by at least 10.2 points ($p < 0.001$). In three out of four Down syndrome cases the gains in IQ were between 10 and 25 points.

Three studies subsequently examined Down syndrome children and found that a formula similar to that used by Harrell et al. (1981) (but without thyroid extract) had no beneficial effect (Bennett et al, 1983; Weathers, 1983; Smith et al., 1984). Similarly, when adult Down syndrome patients were examined, vitamin/mineral supplements failed to change IQ scores (Ellis and Tomporowski, 1983; Coburn et al., 1983; Ellman et al., 1984). It has been argued that the failure of these studies to replicate the original positive findings may reflect the absence of thyroid extract in the subsequent studies. Chanowitz et al. (1985) examined this possibility in a sample of profoundly retarded adults (etiology unstated), but again found no significant improvement in intellectual functioning.

Davis (1987) discussed the results in this area and noted that critical differences may have resulted in the failure to replicate earlier studies. Harrell's subjects were children living at home while several of the follow-up studies used institutionalized adults of low IQ, factors that make a rapid improvement unlikely. These reasonable comments apply to the study of adult subjects, yet there have also been several failures to replicate the initial findings that have used children.

The conclusion that high-dose vitamin therapy does not generally improve the functioning of Down syndrome children seems reasonable, yet Harrell et al. (1981) observed very substantial changes in their sample. The possibility remains that a particular factor may be found that distinguishes a subgroup that responds to supplementation.

Pyridoxal-5-phosphate serves as a major coenzyme in many biochemical reactions. Speculating that there may be a deficiency of vitamin B_6 in Down syndrome, Coleman et al. (1985) were particularly interested in its possible role in the development of myelin and serotonin. In a double-blind study pharmacological doses were administered for the first three years of life (25 mg B_6/kg/day for the first 6 months then 35 mg/kg). Down patients receiving the vitamin were not significantly different from the controls when mental age, height, weight, cranial circumference, and tongue protrusion were measured. Vitamin B_6 did, however, influence auditory evoked potentials. Pueschel et al. (1980) similarly found that vitamin B_6 did not increase the mental age of Down syndrome patients.

VITAMIN AND MINERAL SUPPLEMENTS AND THE BEHAVIORAL PROBLEMS OF CHILDREN

Thiessen and Mills (1975) described a controlled study of children with learning disorders. However, the study was not double-blind, the treatments were not randomly allocated, there was no statistical analysis, and the control group was studied for less than half the time of the experimental group. These workers gave children with severe reading and spelling difficulties 3 g vitamin C, 3 g niacinamide, 250 mg vitamin B_6, and 250 mg panthothenic acid on a daily basis for 9 months to a year and a half. They concluded that reading and spelling were not altered, although hyperactivity, sleep disturbances, and some perceptual dysfunctions improved. Such uncontrolled studies at best suggest hypotheses that deserve to be more systematically examined.

In a well-controlled study, Kershner and Hawke (1979) gave 20 learning-disabled children large doses of vitamins B_6, C, niacinamide, and calcium pantothenate for 6 months. The addition of these vitamins to the diet failed to improve intellectual, perceptual, and behavioral measures. The authors caution, however, that the sweeping generalization that high doses of vitamins are ineffective may not be warranted. Learning disabilities can be the reflection of a range of aberrant mechanisms, and many more well-designed studies are needed to establish the efficacy or otherwise of supplementing particular subgroups with micronutrients. Children need to be carefully described in terms of both behavioral and biochemical parameters, as it is improbable that all will respond equally.

Coleman et al. (1979) studied a group of six hyperkinetic children with low levels of blood serotonin given either methylphenidate or pyridoxine. The treatments failed to reach statistical significance, perhaps not surprisingly in view of the small sample size. However, the trend was for both methylphenidate and pyridoxine to be better than a placebo, a finding that should be further examined.

Hard evidence that children with behavioral problems will benefit from vitamin supplementation does not exist. There are, however, sufficient clinical reports of improvements that it is unwise to simply dismiss the possibility that benefits may result when vitamin/mineral supplementations are given to carefully selected groups of children.

VITAMIN STATUS AND ADULT BEHAVIOR

With vitamin deficiency psychological symptoms such as depression, hysteria, and hypochondria may appear earlier than the symptoms of an outright deficiency disease: this has been observed in the case of thiamine (Brozek, 1957), riboflavin (Sterner and Price, 1973), and vitamin C but not vitamin A deficiency (Kinsman and Hood, 1971). Numerous investigators reported an association between nutritional deficiencies, particularly vitamins B_{12} and folate, and psychiatric syndromes, including depression and dementia (Hunter et al., 1967; Botez et al., 1977; Carney and Sheffield, 1978; Abou-Saleh and Coppen, 1986; Hector and Burton, 1988; Sommer and Wolkowitz, 1988). Some workers hypothesized that cognitive impairment and organic psychosis are associated with B_{12} deficiency (Hector and Burton, 1988) whereas depression is associated with folate deficiency (Carney and Sheffield, 1978; Shorvon et al., 1980). Bell et al. (1990) examined geriatric patients of whom only 3.7% were B_{12}- and 1.3% folate-deficient. Nevertheless, those with below median levels of both vitamins had poorer mental state scores than those with median levels of one of these vitamins. The severity of depression was negatively correlated with folate level whereas those with an organic psychosis and a family history of the disorder had lower B_{12} levels. Botez et al. (1984) selected a group of 49 patients with low folate levels. After 7 to 11 months of folate supplementation the patients were less easily fatigued and distracted and the scores on all the subtests of the Wechsler Intelligence Scale increased, particularly those measuring nonverbal rather than verbal skills.

The elderly as a group have a higher risk of micronutrient deficiency than young adults (Exton-Smith and Scott, 1968). Goodwin et al. (1983) correlated biochemical indices of vitamin status and cognitive functioning in the elderly. They reported significant inverse correlations between folate, riboflavin, and folate status and the ability to think abstractly. Chome et al. (1986) followed up these findings and compared elderly having a deficiency of at least one vitamin with those who did not. The deficient group produced poorer scores in tests of mood. Supplementation failed to alter psychological functioning, although the authors suggest that this may have reflected a small sample size.

Wernicke's disease is a neurological disorder due to thiamine deficiency, characterized by nystagmus, ataxia, confusion, and recent memory loss. Treatment with B vitamins may result in complete recovery (Escobar et al., 1983). However, Korsakoff's dementia, in which new long-term memories are not formed, often persists after treatment or spontaneous recovery from Wernicke's disease. The nutritional complications associated with alcoholism are the most common etiology of Korsakoffs dementia in developed countries. There are, however, reports that Wernicke's disease can be induced by intravenous feeding in hospital (Nadel and Burger, 1976). In such cases the body store of thiamine is depleted as it is needed to metabolize carbohydrate.

GENERAL CONCLUSION

An increasing number of well-designed studies have found that vitamin and mineral supplements benefit psychological functioning in those with a poor diet. In addition, many uncontrolled studies suggest relationships between micronutrients and behavior which should be more systematically examined.

A conservative conclusion is that the data justify further exploration of the possibility that subclinical deficiencies of vitamins and minerals exist in Western societies, and that these may adversely affect behavior and learning capacities. The assumption that the majority of individuals consume adequate levels of vitamins and minerals needs to be experimentally examined. A more specific conclusion must await the findings of research.

Even if future work confirms the hypothesis that subclinical deficiencies of minerals and vitamins exist, improving the diet or giving a vitamin supplement can only improve biological functioning. Whether a child's school performance or behavior is markedly changed will depend on the interaction of changed biology with the school, peer group, and family. In many instances psychological and social influences may prove more influential than nutritional factors.

There is little doubt that many in the general population find simple solutions to complex problems concerning their children very attractive. Although dietary supplementation is potentially a simple solution, at best it is unlikely to offer more than a small part of the answer to any psychological question. Human behavior reflects the summated influence of a multitude of factors: in the majority of cases an improvement of the existing Western diet can be expected to have, at the most, a small impact.

REFERENCES

Adler S. Megavitamin treatment for behaviorally disturbed and learning disabled children. J Learn Dis 1979; 12:678–81.

Abou-Saleh MT, Coppen C. The biology of folate in depression: Implications for nutritional hypotheses if the psychoses. J Psychiatr Res 1986; 20:91–101.

Bell IR, Edman JS, Marby DW, Satlin A, Dreier T, Liptzin B, Cole JO. Vitamin B-12 and folate status in acute geropsychiatric inpatients: Affective and cognitive characteristics of a vitamin nondeficient population. Biol. Psychiat 1990; 27:125–37.

Bennett FC, McClelland s, Kreigsmann ED, Andrus LB, Sells CJ. Vitamin and mineral supplementation in Down's syndrome. Pediatrics 1983; 72:707–713.

Benton D, Buts JP. Vitamin/mineral supplementation and intelligence. Lancet 1990; 335:1158–60.

Benton D, Cook R. Vitamin and mineral supplements improve the intelligence scores and concentration of six year old children. Person Individ Diff 1991; (in press).

Benton D, Roberts G. Effect of vitamin and mineral supplementation on intelligence of a sample of schoolchildren. Lancet 1988; 1:140–143.

Boggs UR, Scheaf A, Santoro D, Ritzman R. The effects of nutrient supplements on the biological and psychological characteristics of low IQ preschool children. J Orthomol Psychiat 1965; 14:97–127.

Botez MI, Botez T, Maag U. The Wechsler subtests in mild organic brain damage associated with foalte deficiency. Psychol Med 1984; 14:431–437.

Botez MI, Fontaine F, Botez T, Bachevalier J. Folate-responsive neurological and mental disorders: Report of 16 cases. Eur Neurol 1977; 16:230–246.

Brozek J. Psychological effects of thiamine restriction and deprivation in normal young men. Am J Clin Nutr 1957; 5:109–118.

Carney MWP, Sheffield MT. Serum folic acid and B-12 in 272 psychiatric inpatients. Psychol Med 1978; 8:139–144.

Chanowitz J, Ellman G, Silverstein CI, Zingarelli G, Ganger E. Thyroid and vitamin-mineral supplement fail to improve IQ of mentally retarded adults. Am J Ment Def 1985; 90:217–219.

Chome J, Paul T, Pudel V, Bleyl H, Heseker H, Huppe R, Kubler W. Effects of suboptimal vitamin status on behavior. Biblthca Nutr Dieta 1986; 38:94–104.

Coburn SP, Schaltendbrand WE, Mahuren JD, Clausman RJ, Townsend D. Effect of megavitamin treatment on mental performance and plasma vitamin B-6 concentrations in mentally retarded young adults. Am J Clin Nutr 1983; 38:352–355.

Coleman M, Sobel S, Bhagavan HN, Coursin D, Marquardt A, Guay M, Hunt C. A double blind study of vitamin B_6 in Down's syndrome infants. J Ment Defic Res 1985; 29:233–240.

Coleman M, Steinberg G, Tippett J, Bhagavan HN, Coursin DB, Cross M, Lewis C, DeVeau L. A preliminary study of the effect of pyridoxine administration in a subgroup of hyperkinetic children: A double-blind crossover comparison with methylphenidate. Biol Psychiat 1979; 14:741–751.

Crombie IK, Todman J, McNeill G, Florey C, Du V, Menzies I, Kennedy RA. Effect of vitamin and mineral supplementation on verbal and non-verbal reasoning of school-children. Lancet 1990; 335:744–747.

Davis DR. The Harrell study and seven follow-up studies: A brief review. J Orthomol Med 1987; 2:111–114.

Ellis NR, Tomporowski PD. Vitamin/mineral supplements and intelligence of institu-tionalized mentally retarded adults. Am J Ment Def 1983; 88:211–214.

Ellman G, Silverstein CI, Zingarelli G, Schafer WP, Silverstein L. Vitamin-mineral supplement fails to improve IQ of mentally retarded young adults. Am J Ment Def 1984; 88:688–691.

Escobar A, Aruffo C, Rodriguez-Carbajal J. Wernicke's Encephalopathy. A case report with neurophysiologic and CT-scan studies. Acta Vitaminol Enzymol 1983; 5:125–131.

Exton-Smith AN, Scott DL (Eds.). Vitamins in the elderly. Bristol: John Wright and Son, 1968.

Goodwin JS, Goodwin JM, Garry PJ. Association between nutritional status and cognitive functioning in a healthy elderly population. J Am Med Assoc 1983; 249:2917–2921.

Greenwood CT, Richardson DP. Nutrition during adolescence. Wld Rev Nutr Diet 1979; 33:1–41.

Harrell RF. Mental responses to added thiamine. J Nutr 1946; 31:283–298.

Harrell RF, Capp RH, Davis DR, Peerless J, Ravitiz LR. Can nutritional supplements help mentally retarded children? Proc Nat Acad Sci USA 1981; 78:574–578.

Hector M, Burton JR. What are the psychiatric manifestations of vitamin B-12 deficiency? J Am Geriatr Soc 1988; 36:1105–1112.

Heseker H, Kubler, W, Westenhofer J, Pudel V. Psychische Veranderungen als Fruhzeichen einer suboptimalen Vitaminversorgung. Ernahrungs-Umschau 1990; 37:87–94.

Hunter R, Jones J, Jones TG, Matthews DM. Serum B-12 and folate concentrations in mental patients. Br J Psychiat 1967; 113:1291–1295.

Kershner J, Hawke W. Megavitamins and learning disorders: A controlled double-blind experiment. J Nutr 1979; 109:819–826.

Kinsman RH, Hood J. Some behavioral effects of ascorbic acid deficiency. Am J Clin Nutr 1971; 24:455–464.

Nadel A, Burger PC. Wernicke encephalopathy following prolonged intravenous therapy. J Am Med Assoc 1976; 235:2403–2405.

Nelson M, Naismith DJ, Burley V, Gatenby S, Geddes N. Nutrient intake vitamin/mineral supplementation and intelligence in British schoolchildren. Br J Nutr 1990; 64:13–22.

Pueschel SM, Reed RB, Cronk CE, Goldstein BI. 5-Hydroxytryptophan and pyridoxine. Am J Dis Child 1980; 134:838.

Sandstead HH, Carter JP, House FR, McConnell F, Horton KB, Van der Zwaag R. Nutritional deficiencies in disadvantated preschool children. Am J Dis Child 1971; 121:455–463.

Schoenthaler S. Malnutrition and maladaptive behavior: Two correlational analyses and a double-blind placebo-controlled challenge in five states. In: Essman WB, ed. Nutrients and brain function. Basel: Karger, 1987, pp. 198–218.

Schoenthaler SJ, Amos SP, Doraz WE, Kelly MA, Wakefield J. Controlled trial of vitamin-mineral supplementation on intelligence and brain function. Person Individ Diff 1991; 4:343–350.

Shorvon, SD, Carney MWP, Chanarin I, Reynolds RH. The neuropsychiatry of mega-loblastic anemia. Br Med J 1980; 281:1036–1038.

Smith GF, Spiker D, Peterson CP, Cicchetti D, Justine P. Use of megadoses of vitamins with minerals in Down syndrome. J Pediatr 1984; 105:228–234.

Sommer BR, Wolkowitz OM. RBC folic acid levels and cognitive performance in elderly patients: A preliminary report. Biol Psychiat 1988; 24:352–354.

Sterner RT, Price RW. Restricted riboflavin: Within subject behavioral effects in humans. Am J Clin Nutr 1973; 26:150–160.

Thiessen I, Mills L. The use of megavitamin treatment in children with learning disabilities. Orthomol Psychiat 1975; 4:228–296.

Weathers C. Effects of nutritional supplementation on IQ and certain other variables associated with Down syndrome. Am J Ment Def 1983; 88:214–217.

Williams RJ. Biochemical individuality. New York: John Wiley and Sons, 1956, pp. 1–214.

BIRTH DEFECTS

11

Importance of Vitamin Status to Pregnancy Outcomes

Adrianne Bendich

Hoffmann-La Roche Inc.
Nutley, New Jersey

INTRODUCTION

Infant mortality, defined as death within the first year of life, occurs at an unexpectedly high rate of over 10 infants per 1000 born in the USA, ranking the USA only 19th as compared to other industrialized nations. In addition, thousands of infants are born yearly with low birth weights and concomitant lifetime disabilities (Wegman, 1987).

Birth defects are the major cause of infant morbidity and mortality in the USA (Oakley, 1986). Thirty percent of all admissions to pediatric hospitals can be traced to adverse pregnancy outcomes. Currently, birth defects are the fifth leading cause of years of potential life lost. In addition to the devastating physical and psychological effects, the total expenditures associated with birth defects are approximately $1.4 billion each year (National Center for Health Statistics, 1987).

Although the etiology of the majority of congenital malformations is not known, there is growing awareness that certain environmental factors such as dietary essential nutrients may affect the incidence of major classes of birth defects including neural tube defects (NTD) and cleft lip/cleft palate. As the next chapter by Drs. Schorah and Smithells clearly indicates, multivitamin supplementation in the months preceding and following conception significantly reduced the risk of having a second child with a neural tube birth defect.

In addition to the elegant studies of Smithells and Schorah involving recurrence of NTD, there is growing evidence that micronutrient status may also alter the rate of first-time occurrence of NTD and other adverse pregnancy outcomes.

The prepregnancy nutritional status of the woman is in many cases predictive of infant birth weight (Paige and Davis, 1986) and low birth weight is closely associated with many of the major congenital abnormalities. Additionally, there are women who are at greater risk for nutritionally related adverse pregnancy outcomes because of their use of prescription drugs or life-style habits which alter micronutrient status. The objectives of this chapter are (1) to review the evidence that vitamin nutriture affects the risk of first time occurrence of NTD; (2) to examine the association of low vitamin status (principally folic acid) and increased risk of birth defects in the offspring of women taking anticonvulsants; (3) to evaluate the findings of decreased risk of recurrence of cleft lip/cleft palate in multivitamin supplemented women; (4) to discuss the vitamin status of women of childbearing potential, including the impact of oral contraceptive use and cigarette smoking; and (5) to suggest recommendations based on the evidence as well as on the basis of safety considerations.

NEURAL TUBE BIRTH DEFECTS

The embryonic neural tube forms the brain and spinal cord. The closure of the tube occurs during the third week postconception (Fig. 1). If the upper portion of the tube fails to close, the brain does not form, leading to a condition termed anencephaly; miscarriage, stillbirth, or death shortly after birth are the most common consequences. If the lower neural tube does not close properly, loss of nerve function occurs below the opening in the spine (spina bifida). Paralysis and loss of bladder and bowel functions are generally found.

There are two general categories of these lesions: open (neural tissue exposed to the surface) or closed (lesions are covered by skin). Open lesions occur between the 17th and 30th day postconception and include anencephaly in which the brain may be absent or rudimentary. Closed lesions occur later and include encephaloceles, in which the brain protrudes through the skull, hydrocephalus, and various caudal lesions. Spina bifida, which results in paralysis below the opening in the spinal cord, can result from open or closed lesions (Lemire, 1988).

Nutritional status has been suggested as the most important environmental factor affecting the risk of NTDs. There is a greater incidence of NTDs in lower socioeconomic groups, which may reflect poorer diet. There is a higher incidence of NTD in infants conceived in the spring, when fresh foods are less available. The incidence of NTD is higher on the east vs. the west coasts of the USA, Canada, and Britain. In Canada and the USA, the incidence varies threefold from east to west. Newfoundland currently has a high incidence of NTDs, 3 per 1000 and the rate declines to 1 per 1000 in western Canada. Northern parts of the British Isles have one of the highest rates of incidence (7 per 1000; recurrence

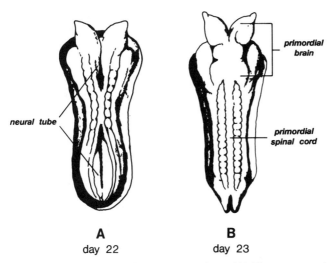

Figure 1 Development of the human embryo. (A) The open neural tube seen on day 22 of pregnancy, and (B) the closed neural tube, seen on day 23, indicating the formation of the primordial brain and spinal cord. If the neural tube fails to close in the area of the primordial brain, anencephaly results. If the tube fails to close in the area of the primordial spinal cord, spina bifida results.

risk can be more than 5%) while Japan has the lowest rate of NTD of less than 1 per 1000 births. The USA prevalence rate is 1 (in California) to 3 per 1000 (in Massachusetts) with a recurrence risk of 3%. These geographic patterns suggest that the causes of NTD include strong environmental components such as nutritional status (Lemire, 1988).

NTDs occur so early following conception that most women are unaware of their pregnancy. Thus, the potential for micronutrients to affect early embryonic events is dependent on an optimal nutritional status of the woman at the time of conception. Preconceptional nutritional status is especially critical because approximately 40% of all pregnancies are unplanned and 95% of NTD are first-time occurrences.

In 1984, Winship et al. published the first case-controlled study associating the intake of folic acid-containing supplements during the 3 months before the last menstrual period with a lowered risk of central nervous system defects in offspring. The odds ratios were below 1.00 in the groups that took folic acid alone or as a component of a multivitamin supplement; the associations did not reach statistical significance.

Recently, between 1988 and 1989, four important epidemiological studies examined the association of preconceptional and early postconceptional vitamin status and risk of occurrence of NTD. The first study was conducted by investigators from the Centers for Disease Control (CDC) using a population from the greater Atlanta area (Mulinare et al., 1988). The second study, by the National Institute of Child Health and Human Development (NICHHD), examined outcomes of pregnancies from California and Illinois (Mills et al., 1989). The third investigation was undertaken in western Australia (Bower and Stanley, 1989) and the fourth mainly involved women from Massachusetts (Milunsky et al., 1989).

CDC Study

The first major epidemiological study of multivitamin supplement use and occurrence of NTD was published by Mulinare et al. (1988). This population-based, retrospective, case control study evaluated the association between multivitamin use and NTD among women who had not previously had an infant with NTD. The study involved the comparison of three groups: (1) 347 women in the Atlanta area who gave birth to infants with NTD between 1968 and 1980; (2) a control group of 2829 randomly selected women whose infants were born without birth defects during the same period; and (3) to account for recall bias, a second control group of mothers whose infants had serious birth defects other than NTD during that period.

Mothers were interviewed by telephone and asked to recall whether they had taken a multivitamin supplement for each of the 3 months before conception through the first 3 months of pregnancy (defined as the periconceptional period in this study). Mothers who used multivitamins or prenatal vitamins through this 6-month period (14% of the population) were compared with those who did not take any supplemental vitamins during this time.

The women in this study were representative of individuals living in metropolitan areas and the surrounding suburbs and presumably ate typical diets. Nevertheless, the results of the study showed that women who took multivitamins for 3 months before and 3 months after conception were 60% less likely to have an infant with NTD than women who did not take multivitamin supplements.

The protective effect of supplemental multivitamins was greatest when they were taken in the 3-month period prior to conception and during the first 3 months of pregnancy. When periconceptional multivitamin users were compared with early postconceptional (3rd–6th month) and late postconceptional multivitamin users (7th–9th month), the greatest protection from NTD occurred with periconceptional multivitamin usage. Some protective benefits were observed when supplemental vitamins were taken during the period immediately after conception. Since NTD occur very early in pregnancy, it is not surprising that multivitamin supplements taken during the last third of pregnancy did not protect against NTD.

NICHHD Study

In contrast to the CDC study in which multivitamin supplement use and pregnancy could have occurred up to 16 years before enrollment, the Mills et al. (1989) NICHHD study interviewed women within 5 months of birth or pregnancy outcome. However, 14.5% of normal controls in the CDC study recalled supplement use, which is almost equivalent to the recall rate of 14.8% in the NICHHD study. If one assumes a difficulty in remembering the use of supplements which occurred many years in the past, then the CDC control group should have had a significantly lower recall rate than the NICHHD group. Even though recall may have been more accurate in the Mills study, their study population differed significantly from the women involved in the CDC study discussed above (Table 1).

Fifty-one percent of the NTD cases in the NICHHD paper were diagnosed by the 35th week of pregnancy. Amniocentesis and/or ultrasound are not per-

Table 1 Comparisons Between the CDC and NICHHD Studies

CDC study (Mulinare et al., 1988)	NICHHD study (Mills et al., 1989)
More statistical power—used 10 controls/ NTD case	Used two controls/NTD case
Rate of NTD in Atlanta population was 1.26/1000 births	Rate of NTD in California is 0.3–0.5/1000 births, the lowest in the USA
Examined anencephaly and spina bifida in their definition of NTD	Examined many more types of NTD and excluded some NTD-associated defects which may have been included in the CDC study
Used only live birth or stillbirth data; no abortions	Used live births, ultrasound, amniocentesis without need for birth; i.e., aborted fetuses were counted
Periconceptional period defined as multivitamin usage assessed for 3 months before until 3 months after confirmed pregnancy	Periconceptional period defined as multivitamin usage 30 days before until 45 days after confirmed pregnancy
Regular user defined as taking multivitamins 3x/week over a 6-month period	Regular user defined as taking multivitamin 6x/week and/or eating fortified cereals; length of intake period not discussed
7% of NTD used multivitamins vs. 15% in controls	15% of NTDs and controls used multivitamins
Included maternal age, smoking history, and chronic illnesses of mothers as confounding variables for statistical analysis	Confounding variables are not defined. Especially important is maternal age

formed during every pregnancy, but only in high-risk pregnancies, predominantly of medically insured women. Women from less economically (and perhaps less nutritionally) advantaged backgrounds may not have been included in this study. It is also possible that the NTD group from NICHHD had risk factors (such as mother's age) which are not affected by multivitamin supplementation. The use of prenatal screening procedures may have biased this study against finding a multivitamin effect.

Although Mills et al. (1989) conclude that vitamin supplements did not lower the risk of NTD, an equally valid conclusion could be that preconceptional supplementation for 30 days is not sufficient to protect against NTD. In the CDC study, preconceptional supplementation for 3 months was associated with significantly lowered risk. Similarly, in the recurrence of NTD studies by Smithells et al. (1981), preconceptional supplementation of an average of 110 days was associated with a significant reduction in NTD.

Western Australia Study

Both the CDC and NICHHD studies lacked information on dietary intake as well as biochemical indicators of vitamin status (enzymatic assays and/or serum/red blood cell vitamin levels). In contrast to these studies, Bower and Stanley (1989) carefully examined the diets and supplement use of 77 cases of NTD, compared to 77 control subjects with infants with birth defects other than NTD (control group 1), and with 154 control subjects with no birth defects (control group 2). All women were from western Australia and were entered into the study following their pregnancy outcomes. Participants completed a food frequency questionnaire which contained questions on the frequency of intake of 105 foods eaten during the 3 months before conception and following 9 months of pregnancy (12 months in total). Folate-containing foods were stressed, and intakes of fiber, riboflavin, carotene, calcium, and vitamin C could also be estimated fairly accurately based on the questionnaire. Information on drug and vitamin supplement use were also included. The concentrations of folic acid and the other vitamins in the multivitamins used by participants were included in the calculations of total folate and other vitamin intakes. Serum and red blood cell folic acid levels were determined following pregnancy. Over 85% of all interviews occurred within 65 weeks of the last menstrual period before conception.

Folic acid status is reflected in the serum and red blood cell folic acid levels (normal levels are approximately >4.5 and >300 ng/ml, respectively). Serum folate reflects recent dietary intake and falls rapidly when folate-depleted diets are consumed experimentally, whereas red blood cell folate levels, which reflect long-term folate status, are not decreased significantly until 16–18 weeks on a folate-deficient diet. In addition to red blood cells, white blood cells, specificially neutrophils, respond to folate intakes with morphological changes. The nucleus of the neutrophil becomes hypersegmented and the degree of hypersegmentation is inversely related to the folate status. Serum folate levels below 4.5 ng/ml and red blood cell folate levels below 250 ng/ml are associated with neutrophil hypersegmentation. Following depletion of red blood cell folate, megaloblastic red cells first appear in the bone marrow and then in the blood, resulting in megaloblastic anemia. Neutrophil hypersegmentation precedes the appearance of megaloblastic red blood cells in the circulating blood. Thus, megaloblastic anemia represents a very late stage in severe folate deficiency and low serum, neutrophil, and red cell levels correspond to early signs of compromised folate status (Pietrzik, 1989).

In the Bower and Stanley study (1989), the use of vitamin supplements containing folic acid during the first 6 weeks of pregnancy was reported by 15% of cases and 21 and 15% of control groups 1 and 2, respectively. Total folate intake (total folate includes sources from food and supplements) was calculated and divided into quartiles, where the lowest intake group was in the first quartile and was assigned a relative risk of 1.00. As the total folate intake increased, the risk of NTD decreased significantly (46% reduced risk).

Risk ratios were also developed which compared the degree of risk reduction based on free folate. The folate in vitamin supplements is the free folic acid. As can be seen in Tables 2 and 3, increased intakes of free folic acid during the first 6 weeks of pregnancy was associated with a 75% reduction in risk and was

Table 2 Total Folate Intake and Risk of NTD

Quartiles total folate (μg/day)	Odds ratios
20.0– 178.4	1
178.5– 239.6	0.97
239.7– 350.1	0.64
350.2–1787.0	0.54

Source: Bower and Stanley, 1989.

Table 3 Free Folate Intake and Risk of NTD

Quartiles free folic acid (μg/day)	Odds ratios
8– 79.8	1
79.9– 115.4	0.54
115.5– 180.5	0.40
180.6–1678.0	0.25

Source: Bower and Stanley, 1989.

thus more protective than food folates (conjugated folate). This suggests that women at risk for NTD may have a reduced ability to deconjugate food folates and form free folic acid, the form of the vitamin which is most readily transported across cell membranes (Yates et al., 1987). Risk of NTD was also reduced as intakes of vitamin C, carotene (Table 4), and fiber increased.

Not unexpectedly, intake, serum, and red blood cell folate levels measured following pregnancy were not related to risk of NTD.

The results of the western Australia study are in accord with the findings of the CDC study. In both, the rate of NTD in the populations studied was approximately 2 NTD/1000 births. Supplementation (with multivitamins or folic acid-containing supplements) was associated with a risk reduction of approximately 50% in both the CDC and this study. More specific information concerning the type of supplements used by the women in the western Australia study is required before further interstudy comparisons can be made.

Boston Study

The fourth study, unlike the three described above, is a prospective one involving over 22,000 women who had undergone either maternal serum alpha-fetoprotein analysis or amniocentesis within the first 16 weeks of pregnancy. The study was designed to examine factors affecting adverse pregnancy outcomes and evaluated many parameters, including nutritional components. Approximately 88% of participants were from Massachusetts, 96% were white, and 70% had attended college. Because this was a prospective study, the majority of women were interviewed prior to fetal diagnosis, and recall bias is therefore not a factor in this study. The women were questioned about use of medications, genetic history, illnesses, infections, and vitamin and nutritional supplement use in the 3 months prior to pregnancy as well as during the first 3 months of pregnancy. Multivitamin and single-vitamin supplement uses were determined and a woman was considered a supplement user if she reported taking at least one supplement/week (87% of users took multivitamins 7 days/week). Dietary recall of frequency of intake of 50 foods consumed during the first 8 weeks of pregnancy was evaluated.

Table 4 Vitamin C and Carotene Intake and Risk of NTD (Dependent Variables)

	Quartiles			
	1	2	3	4
	Odds ratios			
Vitamin C	1.00	0.65	0.51	0.18
Carotene	1.00	1.20	0.47	0.31

Source: Bower and Stanley, 1989.

Of the 22,776 women in the study, 49 had pregnancies with NTD. Eleven of the cases occurred in the 3157 women who used no multivitamins, 29 cases occurred in 12,297 women who used multivitamins in the first trimester only, and the remaining 9 cases occurred in 7322 women who used multivitamins before and during the first trimester. As can be seen in Table 5, the risk of NTD was significantly reduced by 64% in the supplemented compared to the nonsupplemented women. The protective effect of supplementation was highly significant in women who supplemented during the first 6 weeks of pregnancy (risk significantly reduced by 32%) compared to unsupplemented or those beginning supplementation after the seventh week of pregnancy.

Women who took multivitamin supplements which did not contain folic acid had no reduction in the risk of NTD. The dietary folate intake was calculated for women who were not supplemented with folic acid during the first 6 weeks of pregnancy. Women with a dietary folate intake of <100 µg/day had a threefold higher incidence of NTD than women with intakes above 100 µg/day.

Women with a family history of NTD who did not use supplements had a prevalence of NTD of 13 per 1000 compared to those who supplemented and had a prevalence of 3.5 per 1000. The 3.7-fold reduction in risk of NTD in this high-risk population was a most significant finding.

Analysis of the Four Epidemiological Studies

In agreement with the Bower and Stanley (1989) and Mulinare et al. (1988) studies discussed above, the Milunsky et al. study (1989) corroborates the findings of the strong association of periconceptional folic acid-containing multivitamin supplement use and significantly decreased risk of NTD.

Tabulation of the major findings of these studies below shows a clear association of decreased risk of NTD in supplemented groups when the expected rate of occurrence is about 1.8 per 1000. The Mills et al. study (1989) did not show a decreased risk in women surveyed from an area with an already considerably lower rate of NTD (California).

Lowered rate, based on large population bases, may not be predictive of lowered risk, which is based on genetic as well as environmental factors. However,

Table 5 Multivitamin Use and Risk of NTD

	None	First trimester only	Before conception and first trimester
Prevalence per 1000 births	3.5	2.4	1.2
Relative risk	1.00	0.68	0.36

Source: Milunsky et al., 1989.

Table 6 Expected vs. Potential Rate of NTD with Periconceptional
Vitamin Supplementation

Study	Expected rate per 1000	Potential rate in supplemented groups, per 1000[a]
Mulinare et al. (1988)	1.8	0.9–1.0
Bower and Stanley (1989)	1.8	1.0
Milunsky et al. (1989)	2.2	1.2
Mills et al. (1989)	0.9	0.9

[a] Potential decreases in rate of NTD are based on the extrapolation from the reduction
in risk seen in the supplemented groups from each study and may not be applicable
to larger population groups.

reduction in risk translates to lower rates of NTD in the population groups
examined in three of the four epidemiological studies (Table 6).

The reproducibility of the results between the studies is also seen in the
approximately 60% decrease in risk found in each of the three studies outlined
in Table 7. Based on the premise that environmental and genetic factors contribute
to the NTD syndrome, the cumulative data indicate consistent, strong, protective
environmental components, namely, folic acid/multivitamin supplementation.

Similar findings have also been seen in the Smithells et al. (1981), Laurence
et al. (1981), and Biale and Lewenthal (1984), and most recently in the report
by Nevin and Seller (1990) from their intervention studies in very-high-risk
women. For example, rate of recurrence was 13 NTD in 305 infants/ fetuses in
unsupplemented mothers and one NTD in 204 infants/fetuses in the mothers who
took multivitamins during the periconceptional period of 3 months before until

Table 7 Consistency of Odds Ratios in Epidemiological Studies of Reduced
Risk of NTD with Periconceptional Vitamin Supplementation

Study	Cases	Controls	Odds ratios (95% confidence interval)
Mulinare et al. (1988)	171	1,480	0.40 (0.25–0.65)
Bower and Stanley (1989)	77	231	0.38 (0.15–0.94)
Milunsky et al.[a] (1989)	3157	11,675	0.32 (0.15–0.68)

[a] In this study, "cases" represent unsupplemented women and "controls" represent women supplemented preconceptionally as well as during the first 6 weeks of pregnancy.

Table 8 Multivitamin Supplementation
and Recurrence of NTD

	NTD	Pregnancies	%
		Number of	
Unsupplemented	18	320	5.6
Supplemented	1	150	0.7

Source: Smithells, 1989.

3 months after conception (Smithells et al., 1981), and most recently, similar protective findings were reported from a separate cohort of women (Table 8; Smithells, 1989). The consistency of the data from multivitamin supplementation studies is further seen in Table 9 from the recent report from Nevin and Seller (1990).

Laurence et al. (1981), in a placebo-controlled, double-blind study, found that women given 4 mg of folic acid had a lowered recurrence rate of NTD from that found in the placebo group (Table 10); however, the effect was not as dramatic as that seen with multivitamin supplementation. The women in the supplemented group who did have recurrences ($n = 3$) also had the poorest diets.

In a small study, the rate of occurrence of birth defects in women taking anticonvulsants dropped from a predicted level of 150 per 1000 to zero when folic acid supplementation was given periconceptionally to 24 women (Biale and Lewenthal, 1984; discussed in detail in the epilepsy section). These provocative findings await replication in placebo-controlled, double-blind studies.

Two of the four epidemiological studies (Bower and Stanley, 1989; Milunsky et al., 1989) strongly suggest that folic acid is one of the critical essential micronutrients in NTD prevention and that total folate intakes above 350 μg/day were associated with a 50% reduction in risk, while intakes below 240 μg/day did not lower the risk of NTD (Bower and Stanley, 1989) and increased incidence of NTD was associated with intakes of folate below 100 μg/day (Milunsky et

Table 9 Multivitamin Supplementation and Recurrence of NTD,
Results from Northern Ireland, 1976–1989[a]

	NTD	Number of pregnancies	%
Unsupplemented	17	353	4.8
Multivitamins	4	511	0.8

[a] $p = 0.00018$, Fischer's exact test.
Source: Nevin and Seller, 1990.

Table 10   Folic Acid Supplementation and Recurrence of NTD

	NTD	Number of pregnancies	%
Unsupplemented	5	77	6.4
Folic acid supplements	3[a]	109	2.8

[a] Poor diets.
Source: Laurence, 1981.

al., 1989). The inability to metabolize food folates appears to be a potential discriminating factor in the etiology of NTD (Yates et al., 1987; Bower and Stanley, 1989).

EPILEPSY, ANTICONVULSANTS, AND INCREASED RISK OF BIRTH DEFECTS

In the USA, the age-adjusted prevalence of epilepsy is 6.25 per 1000 (Wyngaarden and Smith, 1988). Potentially, 1 in 250–400 pregnant women has epilepsy and a high proportion are exposed to anticonvulsants before and during pregnancy (Gatenby, 1960; Lindhout and Meinardi, 1984). Maternal seizure disorders are frequently reported as pregnancy-associated complications. Women with epilepsy have a higher incidence of offspring with congenital abnormalities than women without epilepsy (Patterson, 1989). The risk of birth defects is increased two to three-fold further in epileptic women taking anticonvulsants, as the majority are known teratogens (Friis, 1983). In a large, multi-institutional study from Japan involving 657 epileptic women, 55 of 638 live births from medicated mothers had malformations while only 3 malformed infants were born to a similar number of unmedicated mothers. Cleft lip/cleft palate occurred at a rate of 31.4 per 1000 in the medicated group compared to the expected rate of 2.7 in the general population. The incidence of miscarriage or stillbirth in the medicated group (13.4%) was twice as high as that seen in the general population (Nakane et al., 1980).

Folate Status and Anticonvulsant Drug Use

The majority of anticonvulsants interfere with folic acid metabolism by reducing folic acid absorption, inhibiting deconjugase enzymes, and/or inhibiting folate transport into tissues, resulting in a suboptimal folate status in nonpregnant epileptics (Krause, 1988; Zhu and Zhou, 1989). Compromised folate status is further exacerbated because of pregnancy when maternal folate progressively declines in nonepileptic and especially chronically treated epileptic women (Dansky et al., 1987). Megaloblastic anemia associated with folic acid deficiency has been documented in several studies in pregnant women taking anticonvulsants (Gatenby, 1960), although the antifolate effects of anticonvulsants are not well recognized by neurologists as a potential component of their teratogenicity (Donaldson, 1989). Whether the teratogenic effects of anticonvulsants such as diphenylhydantoin or valproic acid are direct effects or due to secondary folate deficiency has been examined experimentally as well as clinically.

Experimental Evidence That Folate Supplementation Lessens the Teratogenic Effects of Anticonvulsants

Valproic acid administration to pregnant mice results in a high incidence of neural tube birth defects (exencephaly). Nutritional folate deficiency further increases the rate of exencephaly (Trotz et al., 1986). When folic acid was given concomitantly with a single teratogenic dose of valproate to folate-replete pregnant mice, the rate of exencephaly was reduced by 50% (Trotz et al., 1987).

Administration of phenytoin during early gestation results in fetal abnormalities including skeletal malformations and hydrocephalus. Dietary supplementation with folic acid significantly reduced the skeletal abnormalities seen in the laboratory animals. The combined supplement of folic acid, vitamin B_{12}, vitamin D, nicotinamide, methionine, and threonine significantly reduced the incidence of internal malformations, including hydrocephalus, whereas folic acid alone did not (Zhu and Zhou, 1989).

Epidemiological Evidence of Low Folate Status Associated with Increased Risk of Congenital Malformations

Dansky et al. (1987) evaluated prospectively the relationship between folate status and use of single or multiple antiepileptic drugs, and pregnancy outcomes of 46 epileptic women during 49 pregnancies. Almost half (46%) of the women had below normal serum folate levels and 8% had low red cell folate levels which were inversely correlated with anticonvulsant drug use, especially phenytoin. The risk of adverse pregnancy outcomes, including major congenital malformations associated with low serum folate levels (below 4 ng/ml), was 46.2% compared to 11.8% in women with serum folate above 4 ng/ml ($p < 0.025$). Only two of the women with adverse pregnancy outcomes also had low red blood cell folate levels, suggesting to the authors that a mild folate deficiency without tissue depletion may be sufficient to cause abnormal embryonic development (Fig. 2). This is the second prospective study by this group that has shown a higher rate of spontaneous abortion and major congenital malformations in epileptic women taking anticonvulsants (Dansky et al., 1982, 1985).

Vitamin Supplement Intervention Trial in Women Taking Anticonvulsant Drugs

Although there is a strong association of low folate status and teratogenic effects of certain anticonvulsants, until 1984 there was no published report of an inter-

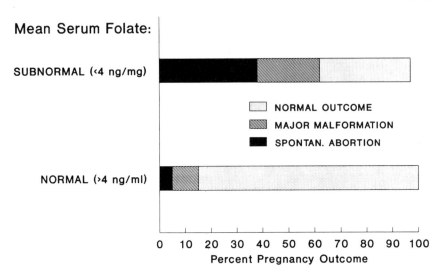

Figure 2 Pregnancy outcomes in women taking antiepileptic drugs: effect of folate status. The rate of spontaneous abortions is inversely related to serum folate levels. The percentage of normal pregnancies is directly related to serum folate levels. (Adapted from Dansky et al., 1987.)

vention trial to determine the effect of folic acid supplementation on the pregnancy outcomes in women taking this class of drugs. Biale and Lewenthal (1984), in a small retrospective study, observed a 15% incidence of congenital defects among 66 newborns of women undergoing long-term anticonvulsant therapy. In a prospective study of 22 women involving 33 pregnancies, all were given 2.5–5 mg folic acid/day preconceptionally and during the entire pregnancy in 26 of the pregnancies, and within the first 40 days and during the remainder of the pregnancy in the 7 remaining pregnancies. No birth defects were seen in the 33 pregnancies. These findings are most provocative and certainly require replication in a larger population-based study. In light of the positive findings and the well-recognized antifolate activities of most anticonvulsants, it would seem unethical to require a placebo group in such a study.

OTHER DRUGS WITH ANTIFOLATE ACTIVITY

Approximately 2 million adults in the USA suffer from inflammatory bowel diseases, Crohn's disease, or ulcerative colitis; the majority of cases are identified between 15 and 35 years of age (Office of Disease Prevention, 1988). One of the most commonly prescribed drugs for the treatment of these chronic digestive system diseases is sulfasalazine.

Table 11 Drugs That Interfere with Folic Acid Metabolism

Drug	Indication
Antiepileptics Phenytoin Phenobarbital Valproic acid and others	Seizure Disorders
Sulfasalazine	Inflammatory bowel diseases; cancer;
Methotrexate	arthritis; psoriasis; antibacterial; anti-
Trimethoprim	malarial; contraception
Oral contraceptives	
Alcohol	

Sulfasalazine has been shown to interfere with folic acid absorption and alter activities of several folate-associated enzymes, resulting in folic acid deficiency in patients receiving this drug chronically (Morgan and Baggott, this volume). A recent compilation of exposures to sulfasalazine in pregnant women has shown a 5.6-fold greater risk of NTD compared to exposures to other drugs (Rosa et al., in press).

Other sulfonamides may indirectly decrease folic acid utilization. Trimethoprim, an antibacterial and antimalarial agent, blocks the formation of the active form of folic acid in cells. Women who are treated with these drugs should be monitored, especially if the possibility of pregnancy exists.

Methotrexate, a well-recognized antifolate, is routinely used for chemotherapy of some cancers. Recently, it was used in the treatment of rheumatoid arthritis at lower dosage levels than those needed to kill tumor cells. Methotrexate is also used in the treatment of psoriasis (Table 11). The folate status of women using this drug and anticipating pregnancy should be carefully monitored.

CLEFT LIP/CLEFT PALATE

There is evidence of potential benefits of vitamins in preventing the serious birth defect, cleft lip/cleft palate. Clefts of the palate and lip occur once in approximately 700–800 births (*Merck Manual*, 1987). A perforation in the palate may involve the hard and/or soft palates. The cleft may vary from involvement of the soft palate only to a complete cleft of the soft and hard palates, the jaw, and the lip. Cleft lip is cosmetically distressing and in some cases interferes with normal speech. Cleft palate interferes with feeding and speech development. The lip and palate develop during the 8th–11th weeks following conception. The embryonic events involved in the formation of cleft lip or cleft palate alone may differ from those involved in the combined defect.

Cleft lip/cleft palate resembles NTD in that both seem to have genetic as well as strong environmental components in their etiologies. In a survey of 480 infants, the greatest incidence of cleft lip/cleft palate occurred when conception was in the late winter, when fresh foods would be least available (Kristoffersen and Rolschau, 1984).

Intervention Studies

Three major intervention studies of the effect of vitamin supplementation on the recurrence of cleft lip/cleft palate have been reported (Table 12). The earliest (Conway, 1958) involved 87 women who had already had one child with cleft lip/cleft palate and were at high risk of recurrence. Of the 87, 48 received no vitamin supplementation during the subsequent 78 pregnancies; five (6.4%) congenital abnormalities including three clefts were seen in this group. Vitamin supplementation was begun during the first trimester of pregnancy in the 39 remaining women who had 59 pregnancies. There were no recurrences in the supplemented group.

Peer et al. (1964) gave a prenatal multivitamin to mothers who had previously given birth to children with cleft palate and/or cleft lip at the first suspicion of pregnancy through the fourth month. The supplement included 5 mg of folate and 10 mg of vitamin B_6. Four cases of cleft palate and/or cleft lip occurred in the vitamin treated group ($n = 176$; 2.3%), vs. 19 in the untreated group ($n = 418$; 4.5%). In a follow-up study of 228 women with 348 pregnancies, there were 11 recurrent oral defects (3.2%) among supplemented mothers (Briggs, 1976).

In 1982, Tolarova reported a greatly reduced rate of recurrence of cleft lip/

Table 12   Impact of Multivitamin Supplementation
on Recurrence of Cleft Lip/Cleft Palate

Study	n	Recurrences	%
Conway, 1958			
supplemented	59	0	–
unsupplemented	78	4	5.1
Peer et al., 1964			
supplemented	176	4	2.3
unsupplemented	418	19	4.5
Briggs, 1976			
supplemented	348	11	3.2
Tolarova et al., 1986			
supplemented	173	3	1.7
unsupplemented	1901	77	4.1

cleft palate in 85 fully supplemented pregnancies (one recurrence), as compared to 212 unsupplemented controls (15 recurrences). The supplement was given for at least 3 months before conception and until at least the end of the first trimester of pregnancy. In 1986, the cumulative findings (including the data in the 1982 study) continued to show a highly significant protective effect of vitamin supplementation in women who had previously had a child with cleft lip/cleft palate ($p < 0.075$) (Tolarova, 1986).

Epidemiological Study

In a case-controlled study examining associations between nutritional status and incidence of clefts, no significant differences in serum or red blood cell folate, vitamin A, or carotene were found between women who had delivered children with or without oral clefts (Niebyl et al., 1985). Since this was a retrospective study, the maternal vitamin status was not measured until following the birth of the affected child and thus may not reflect maternal vitamin status during the early stages of pregnancy when the defect occurs.

SPONTANEOUS ABORTION; ABRUPTIO PLACENTAE

One of the earliest clinical findings of a nutritionally related factor associated with adverse pregnancy outcomes was reported by Hibbard in 1964. The incidence of severe folic acid deficiency as indicated by megaloblastic anemia was 15.6% in the third trimester in women from lower socioeconomic classes. A positive association was found between megaloblastic anemia and the incidence of abruptio placentae. In a series of 98 patients with abruptio placentae, 64 had positive bone marrow biopsies showing megaloblastic red blood cell formation. Marginal folic acid deficiency was documented prospectively in 5.7% of women who later had abruptio placentae, four times the expected rate. A similar association between low folate status and increased rate of spontaneous abortion was reported in this cohort. The incidence of congenital malformations was also greater in the deficient women.

In a cohort of 150 women with spontaneous abortion of unknown etiology, 25% of cases had serum folic acid levels of <2.6 ng/ml; 50% had serum folate <4.1 ng/ml. Intervention with folic acid supplements in 17 women with a history of spontaneous abortions resulted in 15 normal deliveries and 2 pregnancies which had passed the first trimester at the time of the report (Martin et al., 1965).

Streiff and Little (1967) reported that 23 of 63 patients with third trimester bleeding and 15 of 16 patients with abruptio placentae were deficient in folic acid as reflected in serum folate levels below 3 ng/ml and red cell folate levels below 200 ng/ml.

VITAMIN STATUS OF WOMEN

The infant mortality rate of the USA is currently the poorest of the industrialized nations and is directly related to the incidence of birth defect-associated deaths. The vitamin status of women of childbearing age in the USA, especially the folic acid status, does not approach recommended levels for the majority of this population group (U.S. RDA is 400 μg/day). Data from the most recent survey of the U.S. population (NHANES II) showed that over 35% of adults consumed 101–200 μg/day of folic acid whereas over 60% of black females consumed less than 200 μg/day and 25% had intakes below 101 μg/day (Subar et al., 1989). In a separate survey by the USDA, approximately 70% of low-income women consumed less than 200 μg/day of folate (Table 13; Nutrition Monitoring Division, 1989). The 1989 food consumption survey indicates that women in low socio-economic levels have even poorer diets than median-income women. Women from low socioeconomic levels also have a significantly higher infant mortality rate than middle class women.

Of equal importance, especially with regard to NTD, is the evidence that maternal capability to deconjugate food folate may be impaired, resulting in a low-folate status. The impairment may be due to genetic defects and/or hormonal regulation (Yates et al., 1987). In either case, the absorption and metabolism of free folic acid, as found in multivitamins or folic acid supplements, is not affected by this defect. Thus, ingestion of free folic acid may overcome many aspects of diet-associated folate deficiency.

Effects of Oral Contraceptive Use

Of the women who use birth control measures (50%), approximately 16% use oral contraceptives (OC) as their method of birth control (Bachrach and Mosher, 1985). A significant proportion of women become pregnant within the first few

Table 13 Percentage of Low-Income Women with Nutrient Intakes Below the 1980 RDA

	RDA levels (% of women)	
	Below 70%	Below 50%
Folic acid	88	70
Vitamin B$_6$	78	52
Vitamin E	59	39
Vitamin A	50	34
Vitamin C	36	21
Vitamin B$_{12}$	24	10

Source: Nutrition Today, 1989; data from CSFII 1986.

months of cessation of OC use. Several researchers have found significantly reduced serum as well as red cell folate levels in women taking OC, which has been attributed to impaired folate metabolism (Rhode et al., 1983). OC use for 2 years was associated with a significantly lower folate status than OC use for 1 year, suggesting a duration effect. After discontinuation of OC, serum folic acid levels rose consistently during the following 3 months, even though there was no change in diet. However, serum folate was still below 4 ng/ml in many women, which strongly suggests a folate deficiency (Streiff, 1970; Shojania et al., 1971).

The synthetic female hormones used in OC have been shown in vitro to inhibit the intestinal conjugase enzyme required for absorption of conjugated folates found in foods but not the free folic acid used in supplements (Streiff, 1970); however there are data indicating that estrogen increases uterine conjugase activity and thus uterine folate levels (Krumdieck et al., 1975). OC may thus alter absorption of food folates, increase clearance of folic acid from the serum, and/ or increase the rate of urinary excretion while enhancing the levels in the target tissue (Streiff, 1970; Shojania et al., 1975). Subclinical intestinal malfunctions may also be exacerbated by OC-associated folic acid deficiency (Toghill and Smith, 1971).

Wynn (1975) reviewed the vitamin status of women taking OC. Pyridoxine (vitamin B_6) deficiency has been reported in association with OC use. The requirements for pyridoxine are increased because of the consequent alteration in metabolism of tryptophan by estrogen and other OC hormones. Reductions in serum and white blood cell ascorbic acid and serum vitamin B_{12} and beta-carotene have also been reported in women taking OC.

Women who become pregnant shortly after termination of OC use may be at risk of low folate (and other vitamins) during the critical period of organogenesis.

Effects of Cigarette Smoking

Approximately 32% of U.S. women of childbearing age smoke, and a recent survey showed that 45% of pregnant women participating in WIC programs in Missouri were smokers. Data from 127,512 pregnant women enrolled in WIC programs in this state from 1979 to 1985 demonstrated a 2.5 times greater risk of having low-birthweight infants for smokers compared to nonsmokers (Mayer et al., 1990). Women who smoke tend to have poorer diets, a higher incidence of low-birthweight infants and an increased rate of ectopic pregnancies compared to nonsmokers. Ectopic pregnancy is the primary cause of maternal mortality in the first trimester (Handler et al., 1989). Smokers have approximately twice as many spontaneous abortions and 30% more fetal deaths than nonsmokers; however, the overall incidence of birth defects in live births was not found to be greater in smokers in one study (Malloy et al., 1989), whereas a higher incidence of cleft lip/cleft palate in smokers was reported in another study (Ericson et al., 1979).

In a survey study of approximately 200 women, smokers consumed significantly less fiber, minerals, and vitamins than nonsmokers. Specifically, dietary intakes of free and conjugated folate, carotene, vitamin D, thiamin, niacin, vitamins C, E, and B_6 were significantly lower (Haste et al., 1990). As the number of cigarettes smoked per day increased, the folate intake decreased (Rogozinski et al., 1983). Female cigarette smokers have significantly lower serum and red blood cell folate levels and lower serum vitamin C and carotene levels compared to nonsmokers (Witter et al., 1982; Palan et al., 1989). As mentioned above, OC users have lower serum beta-carotene levels than non-OC users; however, cigarette smoking in OC users lowers these levels even further (Palan et al., 1989).

Effects of Alcohol

Abuse of drugs and alcohol is continuing to rise in pregnant women. Alcohol abuse during pregnancy is associated with significantly higher rates of low birthweight, stillbirth, spontaneous abortion, and fetal alcohol syndrome (Little et al., 1989). In addition to the substitution of alcohol for nutrient-dense foods and the direct effects of alcohol on the fetus, alcohol interferes with folic acid absorption (Halsted, 1989).

Nutritional Status of Women Early in Pregnancy

In a comprehensive review of all causes of infant mortality occurring during 1980, the most significant predictor of neonatal death was infant birthweight (CDC, 1990). The risk of death for infants with birthweights less than 1500 g was 431 deaths/1000 live births compared to a risk of 2.1 deaths/1000 live births for infants weighing more than 2500 g. Other critical risk factors were maternal age, education, and prenatal care. Prepregnancy weight status of the mother is a well-established predictor of infant birthweight (Paige and Davis, 1986).

Neonatal mortality rates are more than one and one-half times higher in teen pregnancies than all other pregnancies (ADA, 1989). Teenagers are more likely to be underweight at the beginning of pregnancy than older women. Poor teenagers may be at even greater risk of being underweight and consequently having multiple periconceptional micronutrient deficiencies. The dietary patterns of pregnant adolescents participating in the WIC program that provides supplemental food still demonstrated that more than 20% of participants had less than 100% of the RDA for at least 11 of 16 nutrients studied (ADA, 1989).

In a recent study of 265 women from all social classes in England, Schofield et al. (1989) found that a significant proportion of women during the first trimester had dietary intakes below recommended levels of iron, calcium, ascorbic acid, and folic acid. Folate intake was approximately one-fifth of the British RDA in all groups. The lowest intakes were in the lowest socioeconomic groups.

In most instances of major congenital malformations, fetal growth is retarded, resulting in low birthweight (Wald et al., 1980). Specific deficiencies of folate, pantothenate, and vitamin B_{12} were found in low-birthweight infants compared to normal-weight infants, all of whom were born to mothers with no overt signs of malnutrition (Baker et al., 1977). Smithells et al. (1976) analyzed the first-trimester serum and red blood cell folate and serum vitamin C levels of 959 pregnant women and found that the six women who had NTD also had significantly lower red blood cell folate and serum vitamin C levels than the other 953 women. Like Smithells, Hall (1972) found no association between serum folate levels and risk of NTD.

Recently, in a prospective study of 97 women undergoing amniocentesis, it was shown that vitamin B_{12} levels were lower than normal in the amniotic fluids from fetuses with NTD as well as from fetuses with other related birth defects and from fetuses of women with previous NTD but carrying a normal fetus. The amniotic vitamin B_{12} carrier protein concentrations were higher in these groups than in controls. The authors suggest that the low vitamin B_{12} status may adversely affect folic acid utilization, since vitamin B_{12} is required for the formation of the active form of folic acid within cells. Supplemental folic acid could overcome the secondary deficiency caused by low levels of vitamin B_{12} (Gardiki-Kouidou and Seller, 1988). Future studies should include serum levels of these vitamins and carrier proteins.

Vitamin/Mineral Supplementation and Occurrence of Birth Defects: Intervention Trial

As discussed above, the limited data from intervention trials in high-risk women (recurrence of NTD and cleft lip/cleft palate) as well as the majority of findings from the epidemiological studies on occurrence of NTD point to a strong potential protective effect of folic acid-containing multivitamins. However, to determine a cause-and-effect relationship, a double-blind, placebo-controlled study is required. In terms of public health issues, the trial should include documentation of occurrence of all congenital malformations.

The World Health Organization is sponsoring a placebo-controlled, double-blind study in Hungary to determine the effect of multivitamin/mineral supplementation on the occurrence of all classes of adverse pregnancy outcomes. The supplementation is one part of the Optimal Family Planning Programme involving women aged 18–35. Supplementation commences on the first days of the menstrual period during the third month of baseline, nonpregnant period and continues (whether or not pregnancy occurs) until 12 weeks of gestation. Thus the minimal preconceptional supplementation period is 4 weeks. The placebo in the study contains low levels of vitamin C, calcium, copper, manganese, zinc, and lactose. The supplement contains RDA or higher levels of vitamins A, B_1, B_2, B_6, B_{12}, C, D, and E, folic acid, nicotinamide, pantothenate, calcium, phosphorus, magnesium, iron, copper, manganese, and zinc (Czeizel and Rode, 1984).

The expected rate of NTD in Hungary is approximately 2 per 1000 births (Czeizel, 1983). To establish a statistically and biologically significant reduction of NTD risk, approximately 10,000 pregnancies are expected to be evaluated. In 1989, Czeizel and Fritz reported that 1302 pregnancies had been studied— 599 supplemented and 703 placebo controls. No cases of NTD were found in the supplemented group and three cases were seen in the placebo group. Three cases of cleft lip with or without cleft palate were seen in the supplemented group and one case was found in the placebo group. No other birth defects were discussed in the brief report. In 1990, Czeizel reported (manuscript in preparation) that no incidences of NTD were seen in 1352 pregnancies in the supplemented group and four NTD occurred in 1371 pregnancies in the unsupplemented group. Four cases of congenital cardiovascular malformations were seen in the supplemented group whereas 12 cases were found in the unsupplemented group; four cases of cleft lip/cleft palate were found in the supplemented group and three in the unsupplemented group. Because of the small number of congenital malformations, the statistical significance of these results can be dramatically altered by a single birth defect in either group. Thus, this intervention trial will continue for several years before the promising results can be fully verified.

SAFETY OF VITAMIN AND MINERAL SUPPLEMENTS

It is well established that pregnancy increases the essential nutrient requirements of women (Food and Nutrition Board, 1989). In many instances, the increased requirements cannot be easily met by the diet and most physicians recommend prenatal vitamin/mineral supplements containing the U.S. RDA levels of vitamins for pregnant women (Newman et al., 1987). Olson (1988) recently reviewed the safety of prenatal supplements and found them safe and necessary for most pregnant women. The results of the studies involving NTD, cleft lip/cleft palate, and other birth defects discussed above strongly suggest that essential nutrient requirements may be even more critical during the periconceptional period, before prenatal supplements are ordinarily given. The safety of consuming a single multivitamin containing the U.S. RDA levels of micronutrients is well recognized. The concentration of vitamin A, 5000 IU in multivitamins for adults and 8000 IU for pregnant women, has been accepted as safe by numerous organizations, including the Teratology Society and the International Vitamin A Consultative Group (Bendich and Langseth, 1989).

CONCLUSIONS

The cumulative data from this and the following chapter by Schorah and Smithells show a consistent association of periconceptional multivitamin supplementation with lowered risk of NTD in high-risk women as well as in women with no history of NTD. Similar findings of lowered risk of recurrence of cleft lip/cleft palate is seen in women who took supplements prior to the formation of the embryonic orofacial area.

There is also a strong, recurrent association of compromised folate status with increased risk of several adverse pregnancy outcomes. Dietary intakes of less than 100 μg/day were associated with a threefold higher risk of occurrence of NTD in the prospective study by Milunsky et al. (1989) and total folate intakes above 350 μg/day were associated with a 50% reduction in risk of NTD in the retrospective study by Bower and Stanley (1989) whereas intakes below this level did not lower the risk. Serum folate levels of less than 4 ng/ml were associated with an increased risk of congenital malformations in women taking antiepileptics (Dansky et al., 1987) and similar serum levels (below 4.1 ng/ml) were seen in women with increased risks of spontaneous abortion (Martin et al., 1965). Cessation of oral contraceptive use for 3 months did not return serum levels of all women to above 4.0 ng/ml. Serum folate below 4.5 ng/ml is associated with early signs of folate deficiency, including neutrophil hypersegmentation (Pietrzik, 1989).

The low serum folate levels are clearly linked to the low dietary intakes in the majority of women. The possibility of an additional depression in status due to metabolic defects has yet to be clearly established, but the data from several studies tend to indicate that free folic acid may be a better source of the vitamin than conjugated forms, especially in populations at risk for birth defects.

Although folic acid seems to be the most critical vitamin, most intervention studies were carried out with multivitamin supplements containing folic acid. Additionally, many of the epidemiological studies point to a potential marginal status for a number of vitamins in several populations of women examined. Thus, the use of multivitamin supplements containing folic acid in the intervention studies seems prudent. Micronutrient interactions, such as between folic acid and vitamins B_6, B_{12}, or vitamin C, which may be involved in the mechanisms of neural tube formation, require further investigations.

RECOMMENDATIONS

Family planning is probably the most critical responsibility given to parents. Women have been educated to visit their physician if they suspect pregnancy following the second missed menstruation. As can be clearly seen, lowering the risk of birth defects which are initiated during the first 20–60 days of pregnancy cannot be accomplished if the woman is seen only after the event. It is therefore strongly recommended that physicians and health providers who counsel women of childbearing potential discuss the results of the recent studies and suggest the use of a single-multivitamin supplement containing (400 μg of) folic acid daily if they are contemplating pregnancy. Women using any antifolate drugs must be carefully monitored prior to conception. Since almost half of all pregnancies are unplanned, a more general recommendation of supplementation for all women of childbearing potential may be most effective. As most elegantly stated by Holmes (1988) in the editorial accompanying the Mulinare et al. paper (1988), "the biggest challenge from the observation of Mulinare et al. about the benefits of taking vitamins is to get women of childbearing age to hear and follow this simple advice."

On a public health basis, the recent decrease of the RDA for folic acid from 400 μg (Food and Nutrition Board, 1980) to 180 μg/day for women of childbearing age should be reversed, based upon the data from the Bower and Stanley (1989) and Milunsky et al. (1989) studies. The rationale that 180 μg is "typically consumed in the U.S. and Canada by adults who show no evidence of poor folate status" does not appear to be valid. The philosophy of choosing an RDA level based on the intakes of "apparently healthy people" (Food and Nutrition Board, 1989) does not take into account the prepregnant women who may be at greater risk for NTD or other birth defects if she consumes 180 μg of folate from foods as a minimal daily average. Furthermore, it is quite likely, based on data from national surveys, that intake may fall well below this level during the crucial period of embryogenesis. Yet she may be "apparently healthy." National nutrition policies should consider all cases of need and not be based merely on mean intakes of the population.

REFERENCES

American Dietetic Association (ADA). Position of the American Dietetic Association: Nutrition management of adolescent pregnancy. J Am Diet Assoc 1989; 89:104–109.

Bachrach CA, Mosher WP. Use of contraception in the United States, 1982. In: Advance data from vital health and statistics, 1985:85–1250.

Baker H, Thind IS, Frank O, DeAngelis B, Caterini H, Louria DB. Vitamin levels in low-birth-weight newborn infants and their mothers. Am J Obstet Gynecol 1977; 129:521–524.

Bendich A, Langseth L. Safety of vitamin A. Am J Clin Nutr 1989; 49:358–371.

Biale Y, Lewenthal H. Effect of folic acid supplementation on congenital malformations due to anticonvulsive drugs. Eur J Obstet Gynecol Reprod Biol 1984; 18:211–216.

Bower C, Stanley FJ. Dietary folate as a risk factor for neural-tube defects: Evidence from a case-control study in western Australia. Med J Aust June 5, 1989; 150:613–619.

Briggs M. Vitamin supplementation as a possible factor in the incidence of cleft lip/palate deformities in humans. Clin Plast Surg 1976; 3:647–652.

Centers for Disease Control (CDC). National Infant Mortality Surveillance (NIMS). MMWR 1989; 38:6–8.

Conway H. Effect of supplemental vitamin therapy on the limitation of incidence of cleft lip and cleft palate in humans. Plast Reconstruct Surg 1958; 22:450–453.

Czeizel A. To the editor: Bri Med J 1983; 2:429.

Czeizel A, Fritz G. To the editor: J Am Med Assoc September 22/29, 1989; 262:1634.

Czeizel A, Rode K. Trial to prevent first occurrence of neural tube defects by periconceptional multivitamin supplementation. Lancet 1984; 2:40.

Dansky LV, Andermann E, Rosenblatt D, Sherwin Al, Andermann F. Anticonvulsants, folate levels, and pregnancy outcome: A prospective study. Ann Neurol 1987; 21:176–182.

Dansky L, Andermann E, Andermann F, et al. Maternal epilepsy and congenital malformations: Correlation with maternal plasma anticonvulsant levels during pregnancy. In: Janz D, Dam M, Richens A, et al, eds. Epilepsy, pregnancy and the child. 1982, 251–258.

Dansky L, Andermann E, Andermann F, et al. Pregnancy outcome in relation to maternal plasma antiepileptic (AED) levels and folate (abstract). Can J Neurol Sci 1985; 12:182.

Donaldson JO. Nuerology of pregnancy, 2nd ed., 1989.

Ericson A, Kallen B, Westerholm P. Cigarette smoking an etiologic factor in cleft lip and palate. Am J Obstet Gynecol 1979; 125:348.

Food and Nutrition Board: Committee on Dietary Allowances. Recommended Dietary Allowances, 9th rev. ed., 1980.

Food and Nutrition Board: Subcommittee on the Tenth Edition of the RDA's. Recommended Dietary Allowances, 10th ed., 1989.

Friis ML. Antiepileptic drugs and teratogenesis. Acta Neurol Scand 1983; Suppl. 94:39–43.

Gardiki-Kouidou P, Seller MJ. Amniotic fluid folate, vitamin B_{12} and transcobalamins in neural tube defects. Clin Genet 1988; 33:441–448.

Gatenby PBB. Anticonvulsants as a factor in megaloblastic anemia in pregnancy. Lancet 2:1004–1005.

Hall MH. Folic acid deficiency and congenital malformation. J Obstet Gynaecol 1972; 79:159–161.

Halsted CH. The intestinal absorption of dietary folates in health and disease. J Am Coll Nutr 1988; 8:650–658.

Handler A, Davis F, Ferre C, Yeko T. The relationship of smoking and ectopic pregnancy. Am J Public Health 1989; 79:1239–1242.

Haste FM, Brooke OG, Anderson HR, Bland JM, Shaw A, Griffin J, Peacock JL. Nutrient intakes during pregnancy: Observations on the influence of smoking and social class. Am J Clin Nutr 1990; 51:29–36.

Hibbard BM. The role of folic acid in pregnancy. With particular reference to anaemia, abruption and abortion. J Obstet Gynaecol Br Commonwealth 1964; 71:529–542.

Holmes LB. Does taking vitamins at the time of conception prevent neural tube defects? J Am Med Assoc December 2, 1989; 260:3181.

Horn E. Iron and folate supplements during pregnancy: Supplementing everyone treats those at risk and is cost effective. Br Med J 1988; 297:1325, 1327.

Krause KH, Berlit P, Bonjour JP, Schmidt-Gayk H, Schellenberg B, Gillen J. Vitamin status in patients on chronic anticonvulsant therapy. Int J Vit Nutr Res 1982; 52:375–385.

Kristoffersen K, Rolschau J. Vitamin Supplements and Intrauterine Growth. In: Briggs MH, ed. Recent vitamin research, 1984, Chap 4.

Krumdieck CL, Boots LR, Cornwell PE, Butterworth CE Jr. Estrogen stimulation of conjugase activity in the uterus of ovariectomized rats. Am J Clin Nutr 1975; 28:530–534.

Laurence KM, James N, Miller NH, Tennant GB, Campbell H. Double-blind randomised controlled trial of folate treatment before conception to prevent recurrence of neural tube defects. Br Med J 1981; 282:1509–1511.

Lemire RJ. Neural tube defects. J Am Med Assoc January 22/29, 1988; 259:558–562.

Lindhout D, Meinardi H. Spina bifida and in-utero exposure to valproate. Lancet 1984; 2:396.

Little BB, Snell LM, Gilstrap LC III, Gant NF, Rosenfeld CR. Alcohol abuse during pregnancy: Changes in frequency in a large urban hospital. Obstet Gynecol 1989; 74:547–550.

Malloy MH, Kleinman JC, Bakewell JM, Schramm WF, Land GH. Maternal smoking during pregnancy: No association with congenital malformations in Missouri 1980–83. Am J Public Health 1989; 79:1243–1246.

Martin RH, Harper TA, Kelso W. Serum folic acid in recurrent abortions. Lancet 1965; 1:670–672.

Mayer JP, Hawkins B, Todd R. A randomized evaluation of smoking cessation interventions for pregnant women at a WIC clinic. Am J Public Health 1990; 80:76–78.

Merck Manual of Diagnosis and Therapy, 15th ed., 1987.

Mills JL, Rhoads GG, Simpson JL, Cunningham GC, Conley MR, Lassman MR, Walden ME, Depp R, Hoffman HJ, National Institute of Child Health and Human Development Neural Tube Defect Study Group. The absence of a relation between the periconceptional use of vitamins and neural-tube defects. New Engl J Med August 17, 1989; 321:430–435.

Milunsky A, Jick H, Jick SS, Bruell CL, MacLaughlin DS, Rothman KJ, Willett W. Multivitamin/folic acid supplementation in early pregnancy reduces the prevalence of neural tube defects. J. Am Med Assoc 1989; 262:2847–2852.

Mulinare J, Cordero JF, Erickson JD, Berry RJ. Periconceptional use of multivitamins and the occurrence of neural tube defects. J Am Med Assoc 1988; 260:3141–3145.

Nakane Y, Okuma T, Takahashi R, Sato Y, Wada T, Sato T, Fukushima Y, Kumashiro H, Ono T, Takahashi T, Aoki Y, Kazamatsuri H, Inami M, Komai S, Seino M, Miyakoshi M, Tanimura T, Hazama H, Kawahara R, Otsuki R, Hosokawa K, Inanaga K, Nakazawa Y, Yamamoto K. Multi-institutional study on the teratogenicity and fetal toxicity of antiepileptic drugs: A report of a collaborative study group in Japan. Epilepsia 1980; 21:663–680.

National Center for Health Statistics. Advance report of final mortality statistics, 1985. Monthly Vital Statistics 1988; 36:88–1120.

Nevin NC, Seller MJ. Prevention of neural-tube-defect recurrences. Lancet 1990; 1:178–179.

Newman V, Lyon RB, Anderson PO. Evaluation of prenatal vitamin-mineral supplements. Clin Pharmacol 1987; 6:770–777.

Niebyl EJR, Blake DA, Rocco LE, Baumgardner R, Mellits ED. Lack of maternal metabolic, endocrine, and environmental influences in the etiology of cleft lip with or without cleft palate. Cleft Palate J 1985; 22:20–28.

Nutrition Monitoring Division Human Nutrition Information Service. Nationwide food consumption survey: CSF II—Continuing survey of food intakes by individuals—1986

Low-income women 19–50 years and their children 1–5 years, 4 days, 1986. Nutr Today September/October 1989; 35–38.

Oakley GP Jr. Frequency of human congenital malformations. Clin Perinatol 1986; 13:545–554.

Office of Disease Prevention and Health Promotion. Digestive Diseases. In: Disease prevention/health promotion: The Facts. 1988, Chap 26, 289–299.

Olson RE. Safety of vitamin and mineral supplements for mother and child. In: Berger H, ed. Vitamins and minerals in pregnancy and lactation. Nestle Nutrition Workshop Series, Vol. 16175, 1988.

Paige DM, Davis LR. Fetal growth, maternal nutrition, and dietary supplementation. Clin Nutr 1986; 5:191–199.

Palan PR, Romney SL, Vermund SH, Mikhail MG, Basu J. Effects of smoking and oral contraception on plasma beta-carotene levels in healthy women. Am J Obstet Gynecol 1989; 161:881–885.

Patterson RM. Seizure disorders in pregnancy. Med Clin North Am 1989; 73:661–665.

Peer LA, Gordon HW, Bernhard WG. Effect of vitamins on human teratology. Plastic Reconstruct Surg 1964; 34:358–362.

Pietrzik K. Folate deficiency: Morphological and functional consequences. In: Somogyi JC, Hejda S (eds). Nutrition in the Prevention of Disease. Bibl Nutr Dieta. Basel, Karger, pp. 123–130, 1989.

Rhode BM, Cooper BA, Farmer FA. Effect of orange juice, folic acid, and oral contraceptives on serum folate in women taking a folate-restricted diet. J Am Coll Nutr 1983; 2:221–230.

Rogozinski H, Ankers C, Lennon D, Wild J, Schorah C, Sheppard S, Smithells RW. Folate nutrition in early pregnancy. Human Nutr: Appl Nutr 1983; 37A:357–364.

Rosa FW, Gallo-Torres H, Biriell C, Bem JL. Neural tube defects with sulfasalazine management of maternal chronic inflammatory bowel disease, 1990, in press.

Schofield C, Stewart J, Wheeler E. The diets of pregnant and postpregnant women in different social groups in London and Edinburgh: calcium, iron, retinol, ascorbic acid and folic acid. Br J Nutr 1989; 62:363–377.

Schorah CJ. Importance of an adequate folate nutrition in embryonic and early fetal development. In: Berger H, ed. Vitamins and minerals in pregnancy and lactation. Nestle Nutrition Workshop Series, Vol. 16175167–176, 1988.

Schorah CJ, Wild J, Hartley S, Sheppard S, Smithells RW. The effect of periconceptional supplementation on blood vitamin conceptrations in women at recurrence risk for neural tube defects. Br J Nutr 1983; 49:203–211.

Shojania M, Hornady GJ, Barnes PH. The effect of oral contraceptives on folate metabolism. Am J Obstet Gynecol 1971; 111:782–791.

Shojania AM, Hornady GJ, Scabtta D. The effect of oral contraceptives on folate metabolism. III. Plasma clearance and urinary folate excretion. J Lab Clin Med 1975; 85:185–190.

Smithells RW, Sheppard S, Schorah CJ, Seller MJ, Nevin NC, Harris R, Read AP, Fielding DW. Apparent prevention of neural tube defects by periconceptional vitamin supplementation. Arch Dis Child 1981; 56:911–918.

Smithells RW, Sheppard S, Wild J, Schorah CJ. Prevention of neural tube defect recurrences in Yorkshire: Final report. Lancet August 26, 1989; 2:498–499.

Smithells RW, Sheppard S, Schorah CJ. Vitamin deficiencies and neural tube defects. Arch Dis Child 1976; 51:944–948.

Streiff RR. Folate deficiency and oral contraceptives. J Am Med Assoc 1970; 214:105–108.

Streiff RR, Little AB. Folic acid deficiency and pregnancy. N Engl J Med 1967; 276:776–779.

Subar AF, Block G, James LD. Folate intake and food sources in the US population. Am J Clin Nutr 1989; 50:508–516.

Toghill PJ, Smith PG. Folate deficiency and the pill. Br Med J 1971; 1:608–609.

Tolarova M. Cleft lip and palate and isolated cleft palate in Czechoslovakia. In Marmuthu KM, Gopinath PM, eds. Recent trends in medical genetics. Conference, Madras, India, December 8–10, 1983. Advances in the biosciences, Vol. 56175251–268, 1986.

Tolarova M. Periconceptional supplementation with vitamins and folic acid to prevent recurrence of cleft lip. Lancet July 24, 1982; 2:217.

Trotz M, Wegner CHR, Nau H. Teratology 1986; 33:35A.

Trotz M, Wegner Chr, Nau H. Valproic acid-induced neural tube defects: Reproduction by folinic acid in the mouse. Life Sci 1987; 41:103–110.

Wald N, Cuckle H, Boreham J. Small biparietal diameter of fetuses with spina bifida: implications for antenatal screening. Br J Obstet Gynaecol 1980; 87:219.

Wegman M. Annual summary of vital statistics—1986. Pediatrics 1987; 80:826.

Winship KA, Cahal DA, Weber JCP, Griffin JP. Maternal drug histories and central nervous system anomalies. Arch Dis Child 1984; 59:1052–1060.

Witter FR, Blake DA, Baumgardner R, Mellits ED, Niebyl JR. Folate, carotene and smoking. Am J Obstet Gynecol 1982; 144:857.

Wyngaarden JB, Smith LH. Cecil textbook of medicine, 18th ed., Vol. 2, pp. 2217–2229, 1988.

Wynn V. Vitamins and oral contraceptive use. Lancet 1975; 1:561–564.

Yates JRW, Ferguson-Smith MA, Shenkin A, Guzman-Rodriguez R, White M, Guthrie D. Is disordered folate metabolism the basis for the genetic predisposition to neural tube defects? Clin Genet 1987; 31:279–287.

Zhu MX, Zhou SS. Reduction of the teratogenic effects of phenytoin by folic acid and a mixture of folic acid, vitamins, and amino acids: A preliminary trial. Epilepsia 1989; 30:246–251.

12

A Possible Role for Periconceptional Multivitamin Supplementation in the Prevention of the Recurrence of Neural Tube Defects

Christopher J. Schorah and Richard W. Smithells

University of Leeds
Leeds, England

INTRODUCTION

It is over half a century since Hale (1933) showed that a maternal micronutrient deficiency could lead to a congenital malformation. In the intervening years much information has been generated concerning the role of nutrition in embryonic and fetal development. The work is mostly in animals, but there are a few investigations in humans. We can conclude from these studies, perhaps not unexpectedly, that extreme nutritional deprivation will affect pregnancy in a number of ways, including the induction of congenital malformations. What is still uncertain is whether lesser degrees of undernutrition, which are likely to be encountered in human pregnancy, can also disturb embryogenesis. One of the most intensive areas of study has been the hypothesis that vitamin deficiencies, particularly of folic acid, could contribute to the causation of certain defects of the central nervous system (CNS) known collectively as neural tube defects (NTD). For the purpose of this chapter NTD includes the following lesions: anencephalus, craniorachischisis, spina bifida, meningocele, meningomyelocele, myelocele, and encephalocele, but not isolated hydrocephalus or spina bifida occulta.

There is substantial evidence to implicate deficiencies of certain vitamins in the etiology of NTD in humans and to indicate that appropriate vitamin supplementation leads to a reduction in the rate of recurrence of these conditions. However, even after 25 years of research, we are aware that the link has not been established beyond doubt. The results of current randomized trials, which should be available in 2–3 years, may resolve the issue but, as we indicate in this chapter, problems associated with these studies could make their interpretation difficult. This chapter attempts, therefore, to evaluate critically the available evidence for the role of micronutrient deficiencies in the etiology of NTD. It must be emphasized that NTD are believed to be of multifactorial origin, and the hypothesis explored here is simply that deficiency of one or more micronutrients is one contributory factor.

STUDIES IN ANIMALS

The literature on experimental animal teratogenesis is vast. However, this work is of uncertain relevance to human teratology. It is unwise to extrapolate findings in the experimental animal to man for at least two reasons. First, there are huge interspecies differences in susceptibility to congenital malformations induced by dietary manipulation, differences being found even between different strains of a single species (Seller, 1983a). This also applies to the dietary requirements for different vitamins. Second, much of the experimental work in animals has involved severe deficiencies, or very large doses of micronutrients, conditions which are scarcely ever applicable to humans. Indeed, vitamin-deficient diets have often been augmented by the administration of vitamin antagonists to produce malformations in the experimental animal. There are several reviews covering this area (Kalter and Warkany, 1959; Hurley, 1977) and these will be summarized briefly with reference to CNS malformations.

Vitamin A deficiency has produced hydrocephalus in rabbits but not NTD (Lamming et al., 1954; Millen and Woollam, 1956). In contrast, excessive administration of vitamin A and its metabolites at specific times during pregnancy has produced NTD in a number of species (Cohlan, 1954; Marin-Padilla and Ferm, 1965; Palludan, 1966). An interesting paradox with vitamin A was discovered by Seller (1983a) using the curly tail mouse, a strain which is genetically susceptible to NTD. Administration of vitamin A on the 8th day of pregnancy significantly increased the prevalence of NTD in this species, whereas the same dose administered on day 9 significantly reduced the number of fetuses with the condition. This work not only highlights how a particular nutrient might be both a teratogen and an antiteratogen, but also indicates how critical is the timing of the intervention. NTD has also been produced by deficiencies of vitamin E, B_6, B_{12}, and pantothenic acid (Lefebvres-Boisselot, 1951; Cheng et al., 1960; Woodard and Newberne, 1966; Curley et al., 1968). Hydrocephalus has been induced by folic acid deficiency alone (Richardson and Hogan, 1946; Hogan et al., 1950). However, addition of antibiotics (to prevent intestinal bacterial synthesis of folic acid) and folate antimetabolites have been required to produce

NTD (Nelson et al., 1955, 1956). Such treatment at a critical point in embryogenesis was reported by Nelson to be highly teratogenic to the CNS (Nelson, 1957). Folic acid is of special interest because its administration has been reported to reduce the prevalence of spontaneous NTD in the golden hamster (Moffa and White, 1983) and of experimental CNS malformations induced by teratogens such as the anticonvulsants valproate and phenytoin (Trotz et al., 1985; Zhu and Zhou, 1989) and pyrimethamine (Horvath et al., 1988). However, folic acid therapy has not reduced NTD caused by other teratogenic insults such as arsenate, heat, and alcohol (Graham and Ferm, 1985; Ferm and Hanlon, 1986). One of the highest prevalences of CNS malformations occurs in the zinc-deficient rat (Rogers et al., 1985). There is also a link here with folic acid. Zinc and folic acid are found in similar foods, are associated in plasma (Cherry et al., 1981), and are linked metabolically (Tamura et al., 1978, 1987; Canton et al., 1989). In addition, combined deficiencies of zinc and folic acid potentiate teratogenesis in the rat (Bremert et al., 1989). However, the CNS malformations in zinc deficiency are predominantly hydrocephalus (Hurley and Swenerton, 1966) and it has been suggested that the developmental defect is a closure of the aqueduct, with true NTD being relatively rare (Seller, 1983a).

Overall, animal work points to vitamin A, folic acid, and possibly zinc as the micronutrients most associated with NTD.

ASSOCIATIONS BETWEEN MICRONUTRIENT DEFICIENCY AND NTD IN MAN

The true incidence of NTD (prevalence immediately after the normal time of closure of the neural tube) is impossible to ascertain because spontaneous abortion (Creasy and Alberman, 1976, MacHenry et al., 1979) and, more recently, therapeutic abortion of malformed fetuses considerably reduce the numbers of NTD by term. However, epidemiological studies (mostly undertaken in the UK before the introduction of therapeutic abortion) show a number of fairly constant features in population patterns of NTD which apply less strikingly or not at all to other birth defects (Leck, 1974). There are both geographic and social class variations in the prevalence of the defects in the UK (Table 1) which suggest an association with poverty. This association has been incorporated into a variety of theories of the causation of NTD. The theory of infection (Record, 1961) is consistent with greater overcrowding in poorer families; the theory of soft water (Stocks, 1970) is consistent with the concentration of unskilled workers in the UK in softwater areas; the potato blight theory (Renwick, 1972) is consistent with the consumption of cheap food by the poor. Poor nutrition has been shown to be more prevalent in areas and social classes at increased risk of NTD (Smithells et al., 1976, 1977; Hurley, 1981; Soltan and Jenkins, 1982; Rogozinski et al.,

Table 1   Geographic and Social Class Variations in the Prevalence of NTD

Area	NTD/1000 births	Ref.
London	2.95	Carter and Evans (1973)
Birmingham	4.77	Leck et al. (1968)
Glasgow	5.63	Wilson (1970)
South Wales	7.01	Richards and Lowe (1971)
Belfast	8.70	Elwood and Nevin (1973)
Class	Anencephaly/1000 births	
Professional (I)	0.1	
Skilled (III)	2.4	Fedrick (1970)
Unskilled (V)	3.9	
Unmarried	3.1	

1983; Al-Awadi et al., 1984; Hall, 1986; Whichelow and Erzinglioglu, 1990) and these findings are consistent whether dietary intakes or the blood levels of micronutrients are assessed (Table 2).

Extreme deficiencies of micronutrients in humans are unusual and reports of their effect on the fetus extremely rare. As far as we are aware there are no reports of deficiencies or excesses of single micronutrients leading to NTD. Severe deficiencies of folic acid sufficient to cause megaloblastic anemia in later pregnancy have been associated with CNS malformations, particularly hydrocephalus (Fraser and Watt, 1964). However, others (Pritchard et al., 1970) found no such association. These variable findings in published reports may be explained by the fact that folate deficiency anemia in later pregnancy may not necessarily reflect a deficiency at the time of embryogenesis and closure of the neural tube. A high prevalence of NTD was also noted after gastric bypass surgery for obesity (Haddow et al., 1986) and these patients often have very low levels of iron, folic acid, thiamine, and vitamin B_{12} unless supplements are given (Amaral et al., 1985). A further piece of evidence linking NTD and folate metabolism comes from the use of the folate antagonist aminopterin as an abortifacient. It was sometimes successful in inducing abortions but also produced malformations including those of the neural tube (Thiersch, 1952).

The effects of severe general malnutrition on pregnancy during the Dutch hunger winter of 1944–1945 were studied by Stein et al. (1975). During that winter there was a severe, if relatively short and balanced, deficiency of nutrients lasting 3–6 months. The most striking effect of this famine was a general decrease in the number of births and the birthweight of infants, but an increase in the number of infants with NTD was also noted in the cohort of pregnancies conceived

Table 2 Intake and Blood Levels of Micronutrients Analyzed According to Social Class

		Professional, I and II	Skilled non-manual, III	Semi- and unskilled, IV & V
Vitamin C	Intake (mg/day)	83	62	55***
	Leukocyte (μg/10[8] cells)	37	35	33***
Riboflavin	Intake (mg/day)	1.9	1.4***	1.3***
	Saturation index[a]	1.20	1.24***	1.26***
Folic acid	Intake (μg/day)	177	145*	139***
	Red cell (μg/liter)	249	218**	220**
Retinol	Intake (μg/day)	1235	975	769***
	Plasma (μg/dl)	72	67*	67**

[a] The higher the index the greater the deficiency.
Significantly different from social class I and II. * $p < 0.05$. ** $p < 0.01$. *** $p < 0.001$.

at the height of the famine. This appeared to be the only irreversible effect on the infants born or conceived during the famine. Later studies of these children when adults did not reveal any effects of prenatal exposure to famine on mental performance, physical stature, or health parameters.

Because of the multifactorial basis of NTD, associations between poor nutrition and NTD prevalence in a general pregnant population are likely to be less informative than studies of NTD-affected pregnancies or of women who have had such a pregnancy. When this is done the findings are consistent with nutrient deficiencies, particularly folic acid, being implicated in the etiology of the condition. Evidence of poor nutrition in women who have NTD-affected infants has been reported by Laurence et al. (1983). In their South Wales Study, NTD recurrences affected only infants born to women who had a poor diet. Hibbard and Smithells (1965) showed that women who gave birth to infants with malformations, especially NTD, had a much higher prevalence of raised FIGLU excretion after histidine load (suggesting folate deficiency) than normal controls. However, these tests were carried out in the period immediately postpartum and do not necessarily reflect events early in pregnancy, when the neural tube closes. Poor folate intake in early pregnancy has been associated with NTD in a recent case control study (Bower and Stanley, 1989). Evidence closer to the time of neural tube closure also comes from a large prospective study in which blood vitamin levels were measured in over 1000 women in the first trimester of preg-

Table 3 Mean Maternal Blood Vitamin Levels in the First Trimester of 7 NTD and 7 CVS[a] Affected Pregnancies Compared with All Pregnancies[b]

Pregnancy	Serum folate (μg/liter)	Red cell folate (μg/liter)	Leukocyte vitamin C (μg/10^8 cells)	Riboflavin saturation index[c]
All[b]	6.3	228	34.5	1.23
NTD	4.6	136***	21.5*	1.30
CVS	6.1	239	30.0	1.22

[a] Cardiovascular system malformation.
[b] Approximately 1000 women who were not taking vitamin supplements.
[c] The higher the index the greater the deficiency.
Significantly different from all pregnancies (1 sample t-test). * $p < 0.05$. *** $p < 0.001$.

nancy (Smithells et al., 1976). Subsequently, seven of these were found to have a fetus with NTD and in these women the levels of red cell folate (but not serum folate) and white cell vitamin C were significantly lower than in the rest of the population (Table 3). Serum vitamin B_{12} was low when the lesion was anencephaly (Schorah et al., 1980), but this was not confirmed (Molloy et al., 1985).

Of relevance to the association between poor maternal folate nutrition and NTD-affected pregnancies is the evidence that anticonvulsant therapy in early pregnancy may increase the rate of malformations of the CNS including NTD. Both animal experiments and studies in humans have suggested that the association may be causal, especially for valproate and phenytoin (Bruckner et al., 1983; Strickler et al., 1985; Lindhout and Schmidt, 1986; Anon., 1988). The link with folate arises from reports that both these anticonvulsants can decrease blood folate concentrations, possibly by decreasing folate absorption (Hendel et al., 1984; Engelsen et al., 1984; Dansky et al., 1987). In an uncontrolled study, Biale and Lewenthal (1984) reported a reduction in all malformations in women on anti-convulsant therapy given folate during pregnancy, and Chatot et al. (1984) found a variety of vitamins able to protect rat embryos from the teratogenic effect of serum taken from women on anticonvulsant therapy.

Finally, retrospective studies of the relationship between the prevalence of NTD and periconceptional vitamin use have produced conflicting results. Four case control studies were reported—three from the USA and one from the UK—in which maternal vitamin intake before and after conception was compared between mothers of infants/fetuses with NTD and appropriate controls. Three of these showed a three- to fourfold difference, NTD being associated with a lower rate of vitamin intake (Winship et al., 1984; Mulinare et al., 1988; Milunsky et al., 1989). No such effect was seen in the other (Mills et al., 1989). Winship et al. (1984) obtained information about vitamin intake from general practitioner records, which avoided recall bias, but their numbers were small. The other three studies asked the mothers to recall their vitamin use during the weeks immediately before and after conception.

The study of Mulinare et al. (1988) may be criticized on the grounds that some of the mothers were asked to recall vitamin intake very many years previously. Comparison was made between periconceptional users (those who took vitamins throughout the 3 months before and the 3 months after conception) and those who did not use vitamins in this period: mothers taking vitamins for a shorter period within these 6 months were excluded from analysis. Mills et al. (1989) classified as "nontakers" of vitamins those who started taking them after conception. As a study (Sheppard et al., 1989) suggests that vitamins started during pregnancy but before the time of neural tube closure have a protective effect, this misclassification will tend to reduce any true difference between takers and nontakers.

The best study is probably that of Milunsky et al. (1989). These authors interviewed during early pregnancy mothers who had had either amniocentesis or estimation of serum alpha-fetoprotein. Recall time was therefore very short, and in most cases pregnancy outcome was unknown, thus avoiding recall bias. They showed that vitamins started before conception or within the first 6 weeks of pregnancy were associated with a lower NTD rate than vitamins started after the 6th week or not taken at all. They also showed that low dietary folate increased the risk of NTD, and that multivitamins containing folic acid were effective whereas those without were probably not.

A factor which may contribute to the difference between the results of Mills et al. (1989) and those of the other three studies may be the difference in NTD birth prevalences in the populations from which the mothers were drawn. The rates per 1000 pregnancies were 0.96 (Mills et al., 1989), 1.8 (Mulinare et al., 1988, reported by Khoury et al., 1982), 2.0 (Winship et al., 1984; approximate value for UK in 1981), and 3.5 (Milunsky et al., 1989). The study showing no effect of vitamin supplements was undertaken in the area with the lowest NTD prevalence. As we indicate later (see "Current Studies"), the greater the prevalence of NTD, the more convincing is the evidence of prevention by periconceptional vitamin supplements.

Overall, these findings on poor nutrition and NTD in humans are not conclusive but point to an association between undernutrition and NTD which could be causal. The closest association appears to be with folic acid, but other micronutrients such as zinc cannot be excluded. The best way to determine whether the association is causal is to correct the nutritional problems by appropriate vitamin and/or mineral supplements before closure of the neural tube and to see whether this reduces the prevalence of NTD. It was the accumulated evidence implicating vitamin deficiency in the etiology of NTD which led us to undertake such an intervention study using a multivitamin preparation.

MULTIVITAMIN INTERVENTION STUDIES

We had planned originally to undertake a randomized, placebo-controlled trial, but ethical committees were unwilling to allow us to proceed unless the women were fully informed about the type of therapy they were to receive (i.e., not blind). In the event, and with the wisdom of hindsight probably wrongly, we instigated a nonrandomized trial in volunteers.

The risk of NTD is increased about 10-fold in women who have previously had an affected infant or fetus (and is greater in those who have had more than one). We therefore decided to recruit for supplementation women who had had at least one previous NTD-affected pregnancy and who were not pregnant at the time of entering the trial (in order that vitamin supplementation could be started well before neural tube closure on the 26th day of embryonic life). Patients were recruited in Northern Ireland, southeastern England, Yorkshire, Lancashire, and Cheshire. All women who met the above criteria were invited to take part. Vitamin supplementation was given as Pregnavite Forte F (Bencard), 3 tablets daily, which provides approximately the RDA for most vitamins and some minerals for the 2nd and 3rd trimesters of pregnancy (Table 4). The supplement does not contain vitamin B_{12} or zinc. Volunteers were asked to take the supplements for at least 28 days before conception and to continue until the date of the second missed period, i.e., well after the time of neural tube closure. Women conceiving less than 28 days after starting supplementation or starting supplementation after conception but before closure of the neural tube or failing to take tablets for more than 1 day were regarded as partially supplemented. Women who were pregnant when referred to the centers undertaking the study entered a control group of unsupplemented women. Full details of the studies have been reported (Smithells et al., 1980, 1981, 1983).

Table 4 Daily Supplements Provided by Three Tablets of Pregnavite Forte F (Bencard)

Retinol (mg)	1.2
Vitamin D (μg)	10
Thiamin (mg)	1.5
Riboflavin (mg)	1.5
Pyridoxine (mg)	1.0
Nicotinamide (mg)	15
Folic acid (μg)	360
Ascorbic acid (mg)	40
Iron (ferrous sulfate mg)	75.6
Calcium phosphate (mg)	480

Table 5 Overall Results of the Multivitamin Intervention Studies

(a) Pregnancy outcome (examined fetuses) in supplemented and unsupplemented mothers (1976–1981; cohorts 1 and 2)

	Number of infants	
	Normal	NTD
Fully supplemented	426	3
Unsupplemented	486	24

$p < 0.01$, Fishers exact test.

(b) Pregnancy outcome (examined fetuses) in supplemented and partially supplemented mothers (1976–1984, cohorts 1, 2, and 3)

	No. of previous NTD	Number of infants		
			NTD	
		Normal	Found	Expected[a]
Fully supplemented	1	1005	10	40
	$\geqslant 2$	88	4	9
Partially supplemented	1	195	1	8
	$\geqslant 2$	16	1	2

[a] Assumes 4% recurrence rate after 1 previous NTD, 10% after 2. Seller and Nevin (1984).

The combined results of these studies are shown in Table 5. The data are presented in two ways. Table 5a shows the results in the first two cohorts when a similar number of unsupplemented mothers were recruited. As an increasing proportion of mothers at recurrence risk were recruited, the number remaining unsupplemented was reduced. Table 5b shows our overall experience at the close of the multicenter study without an unsupplemented control group. These results are subdivided according to the number of previous NTDs, and recurrence rates are compared with observed recurrence rates of 4% after one previous NTD and 10% after two (Seller and Nevin, 1984). These are contemporary population recurrence figures in the regions where vitamin intervention trials were undertaken, but before the trials made a significant impact on overall recurrence rates. The population recurrence rates may be an underestimate as amniocentesis data were used. Also included in Table 5b are the results for partially supplemented mothers. The difference between recurrence rates in the supplemented and either the unsupplemented controls or the expected rates are striking, indicating a four-to eightfold reduction in risk. Our experience with the partially supplemented women is similar to that with the fully supplemented.

In spite of the apparent preventive effect of vitamin supplementation, the fact that the trial was not randomized has raised the possibility that factors other than vitamin supplementation could account for the findings (Knox, 1983; Oakley et al., 1983; Elwood, 1983; Wald and Polani, 1984). Possible interpretations of the difference in recurrence rates include the following:

(1) Supplemented mothers aborted more NTD fetuses than did controls (Creasy and Alberman, 1976; MacHenry et al., 1979). The combined data from our studies suggest that the proportion of pregnancies that end in spontaneous abortion was similar in the two groups (supplemented 10.7%, unsupplemented 8.1%). The slightly higher value in the supplemented group is probably due to the fact that these mothers entered the study before conception and even very early abortions are recorded. Most unsupplemented mothers were already pregnant when they first came to our attention. Forty-three of the spontaneously aborted fetuses were examined (approximately half). One of these had an NTD and that was in an unsupplemented pregnancy. It seems unlikely that our findings can be explained by selective abortion of NTD.

(2) Some unknown factor other than vitamin supplementation has reduced NTD in the treated group. This is a very difficult hypothesis to test except by a randomized study. Women were asked to avoid oral contraceptives (OC) for 28 days prior to conception because of the recognized ability of OCs to depress plasma vitamin levels, but there is no evidence that OC use is associated with NTD. All the fully supplemented women in the study had planned pregnancies; this would not be true of all unsupplemented pregnancies. Fully supplemented women would, on average, be more prepared for their pregnancy. Again, however, there is no evidence that this leads to a reduction in NTD recurrence. Indeed, similar pregnancy preparation applied to the studies in the potato avoidance trials designed to test the potato blight hypothesis of Renwick (1972), but potato avoidance did not prevent NTD recurrence (Nevin and Merrett, 1975). Finally, some women in our partially supplemented group did not attend for supplements until after conception. NTD recurrence in this group was very low, yet their pregnancies were largely unplanned.

(3) Supplemented women were at lower prior risk of NTD recurrence than were unsupplemented women. Apart from the number of previous NTD pregnancies (Carter and Roberts, 1967) and geographic and secular differences (which in the intervention studies were eliminated by the use of contemporary controls in each area), there is no evidence to suggest that any particular subgroup within the population has a higher or lower *recurrence* risk than another. However, it is possible that factors affecting *occurrence* risk might also be expected to modify

the *recurrence* rate. Such factors include social class (Nevin et al., 1981) (Table 1); spontaneous abortion immediately prior to the study pregnancy (Smithells and Chinn, 1965; Clarke et al., 1975), and the length of fallow period between the previous pregnancy and the study pregnancy (Clarke et al., 1975). We analyzed the data from our intervention studies to assess the influence of these factors and the number of previous NTDs on the recurrence rates and the outcome of supplementation (Wild et al., 1986). The analysis shows that recurrence risk of NTD is apparently increased by the number of previous NTD, area of residence, immediately prior miscarriage, and interpregnancy interval, but only for number of previous NTD is the change significant. However, and most important, none of these factors contributed any significant differential risk as between supplemented and unsupplemented mothers. The only significant difference between the groups remains that one received a multivitamin supplement and the other did not. The relative risks (i.e., the effect of these factors on recurrence rates) and the risk ratios (the distribution of the factors between the unsupplemented and supplemented groups) are shown in Table 6.

(4) Unidentified factors affecting recurrence risk could be underrepresented in the supplemented group as an accidental consequence of using volunteers. Two other studies of NTD recurrence used volunteers and have therefore, like us, studied a self-selected group: the potato avoidance trial (Nevin and Merrett, 1975) and a folate supplementation trial (Laurence et al., 1983). Laurence found

Table 6 Effect of Possible Factors on Risk of Recurrence of Neural Tube Defect in All Mothers (Supplemented and Unsupplemented) in the Multivitamin Study and the Differential Risk Between the Unsupplemented and Supplemented Groups (Risk Ratio)

Factor	Relative risk of the factor	Differential risk between unsupplemented and supplemented group due to factor (risk ratio)[a]
Two or more previous NTD	2.51	1.003
Social class (IIIM, IV, V)	0.94	0.992
Residence in Northern Ireland	1.35	1.040
Immediately prior spontaneous abortion	2.18	1.032
Immediately prior therapeutic abortion	0.86	1.010
Fallow period <1 year following abortion	3.45	0.922
Vitamin supplements	0.15	—

[a] Values greater than unity indicate increased risk of NTD in the unsupplemented compared with the supplemented group due to the factor, those less than 1 the reverse.

a recurrence rate of 6.9% in his placebo group and Nevin found a similar recurrence rate in those avoiding potato. If self-selection was responsible for decreased recurrence in the multivitamin trial, then one might have expected to find a reduced recurrence rate in these other studies as they were selected by similar criteria.

The evidence against selection bias reducing risk is strengthened by data from Yorkshire and Northern Ireland (Seller and Nevin, 1984; Smithells et al., 1989; Nevin and Seller, 1990). Here attempts have been made to supplement all high-risk women and to know the outcome of all high-risk pregnancies. As a result, the proportion of high-risk women in these two areas who have been fully supplemented has increased, while unsupplemented pregnancies have decreased. If the procedure of recruitment led to the selection for supplementation of a group at low recurrence risk, then as the numbers in this group increased at the expense of the unsupplemented, either those left unsupplemented would show an increase in recurrence rate or more recurrences would occur in the supplemented group. In neither region have these occurred (Table 7).

Table 7 Outcome of Pregnancy in the Multivitamin Studies in Yorkshire and Northern Ireland Divided by Cohort

Factor	Years of cohort[a]					
	Northern Ireland[b]			Yorkshire		
	1977–79	1980–81	1982–89	1977–80	1981–84	1985–87
Total no. of fetuses[c]	183	232	531	263	134	126
No. unsupplemented (%)	126(69)	117(50)	110(21)	216(82)	61(46)	43(34)
No. of unsupplemented recurrences (%)	6(4.8)	6(5.1)	5(4.6)	13(6.0)	3(4.9)	2(4.7)
No. of supplemented recurrences (%)	0(0.0)	1(0.9)	3(0.7)	1(2.1)	0(0.0)	0(0.0)
Overall recurrence rate (%)[d]	3.3	3.0	1.5	5.3	2.2	1.6

[a] Cohort dates in NI were determined by preparation of data for publication and in Yorkshire by change in approach to ascertainment. Recurrence rates were not calculated until the cohorts were closed.

[b] From Seller and Nevin (1984), Nevin and Seller (1990), and unpublished data, personal communication.

[c] Includes all examined fetuses, including partially supplemented.

[d] Recurrence rate in NI at the start of the study 4.2% (Seller and Nevin, 1984).

In addition, if selection bias accounted for the low recurrence rate in the supplemented group, as the relative proportions of the supplemented and unsupplemented groups changed, the overall recurrence rate in the two groups together should have remained unchanged. It has, in fact, decreased at a rate unlikely to be the result of a simple secular trend. Changes have occurred at different times in the two regions associated with increases in the proportion of women supplemented (Table 7). There is no good evidence that the secular fall in NTD prevalence (Leck, 1983) was followed by any major change in recurrence rates and certainly not of the order of the decrease observed in Yorkshire and Northern Ireland (Seller and Hancock, 1985; Czeizel, 1988).

Critical analysis of the intervention studies has not weakened the most direct and straightforward interpretation of the findings, namely, that periconceptional multivitamin supplements cause a significant decrease in the risk of NTD in the offspring of women who have had one or more previous affected pregnancies.

CURRENT STUDIES

Randomized, controlled studies are currently being conducted both in women who are at risk of recurrence (Wald and Polani, 1984; Lenehan et al., 1988) and those who are not (Czeizel and Rode, 1984). It has been argued that even if vitamins prevent NTD recurrences, they do not necessarily prevent first occurrence. For this reason, the study of Czeizel and Rode is of particular interest, especially as NTD recurrences represent only a small minority of all NTDs.

Randomized studies are to be welcomed in the hope that they may finally resolve the issue. However, these are not without difficulties. First, many women at recurrence risk are now aware of the potential benefit that can be offered by multivitamin therapy and may well purchase multivitamin preparations from health food stores or pharmacists. Second, the fortification of certain breakfast cereals with folic acid in the UK has significantly increased the intake of this vitamin in women of childbearing age, including those at high risk of NTD (unpublished work). Third, these will inevitably take a long time, and each can only determine the effect of the chosen supplement in the particular study population at the particular time it is in progress.

Finally, the decreasing prevalence of NTD which has occurred during the last 15 years in many European countries (Leck, 1983) may well make vitamin supplements of lesser importance in areas of low risk. For example, experience in Northern Ireland (an area of high risk) and southeastern England (an area of low risk) suggest that multivitamin supplementation has continued to reduce NTD recurrence in Northern Ireland but has become less effective in southeastern England (Seller and Nevin, 1984; Nevin and Seller, 1990). The findings of the retrospective studies of preconceptional vitamin supplementation and NTD prevalence suggest that this is also true for women at occurrence risk. The combination of these four factors may mean that randomized intervention studies in low-risk areas could reveal low rates of recurrence in all groups, including placebo, and therefore fail to confirm a beneficial effect at times and in areas of high prevalence.

RECOMMENDATIONS FOR PERICONCEPTIONAL VITAMIN SUPPLEMENTATION: TO WHOM, WHEN, AND WHICH VITAMINS

We believe that the balance of evidence strongly favors a role for multivitamin supplementation in the prevention of NTD and that supplementation of women at risk of NTD recurrence should now become routine. However, the suggestion of decreased effectiveness in areas of low prevalence (Seller and Nevin, 1984; Nevin and Seller, 1990) raises doubts about the introduction of the practice in such areas.

If vitamins are to be prescribed for women at recurrence risk, we also need to consider when and which vitamins. Our vitamin supplementation protocol was designed to ensure increased blood vitamin levels at the time of closure of the neural tube and this was achieved (Schorah et al., 1983). However, experience with partially supplemented women suggests that 28 days of preconceptional supplementation may not be necessary. On balance we consider that women should be encouraged to start supplementation before pregnancy but evidence suggests that it may be effective if started up to the 20th day after conception. However, we have three recurrences in 13 examined infants/fetuses when supplements were started 27–41 days postconception, after the usual time for closure of the neural tube (Sheppard et al., 1989). At best this shows the introduction of supplements to be ineffective at this time; at worst it could imply a teratogenic effect, broadly analogous to the effect of vitamin A administration in the curly tail mouse (Seller, 1983a).

Considering which vitamins should be given, there is more evidence to implicate folic acid than any other vitamin. Its role in pyrimidine and purine base synthesis implicates it in DNA metabolism and cell division, and folate supplements are reported to increase placental RNA and DNA levels (Rolschau et al., 1985). Laurence et al. (1983) provided some evidence that periconceptional folic acid therapy alone provides protection against NTD recurrence.

However, undernutrition in humans is rarely limited to a single nutrient and several micronutrients are often required in a single metabolic process. For example, at least five micronutrients are required for the metabolism of folic acid (Schorah, 1988). The individual ingredients of a multivitamin preparation are therefore likely to act together in correcting a dietary or a metabolic deficiency. Chatot et al. (1984) reported that malformations induced in rat embryos cultured in sera from women on anticonvulsant therapy could be prevented by combinations of nutrients, but the effective antidote was not the same in all sera, even when they contained the same anticonvulsant drug. For these reasons and because of the apparent effectiveness of the treatment, our recommendation would be to continue with a formulation such as Pregnavite Forte F unless future research shows us a better alternative.

Any medication in early pregnancy should be given only with serious consideration of the possibility of harmful effects. This would be especially important if the treatment were to be extended to the general population where reduced risk of NTD would mean that a much larger proportion would not need or benefit from the treatment. Vitamin A in doses greater than 10-fold that provided by Pregnavite Forte F has been reported to be harmful in early pregnancy (Bernhardt and Dorsey, 1974; Stange et al., 1978; Rosa, 1983), but there are no reports of vitamins taken at the RDA for pregnancy (intakes which can be obtained without supplementation of the diet) producing harmful effects. It is, however, difficult to identify treatments which might be associated with a small increase in risk to the fetus and we must continue to seek diligently for evidence of harm, even though in over 1000 supplemented pregnancies in the multivitamin intervention studies we have observed none.

AREAS REQUIRING FURTHER INVESTIGATION

We have already suggested that research to pinpoint the protective ingredients in multivitamin supplements should continue, not least because recurrences may still occur in some fully supplemented women. Current trials (Wald and Polani, 1984; Czeizel and Rode, 1984; Lenehen et al., 1988) may shed light on this. However, once it is accepted that multivitamin therapy is effective for preventing NTD, therapeutic trials to identify the most effective combinations become ethically difficult. An alternative approach to this problem would be metabolic studies in individuals either with NTD or at high risk of an affected pregnancy. These investigations would be directed at identifying disturbances in vitamin metabolism that might be causal. This also offers the potential advantage of developing a screening test which could identify those at risk of NTD-affected pregnancies and reduce the number that would require vitamin supplementation. This approach would not be helpful if the cause was simply a dietary deficiency of nutrients, but there is little doubt that human NTDs result from an interaction of genetic and environmental factors, as was clearly shown in the curly tail mouse by Seller (1983a).

There is clear evidence of racial differences in predisposition to NTD. The Irish are at high risk and black populations at low risk of NTD, and this differential risk is maintained in migrant populations (Stevenson et al., 1966; Naggan and MacMahon, 1967; Leck, 1969; Elwood and Nevin, 1973). The prevalence of NTD in dizygotic co-twins is similar to that in siblings, while that in monozygotic co-twins is higher. The genetic contribution to NTD appears to be polygenic

(Janerich and Piper, 1988). However, the rate of decline in NTD prevalence seen recently in the UK (Leck, 1983) has been too rapid to have a purely genetic explanation. A multifactorial etiology for NTD with interaction between environmental and genetic factors implies that a relatively rapid fall in prevalence must reflect environmental changes, and that genetic factors contribute more to the residual cases, which will therefore be less responsive to modification of the environment. The varying response to supplements in the intervention studies, especially in different regions (Seller and Nevin, 1984), is consistent with this concept.

Interaction between environmental and genetic factors could occur through inborn errors of micronutrient metabolism. These need not be severe enough to induce clinical problems in the mother, but could affect the fetus because of increased maternal requirements in pregnancy or because the genetic error affects transfer of the vitamin to the fetoplacental unit. Metabolic differences between individuals in the handling of folic acid have been reported in the general population, especially in pregnancy (Schorah, 1988). If such lesions are implicated in NTD, then it ought to be possible to identify disturbances of vitamin metabolism in those at high risk of NTD or in the affected subjects themselves. Such metabolic lesions may be difficult to identify as they will be partial and may primarily affect metabolic processes which predominate in the placenta or the embryo. Nevertheless, there is increasing evidence that disturbances of both folate and B_{12} metabolism exist in population groups at high NTD risk. A significantly higher than expected proportion of red cell folate and leukocyte vitamin C values in women who have had one NTD-affected pregnancy fall below the 5th percentile (Schorah et al., 1983). Yates and colleagues (1987) reported that women at very high risk (two or more previous NTDs) have significantly lower mean red cell folate values than controls, and women with three or four previous NTDs had even lower red cell folate levels. They also found a significant relationship between dietary and red cell folate in the controls but not in the high-risk groups, a finding that we subsequently confirmed (unpublished observations).

We have also done some preliminary measurements of folic acid uptake by trophoblast cells grown in tissue culture and find that the initial rate of uptake is more rapid in trophoblast tissue taken from normal pregnancies than in cells from an NTD-affected pregnancy (Habibzadeh et al., 1990). High levels of vitamin B_{12}-binding proteins (transcobalamins I and II) in the amniotic fluid of pregnant women who have had previous NTD-affected pregnancies have been reported (Magnus et al., 1986; Gardiki-Kouidou and Seller, 1988). This suggests a possible abnormality of vitamin B_{12} metabolism in placental or fetal tissue in these high-risk groups. This could affect folic acid metabolism because of the metabolic interrelationship of the two vitamins (Scott and Weir, 1981).

These suggestions of impaired vitamin metabolism in NTD are important areas for future research, not only because they may lead to ways of identifying women at risk of NTD but also because they may identify the metabolic cause(s) of the malformation. In suggesting the need for further study of vitamin metabolism we complete the circle and return to the findings of Hibbard and Smithells (1965) who, by showing raised FIGLU excretion in women at the end of an NTD-affected pregnancy, first suggested the possibility of disturbed folate metabolism in this condition. The presence of a metabolic lesion does not mean that dietary factors are unimportant. On the contrary, the success of the vitamin intervention study could result from the dietary correction of a metabolic problem. Dietary deficiencies of the severity seen in malnourished humans are not associated with NTD in most women, but the genetic background varies considerably. It is also worth noting that in many areas of the world where malnutrition is rife, fruit is relatively plentiful, and frank folic acid deficiency is rare outside later pregnancy.

CONCLUSION

There is substantial evidence of an association between NTD and vitamin deficiency (dietary or metabolic). The central issue is whether this association is causal. Hill (1965) identified criteria which help to determine whether an association is likely to be causal, and on all but one of these the hypothesis that vitamin insufficiency contributes to the causation of NTD stands up to scrutiny. The findings from dietary and blood measurements and from metabolic studies in humans are strikingly consistent in indicating that poor nutrition, especially of folic acid, has a role to play in NTD. The implication of folic acid insufficiency is plausible because of its importance in DNA synthesis and cell division. Finally, preventive action in the form of intervention studies has led to dramatic decreases in recurrence rates in groups receiving vitamin supplements during pregnancy, but only if supplements were taken before closure of the neural tube.

Randomized trials may help to resolve the issue, but intervention studies in low-risk areas may be unrewarding for the reasons outlined. Attempts to prevent first occurrence in areas of relatively high prevalence with appropriate randomization may well be the best approach (Czeizel and Rode, 1984) as they also offer the opportunity to test safety, the feasibility of wide-scale supplementation, and the degree of compliance in a large population. The problem of whole-population supplementation may outweigh all others, and this underlines the need for metabolic studies of micronutrient metabolism in high-risk groups. The hope is to pinpoint a disorder which could be used as a marker to identify, perhaps early in life, those who will require supplements before and during pregnancy. It is important to encourage good nutrition, especially in women of childbearing age, but this ideal is difficult to attain, especially among the disadvantaged in society in whom NTD prevalence is highest. The current development of pre-pregnancy counseling clinics provides an opportunity to discuss not only diet but all factors conducive to the eventual birth of a healthy baby.

ACKNOWLEDGMENT

We acknowledge the contributions to these studies of the following colleagues: Dr. Sheila Sheppard, Mrs. Jenny Wild, Dr. Mary Seller, Prof. Norman Nevin, Prof. Rodney Harris, Dr. Andrew Read, Dr. David Fielding, and the late Dr. Stanley Walker.

We also express our gratitude to the following for research support: Action Research for the Crippled Child, Children's Research Fund, Department of Health, Beecham Pharmaceuticals plc.

REFERENCES

Al-Awadi SA, Farag TI, Teebi AS, Naguib KK, El-Khalifa MY. Anencephaly disappearing in Kuwait. Lancet 1984; 2:701–702.

Amaral JF, Thompson WR, Caldwell MD, Martin HF, Randall HT. Prospective hematologic evaluation of gastric exclusion surgery for morbid obesity. Ann Surg 1985; 201:186–193.

Anon. Valproate spina bifida and birth defect registries. Lancet 1988; 2:1404–1405.

Biale Y, Lewenthal J. Effect of folic supplementation on congenital malformations due to anticonvulsive drugs. Eur J Obstet Gynecol Reproduct Biol 1984; 18:211–216.

Bower C, Stanley FJ. Dietary folate as a risk factor for neural tube defects: evidence from a case-control study in Western Australia. Med J Aust 1989; 150:613–619.

Bernhardt IB, Dorsey DJ. Hypervitaminosis A and congenital renal anomalies in a human infant. Obstet Gynecol 1974; 43:750–755.

Bremert JC, Dreosti IE, Tulsi RS. Teratogenic interaction of folic acid and zinc deficiencies in the rat. Nutr Rep Int 1989; 39:383–390.

Bruckner A, Lee YJ, O'Shea KS, Henneberry RC. Teratogenic effects of valproic acid and diphenylhydantoin on mouse embryos in culture. Teratology 1983; 27:29–42.

Canton MC, Cottor BM, Cremin FM, Morrissey PA. The effect of dietary zinc deficiency on pancreatic gamma-glutamyl hydrolase activity and on absorption of pteroylpolyglutamate. Br J Nutr 1989; 62:185–193.

Carter CO, Evans K. Spina bifida and anencephalus in Greater London. J Med Genet 1973; 10:209–234.

Carter CO, Roberts JAF. The risk of recurrence after two children with central nervous system malformations. Lancet 1967; 1:306–308.

Chatot CL, Klein NW, Clapper ML, Resor SP, Singer WD, Russman BS, Holmes GL, Mattson RH, Cramer JA. Human serum teratogenicity studied by rat embryo culture: Epilepsy, anticonvulsant drugs and nutrition. Epilepsia 1984; 25:205–216.

Cheng DW, Bairnson TA, Rao AN, Subbammal S. Effects of variations of rations on the incidence of teratogeny in vitamin E deficient rats. J Nutr 1960; 71:54–60.

Cherry FF, Bennett EA, Bazzano GS, Johnson LK, Fosmire GJ, Batson HK. Plasma zinc in hypertension/toxemia and other reproductive variables in adolescent pregnancy. Am J Clin Nutr 1981; 34:2367–2375.

Clarke C, Hobson D, McKendrick OM, Rogers SC, Sheppard PM. Spina bifida and anencephaly: Miscarriage as possible cause. Br Med J 1975; 4:743–746.

Cohlan SQ. Congenital anomalies in the rat produced by excessive intake of vitamin A during pregnancy. Pediatrics 1954; 13:556–567.

Creasy MR, Alberman ED. Congenital malformations of the central nervous system in spontaneous abortions. J Med Genet 1976; 13:9–16.

Curley FJ, Ingalls TH, Zappasodi P. 6-Aminonicotinamide induced skeletal malformations in mice. Arch Environ Health 1968; 16:309–315.

Czeizel A. Neural tube defects. J Am Med Assoc 1988; 259:3562.

Czeizel A, Rode K. Trial to prevent first occurrence of neural tube defects by periconceptional multivitamin supplementation. Lancet 1984; 2:40.

Dansky LV, Andermann E, Rosenblatt D, Sherwin AL, Andermann F. Anticonvulsants, folate levels and pregnancy outcome. Ann Neurol 1987; 21:176–182.

Elwood JM. Can vitamins prevent neural tube defects? Can Med Assoc J 1983; 129:1088–1092.

Elwood JH, Nevin NC. Factors associated with anencephalus and spina bifida in Belfast. Br J Prev Soc Med 1973; 27:73–80.

Engelsen B, Strandjord R, Gjerde IO, Markestad T, Ulstein M, Evjen OK. Folate concentrations in pregnancies in women on antiepileptic drug therapy. Acta Neurol Scand 1984; 69 (Supp 98):83–84.

Fedrick J. Anencephalus: Variation with maternal age, parity, social class and region in England, Wales and Scotland. Ann Hum Genet 1970; 34:31–38.

Ferm VH, Hanlon DP. Arsenate-induced neural tube defects not influenced by constant rate administration of folic acid. Pediatr Res 1986; 20:761–762.

Fraser JL, Watt HJ. Megaloblastic anemia in pregnancy and the puerperium. Am J Obstet Gynecol 1964; 89:532–534.

Gardiki-Kouidou P, Seller MJ. Amniotic fluid folate, vitamin B_{12} and transcobalamin in neural tube defect. Clin Genet 1988; 33:441–448.

Graham JM, Ferm VH. Heat induced and alcohol induced neural tube defects, interactions with folate in the golden hamster model. Pediatr Res 1985; 19:247–251.

Habibzadeh N, Smithells RW, Schorah CJ. Folic acid metabolism in placental cells associated with neural tube defects. In: Curtius HC, Ghisla S, eds. Chemistry and biology of pteridines. Berlin: Walter de Gruyter, 1990: 1257–1261.

Haddow JE, Hill LE, Kloza EM, Thanhauser D. Neural tube defects after gastric bypass. Lancet 1986; 1:1330.

Hale F. Pigs born without eyeballs. J Hered 1933; 24:105–106.

Hall JG. Neural tube defect among the Sikh population of British Colombia. Proc Greenwood Genetic Cent 1986; 5:129–131.

Hendel J, Dam M, Gram L, Winkel P, Jorgensen I. The effects of carbamazepine and valproate on folate metabolism in man. Acta Neurol Scand 1984; 69:226–231.

Hibbard ED, Smithells RW. Folic acid metabolism and human embryopathy. Lancet 1965; 1:1254.

Hill AB. The environment and disease: association or causation. Proc Roy Soc Med 1965; 58:295–300.

Hogan AG, O'Dell BL, Whitley JR. Maternal nutrition and hydrocephalus in newborn rats. Proc Soc Exp Biol Med 1950; 74:293–296.

Horvath C, Compagnon A, Petter C. Teratogenic effect of pyrimethamine in the rat: in vivo prevention by calcium folinate. C R Soc Biol 1988; 182:158–166.

Hurley LS. Nutritional deficiencies and excesses. In: Wilson JG, Fraser FC, eds. Handbook of teratology, Vol. 1. New York: Plenum Press, 1977, 261–308.

Hurley LS. Zinc deficiency and CNS malformations in humans. Am J Clin Nutr 1981; 34:2864–2868.

Hurley LS, Swenerton H. Congenital malformations resulting from zinc deficiency in rats. Proc Soc Exp Biol Med 1966; 123:692–697.

Janerich DJ, Piper J. Shifting genetic patterns in anencephaly and spina bifida. J Med Genet 1978; 15:101–105.

Kalter H, Warkany J. Experimental production of congenital malformations in mammals by metabolic procedures. Physiol Rev 1959; 39:69–115.

Khoury MJ, Erickson JD, James LM. Etiologic heterogeneity of neural tube defects: Clues from epidemiology. Am J Epidemiol 1982; 115:538–548.

Knox EG. Vitamin supplementation and neural tube defects. Lancet 1983; 2:39.

Lamming GE, Woollam DHM, Millen JW. Hydrocephalus in young rabbits associated with maternal vitamin A deficiency. Br J Nutr 1954; 8:363–369.

Laurence KM, Campbell H, James NE. The role of improvement in the maternal diet and preconceptional folic acid supplementation in the prevention of neural tube defects. In: Dobbing J, ed. Prevention of spina bifida and other neural tube defects. London: Academic Press; 1983, 85–125.

Leck I. Ethnic differences in the incidence of malformations following migration. Br J Prev Soc Med 1969; 23:166–173.

Leck I. Causation of neural tube defects: Clues from epidemiology. Br Med Bull 1974; 30:158–162.

Leck I. Epidemiological clues to the causation of neural tube defects. In: Dobbing J, ed. Prevention of spina bifida and other neural tube defects. London: Academic Press, 1983, 155–218.

Leck I. Record RG, Mckeown T, Edwards JH. The incidence of malformation in Birmingham 1950–59. Teratology 1968; 1:263–280.

Lefebvres-Boisselot J. Role teratogene de la deficience en acide panthothenique chez le rat. Ann Med 1951; 52:225–298.

Lenehan P, MacDonald D, Kirke P. Neural tube defects and vitamin prophylaxis. In. Berger H, ed. Vitamins and minerals in pregnancy and lactation. Nestle Nutrition Workshop Series No. 16. New York: Raven Press, 1988, 177.

Lindhout D, Schmidt D. In utero exposure to valproate and neural tube defects. Lancet 1986; 1:1392–1393.

MacHenry JCRM, Nevin NC, Merrett JD. Comparison of central nervous system malformations in spontaneous abortions in Northern Ireland and southeast England. Br Med J 1979; 1:1395–1397.

Magnus P, Magnus EM, Berg K. Increased levels of apotranscobalamins I and II in amniotic fluid from pregnant women with previous NTD offspring. Clin Genet 1986; 30:167–72.

Marin-Padilla M, Ferm VH. Somite necrosis and developmental malformations induced by vitamin A in the golden hamster. J Embryol Exp Morphol 1965; 13:1–8.

Millen JW, Woollam DHM. The effect of duration of vitamin A deficiency in female rabbits upon the incidence of hydrocephalus in their young. J Neurol Neurosurg Psychiat 1956; 19:17–20.

Mills JL, Rhoads GC, Simpson JL, Cunningham GC, Conley MR, Lassman MR, Walden MC, Depp OR, Hoffman HJ. The absence of a relation between the periconceptional use of vitamins and neural-tube defects. N Engl J Med 1989; 321:430–435.

Milunsky A, Jick H, Jick SS, Bruell CL, MacLaughlin DS, Rothman KJ, Willet W. Multivitamin/folic acid supplements in early pregnancy reduces the prevalence of neural tube defects. J Am Med Assoc 1989; 262:2847–2852.

Moffa AM, White JA. The effect of periconceptional supplementation of folic acid on the incidence of open neural tube defects in golden hamster embryos. Teratology 1983; 27:64A.

Molloy AM, Kirke P, Hillary I, Weir DG, Scott JM. Maternal serum folate and vitamin B_{12} concentrations in pregnancies associated with neural tube defects. Arch Dis Child 1985; 60:660–665.

Mulinare J, Cordero JF, Erickson JD, Berry RJ. Periconceptional use of multivitamins and the occurrence of neural tube defect, J Am Med Assoc 1988; 260:3141–3145.

Naggan L, MacMahon B. Ethnic differences in the prevalence of anencephaly and spina bifida in Boston Massachusetts. New Engl J Med 1967; 227:1119–1123.

Nelson MM. Production of congenital anomalies in mammals by maternal dietary deficiencies. Pediatrics 1957; 19:764–776.

Nelson MM, Wright HV, Asling CW, Evans HM. Multiple congenital abnormalities resulting from transitory deficiency of pteroylglutamic acid during gestation in the rat. J. Nutr 1955; 56:349–370.

Nelson MM, Wright HV, Baird CDC, Evans HM. Effect of a 36 hour period of pteroylglutamic acid deficiency on fetal development in rats. Proc Soc Exp Biol Med 1956; 92:554–556.

Nevin NC, Johnston WP, Merrett JD. Influence of social class on the risk of recurrence of anencephalus and spina bifida. Dev Med Child Neurol 1981; 23:155–159.

Nevin NC, Merrett JD. Potato avoidance during pregnancy in women with a previous infant with either anencephaly and/or spina bifida. Br J Prev Soc Med 1975; 29:111–115.

Nevin NC, Seller MJ. Prevention of neural tube defect recurrences. Lancet 1990; 335:178–179.

Oakley GP, Adams MJ, James LM. Vitamins and neural tube defects. Lancet 1983; 2:798–789.

Palludan B. Swine in teratological studies. In: Bustad LK, McClella RO, eds. Swine in biomedical research. Seattle: Frayn Printing Co, 1966:51–78.

Pritchard JA, Scott DE, Whalley PJ, Haling RF. Infants of mothers with megaloblastic anemia due to folate deficiency. J Am Med Assoc 1970; 211:1982–1984.

Record RG. Anencephalus in Scotland. Br J Prev Soc Med 1961; 15:93–105.

Renwick JH. Hypothesis: Anencephaly and spina bifida are usually preventable by avoidance of a specific unidentified substance present in certain potato tubers. Br J Prev Soc Med 1972; 26:67–72.

Richards IDG, Lowe CR. Incidence of congenital malformations in South Wales 1964–66. Br J Prev Soc Med 1971; 25:59–64.

Richardson LR, Hogan AG. Diet of mother and hydrocephalus in infant rats. J Nutr 1946; 32:459–465.

Rogers JM, Keen CL, Hurley LS. Zinc deficiency in pregnant Long-Evans hooded rats: Teratogenicity and tissue trace elements. Teratology 1985; 31:89–100.

Rogozinski H, Ankers C, Lennon D, Wild J, Schorah C, Sheppard S, Smithells RW. Folate nutrition in early pregnancy. Human Nutr: Applied Nutr 1983; 37A:357–364.

Rolschau J, Date J, Kristoffersen K. Folic acid supplements and intrauterine growth. Acta Obstet Gynecol Scand 1979; 58:343–346.

Rosa FW. Teratogenicity of isotretinoin. Lancet 1983; 2:513.

Schorah CJ. Importance of adequate folate nutrition on embryonic and early fetal development. In: Berger H, ed. Vitamins and minerals in pregnancy and lactation. Nestle Nutrition Workshop Series No. 16. New York: Raven Press, 1988, 167–176.

Schorah CJ, Smithells RW, Scott J. Vitamin B_{12} and anencephaly. Lancet 1980; 1:880.

Schorah CJ, Wild J, Hartley R, Sheppard S, Smithells RW. The effect of periconceptional supplementation on blood vitamin concentrations in women at recurrence risk for neural tube defect. Br J Nutr 1983; 49:203–211.

Scott JM, Weir DG. The methyl folate trap. Lancet 1981; 2:337–338.

Seller MJ. Maternal nutritional factors and neural tube defects in experimental animals. In: Dobbing J, ed. Prevention of spina bifida and other neural tube defects. London: Academic Press, 1983a, 1–14.

Seller MJ. The cause of neural tube defects: some experiments and a hypothesis. J Med Genet 1983b; 20:164–168.

Seller MJ, Hancock PC. Is recurrence rate of neural tube defects declining? Lancet 1985; 1:175.

Seller MJ, Nevin NC. Periconceptional vitamin supplementation and prevention of neural tube defects in southeast England and Northern Ireland. J Med Genet 1984; 21:325–330.

Sheppard S, Nevin NC, Seller MJ, Wild J, Smithells RW, Reed AP, Harris R, Fielding DW, Schorah CJ. Neural tube defect recurrence after "partial" vitamin supplementation. J Med Genet 1989; 26:326–329.

Smithells RW, Ankers C, Carver ME, Lennon D, Schorah CJ, Sheppard S. Maternal nutrition in early pregnancy. Br J Nutr 1977; 38:497–506.

Smithells RW, Chinn ER. Spina bifida in Liverpool. Dev Med Child Neurol 1965; 7:258–268.

Smithells RW, Nevin NC, Seller MJ, Sheppard S, Harris R, Read AP, Fielding DW, Walker S, Schorah CJ, Wild J. Further experience of vitamin supplementation for prevention of neural tube defect recurrences. Lancet 1983; 1:1027–1031.

Smithells RW, Sheppard S, Schorah CJ. Vitamin deficiencies and neural tube defects. Arch Dis Child 1976; 51:944–950.

Smithells RW, Sheppard S, Schorah CJ, Seller MJ, Nevin NC, Harris R, Read AP, Fielding DW. Possible prevention of neural tube defects by periconceptional vitamin supplementation. Lancet 1980; 1:339–340.

Smithells RW, Sheppard S, Schorah CJ, Seller MJ, Nevin NC, Harris R, Read AP, Fielding DW. Apparent prevention of neural tube defects by periconceptional vitamin supplementation. Arch Dis Child 1981; 56:911–918.

Smithells RW, Sheppard S, Wild J, Schorah CJ. Prevention of neural tube defect recurrences in Yorkshire: Final report. Lancet 1989; 2:498–499.

Soltan MH, Jenkins DM. Maternal:fetal plasma zinc concentrations and fetal abnormality. Br J Obstet Gynaecol 1982; 89:56–60.

Stange L, Carlstrom K, Eriksson M. Hypervitaminosis A in early human pregnancy and malformation of the central nervous system. Acta Obstet Gynecol Scand 1978; 57:289–291.

Stein Z, Susser M, Gerhart S, Marolla F. Famine and development. The Dutch hunger winter of 1944–45. London: Oxford University Press, 1975.

Stevenson AC, Johnson HA, Stewart MIP, Golding DR. Congenital malformations: A report of a study of series of consecutive births in 24 centres. Bull WHO 1966; 34:1–125.

Stocks P. Incidence of congenital malformations in the regions of England and Wales. Br J Prev Soc Med 1970; 24:67–77.

Strickler SM, Dansky LV, Miller MA, Seni MH, Andermann E, Spielberg SP. Genetic predisposition to phenytoin induced birth defects. Lancet 1985; 2:746–749.

Tamura T, Kaiser LL, Watson JE, Halstead CH, Hurley LS, Stokstad ELR. Increased methionine synthetase activity in zinc deficient rat liver. Arch Biochem Biophys 1987; 256:311–316.

Tamura T, Shane B, Baer MT, King JC, Margen S, Stokstad ELR. Absorption of mono and polyglutamyl folates in zinc depleted man. Am J Clin Nutr 1978; 31:1984–1987.

Thiersch JB. Therapeutic abortions with folic acid antagonist, 4 amino pteroylglutamic acid administered by the oral route. Am J Obstet Gynecol 1952; 63:1298–1304.

Trotz M, Gansau CH, Nau H. Effect of folic acid deficient diet and folinic acid treatment on the embryo toxicity of valproic acid in the mouse. Teratology 1985; 32:35A.

Wald NJ, Polani PE. Neural tube defects and vitamins: The need for a randomized clinical trial. Br J Obstet Gynaecol 1984; 91:516–523.

Whichelow MJ, Erzinglioglu SW. Is there a north south divide? Regional variations in the diet of British adults. Proc Nutr Soc 1990; 49:76A.

Wild J, Read AP, Sheppard S, Seller MJ, Smithells RW, Nevin NC, Schorah CJ, Fielding DW, Walker S, Harris R. Recurrent neural tube defects, risk factors and vitamins. Arch Dis Child 1986; 61:440–444.

Wilson TS. A study of congenital malformations of the central nervous system among Glasgow births. 1964–68. Hlth Bull (Edinb.) 1970; 28:32–38.

Winship KA, Cahal DA, Weber JCP, Griffin JP. Maternal drug histories and central nervous system anomalies. Arch Dis Child 1984; 59:1052–1060.

Woodard JC, Newberne PM. Relation of vitamin B_{12} and one carbon metabolism to hydrocephalus in the rat. J Nutr 1966; 88:375–381.

Yates JRW, Ferguson-Smith MA, Shenkin A, Guzman-Rodriguez R, White M, Clark BJ. Is disordered folate metabolism the basis for the genetic predisposition to neural tube defects. Clin Genet 1987; 31:279–287.

Zhu MX, Zhou SS. Reduction of teratogenic effects of phenytoin by folic acid and a mixture of folic acid, vitamins and amino acids. A preliminary trial. Epilepsia 1989; 30:246–251.

IMMUNOLOGICAL FUNCTIONS

13

Vitamin E Supplementation and Enhancement of Immune Responsiveness in the Aged

Simin Nikbin Meydani and Jeffrey B. Blumberg

U.S. Department of Agriculture
Human Nutrition Research Center on Aging, Tufts University
Boston, Massachusetts

INTRODUCTION

Vitamin E was first isolated, identified, and synthesized in the 1930s although no overt clinical deficiency was reported in humans until much later when supplemental doses were found effective in treating malabsorption syndromes (Kayden et al., 1965). Recently, several medical uses for pharmacological doses of vitamin E have been developed based on an increased understanding of the damaging effects of free radical-induced events in tissues (Flodin, 1988). Oxidant species, especially those produced by lipid peroxidation, appear to contribute to the etiology and pathology of many disorders including cardiovascular disease, rheumatoid arthritis, reperfusion injury, emphysema, and cancer (Halliwell, 1987). As the body's principal lipid-soluble antioxidant, vitamin E may play an important role in the amelioration and treatment of these and other disorders. Data supporting this contention also raise the possibility that the dietary recommendations for vitamin E should be higher than current estimates if criteria for disease prevention are considered.

Vitamin E has been demonstrated to provide therapeutic benefit in several diseases and has been given for other disorders, although the data are somewhat equivocal or conflicting (Table 1). Vitamin E is effective in the prevention of retrolental fibroplasia in neonates and has been associated with the lowered incidence of this disorder (Johnson et al., 1987). The potential value of pharmacological levels of vitamin E in cardiovascular disease and diabetes mellitus

Table 1 Therapeutic Applications of Vitamin E

Disorder	Efficacy[a]	Selected References
Bronchopulmonary dysplasia	±	Saldanha et al., 1982
Cardiopulmonary bypass	±	Cavarocchi et al., 1986
Chronic cholestasis	+	Sokol et al., 1984
Chronic liver disease	+	Sokol et al., 1985
Contracture around breast implants	+	Baker, 1981
Crohn's disease	+	Harding et al., 1982
Cystic fibrosis	+	Stead et al., 1986
Cystic mastitis	+	Ernster et al., 1985
Genetic hemolytic disorders	+	Rachmilewitz et al., 1982
Hyperbilirubinemia	±	Gross, 1979
Intermittent claudication	+	Haeger, 1982
Intraventricular hemorrhage	+	Sinha et al., 1987
Osteoarthritis	±	Machtey and Ouaknine, 1978
Pancreatitis	+	Dutta et al., 1982
Premenstrual syndrome	±	London et al., 1987
Retrolental fibroplasia	+	Johnson et al., 1987
Shock lung syndrome	+	Wolf and Seeger, 1982
Short-bowel syndrome	+	Howard et al., 1982

[a] +, efficacy established; ±, efficacy still equivocal.

has been studied but positive results have yet to be clearly proved by controlled protocols (Bieri et al., 1983). A clinical application for vitamin E in patients with Parkinson's disease is now being tested in long-term studies (Tetrud and Langston, 1989).

Explorations for new uses of vitamin E can now be based on its established antioxidant properties and modulation of the arachidonic acid (AA) cascade in the cell membrane. Clinical and experimental data suggest possible applications of vitamin E treatment for autoimmune disorders (Ayres and Mihan, 1978), idiopathic nocturnal leg cramps (Catchcart, 1972), phrynoderma (Nadiger, 1980), hemodialysis-induced anemia (Ono, 1985), and alcoholism (Tanner et al., 1986).

Considerable evidence now suggests that free radical damage contributes to the pathogenesis of diseases associated with aging such as amyloidosis, atherosclerosis, cancer, cataract, senile dementia, and immune disorders (Harman, 1982). An immunological basis for many age-related diseases was proposed by Walford and Weindruch (1981). Epidemiological data indicate that improved alpha-tocopherol status is associated with a lower incidence of cancer (Menkes et al., 1986; Wald et al., 1987; Knekt et al., 1988) and of infectious disease (Chavance et al., 1984). The efficacy of vitamin E in treating inflammatory diseases has been examined. Therapy with pharmacological doses of alpha-tocopherol appears effective in relieving pain and improving mobility in patients with osteoarthritis (Machtey and Ouaknine, 1978; Blankenhorn, 1986). Laboratory experiments demonstrate a beneficial effect of vitamin E supplementation on the symptoms of adjuvant arthritis, an animal model of rheumatoid arthritis (Yoshikawa et al., 1983; Pletsityi et al., 1987). Thus, a number of practical applications for vitamin E intervention can be envisioned should its efficacy in enhancing immune function be clearly demonstrated in humans.

DIETARY INTAKE, BIOAVAILABILITY, AND SOURCES OF VITAMIN E

The vitamin E content of diets varies widely depending principally on the amount and types of fat consumed. Analyses of balanced adult diets as consumed in the United States indicate average daily intakes of d-alpha-tocopherol between 7 and 9 mg (10.4–13.4 IU) (Witting and Lee, 1975). Total tocopherol intake (including beta- and gamma-tocopherol and alpha-tocotrienol) may be two to three times higher such that d-alpha-tocopherol equivalents (alpha-TE) (1 alpha-TE = 1 mg RRR = alpha-tocopherol) may range from 8 to 11 mg (12–16 IU). The requirement for vitamin E increases when the intake of polyunsaturated fatty acids increases (Horwitt, 1986). Poor vitamin E status in the presence of high polyunsaturated fatty acid intake promotes an acceleration of lipid peroxidation events in blood and tissues.

Alpha-tocopherol has the highest biological activity among the vitamin E compounds, all eight isomers of the tocol and trienol series are widely distributed in nature. Vegetable oils are the richest sources of vitamin E although alpha-tocopherol generally represents less than 10% of their total tocopherol content. Alpha-tocopherol accounts for almost all of the vitamin E activity in foods of animal origin. Due to a large number of factors which influence the vitamin E content of food, e.g., processing, storing, and cooking, no correlation exists between tabular food values and direct analysis of dietary intake (Bauernfeind, 1980). The alpha-tocopherol contents of some animal and vegetable sources are listed in Table 2.

Criteria for adequacy of vitamin E intake are suggested by the National Research Council Recommended Dietary Allowances (RDA) to include a ratio of tocopherol to polyunsaturated fatty acids which protects tissue lipids from peroxidation, permits normal physiological function, and allows for individual variations of tissue lipids (*Recommended Dietary Allowances*, 1989). The vitamin E content in average diets is generally considered satisfactory as there is no significant clinical or biochemical evidence that vitamin E status of the U.S. population is inadequate. Hence, the RDA has established "an arbitrary but practical allowance for male adults of 10 mg of alpha-TEs per day (and) because women are generally smaller, their allowance is 8 mg/day."

Table 2 Alpha-Tocopherol Content (μg/g) of
Selected Food Items

Animal origin[a]		Vegetable oils	
beef	5–8	Coconut	11
pork	4–6	Corn	159
chicken	2–4	Cottonseed	440
halibut	4–13	Olive	100
cod	15–33	Peanut	189
shrimp	6–19	Rapeseed	236
butter	10–33	Safflower	396
lard	2–30	Sunflower	487
eggs	8–12	Wheat germ	1194

[a] Range.
Source: Adapted from Bauernfeind, 1980.

Vitamin E from foods is absorbed along with other dietary lipids into the lymphatic system in association with chylomicrons. The absorption efficiency of tocopherols ranges from 20 to 40%. In order to double plasma tocopherol levels vitamin E supplements must be 10-fold or more that of normal dietary intake ranges (Blumberg, 1987). As discussed above, because of the lipid-soluble thus hydrophobic nature of the tocopherol molecule, considerable malabsorption with possible deficiency of the vitamin occurs with pathological conditions that cause fat malabsorption. The recent synthesis of deuterated vitamin E compounds allows for quantitative in vivo assessments of tocopherol bioavailability and activity. The use of this approach indicates that the half-time for tocopherol turnover varies among tissues and ranges from 7.6 days in the lung to 76 days in the spinal cord of rats (Burton et al., 1988). Interestingly, Burton et al. (1988) observed a selective accumulation of the naturally occurring d-stereoisomer species in all tissues examined, indicating a discriminative effect.

NUTRITION AND THE IMMUNE SYSTEM

Examination of the immune system is a useful approach to the study of nutrition and aging. The synthesis of antibodies, complement, and other proteins and the clonal proliferation of immunocompetent cells requires the ready availability of nutrient substrates. Since malnutrition impairs immunity, one can postulate that nutritional problems may contribute to declining immunity in old age and associated disease processes. If this hypothesis is correct, the appropriate modification of nutritional status should improve immunity and reduce the burden of illness in the elderly.

The protective responses of the immune system require collaborations among at least four principal cell types. B lymphocytes make and secrete immunoglobulin antibodies. Cytotoxic or killer T lymphocytes and natural killer cells bind to and destroy antigen-bearing cells found in tumors and virally infected target cells. Helper T cells release lymphokines that promote the proliferation and functional maturation of both T and B lymphocytes. Antigen-presenting cells, including those of the macrophage (MO) and dendritic series, are not themselves specific for any particular antigen but can ingest and process antigenic particles and then display the resulting fragments in a form which is stimulatory for T cells.

Cell-mediated immunity is that specific immune response to antigens mediated by lymphocytes and MO with minor partipation by other cell types. Cellular immunity is responsible for delayed-type hypersensitivity (DTH) skin test, foreign graft rejection, resistance to many pathogenic microorganisms, and tumor immunosurveillance. The humoral immune system primarily involves B-cell production of immunoglobulins and other humoral constituents such as complement proteins. Cells of the immune system are highly dependent on a functioning cell membrane for secretion of lymphokines and antibodies, antigen reception, lymphocyte transformation, and contact cell lysis. The established role of vitamin E in the maintenance of membrane integrity and its antioxidant property make alpha-tocopherol a potentially critical nutrient in the regulation of immune function.

ROLE OF AA METABOLITES IN CONTROL OF THE IMMUNE SYSTEM

AA metabolites, prostaglandins (PGs), hydroxyeicosatetraenoic acid (HETE), and leukotrienes (LTs) are produced by most cells including human peripheral blood mononuclear cells (PBMC) and mouse splenocytes in response to stimulation by mitogens or antigens. PGs can inhibit T-cell proliferation and thus cell-mediated immune functions (Goodwin et al., 1974; Webb et al. 1980). Likewise, inhibition of PG synthesis in vitro enhances T-cell proliferation (Goodwin et al., 1974; Muscoplat et al, 1978; Webb et al, 1980; Metzger et all, 1980; Fisher and Bostic-Bruton, 1982; Rola-Pleszczynski, 1985). Cellular and humoral immune responses are under negative control by PG. In vitro, protstaglandin E_2 (PGE$_2$) inhibits T-cell proliferation (Goodwin et al., 1974; Webb et al, 1980), lymphokine production (Gordon et al., 1976), and the generation of cytotoxic cells (Plaut, 1979).

In addition to PGE$_2$ other products, i.e., LT and HETE, have been shown to inhibit proliferation in mouse splenocytes (Goodman and Weigle, 1980; Rola-Pleszczynski, 1985). This effect may be mediated by decreased T-helper and increased T-suppressor/cytotoxic cell proliferation (Rola-Pleszczynski et al., 1982; Gualde et al., 1985; Payan et al., 1984).

EFFECT OF AGING ON THE IMMUNE SYSTEM

Considerable evidence indicates that aging is associated with altered regulation of the immune system (Siskind, 1980). Well-documented, age-related functional changes have been defined for both humoral and cell-mediated responses (Siskind, 1980; Makinodan, 1981; Hausman and Weksler, 1985). Although the major alterations have been demonstrated in the T lymphocytes (Makinodan, 1981; Miller, 1989), recent observations (Rosenstein et al., 1980; Bartocci et al., 1982) indicate that supressive factors from MO contribute to the age-associated changes in T cells.

Cooperation between MO and lymphocytes is essential in antigen recognition, lymphocytes differentiation, and eventual antibody production, and development of the effector state of cellular immunity or the delayed hypersensitivity phase (Unanue, 1980). In addition to presenting·antigen, MO secrete interleukin 1 (IL-1) which induces the production of the T-cell growth factor IL-2 by the activated T cells. MOs have high levels of AA in their phospholipids and upon stimulation, mouse peritoneal MOs release up to 50% of their AA content in the form of oxygenated metabolites, i.e., PG, HETE, and LT (Humes et al., 1977; Scott et al., 1982; Bonney et al., 1985). These compounds, in addition to their effects on biological activities of MO, suppress lymphocyte proliferation and lymphokine synthesis (Goodwin et al., 1974; Gordon et al., 1976; Webb et al., 1980; Gualde et al., 1984; Rola-Pleszczynski, 1985). Other oxidative metabolites of activated MO such as H_2O_2 have also been shown to suppress lymphocyte proliferation (Metzger et al., 1980; Fisher and Bostic-Bruton, 1982; Lipsky, 1984). Therefore, MO can affect lymphocyte proliferation in two ways: (1) by producing enhancing factors such as IL-1 which stimulate helper T cells to synthesize IL-2 and (2) by producing suppressive factors such as eicosanoids and hydrogen peroxide (H_2O_2) which inhibit IL-2 production and lymphocyte proliferation.

Several groups have shown that antigen (Miller and Stutman, 1981; Thoman and Weigle, 1982) and mitogen (Gillis et al., 1981; Thoman and Weigle, 1982; Chang et al., 1982) stimulated IL-2 production declines with age and contributes to the T-cell-mediated defects observed with aging in rats, mice, and humans. Furthermore, IL-2 reconstitution in vitro (Chang et al., 1982) and in vivo (Thoman and Weigle, 1985) improves cell-mediated lymphocyte responses of aged mice. Chang et al. (1982) showed that changes in both MO and T lymphocytes were responsible for decreased IL-2 production. Rosenberg et al. (1983) demonstrated that cell-cell interaction and cooperation via lymphokines and other regulatory molecules is impaired in aged mice and that increased MO number in the aged rat spleen might have a suppressive effect. Chang et al. (1982) also showed that MO from old mice decreased IL-2 production by spleen lymphocytes from young mice.

The suppressive effect of MO from aged mice has been attributed to either a decrease in IL-1 production (Chang et al., 1982) or an increase in suppressive factors. Increased PGE_2 production by MO from aged rats (Bash, 1983) and mice (Bartocci et al., 1982; Meydani et al., 1986a) has been reported. Furthermore, Rosenstein and Strausser (1980) were able to achieve substantial enhancement of aged spleen cell responsiveness in vitro and in vivo with indomethacin, an inhibitor of cyclooxygenase, the enzyme involved in PGE_2 production. Bartocci et al. (1982) also showed that decreasing MO production of PGE_2 with aspirin results in enhanced tumor rejection in aged mice. Splenocytes from aged mice synthesize more PGE_2 and accumulate less IL-2 in concanavalin A (Con A)-stimulated mitogen cultures than young mice (Meydani et al., 1986a). Goodwin and Messner (1980) demonstrated that phytohemagglutinin (PHA)-stimulated cultures of PBMC from subjects over 70 are more sensitive to inhibition by PGE_2 than are cultures from younger subjects. These investigators also demonstrated that this depressed responsiveness to PHA can be partly reversed by blocking the endogenous production of PGE_2 with indomethacin.

EFFECT OF VITAMIN E ON IMMUNE RESPONSES

Various methods have been developed to experimentally modify the decline of immunological vigor in aging rodents. These methods include dietary manipulation, chemical therapy, genetic manipulation, and cell grafting. Although several studies report encouraging effects of calorie restriction on life span and immune functions of long- and short-lived rodents (Masoro, 1985), the effect of individual dietary components with known or potentially important roles in the immune system has been largely overlooked.

Tissue culture and animal studies have shown that vitamin E is essential for normal function of the immune system. Moreover, the level of vitamin E intake higher than currently recommended may be required for optimal function of the immune system (Bendich et al., 1986; Reddy et al., 1987; Jensen et al., 1988). The role of vitamin E supplementation in enhancement of the immune response of young animals has been reviewed (Tengerdy, 1980; Meydani and Blumberg, 1991a). Briefly, Tengerdy first reported that chickens given 100 mg/kg vitamin E had significantly increased generation of anti-sheep red blood cell (SRBC) antibodies and plaque-forming cells (PFC) (Tengerdy and Brown, 1977). Mice fed diets containing 60–100 mg/kg of vitamin E had significantly increased humoral immune responses as measured by PFC and antibody responses to SRBC and tetanus toxoid (Tengerdy, 1980). Vitamin E deficiency decreases the PFC response to SRBC in mice, an effect restored to normal by vitamin E but not by the synthetic antioxidant N-N-diphenyl-p-phenylenediamine (Tengerdy, 1980). Corwin and Shloss (1980) found that vitamin E and 2-mercaptoethanolamine are both mitogenic in vitro. Vitamin E supplementation in mice enhanced the proliferative response of lymphocytes to suboptimal doses of Con A. Pigs supplemented with vitamin E show enhanced proliferation of peripheral blood lymphocytes to PHA (Larsen and Tollersrud, 1981), whereas vitamin E deficiency in dogs decreases the blastogenic response of lymphocytes to Con A (attributable to a serum factor that could be washed from the cell surface of depressed lymphocytes) (Langweiler and Schultz, 1981). In mice, dietary vitamin E was shown to enhance helper T-cell activity (Tanaka et al., 1979). Reddy et al. (1986) showed that serum from tocopherol-supplemented calves inhibited infectious bovine rhinotracheitis viral replication more effectively in tissue culture than serum from unsupplemented calves. These findings suggest that vitamin E supplementation might be beneficial in increasing resistance to this cattle disease and possibly other viral infections.

Bendich et al. (1986) demonstrated that while a diet containing 15 mg/kg of vitamin E was adequate to prevent myopathy in rats, optimal lymphocyte proliferation to PHA and Con A was obtained only with much higher levels of vitamin E (50–200 mg/kg). Eskew et al. (1985) showed that the vitamin E required for optimal immune response is higher under conditions where lipid peroxidation and oxidative stress are increased.

EFFECT OF VITAMIN E ON IMMUNE RESPONSE OF AGED ANIMALS

One of the biological changes associated with aging is an increase in free radical formation with subsequent damage to cellular processes. Numerous studies have expounded on the free radical theory of aging and the role of antioxidants, including vitamin E, on the life expectancy of rodents (see Blumberg and Meydani, 1986). Oxygen metabolites, especially H_2O_2 produced by activated MO, depress lymphocyte proliferation. Free radical formation associated with aging may be an underlying factor in the depressed immune response observed in aged rodents. Tocopherol decreases H_2O_2 formation in polymorphonuclear white blood cells (Baehner et al., 1977).

It was suggested by Harman (1982) that vitamin E and other antioxidants may increase longevity by influencing the immune system and reducing age-related diseases. As mentioned earlier, an immunological basis for many age-associated diseases was proposed by Walford et al. (1981). Vitamin E supplementation has been shown to be protective against some of these diseases in animals. For example, Ip (1985) showed that vitamin E deficiency increases 7,12-dimethylbenz[a]anthracene (DMBA)-induced mammary adenocarcinomas and decreases the effectiveness of selenium supplementation in reducing DMBA-induced carcinogenesis. Horvath and Ip (1983) showed that vitamin E supplementation decreased lipid peroxidation and potentiated the prophylactic action of selenium against mammary carcinogenesis. Ip (1982) also showed that vitamin E deficiency increases the risk of development of mammary tumors, especially in rats fed diets high in polyunsaturated fatty acids. The protective effect of vitamin E appears to be due to its antioxidant effect rather than its effect on enzymes involved in DMBA detoxification. Meydani et al. (1986b) found that while 40% of old mice fed 30 mg/kg vitamin E had kidney amyloidosis, a common age-related immunopathological feature, none of the old mice fed 500 mg/kg vitamin E had evidence of amyloid deposits. An increase in the average life span of short-lived autoimmune-prone NZB/NZW mice receiving vitamin E supplements was reported by Harman (1980).

These observations prompted the evaluation of the effect of vitamin E supplementation on the cell-mediated immune response of aged mice. Supplementation with 500 mg/kg dietary dl-alpha-tocopheryl acetate in 24-month-old mice for 6 weeks significantly increased splenocyte proliferation to Con A and lipopolysaccharide (LPS) but not to PHA relative to 24-month-old control animals fed 30 ppm of the vitamin. In addition, vitamin E supplementation significantly increased DTH to 2,4-dinitro-7-fluorobenzene. This immunostimulatory effect of vitamin E was associated with increased production of IL-2 and decreased production of PGE_2 (Meydani et al., 1986a). No stimulatory effect of vitamin E was noted on natural killer cell (NK)-mediated cytotoxicity; however, when the mice were immunized with sheep red blood cell (SRBC) (a condition associated with increased oxidative stress) prior to assessment, the supplemented mice had a greater NK-mediated cytotoxicity (Meydani et al., 1988).

EFFECT OF VITAMIN E ON IMMUNE RESPONSES OF ELDERLY SUBJECTS

Studies of the effects of vitamin E on the immune response in humans are limited, especially as they relate to the elderly. Ziemlanski et al. (1986) supplemented 20 institutionalized elderly women (63–93 years) with 100 mg dl-alpha-tocopheryl acetate twice daily and assessed serum protein and immunoglobulin concentrations after 4 and 12 months. Vitamin E increased total serum protein with the principal effect on alpha-2- and beta-2-globulin fractions occurring at 4 months. No significant effects were noted on levels of immunoglobulins and complement component C3 although another group that received vitamin C (400 mg daily) along with vitamin E displayed significant increases in IgG and C3 levels.

Harman and Miller (1986) supplemented 103 elderly patients from a chronic care facility with 200 or 400 mg alpha-tocopheryl acetate daily but did not see any beneficial effect on antibody development against influenza virus vaccine. Unfortunately, data on the health status, medication use, antibody levels, and other relevant parameters were not reported.

Meydani et al. (1990) using a double-blind, placebo-controlled trial showed that vitamin E supplementation significantly improved in vivor and in vitro immune indices of older adults. Healthy elderly (60 years and older) were supplemented with 800 mg/day of dl-alpha-tocopheryl acetate or placebo for 30 days. Blood samples were collected before and after supplementation for measurement of different biochemical and immunological parameters. Plasma and WBC vitamin E levels increased three fold. DTH, an in vivo indicator of cell-mediated immunity, was also measured before and after supplementation using Multitest CMI, which administers seven recall antigens simultaneously and uniformly.

A marked improvement was seen in DTH following vitamin E supplementation (Fig. 1). In vitro both IL-2 production (Fig. 2) and lymphocyte proliferation were significantly improved by vitamin E supplementation. The increase in immunological parameters was associated with a 34% decrease in PGE_2 synthesis by PBMC ($p < 0.0004$) and a 56% decrease in plasma lipid peroxide levels ($p < 0.001$). Significantly more subjects in the vitamin E group showed a reduction in plasma lipid peroxides and PGE_2 production by PBMC than controls (Table 3). In view of the known immunosuppressive effect of PGE_2 on immune function, it is plausible that the immunostimulatory effect of vitamin E is due to a reduction

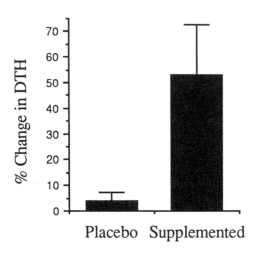

Figure 1 Effect of vitamin E supplementation (Suppl.) on delayed-type hypersensitivity skin test in elderly subjects. Data represent percent change in cumulative score (the sum of induration diameter of all positive responses, i.e., induration diameter ≥ 2 mm). Percent change for each subject was calculated as:

(postsuppl. value − presuppl. value × 100)/presuppl. value.

Percent change in supplemented group is significantly higher than that in placebo group at $p = 0.04$ by Wilcoxon signed rank test. (Reprinted from Meydani et al. (1990) with permission from the American Journal of Clinical Nutrition.)

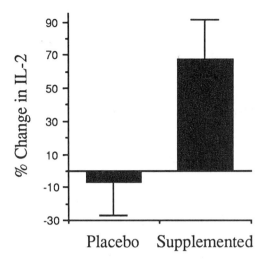

Figure 2 Effect of vitamin E supplementation on Il-2 production. Data represent percent change in Il-2 production in response to Con A (10 μg/ml). Percent change for each subject was calculated as in Fig. 1. Percent change in supplemented group is significantly higher than that in placebo group at p = 0.025 by Wilcoxon signed rank test.

in PGE_2 synthesis and a concomitant increase in IL-2 production. Epidemiological studies (Chavance, 1968) indicate a lower incidence of infectious disease in elderly subjects with high plasma tocopherol levels. Population groups maintaining high plasma tocopherol levels have also been noted to possess a lower incidence of cancer (Menkes et al., 1986; Trickler and Shklar, 1987). Furthermore, Christou et al. (1989) showed that a significant correlation exists in preoperative patients between DTH and mortality from sepsis. Improved DTH response in hospitalized patients has been shown to decrease sepsis and mortality (Fletcher et al., 1986). Wayne et al. (1990) showed that healthy elder subjects

Table 3 Percent of Subjects Showing Decreased Production of Plasma Lipid Peroxide and PBMC PGE_2

Parameter	Placebo (N = 14)	Vitamin E (N = 18)	p^a
	%		
Plasma lipid peroxide	64	94	0.009
PBMC PGE_2	42	88	0.009

[a] Analyzed by chi-square.

who were anergic when tested for DTH had significantly higher mortality from all causes in subsequent years.

As mentioned above, it has been demonstrated that a higher than standard intake of tocopherol is necessary to promote optimal immune responsiveness in young rodents (Bendich et al., 1986). Although our study (Meydani et al., 1990) suggests that many elderly might benefit from a supplementary intake of vitamin E, such public health recommendations should be deferred pending longer term investigations which include a range of levels of tocopherol. Nevertheless, it is encouraging to note that a single nutrient supplement can enhance immune responsiveness in healthy elderly consuming the recommended level of all other nutrients.

SAFETY AND TOXICITY OF VITAMIN E

Oral alpha-tocopherol and its esters possess very low toxicity according to extensive acute and chronic animal studies, six double-blind placebo-controlled studies performed with normal adults, and several large but less well-controlled trials (reviewed by Bendich and Machlin, 1988). Additional evidence of safety can be inferred from the frequent use of higher than RDA levels of vitamin E supplements, a relatively popular practice in the United States. Although minor side effects, such as breast soreness, fatigue, and gastrointestinal symptoms, have been reported from individual cases and uncontrolled studies, most of these reactions have not been observed in well-controlled studies (Bendich and Machlin, 1988). In our studies (Meydani et al., 1991b), supplementation of elderly subjects with 800 mg of vitamin E for 30 days had no effect on liver enzymes, blood cell counts and white blood cell differential counts, plasma levels of other nutrients, serum thyroid hormone levels (T3 and T4), or urinary creatinine levels. Furthermore, none of the subjects complained of any side effects. It is important to note that a synergistic drug-nutrient interaction may occur between oral vitamin K antagonists such as the anticoagulant warfarin and doses of vitamin E greater than 1200 IU/day (Corrigan, 1982). Prolonged bleeding time, ecchymosis, and depressed vitamin K–dependent clotting factors observed at these high intakes are not noted with lower doses of vitamin E (Corrigan and Ulfers, 1981). Patients with vitamin K deficiency resulting from malabsorption syndromes or dietary deficiency should avoid high doses of vitamin E, as this could increase risk of bleeding.

SUMMARY

Dietary antioxidants appear to play an important protective role against several functional changes associated with the aging process. Studies in both animals and healthy humans indicate that vitamin E can enhance immune responsiveness in the aged. The evidence for alpha-tocopherol's immunomodulatory capacity is compelling and also attractive because of the established safety of the vitamin. Moreover, nutritional intervention represents an especially practical approach for delaying or reversing the decline of immune responsiveness with age. It seems reasonable to postulate that any factor which could beneficially alter this age-related change may also positively affect the development of many chronic diseases common among the elderly. Although further studies are necessary to confirm and expand on the research conducted to date, enhancing vitamin E status may improve immunocompetence and promote the realization of a more productive and fuller life span for the elderly.

REFERENCES

Ayres S, Jr, Mihan R. Is vitamin E involved in the autoimmune mechanism? Cutis 1978; 21:321.

Baehner BL, Boxer LA, Allen JM, Davis J. Auto-oxidatin as a basis for altered function by polymorphonuclear leukocytes. Blood 1977; 50:327.

Baker JL. The effectiveness of alpha-tocopherol (vitamin E) in reducing the incidence of spherical contracture around breast implants. Plast Reconstruct Surg 1981; 68:696.

Bartocci A, Maggi FM, Welker RD, Veronese F. Age-related immunosuppression: Putative role of prostaglandins. In: Powles TJ, Backman RS, Honn KV, Ramwell P, eds. Prostaglandins and cancer. New York: Alan R. Liss, 1982, 725.

Bash JA. Cellular immunosenescence in F344 rats; decline in responsiveness to phytohemagglutinin involves changes in both T cells and macrophages. Mech Aging Dev 1983; 21:321.

Bauernfeind J. Tocopherols in foods. In: Machlin L, ed. Vitamin E: A comprehensive treatise. New York: Marcel Dekker, 1980, 99.

Bendich A, Garbiel E, Machlin LJM. Dietary vitamin E requirement for optimum immune response in the rat. J Nutr 1986; 116:675.

Bendich A, Machlin L. Safety of oral intake of vitamin E. Am J Clin Nutr 1988; 48:612.

Bieri JG, Corash L, Hubbard VS. Medical uses of vitamin E. N Engl J Med 1983; 308:1063.

Blankenhorn G. Efficacy of Spondyvit® (vitamin E) in activated arthroses. A multicenter, placebo-controlled, double-blind study. Z Orthop 1986; 23:340.

Blumberg J, Meydani SN. Role of dietary antioxidants in aging. In: Munro H, Hutchinson M, eds. Bristol-Myers nutrition symposia: Nutrition and aging, Vol. 5. New York: Academic Press, 1986, 85.

Blumberg JB. Vitamin E requirements during aging. In: Hayaishi O, Miro M, eds. Clinical and nutritional aspects of vitamin E. Amsterdam: Elsevier 1987, 53.

Bonney RJ, Opas EE, Humes JL. Lipoxygenase pathway of macrophages. Fed Proc 1985; 44:2933.

Boyum AI. Isolation of mononuclear cells and granulocytes from human blood. Scand J Clin Lab Invest 1968; 97(suppl 21):77.

Burton GW, Ingold KU, Foster DO, Cheng SC, Webb A, Hughes L, Lusztyk E. Comparison of free α-tocopherol and α-tocopheryl acetate as sources of vitamin E in rats and humans. Lipids 1988; 23:834.

Catchcart RF. Leg cramps and vitamin E. J Am Med Assoc 1972; 219:216.

Cavarocchi NC, England MD, O'Brien JF, Solis E, Rosso P, Schaff HV, Orszulak TA, Pluth JR, Kaye MP. Superoxide generation during cardiopulmonary bypass: Is there a role for vitamin E? J Surg Res 1986; 40:519.

Chang MP, Makinodan T, Peterson WJ, Strehler BL. Role of T cells and adherent cells in age-related decline in murine interleukin 2 production. J Immunol 1982; 129:2426.

Chavance M, Brubacher G, Herberth B, Vernes G, Mistacki T, Dete F, Fournier C, Janot C. Immunological and nutritional status among the elderly. In: Chandra RK, ed. Nutrition, immunity, and illness. New York, Pregamon Press, 1985, 137.

Christou NV, Tellado-Rodrigues J, Chartrand L, Giannas B, Kapadia B, Meakins J, Rode H, Gordon J. Estimating mortality risk in preoperative patients using immunologic, nutritional, and acute-phase response variables. Ann Surg 1989; 210:69.

Corrigan JJ, Ulfers LL. Effect of vitamin E on prothrombin levels in warfarin-induced vitamin K deficiency. Am J Clin Nutr 1981; 34:1701.

Corrigan JJ, Jr. The effect of vitamin E on warfarin-induced vitamin K deficiency. Ann NY Acad Sci 1982; 292:361.

Corwin LM, Shloss J. Role of antioxidants on the stimulation of the mitogenic response. J Nutr 1981; 110:2497.

Dutta SK, Bustin MP, Russell RM, Costa BS. Deficiency of fat-soluble vitamins in treated patients with pancreatic insufficiency. Ann Intern Med 1982; 97:549.

Ernster VL, Goodson WH, Hunt TK, Petrakis NL, Sicles EA, Miike R. Vitamin E and benign breast "disease": A double-blind, randomized clinical trial. Surgery 1985; 97:490.

Eskew ML, Scholz RW, Reddy CC, Todhunter DA, Zarkower A. Effects of vitamin E and selenium deficiencies on rat immune function. Immunology 1985; 54:173.

Fisher RI, Bostic-Bruton F. Depressed T-cell proliferative responses in Hodgkin's disease: Role of monocyte-mediated suppression via prostaglandins and hydrogen peroxide. J Immunol 1982; 129:1770.

Fletcher JD, Koch GA, Endres E, et al. Anergy and the severely ill surgical patient. Aust NZ J Surg 1986; 56(2):17.

Flodin NW. Vitamin E. In: Pharmacology of micronutrients. New York: A. R. Liss, 1988, 59.

Gillis S, Kojak R, Durante, and Weksler ME. Immunological studies of aging. Decreased production of and response to T cell growth factor by lymphocytes from aged humans. J Clin Invest 1981; 67:937.

Goodman MG, Weigle WO. Modulation of lymphocyte activation I. Inhibition by an oxidation product of arachidonic acid. J Immunol 1980; 125:593.

Goodwin JS, Messner RP, Peake GT. Prostaglandin suppression of mitogen stimulated leukocytes in culture. J Clin Invest. 1974; 54:368.

Goodwin JS, Messner RP. Sensitivity of lymphocytes to prostaglandin E_2 increased in subjects over age 70. J Clin Invest 1980; 332:260.

Gordon D, Bray M, Morley J. Control of lymphokine secretion by prostaglandins. *Nature* 1976; 262:401.

Gross SJ. Vitamin E and neonatal bilirubinemia. Pediatrics 1979; 64:321.

Gualde N, Mexmain S, Aldigier JC, Goodwin JS, Rigaud M. Effect of eicosatetraenoic acids on lymphocyte proliferation in vitro. In: Thaler-Dao Acrastes de Paulet H, Paoleti R, eds., Icosanoids and cancer. New York; Raven Press, 1984, 155.

Gualde N, Atlur D, Goodwin JS. Effect of lipoxygenase metabolites of arachidonic acid on proliferation of human T cells and T cell subsets. J Immunol 1985; 134:1125.

Haeger K. Longterm study of α-tocopherol in intermittent claudication. Ann NY Acad Sci 1982; 393–369.

Halliwell B. Oxidants and human disease: Some new concepts. FASEB J. 1987; 1:358.

Harding AE, Muller DPR, Thomas PK, Wilison HJ. Spinocerebellar degeneration secondary to chronic intestinal malabsorption: A vitamin E deficiency syndrome. Ann Neurol 1982; 12:419.

Harman D. Free radical theory of aging: Beneficial effect of antioxidants on the lifespan of male NZB mice; role of free radical pathogenesis of systematic lupus erythematosus. Age 1980; 3:64.

Harman D. Nutritional implications of the free radical theory of aging. J Am Coll Nutr 1982; 1:27.

Harman D, Miller RW. Effect of vitamin E on the immune response to influenza virus vaccine and incidence of infectious disease in man. Age 1986; 9:21.

Hausman PB, Weksler ME. Changes in the immune response with age. In: Finch CE, Schneider EL, eds. Handbook of biology of aging, 2nd ed. New York: Van Nostrand Reinhold, 1985; 414.

Horvath PM, Ip C. Synergistic effect of vitamin E and selenium in the chemoprevention of mammary carcinogenesis in rats. Cancer Res 1983; 43:5335.

Horwitt M. The promotion of vitamin E. J Nutr 1986; 116:1371.

Howard L, Ovesen L, Satya-Murti S, Chu R. Reversible neurological syndrome. Am J Clin Nutr 1982; 36:1243.

Humes JL, Bonney RJ, Pebes L, et al. Macrophage synthesize and release prostaglandins in response to inflammatory response. Nature 1988; 269:149.

Ip C. Dietary vitamin E intake and mammary carcinogenesis in rats. Carcinogensis 1982; 3:1453.

Ip C. Attenuation of the anticarcinogenic action of selenium by vitamin E deficiency. Cancer Lett 1985; 25:325.

Jensen M, Fossum C, Ederoth M, Hakkarainen RVJ. The effect of vitamin E on the cell-mediated immune response in pigs. J Vet Med 1988; B35:549.

Johnson LH, Quinn GE, Abbasi S, Bowen FW. Vitamin E and retinopathy of prematurity. J Am Coll Nutr 1987; 6:85A.

Kayden HJ, Silber R, Kossman CE. The role of vitamin E deficiency in the abnormal autohemolysis of acanthocytosis. Trans Assoc Am Physicians 1965; 78:334.

Knekt P, Aromaa A, Maatela J, Aaran R, Nikkari T, Hakama M, Hakulinen T, Petro R Saxen E, Teppor L. Serum vitamin E and risk of cancer among Finnish men during a 10-year follow-up. Am J Epidemiol 1988; 127:28.

Langweiler M, Schultz RD, Sheffy BE. Effect of vitamin E deficiency on the proliferative response of canine lymphocytes Am J Vet Res 1981; 42;1681.

Larsen HJ, Tollersrud S. Effect of dietary vitamin E and selenium on the phytohaemagglutinin response of pig lymphocytes. Res Vet Sci 1981; 31:301.

Lipsky PE. Immunosuppression by D-penicillamine in vitro. Inhibition of human T-lymphocyte proliferation by copper- or ceruloplasmin-dependent generation of hydrogen peroxide and protection by monocytes. J Clin Invest 1984; 73:53.

London RS, Murphy L, Kitlowski KE, Reynolds MA. Efficacy of alpha-tocopherol in the treatment of premenstrual syndrome. J Reprod Med 1987; 32:400.

Machtey I, Ouaknine L. Tocopherol in osteoarthritis: A controlled pilot study. J Am Geriat Soc 1978;26:328.

Makinodan T. Cellular basis of immunologic aging. In: Schimke RT, ed. Biological mechanisms in aging. USDA, NIH, 1981; 488.

Masoro EJ. Nutrition and aging: A current assessment. J Nutr. 1985; 115:842.

Menkes MS, Comstock GW, Vuilleumier JP, Helsing KJ, Rider A, Brookmezer R. Serum β-carotene vitamins A and E, selenium, and the risk of lung cancer. N Engl J Med 1986; 315:1250.

Metzger Z, Hoffeld JT, Oppenheim JJ. Macrophage mediated suppression. I. Evidence for participation of both hydrogen peroxide and prostaglandins in suppression of murine lymphocyte proliferation. J Immunol 1980; 124:983.

Meydani SN, Meydani M, Verdon CP, Blumberg JB, Hayes KC. Vitamin E supplementation suppresses prostaglandin E_2 synthesis and enhances the immune response of aged mice. Mech Aging Dev 1986a; 34:191.

Meydani SN, Cathcart ES, Hopkins RE, Meydani M, Hayes KC, Blumberg JB. Antioxidants in experimental amyloidosis of young and old mice. In: Glenner GG, Asserman EP, Benditt E, Calkins E, Cohen DS, Zucker-Franklin D, eds. Fourth Int. Symposium of amyloidosis. New York: Plenum Press, 1986b, 683.

Meydani SN, Yogeeswaran G, Liu S, Baskar S, Meydani M. Fish oil and tocopherol induced changes in natural killer cell mediated cytotoxicity and PGE_2 synthesis in young and old mice. J Nutr 1988; 118:1245.

Meydani SN, Blumberg JB. (1991a). Vitamin E and the immune response. In: Cunningham-Rundles S, ed. Nutritional modulation of immune response. New York: Marcel Dekker, 1980a, in press.

Meydani SN, Barklund P, Liu S, Meydani M, Miller RA, Cannon JG, Morrow FD, Rocklin R, Blumberg JB. Vitamin E supplementation enhances cell-mediated immunity in healthy elderly. Am J Clin Nutr 1990; 52: 557.

Meydani SN, Morrow F, Meydani M, Blumberg JB. Safety assessment of short-term supplementation with vitamin E in healthy older adults. Am J Clin Nutr 1991b (in press).

Miller, RA. The cell biology of aging: Immunological models. J Gerontol 1989; 44:b4.

Miller RA, Stutman O. Decline in aging ice, of the anti-TNP cytotoxic response attributable to loss of Cyt-2-, IL-2-producing helper cell function. Eur J Immunol 1981; 1:751.

Muscoplat CC, Rakich PM, Thoen CO, et al. Enhancement of lymphocyte blastogenic and delayed hypersensitivity skin responses by indomethacin. Infec Immunol 1978; 20:627.

Nadiger HA. Role of vitamin E in the aetilogy of phryoderma (follicular hyperkatosis) and it interrelationship with B-complex vitamins. Br J Nutr 1980; 44:211.

Ono K. Effects of large dose vitamin E supplementation on anemia in hemodialysis patients. Nephron 1985; 40:440.

Payan DG, Missirian-Bastian A, Goetzl EJ, Human T-lymphocyte subset specificity of the regulatory effects of leukotriene B_4. Proc Natl Acad Sci USA 1984; 81:3501.

Plaut M. The role of cyclic AMP in modulating cytotoxic T lymphocytes. J Immunol 1979; 123:692.

Pletsityi K, Nikushkin E, Askerov M, Ponomareva L. Inhibition of development of adjuvant arthritis in rats by vitamin E. Bull Exp Biol Med 1987; 103:49.

Rachmilewitz EA, Kornberg A, Acker M. Vitamin E deficiency due to increase consumption in β-thalassemia and Gaucher's disease. Ann NY Acad Sci. 1982; 393:336.

Recommended Dietary Allowances. Food and Nutrition Board, Commission on Life Sciences, National Research Council, National Academy Press, 1989, 99.

Reddy PG, Morrill JL, Frey RA. Vitamin E requirements of dairy calves. J Dairy Sci 1987a; 70:123.

Rola-Pleszcynski M, Borgeat P, Sirois P. Leukotriene B₄ induces human suppressor lymphocytes. Biochem Biophys Res Commun 1982; 198:1531.

Rola-Pleszczynski M. Immunoregulation by leukotrienes and other lipoxygenase metabolites. Immunol Today 1985; 6:302.

Rosenberg JS, Gilman SC, Feldman JD. Effect of aging on cell cooperation and lymphocyte responsiveness to cytokines. J Immunol 1983; 130:1754.

Rosenstein MM, Strauser HR. Macrophage induced T-cell mitogen suppression with age. J. Reticuloendoth Soc 1980; 27:159.

Saldanha RL, Cepeda EE, Poland RL. The effect of vitamin E prophylaxis on the incidence and severity of bronchopulmonary dysplasia. J Pediatr. 1982; 101:89.

Scott WA, Pawlowski NA, Andreach M, Cohen ZA. Resting macrophages produce distinct metabolites from exogenous arachidonic acid. J Exp Med 1982; 155:535.

Sinha S, Toner N, Davies J, Bogle S, Chiswick M. Vitamin E supplementation reduces frequency of periventricular hemorrhage in very preterm babies. Lancet 1987;1:446.

Siskind GW. Immunological aspects of aging: An overivew. In: Schimke RT, ed. Biological mechanisms in aging. USDA, NIH, 1980, 455.

Sokol RJ, Heubi JE, Iannaccone ST, Bove KE, Balistreri WF. Vitamin E deficiency with normal serum vitamin E concentrations in children with chronic cholestasis. N Engl J Med 1984; 310:1209.

Sokol RJ, Balistreri WF, Hoffnagle JH, Jones EA. Vitamin E deficiency in adults with chronic liver disease. Am J Clin Nutr 1985; 41:66.

Stead RJ, Muller DPR, Mathews S, Hodson ME, Batten JC. Effect of abnormal liver function on vitamin E status and supplementation in adults with cystic fibrosis. Gut 1986; 27:714.

Tanaka J, Fuyiwara H, Torisu M. Vitamin E and immune response enhancement of helper T cell activity by dietary supplementation of vitamin E in mice. Immunology 1979; 38:727.

Tanner AR, Bantock I, Hinks L, Lloyd B, Turner NR, Wright R. Depressed selenium and vitamin E levels in an alcoholic population: Possible relationship to hepatic injury through increased lipid peroxidation. Dig Dis Sci 1986; 31:1307.

Tengerdy P, Brown JC. Effect of vitamin E and A on humoral immunity and phagocytosis in E. coli infected chickens. Poultry Sci 1977; 56:957.

Tengerdy RP. Effect of vitamin E on immune responses. Basic Clin. Nutr 1980; 1:429.

Tetrud JW, Langston JW. The effect of Deprenyl (selegiline) on the natural history of Parkinson's disease. Science 1989; 245:519.

Thoman ML, Weigle WO. Cell-mediated immunity in aged mice: an underlying lesion in IL-2 synthesis. J Immunol 1982; 128:2351.

Thoman ML, Weigle WO. Reconstitution of in vivo cell-mediated lympholysis response in aged mice with interleukin 2. J Immunol 1985; 134:949.

Trickler D, Shklar G. Prevention by vitamin E of experimental oral carcinogenesis. J Natl Cancer Inst 1987; 78:1615.

Unanue ER. Cooperation between mononuclear phagocytes and lymphocytes in immunity. N Engl J Med 1980; 303:977.

Wald NJ, Thompson SG, et al. Serum vitamin E and subsequent risk of cancer. Br J Cancer 1987; 56:69.

Walford RL, Weindruch RH, Gottesman SRS, et al. The immunopathology of aging. In: Eisdorfer C, Starr B, Christo Falo VJ, eds. Ann Rev Gerontol Geriatr, Vol 2. New York: Springer, 1981, 1–48.

Wayne SJ, Rhyne RL, Gany PJ, Goodwin JS. Cell-mediated immunity as a predictor of morbidity and mortality. J Gerontol 1990; 45:M45.

Webb DR, Rogers TJ, Nowowiejski I. Endogenous prostaglandin synthesis and the control of lymphocyte function. Proc NY Acad Sci 1980; 332:260.

Witting LA, Lee L. Dietary levels of vitamin E and polyunsaturated fatty acids and plasma vitamin E. Am J Clin Nutr 1975; 28:571.

Wolf HRD, Seeger HW. Experimental and clinical results in shock lung treatment and vitamin E. Ann NY Acad Sci 1982; 393:392.

Yoshikawa T, Tanada H, Kondo M. Effect of vitamin E on adjuvant arthritis in rats. Biochem Med 1983; 29:227.

Ziemlanski S, Wartanowicz M, Klos A, Raczka A, Klos M. The effects of ascorbic acid and alpha-tocopherol supplementation on serum proteins and immunoglobulin concentrations in the elderly. Nutr. Int 1986; 2:1.

14

Vitamin A Deficiency: Role in Childhood Infection and Mortality

Jean H. Humphrey and Keith P. West, Jr.

Dana Center for Preventive Ophthalmology, Wilmer Eye Institute
Baltimore, Maryland

INTRODUCTION

Vitamin A (VA) deficiency is a long-standing nutritional problem in developing countries, recognized largely by its dramatic, specific, and readily observable ocular manifestation, xerophthalmia. This potentially blinding ocular disease has disappeared from developed countries but continues to plague large numbers of children throughout the world where VA deficiency is endemic (World Health Organization, 1982). Each year in Asia alone more than 5 million children develop xerophthalmia: 10% of these children suffer severe corneal disease of whom half go blind (Sommer et al., 1981).

Concurrent infection, protein-energy malnutrition (PEM), and an excessive risk of mortality attend severe VA deficiency and corneal xerophthalmia (McLaren et al., 1965; Venkataswamy et al., 1979; Menon and Vijayaraghavan, 1980; Sommer, 1982a). Until recently, milder stages of xerophthalmia (night blindness or conjunctival xerosis) were held to confer little health risk per se, serving more as markers for potentially blinding, severe xerophthalmia in the community (World Health Organization, 1976). However, it is increasingly clear that mild xerophthalmia represents a state of moderate to severe systemic VA deficiency with measurable risk in terms of child morbidity (Sommer et al., 1984; Milton et al., 1987) and mortality (Sommer et al., 1983).

A much larger proportion of children in regions of endemic deficiency have clinically normal eyes but marginal or deficient VA status by biochemical (Sommer et al., 1980; Sommer, 1982a; Flores et al, 1984) and functional (Natadisastra et al., 1987) indicators. These children comprise the "base" rather than the "tip" of the iceberg. Evidence from field supplementation trials indicates that subclinical (marginal) VA deficiency predisposes children to a higher risk of mortality (Sommer et al., 1986; Muhilal et al., 1988), presumably due to compromised host resistance leading to increased infection (West et al., 1989). This chapter addresses the evidence to date on the impact of VA deficiency and supplementation on childhood infection and survival.

MANIFESTATIONS OF VA DEFICIENCY

VA deficiency causes multiple abnormalities reflecting its systemic nature, both specific (e.g., ocular signs, low serum retinol levels) and nonspecific (widespread epithelial metaplasia, immunological dysfunction). Many of these changes may help explain causal pathways linking VA deficiency to increased susceptibility to infection.

Ocular Signs

Xerophthalmia encompasses two aspects of ocular disease that reflect different underlying functions of VA: (1) dark maladaptation or night blindness; and (2) metaplasia and keratinization of the conjunctival and corneal epithelium. These

Table 1 Classification of Xerophthalmia and Serum Vitamin A Levels with Minimum Prevalence Criteria for Public Health Significance

Classification	Minimum Prevalence (%)
Night blindness (XN)	1.0
Conjunctival xerosis (X1A)	—
Bitot's spots (X1B)	0.5
Corneal xerosis (X2)	
Corneal ulceration/keratomalacia $<\frac{1}{3}$ corneal surface (X3A)	0.01
Corneal ulceration/keratomalacia $\geq\frac{1}{3}$ corneal surface (X3B)	
Corneal scar (XS)	0.05
Serum vitamin A	
<0.35 μmol/liter (deficient)	5.0
0.35–0.69 μmol/liter (marginal)	
≥0.70 μmol/liter (adequate)	

Source: Adapted from WHO, 1980 revision.

conditions have been classified by the World Health Organization (WHO) by stages of severity, with minimum prevalences that represent public health importance (Table 1).

In VA deficiency, the level of rhodopsin, the visual pigment in the rods of the eye, declines, resulting in night blindness (XN). This function in the visual cycle has been elucidated at the molecular level (Wald, 1955). Night blindness can be diagnosed by dark adaptometry (Russell et al., 1973) but more easily in children by a positive history elicited from a mother (Sommer et al., 1980).

Conjunctival xerosis (reviewed in Wittpenn and Sommer, 1986) presents as a granular, dry patch initially temporal to the limbus, often with progression to the nasal quadrant. These lesions can be covered with clearly visible accumulations of cellular debris and saprophytic bacteria forming Bitot's spots (X1B) (Fig. 1). Night blindness and uncomplicated conjunctival xerophthalmia rarely progress to blindness. However, these stages of "mild" xerophthalmia appear to reflect moderate to severe systemic VA depletion with associated risk of infectious disease (see below).

Corneal involvement initially appears as superficial punctate keratopathy, progressing to xerosis (X2) which can be viewed with a hand light on examination.

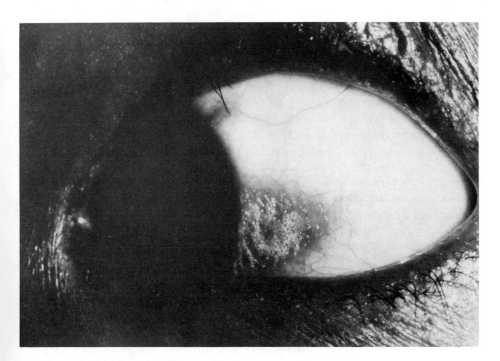

Figure 1   Bitot's spot (X1B).

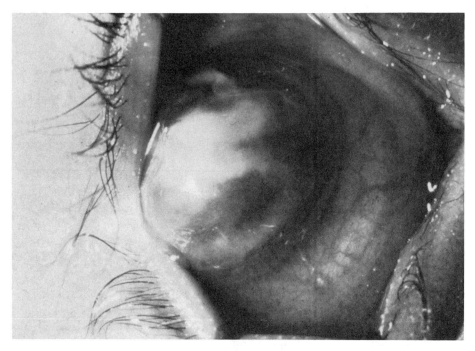

Figure 2 Keratomalacia (X3B).

Corneal ulceration (X3A or X3B depending on severity) may appear as a well-demarcated, "punched-out" defect (Sommer, 1982a,b) that may be shallow or be sufficiently deep to perforate the stroma. A full-thickness ulcer can cause loss of ocular contents and, frequently, prolapse of the iris (forming a descemetocele). The most severe stage, keratomalacia (X3B), involves necrosis of at least one-third of the corneal surface (Fig. 2), usually leaving the eye irreversibly blind. Most corneal xerophthalmia is preceded by infectious illness (e.g., measles, diarrhea, etc.) and moderate to severe PEM (Sommer, 1982a).

Biochemical Alterations

Serum retinol levels are homeostatically controlled, remaining within normal limits over a wide range of hepatic concentrations (Olson, 1986). Only when hepatic stores are nearly depleted do serum VA concentrations fall dramatically. Serum retinol levels <0.35 μmol/liter (<10 μg/dl) may be considered to be "deficient," 0.35–0.69 μmol/liter to be "marginal," and ≥0.70 μmol/liter as "adequate" for classification purposes. Serum determinations are useful for assessing VA status in a population. Vitamin A deficiency is considered an endemic problem in communities where at least 5% of children have ''deficient'' levels (Table 1).

Hematological status is altered in vitamim A deficiency (Hodges, et al., 1978; Lloyd-Puryear et al, 1989). The resulting anemia may respond to vitamin A but not iron (Hodges et al., 1978), partially to vitamin A (Muhilal et al., 1988), or best to both vitamin A and iron (Mejia and Chew, 1988). These findings suggest that hematopoiesis is dependent on adequate nutriture of both micronutrients, though the role of vitamin A has not been fully elucidated. Vitamin A deficiency is associated with depressed iron mobilization from stores, resulting in increased liver ferritin concentrations (Wolbach and Howe, 1925; Mejia et al., 1979) decreased plasma iron levels (Hodges et al., 1978), and decreased incorporation of iron into hemoglobin (Mejia et al., 1979).

Epithelial Changes

VA appears to exert a regulatory effect on cellular growth and differentiation, possibly through modified gene expression at the nuclear level (reviewed by Zile and Cullum, 1983) or through its role in glycoprotein synthesis (DeLuca, 1977). In VA deficiency, cell replication is depressed and differentiated cells undergo morphological changes resulting in loss of ciliae and disrupted microvilli on mucosal surfaces (Wong and Buck, 1971; Biesalski et al., 1986). In the respiratory tract, basal cells differentiate abnormally into stratified squamous epithelium (McDowell et al., 1984). VA-deficient animals exhibit keratinizing metaplasia of epithelia of the trachea (Wolbach and Howe, 1925; Wong and Buck, 1971; DeLuca et al., 1972; McDowell et al., 1984; Strum et al., 1985; Biesalski et al., 1986), salivary gland (Wolbach and Howe, 1925), vagina (Sietsema and DeLuca, 1982), and genitourinary tracts (Wolbach and Howe, 1925), often prior to changes on the ocular surface. Intestinal mucosal cell renewal (Zile et al., 1977) and goblet cell differentiation (Rojanapo et al., 1980 are disturbed, though frank keratinization does not appear to occur in animals (Wolbach and Howe, 1925).

Studies or nonocular epithelial changes in VA deficiency in children are sparse. Limited data suggest that diffuse metaplasia occurs late in deficiency. An early autopsy study of 13 infants, six of whom had keratomalacia and all of whom were severely malnourished, showed pervasive keratinizing metaplasia throughout the respiratory, gastrointestinal, and genitourinary tracts (Blackfan and Wolbach, 1933). Direct evidence of epithelial histopathology in early (prexerophthalmic) VA deficiency in children has been demonstrated only on the ocular surface where loss of goblet cells and disruption of the conjunctival epithelium occur (Natadisastra et al., 1987). The degree to which these lesions develop concurrently in the luminal tracts and break down the ''epithelial barrier'' (and the implications for infection) is presently not known.

Immunological Dysfunction

VA status appears to alter the immune response to infection although animal and, presently sparse, human data are not fully concordant on the magnitude or mechanisms involved in this effect. Specific components of host resistance that may be regulated by VA have been reviewed by several authors (Wolf, 1980; Dennert, 1984; Vyas and Chandra, 1984; Nauss, 1986; Chew, 1987; West et al., 1989).

Cell-Mediated Immunity

Depressed mitogen-induced blast transformation of splenocytes is consistently observed in VA deficient animals (Nauss et al., 1979; Chandra and Au, 1981; Mark et al., 1983; Nauss and Newberne, 1985). Superimposed (viral) infection does not alter this differential response (Nauss and Newberne, 1985). Redistribution of competent lymphocyte subsets to regional lymph nodes may underlie this reduced response (Mark et al., 1983) possibly due to changes in mitogen recognition by T cells in the VA-deficient state. VA repletion quickly returns the splenocyte response to normal (Nauss et al., 1979). Conversely, thymic lymphocyte blast transformation appears to be unaffected by VA deficiency (Nauss et al., 1979; Chandra and Au, 1981). Indian investigators have reported reduced T-cell numbers in mildly VA-deficient children (serum VA below 0.30 μmol/liter), but normal in vitro mitogenic stimulation of T cells (Bhaskaram et al., 1987–88).

Animals exhibit depressed delayed-type hypersensitivity (DTH) early in deficiency before anorexia and growth faltering occur (Smith et al., 1987). However, data on VA-induced changes in DTH in children are inconclusive: an early study in India reported a depressed DTH response among VA-deficient children (Jayalakshmi and Gopalan, 1958) while in Bangladesh VA supplementation had no effect on the DTH reaction to various skin test antigens (Brown et al., 1980).

T-helper cells from VA-deficient animals appear less able to support the humoral arm of immunity. Following VA depletion, T-cell-dependent serum immunoglobulin (Ig) G levels fall earlier and more dramatically than do levels of IgM (Smith and Hayes, 1987). Depressed antigen-specific IgG secretion in VA deficiency has been attributed to an inability of T-helper cells to stimulate activated B cells for clonal expansion and class switching (Carman et al., 1989).

Humoral Immunity

Depressed antibody responses observed in VA-deficient animals following antigenic challenge (Pruzansky and Axelrod, 1955; Harmon et al., 1963; Brown et al., 1980; Sirisinha et al., 1980; Chandra and Au, 1981; Smith and Hayes, 1987; Pasatiempo et al., 1989) may be mediated, in part, by altered T-cell-dependent activation (Carman et al., 1989).

However, T-cell-independent initiation of antibody (Ab) production may also be affected by VA deficiency. The splenic antibody response to the capsular polysaccharide of *Streptococcus pneumoniae*, type III (SSS-III), is restricted primarily to the IgM class. VA deficiency markedly reduced the Ab response to SSS-III challenge in rats (Pasatiempo et al., 1989). Retinol repletion near the time of SSS-III inoculation readily restored the Ab response to normal. Streptococcal infection is known to cause pneumonia, otitis media, and meningitis in infants and children (Hoeprich, 1983).

Few data exist regarding whether VA supplementation enhances humoral immunity in children. In Bangladesh (Brown et al., 1980), children randomized to receive orally 60,000 μg retinol equivalents (RE) VA or placebo at the time of tetanus toxoid immunization showed no differences in antitetanus toxoid antibody responses. A second, small (nonrandomized) trial among severely VA-deficient Bangladeshi children reported low initial serum IgG and IgA levels compared to controls which returned to normal following administration of 30,000–60,000 μg RE of VA by different routes (Faruque et al., 1984). More work is needed to determine the effect vitamin A may have on vaccine efficacy.

Nonspecific Immunity

Vitamin A appears to influence several innate host defense mechanisms. These include lymphocyte trapping and localization in the periphery (McDermott et al., 1982; Takagi and Nakano, 1983), natural killer cell function (Nauss and Newberne, 1985), leukocyte lysozyme activity (Mohanram et al., 1974), and phagocytosis (Rhodes and Oliver, 1980; Ongsakul et al., 1985). Recently, macrophage function was found to be normal in mildly VA-deficient children, although supplementation of these same children with VA (30,000 μg RE) had a nonspecific immunopotentiating effect (enhanced interleukin 1 production) (Bhaskaram et al., 1989).

VA DEFICIENCY AND INFECTIOUS DISEASE

Acute respiratory infection (ARI) (Bulla and Hitze, 1978) and diarrheal diseases (Snyder and Merson, 1982) are the leading causes of preschool childhood mortality in developing countries, jointly accounting for at least 5 million childhood deaths each year (Gwatkin, 1980). The frequent coexistence of both VA deficiency and infectious diseases in populations with high child mortality has prompted study of their causal association.

Respiratory Infection

There is growing epidemiological evidence linking VA deficiency to risk of childhood respiratory infection. Cross-sectional studies routinely report an association between mild xerophthalmia (Tielsch et al., 1986; De Sole et al., 1987) or biochemical VA deficiency (Bloem et al., 1990) and respiratory infection (e.g., history of cough with fever). However, temporality of association cannot be ascertained in such studies.

A cohort study of 3500 Indonesian preschool children followed up quarterly over 18 months found mildly xerophthalmic (XN or X1B) children to have a two-fold higher risk (age- and nutritional status-adjusted) of contracting clinically diagnosed, lower respiratory infection (Sommer et al., 1984). A relative risk of 2 for lower tract infection associated with mild xerophthalmia was also reported from an 18-month longitudinal study in India ($n = 1500$) that employed weekly morbidity reporting (Milton et al., 1987). In a Thai community-based study of 143 children an inverse dose-response relationship was observed between baseline serum retinol level and incidence of respiratory disease (by history). Children whose baseline serum level was below 0.35 μmol/liter were 3.6 times more likely to have reported a respiratory infection during the subsequent 2 months than children with a serum retinol level >0.70 μmol/liter (Bloem et al., 1990). The opposing pathway appears to be operative as well: Indonesian children with lower respiratory infection were twice as likely to develop xerophthalmia over cumulative 3-month periods than disease-free children (Sommer et al., 1987). However, these children may have also been subclinically VA-deficient prior to onset of respiratory infection.

Not all prospective studies have shown a positive relationship between VA deficiency and respiratory infection. In West Bengal (Sinha and Bang, 1976), 310 preschoolers were examined monthly for xerophthalmia and morbidity histories were elicited. No association was found between mild xerophthalmia and upper respiratory infection. However, an exceedingly high prevalence of upper airway infection throughout the year ($\sim$70%) may have overwhelmed any real association.

While the balance of data suggest that VA deficiency predisposes children to respiratory infection, agent-specific effects and mechanisms of action remain unknown. *Hemophilus influenza* and *Streptococcus pneumoniae* are among the most frequently reported bacterial pathogens in children with severe pneumonia (Shann et al., 1984). It is of interest that VA deficiency compromises the specific humoral response to the capsular polysaccharide of *S. pneumoniae* (noted above, Pasatiempo et al., 1989). VA status may also influence risk of ARI through its regulatory role in the synthesis of glycoproteins (Wolf, 1980), which are integral to maintaining epithelial cell surface membranes and mucus production. VA deficiency results in depressed mucus production and a loss of ciliae in the respiratory tract (Wong and Buck, 1971). This may compromise escalation, prolong contact, increase adherence, and promote colonization (Niederman et al., 1983) and tissue invasion by pathogens. Nasal washings from apparently healthy and xerophthalmic (with XN or X1B) Indian children were inoculated in vitro with *Klebsiella pneumoniae* (Chandra, 1988). Bacterial adherence to harvested epithelial cells increased directly with severity of xerophthalmia, indicating that VA deficiency may permit increased bacterial colonization. In turn, this may lead more readily to mucosal penetration and systemic infection.

Diarrhea

Preschool children in developing countries experience an average of three to four episodes of diarrhea each year (Black et al., 1982; Sepulveda et al., 1988; El Samani et al., 1988), frequently totaling 40–50 days (Black et al., 1982). Evidence relating VA deficiency to risk of diarrhea was recently reviewed (Feachem, 1987).

In Indonesia mildly xerophthalmic children (XN or X1B) had a three-fold higher risk of incident diarrhea between quarterly examinations relative to non-xerophthalmic children (Sommer et al., 1984). This association remained after stratification by age and nutritional status. As with respiratory infection, children with a recent history of diarrhea were also twice as likely to later develop xerophthalmia compared to those without diarrhea, providing further evidence of a "vicious cycle" (Sommer et al., 1987).

A case control study in Nepal ($n = 50$ matched pairs) reported that children with Bitot's spots (X1B) were 30 times more likely to have had diarrhea during the previous 4 weeks than contols matched on age, sex, season, and village of residence (Brilliant et al., 1985). However, a prospective study in India found no relationship between preexisting xerophthalmia and incidence of diarrhea (Milton et al., 1987). In Thailand, there was also no relationship between serum retinol level and subsequent risk of diarrhea over a 3-month period (Bloem et al., 1990).

Three studies in Bangladesh suggest that VA deficiency may be a stronger risk factor for *persistent* (lasting more than 2–3 weeks) rather than acute diarrhea. (1) In a series of 4155 children presenting with diarrhea to a clinical research center, night blindness and conjunctival xerosis were more prevalent among cases of persistent (5 and 13%, respectively) than acute (<1 and 5%, respectively) diarrhea (Shahid et al., 1988). (2) A clinic-based study of nearly 3000 children presenting with diarrhea found a positive history of night blindness to be associated with prolonged diarrhea (>7 days, odds ratio = 4.7) and dysentery (odds ratio = 2.6) compared to patients without XN (Stoll et al., 1985). Night-blind children were also more likely to have had *Shigella* isolated from their stool (odds ratios = 1.65), the pathogen most frequently associated with persistent diarrhea in Bangladesh (Black et al., 1982). (3) Finally, a case control study ($n = 46$ pairs) reported a fourfold higher risk of mild xerophthalmia associated with a previous history of protracted diarrhea (Stanton et al., 1986). Lesions in the gut that may contribute to VA deficiency-induced risk of diarrhea are likely to involve mucosal and local immunological dysfunction. Although the intestinal epithelium does not keratinize in VA deficiency (Wolbach and Howe, 1925), cell kinetics are disturbed causing delays in intestinal cell migration from the crypts (Zile et al.,

1976) and mucosal goblet cell losses (Rojanapo et al., 1980) which may lengthen and promote pathogen exposure. Gut-associated lymphoid tissue appears compromised in mounting a local immune response in vitamin A–deficient animals. A reduction in cellularity of Peyer's patches (Majumder et al., 1987) and impaired localization of normal lymphocytes to mesenteric lymph nodes (Craig and Cebra, 1971) have been observed.

VA DEFICIENCY AND CHILDHOOD MORTALITY

Given the apparent, multiplicative role of VA in health and the risks of infection during deficiency, it may be expected that VA deficiency plays a role in mortality of young children. Epidemiological observations suggest that this is true and that it follows a dose-response relationship.

Severe VA Deficiency (Corneal Xerophthalmia)

Potentially blinding corneal xerophthalmia is both an ophthalmic and a medical emergency, with case fatality rates approaching 80–100% if untreated (Stephenson, 1910; Stranski, 1924). These rates probably approximate the risk of keratomalacic children dying in many rural underserved areas of the world. Even with proper treatment, the mortality of severe xerophthalmia (X3A, X3B) is excessive: 29% among hospitalized Tanzanian children (Foster and Sommer, 1987) and 12.5% among treated and recovered Indonesian children within 14 months of discharge from the hospital (Sommer 1982a).

Moderate VA Deficiency (Mild Xerophthalmia)

During the past decade mild xerophthalmia, once thought to be relatively benign, has been linked to an increased risk of child mortality. A prospective study of Indonesian preschoolers found a fourfold higher risk of mortality among children with XN and X1B (93.2 per 1000 per year) vs. their nonxerophthalmic peers (23.2 per 1000 per year) (Sommer et al., 1983). At each preschool age mortality rose directly with the severity of VA deficiency, reflected by the clinical stages of xerophthalmia [XN < X1B < (XN + X1B)]. The association was consistent across baseline weight for height strata, with mild xerophthalmia appearing to exert a stronger effect on mortality than wasting (<90% of Harvard median) Sommer et al., 1983). Cause-specific mortality data were not available. Infections were the most likely causes of death given that (1) respiratory and diarrheal illnesses are the two most common causes of all childhood mortality in developing countries (Gwatkin, 1980), and (2) in this study population, surviving xerophthalmic children were at higher risk of these illnesses compared to normal controls (Sommer et al., 1984). It was estimated that in Indonesia preschool child mortality could be reduced 16% solely by preventing xerophthalmia in the community (Sommer et al., 1983).

Experimental animal data have long implicated VA deficiency as an underlying cause of death. VA-depleted animals often develop infections and die before developing xerophthalmic lesions (Stephenson and Clark, 1920). Raised under germ-free conditions, VA-deficient animals develop classic keratinizing lesions but survive much longer than their equally deficient litter mates reared in a conventional environment (Bieri et al., 1969). Survival of VA-deficient rats in the laboratory can be measurably extended by broad-spectrum antibiotic treatment (Anzano et al., 1979).

VA SUPPLEMENTATION AND CHILD HEALTH

If VA deficiency causally increases risk of infectious disease, then supplementation with VA should improve resistance to infection observed by reduced incidence, duration, or other aspects of severity. Furthermore, such an impact on child health should influence child survival where mortality from infection is high.

VA Supplementation and Morbidity

Developing Countries

Definitive studies of the efficacy of VA in reducing infection have not been carried out in developing countries, although several are currently underway. One randomized clinical trial among 166 children in northeastern Thailand (Bloem et al., 1990) reported 34% fewer episodes of respiratory infection (by history) during the 2 months following receipt of 60,000 μg RE VA. Between 2 and 4 months after intervention, 43% fewer supplemented children reported respiratory infections compared to controls (13% vs. 23.4%, respectively). These differences were not statistically significant. No consistent effect on diarrhea was observed.

Developed Countries

The role of VA supplementation in reducing morbidity in *developed* countries has been investigated in two high-risk groups: very-low-birthweight (VLBW) premature infants and preschool children prone to respiratory infection.

Among VLBW infants, bronchopulmonary dysplasia (Northway et al., 1967) is an important cause of death. Premature infants with BPD tend to have suboptimal VA status (Shenai et al., 1985), attributed to their being deprived of transplacental retinol during the third trimester of pregnancy (Bhatia and Ziegler, 1983). Randomly assigned intramuscular injection of VA (600 μg RE) vs. saline solution to 40 VLBW newborns every other day for the first month of life resulted in elevated plasma retinol levels, a 50% reduction in the incidence of BPD, and a

60% reduction in airway infection (Shenai et al., 1987). Supplemental VA may have promoted normal repair of injured respiratory epithelium, preventing the classic tracheobronchitis and squamous epithelium of BPD.

The role of VA supplementation in reducing susceptibility to infection was studied in Australian children with apparently normal VA status (serum retinol ~45 µg/dl) but prone to respiratory infection (Pinnock et al., 1986). Children randomly assigned to receive an oral dose of 1160 µg RE VA vs. placebo three times per week over an 11-month period had 19% fewer episodes of respiratory symptoms, the entire effect observed in children with a history of lower respiratory infection. However, a second double-masked, randomized trial (Pinnock et al., 1988) in children with a history of respiratory syncytial virus–positive bronchiolitis in infancy (a risk factor for respiratory disease later in life) showed no discernible effect on incidence or duration of respiratory infection from a weekly oral dose of 4.2 mg RE VA (equivalent to 450 µg/day) over 12 months. Thus, low-level VA supplementation plays little if any, role in altering the incidence or course of infection in apparently well-nourished children in developed countries.

The recent Nationwide Continuing Survey of Food Intakes by Individuals (CSFII) in the United States suggests that infants and young children from low-income households may not have adequate vitamin A intake. Among low-income women aged 19–34, one-third consume less than 50% and half less than 70% of their RDA for vitamin A. The impact this low dietary intake may have on the vitamin A status of pregnant and lactating women, fetal stores and breast milk concentrations of vitamin A, vitamin A status of their infant, and any impact on morbidity and mortality have not been studied in these low-income populations.

Impact on Reduced Mortality

Developing Countries

While direct studies of VA supplementation on childhood morbidity are lacking, two community trials, both in Indonesia, investigated the impact of VA supplementation on child mortality in areas where VA deficiency is endemic. A randomized, controlled trial in 450 villages with more than 25,000 preschool children reported that semiannual delivery of 200,000 IU VA (60,000 µg RE, capsular form) by village volunteers reduced mortality by 34% (Sommer et al., 1986). Cumulative mortality in supplemented and control villages diverged following each capsule distribution (approximately 2 and 8 months following baseline examination) (Fig. 3). Although nearly 80% of all program children received a VA capsule every 6 months, further analysis suggested that an even greater impact may have been possible with more complete coverage (Tarwotjo et al., 1987). However, the observed effect was twice the 16% reduction that had been predicted by preventing xerophthalmia alone in the community (Sommer et al., 1983), suggesting that subclinical VA deficiency influenced the risk of mortality.

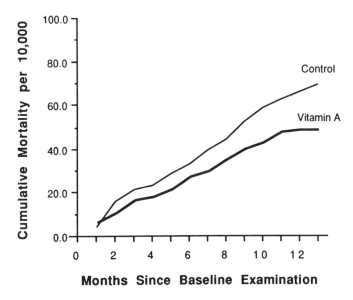

Figure 3 Cumulative 12-month mortality rates for children 1–5 years of age, sexes combined, in vitamin A supplement and control villages, Aceh Province, Indonesia. (Adapted from Sommer et al., 1986; used with permission from West et al., 1989.)

The second trial intervened not with periodic large oral doses but with VA-fortified monosodium glutamate (MSG-A) routinely sold in the market (Muhilal et al., 1988). The reduction in mortality among preschool-aged children in villages with MSG-A approximated that in the large-dose VA trial: 31%. Cumulative mortality curves diverged in a linear fashion throughout the year of follow-up (Fig. 4). MSG fortification also appeared effective in lowering xerophthalmia rates, increasing serum and breast milk retinol levels, increasing hemoglobin concentration, and accelerating linear growth.

These two field trials were carried out in ethnically distinct populations 1200 miles apart where the baseline childhood mortality rates and modes of VA intervention were different. Neither study reliably ascertained causes of death although presumably enhanced survival was mediated through reduced infection. Their results suggest that 30% of the 600,000 rural, preschool child deaths in Indonesia each year could be averted by improved VA nutriture. These studies have stimulated vigorous debate (de L. Costello, 1986; Gray, 1986; Martinez et al., 1986; Sommer and West, 1986) indicating the need for further evidence of the impact of VA on mortality (where risk factors vary from Indonesia) before general acceptance can be expected and public health recommendations made

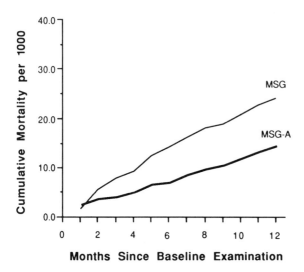

Figure 4 Cumulative 12-month mortality rates for children 1–5 years of age, sexes combined, in villages receiving commercially marketed vitamin A-fortified (MSG-A) and unfortified (MSG) monosodium glutamate, West Java, Indonesia. (Adapted from Muhilal et al., 1988; used with permission from West et al., 1989.)

about the benefits of community-based VA supplementation in child health and survival.

An additional investigation focused on the impact of large-dose VA supplementation on measles mortality. In developing countries measles is still a widespread, devastating childhood illness with case fatality reaching 15% (Koblinsky, 1982). Measles causes a marked deterioration in both protein-energy and vitamin A status (Sanford-Smith and Whittle, 1973; Reddy et al., 1986). The interaction of measles with vitamin A status can be particularly tragic: one-half or more of children presenting with active corneal xerophthalmia report a recent episode of measles (McLaren et al., 1965; Sommer, 1982; Foster and Sommer, 1987). A randomized, clinical trial in Tanzania investigated the impact of VA supplementation on reducing in-hospital mortality due to severe measles among 180 children (Barclay et al., 1987). Half of the children were ranJomly allocated to receive VA (60,000 μg RE, orally) on two successive days while control children received standard care. Mortality was 50% lower in the treated compared to the control group, the entire effect being observed in children below 2 years of age. These studies have lead UNICEF and the World Health Organization to recommend large-dose VA supplementation (60,000 μg RE) for children with measles where case fatality rates exceed 1% or where VA deficiency is endemic (Editorial, 1987).

Developed Countries

A similar trial carried out in London (Ellison, 1932) 55 years before the Tanzania trial showed remarkably consistent results. Six hundred children hospitalized for measles were allocated to receive approximately 6000 μg RE (300 Carr–Price units) plus 2000 IU vitamin D daily or to serve as controls. Mortality was 50% lower in the supplemented group, (3.7 vs. 8.7). No other studies measuring the impact of VA supplementation on reduced mortality among apparently well-nourished, ill, or low-income children have been carried out in developed countries.

INDICATIONS FOR DOSING CHILDREN WITH VA

Indications

Oral VA supplementation with 200,000 IU (60,000 μg RE) is currently recommended for the treatment of xerophthalmia and prevention of VA deficiency in endemic areas (Sommer, 1982b).

Treatment

Any stage of xerophthalmia should be treated with 60,000 μg RE oral VA immediately upon diagnosis, the following day, and again approximately 2 weeks later. For children under 1 year the dose is halved (30,000 μg RE). Children with measles living in areas of endemic VA deficiency or where measles case fatality exceed 1% should receive the full treatment regimen (World Health Organization, 1988) whenever possible.

In addition, children with high-risk conditions such as severe PEM, frequent diarrhea, or lower respiratory infection should be given one large dose of VA (Sommer, 1982b; World Health Organization, 1988). Children undergoing nutritional rehabilitation from PEM should receive supplemental VA to support rapid catch-up growth which may otherwise deplete meager liver stores, cause a drop in serum levels, and precipitate xerophthalmia (Gopalan et al., 1960).

Prophylaxis

In areas where VA deficiency constitutes a problem of public health significance (Table 1), children 12 months of age or older may be prophylactically dosed with 60,000 μg RE vitamin A every 3–6 months. Half this dosage is administered to infants 6–11 months of age. Younger infants may be given 15,000 μg RE once prior to reaching 6 months of age. Mothers of newborns may be given a single, large dose of VA at delivery or within 2 months postpartum to increase breast milk levels of VA, providing extra protection to the breast-fed infant (World Health Organization, 1988). Precautions concerning the administration of large doses of VA to women in the childbearing years have been discussed elsewhere (Underwood, 1986).

Refugee populations and victims of famine are at high risk of both VA deficiency and receiving inadequate VA in their rations. Refugee children below 5 years of age, and other age groups affected by xerophthalmia, should be routinely supplemented with VA until sufficiency of dietary VA has been established (Nieburg et al., 1988).

SAFETY

Severe, acute toxicity after vitamin A supplementation follows abusively high intakes over short periods of time (Bauernfeind, 1980; Bendich and Langseth, 1989). Published accounts of side effects in children following a single ingestion of 165,000–330,000 IU of vitamin A report either no adverse reactions or self-limited side effects (e.g., headache, nausea, vomiting) in 0.7–25% of recipient children, depending on the size of the dose (reviewed in West and Sommer, 1985). A randomized, double-masked, field trial among ~3000 preschool children in the Philippines recently found 6.6 and 1.4% incidence of nausea or vomiting attributable to oral receipt of 60,000 and 30,000 µg RE VA, respectively (Florentino, 1990). Side effects were limited to a 24-hr duration. Further studies are needed to assess the relative efficacy of the 30,000 µg RE dosage to prevent VA deficiency with a view toward lowering the recommendation in the future.

There appears to be minimal risk of toxicity following ingestion of a single dose of 30,000–60,000 µg RE VA for preschool children (1–5 years of age). The high benefit-risk ratio of supplementation was recently reinforced by the World Health Organization (1988). However, measures should always be taken to guard against potential abuse in order to further minimize the risk of acute toxicity. In developing countries reported side effects to date are of concern primarily in terms of affecting community compliance in supplementation programs.

In developed countries, about 200 cases of hypervitaminosis A are reported annually (Bendich and Langseth, 1989), usually due to excessive doses of vitamin A supplements. Most symptoms are usually reversible within days after cessation of dosing.

CONCLUSION

Epidemiological studies indicate that VA deficiency is a risk factor for early childhood respiratory infection, diarrhea, and mortality in developing countries. Laboratory experiments have long pointed to a VA-infection interaction, citing both specific and nonspecific mechanisms of host resistance that are altered and believed to underlie a known high mortality in the VA-deficient state.

VA supplementation (either by periodic large doses or fortification) has been shown to reduce preschool child mortality by approximately one-third. This impact is likely mediated through altered resistance to infection, although direct evidence in human populations is still lacking. Large field trials are presently underway to further investigate the role of VA supplementation in improving child health and survival under different cultural and environmental conditions.

ACKNOWLEDGMENTS

The authors thank Drs. Alan Scott and Alfred Sommer for their helpful comments during preparation of this manuscript, and Ms. Diane Carter for preparing its many drafts.

This chapter was prepared under Cooperative Agreement No. DAN-0045 between the Dana Center for Preventive Ophthalmology of the Wilmer Institute, The Johns Hopkins University; and the Office of Nutrition, Bureau of Science and Technology, U.S. Agency for International Development (USAID), Washington, D.C. Support was also received from Task Force Sight and Life (Roche), Basel, Switzerland and from grant S10-RR-04060 from the National Institutes of Health.

REFERENCES

Anzano MA, Lamb AJ, Olson JA. Growth, appetite, sequence of pathological signs and survival following the induction of rapid, synchronous vitamin A deficiency in the rat. J Nutr 1979; 109:1419–1431.

Barclay AJG, Foster A, Sommer A. Vitamin A supplements and mortality related to measles: A randomized clinical trial. Br Med J 1987; 294:294–296.

Bauernfeind JC. The safe use of vitamin A. A report of the International Vitamin A Consultative Group (IVACG). Washington, DC: Nutrition Foundation, 1980.

Bendich A, Langseth L. Safety of vitamin A. Am J Clin Nutr 1989; 49:358–371.

Bhaskaram P, Jyothi SA, Rao KV. Immune status of children with mild vitamin A deficiency. Annual report of the National Institute of Nutrition, Indian Council for Medical Research, Hyderabad, India, 1987–88.

Bhaskaram P, Sharada K, Sivakumar B, Rao KV, Nair M. Effect of iron and vitamin A deficiencies on macrophage function in children. Nutr Res 1989; 9:35–45.

Bhatia J, Ziegler EE. Retinol-binding protein and prealbumin in cord blood of term and preterm infants. Early Hum Dev 1983; 8:129–133.

Bieri JG, McDaniel EG, Rogers WE, Jr. Survival of germfree rats without vitamin A. Science 1969; 163:574–575.

Biesalski HK, Stofft E, Wellner U, Niederauer U, Bassler KH. Vitamin A and ciliated cells. I. Respiratory epithelia. Zeithschrift fur Ernahrungswissenschaft 1986; 25:114–121.

Black RE, Brown KH, Becker S, Abdul Alim ARM, Huq I. Longitudinal studies of infectious diseases and physical growth of children in rural Bangladesh. II. Incidence of diarrhea and association with known pathogens. Am J Epidemiol 1982; 115:315–323.

Blackfan KD, Wolbach SB. Vitamin A deficiency in infants: A clinical and pathological study. J Pediatr 1933; 3:679–706.

Bloem MW, Wedel M, Egger RJ, Speek AJ, Schrijver J, Saowakontha S, Schreurs WHP. Mild vitamin A deficiency and risk of respiratory infection and diarrhea in preschool and school children in Northeast Thailand. Am J Epidemiol 1990; 131:332–339.

Brilliant LB, Pokhrel RP, Grasset NC, Lepkowski JM, Kolstad A, Hawks W, Pararajasegaram R, Brilliant GE, Gilbert S, Shrestha SR, Kuo J. Epidemiology of blindness in Nepal. Bull WHO 1985; 63:375–386.

Brown KH, Rajan MM, Chakraborty J, Aziz KMA. Failure of a large dose of vitamin A to enhance the antibody response to tetanus toxoid in children. Am J Clin Nutr 1980; 33:212–217.

Bulla A, Hitze KL. Acute respiratory infections: A review. Bull WHO 1978; 56:481–498.

Carman, JA, Smith SA, Hayes CE. Characterization of a helper T lymphocyte defect in vitamin A–deficient mice. J Immunol 1989; 142:388–393.

Chandra RK. Increased bacterial binding to respiratory epithelial cells in vitamin A deficiency. Br Med J 1988; 297:834–835.

Chandra RK, Au B. Single nutrient deficiency and cell mediated immune responses III. Nutr Res 1981; 1:181–185.

Chew BP. Vitamin A and beta-carotene on host defence. J Dairy Sci 1987; 70:2732–2743.

Craig SW, Cebra JJ. Peyer's patches: an enriched source of precursor's for IgA-producing immunocytes in the rabbit. J Exp Med 1971; 134:188–200.

de L Costello AM. Vitamin A supplementation and childhood mortality (letter). Lancet 1986; 2:161.

De Luca L, Maestri N, Bonanni F, Nelson D. Maintenance of epithelial cell differentiation: The mode of action of vitamin A. Cancer 1972; 30:1326–1331.

DeLuca LM. The direct involvement of vitamin A in glycosyl transfer reactions of mammalian membranes. Vitamins and Hormones. New York: Academic Press, Vol. 35, 1977, 1–57.

Dennert G. Retinoids and the immune system: Immunostimulation by vitamin A. In: Sporn MB, ed. The retinoids. Orlando: Academic Press, Vol. 2, 1984, 373–390.

De Sole G, Belay Y, Zegeye B. Vitamin A deficiency in Southern Ethiopia. Am J Clin Nutr 1987; 45:780–784.

Editorial. Vitamin A for measles. Lancet 1987; 1:1067–1068.

Ellison JB. Intensive vitamin A therapy in measles. Br Med J 1932; 2:708–711.

El Samani EFZ, Willett WC, Ware JH. Association of malnutrition and diarrhea in children aged under five years. Am J Epidemiol 1988; 128:93–105.

Faruque SM, Kabir Y, Bashar SAM. Effect of vitamin A supplementation on the serum levels of some immunoglobulins in vitamin A deficient children. Paediatrica Indonesia 1984; 24:249–253.

Feachem RG. Vitamin A deficiency and diarrhoea: A review of the interrelationships and their implications for the control of xerophthalmia and diarrhoea. Trop Dis Bull 1987; 84:R1–R16.

Florentino RF, Tanchoco CC, Ramos AC, Mendoza TS, Natividad ED, Tangco JB,

Sommer A. Tolerance of preschoolers to two dosage strengths of vitamin A preparation. Am J Clin Nutr 1990; 52:694–700.

Flores H, Campos F, Araujo CRC, Underwood BA. Assessment of marginal vitamin A deficiency in Brazilian children using the relative dose response procedure. Am J Clin Nutr 1984; 40:1281–1289.

Foster A, Sommer A. Corneal ulceration, measles, and childhood blindness in Tanzania. 1986; Br J Ophthalmol 71:331–343.

Gopalan C, Venkatachalam PS, Bhavani B. Studies of vitamin A deficiency in children. Am J Clin Nutr 1960; 8:833–840.

Gray RH. Vitamin A supplementation and childhood mortality (letter). Lancet 1986; 2:161–162.

Gwatkin DR. How many die? A set of demographic estimates of the annual number of infant and child deaths in the world. Am J Publ Health 1980; 70:1286–1289.

Harmon BG, Miller ER, Hoefer JA, Ullrey DE, Luecke RW. Relationship of specific nutrient deficiencies to antibody production in swine. J Nutr 1963; 79:263–268.

Hodges RE, Sauberlich HE, Canham JE, Wallace DL, Rucker RB, Mejia LA. Hematologic studies in vitamin A deficiency. Am J Clin Nutr 1978; 31:876–885.

Hoeprich PD, ed. Infectious diseases, 3rd ed., Philadelphia: Harper and Row, 1983.

Jayalakshmi UT, Gopalan C. Nutrition and tuberculosis. I. An epidemiologic study. Indian J Med Res 1958; 46:87–92.

Koblinsky MA. Severe measles and measles blindness. State-of-the-art-paper prepared for United States Agency for International Development, Baltimore, ICEPO, 1982.

Lloyd-Puryear M, Humphrey JH, West KP, Jr, Aniol K, Mahoney F, Mahoney J, Keenum DG. Vitamin A deficiency and anemia among Micronesian children. Nutr Res 1989; 9:1007–1016.

Majumder MSI, Sattar AKMA, Mohiduzzaman M. Effect of vitamin A deficiency on guinea pig Peyer's patches. Nutr Res 1987; 7:539–545.

Mark DA, Baliga BS, Suskind RM. All-trans retinoic acid reverses immune-related hematological changes in the vitamin A deficient rat. Nutr Rep Int, 1983; 28:1245–1252.

Martinez H, Shekar M, Latham M. Vitamin A supplementation and child mortality. Lancet 1986; 2:451–452.

McDermott MR, Mark DA, Befurs AD, Baliga BS, Suskind RM, et al. Impaired intestinal localization of mesenteric lymphoblasts associated with vitamin A deficiency and protein-calorie malnutrition. Immunology 1982; 45:1–5.

McDowell EM, Keenan KP, Huang M. Effects of vitamin A deprivation on hamster tracheal epithelium. Virchows Arch [Cell Pathol] 1984; 45:197–219.

McLaren DS, Shirajian E, Tchalian M, Khoury G. Xerophthalmia in Jordan. Am J Clin Nutr 1965; 17:117–130.

Mejia LA, Chew F. Hemotologic effect of supplementing anemic children with vitamin A alone and in combination with iron. Am J Clin Nutr 1988; 48:595–600.

Mejia LA, Hodges RE, Rucker RB. Role of vitamin A in the absorption, retention and distribution of iron in the rat. J Nutr 1979; 109:129–137.

Menon K, Vijayaraghavan K. Sequelae of severe xerophthalmia: A follow-up study. Am J Clin Nutr 1980; 33:218–220.

Milton RC, Reddy V, Naidu AN. Mild vitamin A deficiency and childhood morbidity—An Indian experience. Am J Clin Nutr 1987; 46:827–829.

Mohanram M, Reddy V, Misha S. Lysozyme activity in plasma and leucocytes in malnourished children. J Nutr 1974; 32:313–316.

Mohanram M, Kukarni KA, Reddy V. Hematologic studies in vitamin A deficient children. Int J Vit Nutr Res 1977; 47:389–393.

Muhilal, Permeisih D, Idjradinata YR, Muherdiyantiningsih, and Karyadi D. Vitamin A-fortified monosodium glutamate and health, growth, and survival of children: A controlled field trial. Am J Clin Nutr 1988; 48:1271–1276.

Natadisastra G, Wittpenn JR, West KP, Jr, Muhilal, and Sommer A. Impression cytology for detection of vitamin A deficiency. Arch Ophthalmol 1987; 105:1224–1228.

Nauss KM. Influence of vitamin A status on the immune system. In: Bauernfeind JC, ed. Vitamin A deficiency and its control. Orlando: Academic Press, 1986, 207–243.

Nauss KM, Newberne PM. Local and regional immune function of vitamin A deficient rats with ocular herpes simplex virus (HSV) infections. J Nutr 1985; 115:1316–1324.

Nauss, KM, Mark DA, Suskind RM. The effect of vitamin A deficiency on the vitro cellular immune response of rats. J Nutr 1979; 109:1815–1823.

Nieburg P, Waldman RJ, Leavell R, Sommer A, DeMaeyer EM. Vitamin A supplementation to refugees and famine victims. Bull WHO 1988; 66:689–697.

Niederman MS, Rafferty TD, Sasaki CT, Merrill WW, Matthay RA, Reynolds HY. Comparison of bacterial adherence to ciliated and squamous epithelial cells obtained from human respiratory tract. Am Rev Respir Dis 1983; 127:85–90.

Northway WH, Jr, Rosan RC, Porter DY. Pulmonary disease following respiratory therapy of hyaline membrane disease: Bronchopulmonary dysplasia. N Engl J Med 1967; 276:357–368.

Olson JA. Physiological and metabolic basis of major signs of vitamin A deficiency. In: Bauernfeind JC, ed. Vitamin A deficiency and its control. Orlando: Academic Press, 1986, 19–67.

Ongsakul M, Sirisinha S, Lamb AJ. Impaired blood clearance of bacteria and phagocytic activity in vitamin A deficient rats. Proc Soc Exp Biol Med 1985; 178:204–208.

Pasatiempo AMG, Bowman TA, Taylor CE, Ross AC. Vitamin A depletion and repletion: Effects of antibody response to the capsular polysaccharide of *Streptococcus pneumoniae*, type III (SSS-III). Am J Clin Nutr 1989; 49:501–510.

Pinnock CB, Douglas RM, Badcock NR. Vitamin A status in children who are prone to respiratory tract infections. Aust Paediatr J 1986; 22:95–99.

Pinnock CB, Douglas RM, Martin AJ, Badcock NR. Vitamin A status of children with a history of respiratory syncytial virus infection in infancy. Aust Paediatr J 1988; 24:286–289.

Pruzansky J, Axelrod AE. Antibody production to diphtheria toxoid in vitamin deficiency states. Proc Soc Exp Biol Med 1955; 89:323–325.

Reddy V, Bhaskaran P, Raghuramulu N, Milton RC, Rao V, Madhusudan J, Krisna KVR. Relationship between measles, malnutrition, and blindness: A prospective study in Indian children. Am J Clin Nutr 1986; 44:924–930.

Rhodes J, Oliver S. Retinoids as regulators of macrophage function. Immunology 1980; 40:467–472.

Rojanapo W, Lamb A, Olson JA. The prevalence, metabolism and migration of goblet cells in rat intestine following induction of rapid, synchronous vitamin A deficiency. J Nutr 1980; 110:178–188.

Russell RM, Multack R, Rosenberg IH, Smith VC, Krill AE. Dark-adaptation testing for diagnosis of subclinical vitamin A-deficiency and evaluation of therapy. Lancet 1973; 2:1161–1163.

Sanford-Smith JH, Whittle HC. Corneal ulceration following measles in Nigerian children. Br J Ophthalmol 1973; 63:720–724.

Sepulveda J, Willett W, Munoz A. Malnutrition and diarrhea. Am J Epidemiol 1988; 127:365–376.

Shahid NS, Sack DA, Rahman M, Alam AN, Rahman N. Risk factors for persistent diarrhoea. Br Med J 1988; 297:1036–1038.

Shann F, Gratten M, Germer S, Linnemann V, Hazlett D, Payne R. Aetiology of pneumonia in children in Goroka Hospital, Papua New Guinea. Lancet 1984; 2:537–541.

Shenai JP, Chytil F, Stahlman MT. Liver vitamin A reserves of very low birth weight neonates. Pediatr Res 1985; 19:892–893.

Shenai JP, Kennedy KA, Chytil F, Stahlman MT. Clinical trial of vitamin A supplementation in infants susceptible to bronchopulmonary dysplasia. J Pediatr 1987; 111:269–277.

Sietsema WK, DeLuca HF. A new vaginal smear assay for vitamin A in rats. J Nutr 1982; 112:1481–1489.

Sinha DP, Bang FB. The effect of massive doses of vitamin A on the signs of vitamin A deficiency in preschool children. Am J Clin Nutr 1976; 29:110–115.

Sirisinha, S, Darip MD, Moongkarndi P, Ongsakul M, Lamb A. Impaired local immune response in vitamin A deficient rats. Clin Exp Immunol 1980; 40:127–135.

Smith SM, Hayes CE. Contrasting impairments in IgM and IgG responses of vitamin A deficient mice. Proc Natl Acad Sci USA 1987; 84:5878–5882.

Smith SM, Levy NS, Hayes CE. Impaired immunity in vitamin A deficient mice. J. Nutr 1987; 117:857–865.

Snyder JD, Merson MH. The magnitude of the global problem of acute diarrhoeal disease: A review of active surveillance data. Bull WHO 1982; 60:605–613.

Sommer A. Vitamin A, xerophthalmia, and diarrhoea (letter). Lancet 1980; 1:1411–1412.

Sommer A. Nutritional blindness: Xerophthalmia and keratomalacia. New York: Oxford University Press, 1982a.

Sommer A. Field guide to the detection and control of xerophthalmia, 2nd ed. Geneva: WHO, 1982b.

Sommer A, West KP, Jr. Vitamin A supplementation and child mortality (letter). Lancet 1986; 2:451–452.

Sommer A, Hussaini G, Muhilal, Tarwotjo I, Susanto D, Saroso JS. History of night-blindness: A simple tool for xerophthalamia screening. Am J Clin Nutr 1980; 33:887–891.

Sommer A, Tarwotjo I, Hussaini G, Susanto D, Soegiharto T. Incidence, prevalence and scale of blinding malnutrition. Lancet 1981; 1:1407–1408.

Sommer A, Tarwotjo I, Hussaini G, and Susanto D. Increased mortality in children with mild vitamin A deficiency. Lancet 1983; 2:585–588.

Sommer A, Katz J, Tarwotjo I. Increased risk of respiratory disease and diarrhea in children with preexisting mild vitamin A deficiency. Am J Clin Nutr 1984; 40:1090–1095.

Sommer A, Tarwotjo I, Djunaedi E, West KP, Jr, Loeden AA, Tilden R, Mele L, and the Aceh Study Group. Impact of vitamin A supplementation on childhood mortality: A randomized controlled community trial. Lancet 1986; 1:1169–1173.

Sommer A, Tarwotjo I, Katz J. Increased risk of xerophthalmia following diarrhea and respiratory disease. Am J Clin Nutr 1987; 45:977–980.

Stanton BF, Clemens JD, Wojtyniak B, Khair T. Risk factors for developing mild nutritional blindness in urban Bangladesh. Am J Dis Child 1986; 140:585–588.

Stephenson M, Clark AB. A contribution to the study of keratomalacia among rats. Biochem J 1920; 14:502–521.

Stephenson S. On sloughing corneae in infants: An account based upon the records of thirty-one cases. Ophthalmoscope 1910; 8:782–818.

Stoll BJ, Banu H, Kabir I, Molla A. Nightblindness and vitamin A deficiency in children attending a diarrhoeal disease hospital in Bangladesh. J Trop Pediatr 1985; 31:36–38.

Stranski E. Klinische beitrage zur frage der aetiologie der keratomalacie. Jahrb Kinderheilkd 1924; 104:183–194. (in German)

Strum JM, Latham PS, Schmidt MC, McDowell EM. Vitamin A deprivation in hamsters. Virchows Arch [Cell Pathol] 1985; 50:43–57.

Takagi J, Nakano K. The effect of vitamin A depletion on antigen-stimulated trapping of peripheral lymphocytes in local lymph nodes of rats. Immunology 1983; 48:123–128.

Tarwotjo I, Sommer A, West KP, Jr, Djunaedi E, Mele L, Hawkins B. Influence of participation on mortality in a randomized trial of vitamin A prophylaxis. Am J Clin Nutr 1987; 45:1466–1471.

Tielsch JM, Sommer A. The epidemiology of vitamin A deficiency and xerophthalmia. Ann Rev Nutr 1984; 4:183–205.

Underwood BA. The safe use of vitamin A by women during the reproductive years. A report of the International Vitamin A Consultative Group (IVACG). The Nutrition Foundation, Washington, DC, 1986.

Venkataswamy G, Cobby M, Pirie A. Rehabilitation of xerophthalmic children. Trop Geogr Med 1979; 31:149–154.

Vyas D, Chandra RK. Vitamin A and immunocompetence. In: Watson RR, ed. Nutrition, disease resistance, and immune function. New York: Marcel Dekker, 1984, 1–34.

Wald G. The photoreceptor process in vision. Am J Ophthalmol 1955; 40:18–41.

West KP, Jr, Sommer A. Delivery of oral doses of vitamin A to prevent vitamin A deficiency and nutritional blindness. Food Rev Int 1985; 1(2):355–418.

West KP, Jr, Howard GR, Sommer A. Vitamin A and infection: Public health implications. Ann Rev Nutr 1989; 9:63–86.

Wittpenn J, Sommer A. Clinical aspects of vitamin A deficiency. In: Bauernfeind JC, ed. Vitamin A deficiency and its control. Orlando: Academic Press, 1986, 177–206.

Wolbach SB, Howe PR. Tissue changes following deprivation of fat-soluble A vitamin. J Exp Med 1925; 42:753–777.

Wolf G. Vitamin A. In: Alfin-Slater R, Kritchensky D, eds. Human nutrition: A comprehensive review—Nutrition and the adult. New York: Plenum Press, 1980, 97–203.

Wong YC, Buck RC. An electron microscopic study of metaplasia of the rat tracheal epithelium in vitamin A deficiency. Lab Invest 1971; 24:55–66.

World Health Organization. A joint WHO/USAID/UNICEF/HKI/IVACG meeting on the control of vitamin A deficiency and xerophthalmia (WHO Technical Report Series, No. 672), Geneva, 1982.

World Health Organization. A joint WHO/UNICEF statement on the expanded programme on immunization—Programme for the prevention of blindness nutrition programme: Vitamin A for measles, 1987.

World Health Organization. Vitamin A supplements: A guide to their use in the treatment and prevention of vitamin A deficiency and xerophthalmia, prepared by a WHO/UNICEF/IVACG Task Force, Geneva, 1988.

Zile MH, Cullum ME. The function of vitamin A: Current concepts. Proc Soc Exp Biol Med 1983; 72:139–152.

Zile MH, Bunge EC, DeLuca HF. Effect of vitamin A deficiency on intestinal cell proliferation in the rat. J Nutr 1977; 107:552–560.

POPULATION GROUPS AND PREVENTIVE NUTRITION

15

Role of Dietary Folate and Oral Folate Supplements in the Prevention of Drug Toxicity During Antifolate Therapy for Nonneoplastic Disease

Sarah L. Morgan and Joseph E. Baggott

University of Alabama at Birmingham
Birmingham, Alabama

INTRODUCTION AND HISTORICAL PERSPECTIVE

Folic acid antagonists have been used extensively to treat neoplastic disorders (Bleyer, 1978; Jackson, 1984) since Farber et al. (1948) demonstrated that aminopterin (4-aminopteroylglutamic acid) would induce remissions in acute leukemia. Two major antifolates, sulfasalazine (salicylazosulfapyridine, SASP)and methotrexate (4-amino-10-methylpteroylglutamic acid, MTX) are now also used in the treatment of a wide variety of nonneoplastic disorders.

One of the earliest uses of an antifolate in nonmalignant disease was by Gubner (1951) and by Gubner et al. (1951), who administered aminopterin (4-aminopteroylglutamic acid) to patients with rheumatoid arthritis, rheumatic fever, and psoriatic arthritis. In these studies there was remission of articular and periarticular inflammation in seven of the eight patients treated. Toxicities such as alopecia, mouth ulcers, sore throat, abdominal cramps, diarrhea, and pancytopenia were noted. One patient with extensive psoriasis had a remission of skin lesions lasting several weeks. Following these observations, aminopterin became an established treatment for psoriasis (Rees et al., 1955). However, methotrexate, which was introduced soon after aminopterin (Farber, 1949), became recognized as a preferable and less toxic therapeutic agent (Edmondson and Guy, 1958; Rees and Bennett, 1986). Methotrexate was approved in the early 1970s by the Food and Drug Administration (FDA) for use in the treatment of psoriasis, and aminopterin became unavailable. Methotrexate is now the most commonly used chemotherapeutic agent for the treatment of severe psoriasis (Hanno et al., 1980; Roenigk et al., 1969; McCullough and Weinstein, 1984). Methotrexate has now been evaluated in a variety of disorders (see Table 1) characterized by chronic inflammation and altered immune mechanisms.

Other drugs having an antifolate effect are used in the treatment of many different types of disorders including malaria, bacterial infection, hypertension, gout, epilepsy, and infection with *Pneumocystis carinii*. These agents, respectively, are pyrimethamine, trimethoprim, triamterene, colchicine, phenytoin, and trimetrexate (Butterworth and Tamura, 1989). Caution should be used when two or more folate antagonists are prescribed at the same time, since they may have additive effects, especially in nutritionally depleted subjects (see section on ''Toxicity of Antifolate Drugs'').

An important goal for the use of antifolates in the treatment of nonneoplastic disease is to maximize clinical effectiveness while minimizing toxicity. This chapter reviews the use of antifolates, especially MTX and SASP in a variety

Table 1   Nonneoplastic Diseases Treated with Methotrexate

Disease:	Ref.
Psoriasis	Roenigk et al. (1969)
	Hanno et al. (1980)
Psoriatic arthritis	Black et al. (1964)
Polymyositis	Arnett et al. (1973)
Dermatomyositis	Giannini and Callen (1979)
	Malaviya et al. (1968)
Reiter's disease	Owen and Cohen (1979)
Wegener's granulomatosis	Capizzi and Bertino (1971)
Sarcoidosis	Lacher (1968)
Bronchial asthma	Mullarkey et al. (1988)
Primary sclerosing cholangitis	Kaplan et al. (1987)
Primary biliary cirrhosis	Kaplan et al. (1988)
Inflammatory bowel disease	Kozarek et al. (1989)
Rheumatoid arthritis	Williams et al. (1985)
	Weinblatt et al. (1985)
	Anderson et al. (1985)
Malaria,	Butterworth and Tamura (1989)
Bacterial infections	
Hypertension	
Epilepsy	
Pneumocystis carinii	
Infection	

of nonneoplastic disorders, including inflammatory bowel disease (IBD), psoriasis, and rheumatoid arthritis (RA), emphasizing the latter. Specifically, antifolates are discussed with regard to (1) efficacy, (2) mechanism of action, and (3) toxicity. In addition, the role of baseline nutritional folate status, nutritional effects of folate antagonists, and the use of folate supplements to ameliorate toxicity are reviewed. In the field of cancer chemotherapy a well-known precedent has been established for the use of citrovorum factor (CF) (folinic acid, leucovorin) "rescue" to counteract toxic manifestations of MTX. It is beyond the scope of this chapter to discuss the apparent paradox of administering a vitamin antagonist and a vitamin at the same time. Nevertheless the successful use of CF rescue provides a rationale for the judicious use of folate supplements to offset certain toxic manifestations associated with the use of MTX in the management of nonneoplastic disease.

CLINICAL USE OF SULFASALAZINE AND METHOTREXATE IN NONNEOPLASTIC DISEASE

Sulfasalazine Therapy for Rheumatoid Arthritis

Sulfasalazine was synthesized in the late 1930s in order to provide an agent with combined sulfonamide and salicylate effects for possible use in the treatment of rheumatoid arthritis (Hirschberg and Paulus, 1987). It is of interest that the use of SASP for arthritis antedates clinical trials with aminopterin for this purpose (Hirschberg and Paulus, 1987). Although both SASP and MTX are now known to interfere with several enzymes involved in folic acid metabolism (see "Folate Status of Patients Receiving Antifolate Therapy for Nonneoplastic Diseases"), SASP was synthesized well before the chemical structure of folic acid was known and before purposeful synthesis of folic acid analogs became possible. Thus, the antifolate effects of SASP were not fully appreciated until after aminopterin and MTX had been evaluated clinically. Sulfasalazine proved effective in clinical trials during the early 1940s, but interest waned until McConkey et al. (1980) conducted an uncontrolled trial in 74 RA patients treated with SASP. Thirty-eight patients (51%) showed improvement and were able to remain on the drug for at least one year. The most common adverse effect noted was dyspepsia; megaloblastic anemia and neutropenia were also reported. In a similar noncontrolled trial, Bird et al. (1982) followed patients on a dose of up to 3.0 g of SASP per day for 6 months. The levels of acute phase reactants in serum decreased in these patients and there was improvement in clinical variables such as grip strength and pain score.

More recently controlled trials of SASP have been conducted. Pullar et al. (1983) compared SASP to placebo and intramuscular gold sodium thiomalate in patients with RA. After 6 months, patients on SASP and gold had similar improvements in laboratory and clinical measures of RA. The placebo group had no significant change in rheumatoid factor levels, pain score, grip strength, and index of disease activity. The major toxic manifestations were nausea and vomiting. An additional study by Pullar et al. (1985) showed that there was a positive dose-response relationship of SASP therapy and clinical improvement, with a dose of >40 mg/kg/day showing greatest benefit.

Pinals et al. (1986) used 3 g of SASP per day, in a 15-week, randomized, parallel, double-blind trial. Compared to placebo, the SASP-treated group had significant improvement in duration of morning stiffness, grip strength in both hands, pain on an analog scale, joint pain/tenderness count and score, and joint swelling count and score. Twenty-eight percent of the SASP patients were withdrawn from the study because of adverse drug reactions including gastrointestinal intolerance, rash or pruritus, elevated liver enzymes, and anemia. Only 2% of the patients in the placebo group were withdrawn for adverse drug reactions. The authors concluded that SASP is an effective drug for the treatment of RA.

The Cooperative Systematic Studies of Rheumatic Diseases Programs (Williams et al., 1988) compared SASP (2 g/day), gold sodium thiomalate (50 mg/week), and placebo in 186 patients with RA in a double-blind, randomized study for 37 weeks. The only significant differences between the SASP, injectable gold, and placebo groups were a decreased sedimentation rate and an improvement in grip strength in the right hand in the SASP and gold-treated groups. The excellent response to placebo was unexplained in this trial since injectable gold has previously been found to be superior to placebo therapy. Sixteen percent of patients were withdrawn from SASP therapy because of skin rash and gastrointestinal intolerance.

Methotrexate Therapy for Rheumatoid Arthritis

Short-Term Trials

While folic acid analog were first used in RA in the 1950s (Gubner, 1951; Gubner et al., 1951), their considerable toxicity and preference of clinicians for corticosteroid therapy dampened enthusiasm for their early use. However, in the 1980s there were numerous controlled clinical trials examining the efficacy of MTX in the treatment of RA. Four major short-term trials have evaluated the efficacy of MTX.

(1) The Cooperative Systematic Studies of Rheumatic Diseases Programs (Williams et al., 1985) studied 189 patients with RA who were entered into a prospective, controlled, double-blind, multicenter trial. One hundred ten patients remained on the trial for 18 weeks, receiving 7.5–15 mg of MTX orally per week. Patients receiving MTX had greater clinical improvement than patients receiving placebo as judged by the following criteria: duration of morning stiff-

ness, grip strength in both hands, 50-foot walking time, pain analog scale, patient assessment of disease, and physician assessment of disease by standard indices. Approximately one-third of the patients receiving MTX were withdrawn from the study for adverse drug reactions.

(2)   Weinblatt et al. (1985) evaluated 28 patients with RA in a 24-week, double-blind, crossover trial which compared MTX in pulsed doses of 7.5–15 mg weekly, with placebo. Significantly greater improvement was noted with MTX treatment compared to placebo, as judged by the number of swollen joints, number of tender/painful joints, joint-swelling index, joint pain/tenderness index, 50-foot walking time, duration of morning stiffness, and patient and physician assessment of disease activity. Most adverse effects of therapy occurred with equal frequency in the 7.5- and 15-mg MTX dose groups; however, nausea was more frequent during high-dose therapy. Fifty-two percent of patients had adverse reactions while taking MTX, compared with 15% of patients with adverse reactions while taking placebo. Immunological studies showed that there were no differences between MTX and placebo in mean rheumatoid factor titers, the levels of circulating immune complexes, and percentage of blood mononuclear cells expressing phenotypic and activation markers. The proliferative response of lymphocytes to mitogens was the same in the placebo and MTX-treated groups.

(3)   Andersen et al. (1985) studied 12 patients treated with weekly pulsed doses of intramuscular MTX (5–15 mg/week), in a double-blind, placeo-controlled, crossover study. After 13 weeks of therapy, the patients on MTX had significant improvement in joint counts for swelling and pain/tenderness, joint scores for swelling and pain/tenderness, duration of morning stiffness, and patient and physician assessment of disease compared to those on placebo. Adverse reactions during MTX treatment included pancytopenia, stomatitis, pruritic skin rash, and proteinuria (one patient each). Rheumatoid factor titers were not statistically different between treatment groups; however, there was a statistically significant decrease in IgG, IgM, and IgA during MTX treatment. There were no differences in absolute lymphocyte count, mononuclear cell subsets or proliferative responses to phytohemagglutinin and pokeweed mitogen between treatment groups.

(4)   Furst et al. (1989) followed 46 patients for 18 weeks in a double-blind, parallel study comparing a 5, 10, or 20 mg/m^2 dose of oral weekly MTX to placebo. A linear dose-response relationship was found for 5 and 10 mg/m^2 of MTX vs. placebo for patient pain and patient global scale, physician global scale, joint tenderness count, and activity of daily living score. Gastrointestinal toxicity occurred in 83, 71, and 62% of the patients on the high-, intermediate-, and low-dose MTX groups, respectively, indicating a dose-response relationship for toxicity. The frequencies of both gastrointestinal toxicity and stomatitis were significantly higher in the MTX arms of the study when compared to the placebo.

Long-Term Trials

There have been several studies of the long-term effectiveness of MTX. Weinstein et al. (1985) followed 21 patients with RA taking low-dose MTX (i.e., 5–15 mg/week, orally for 6 months or longer). Fifteen patients (71%) were able to continue therapy for a mean of 42 months with a mean cumulative dose of MTX of 2021 mg (range: 915–3075 mg). Three patients (14%) had a striking clinical remission and 9 (43%) had marked improvement in symptoms. Adverse reactions included nausea/dyspepsia (7 patients), stomatitis (3 patients), thrombocytopenia, herpes zoster, and acute hepatitis (1 patient each). Two patients discontinued MTX permanently because of severe gastrointestinal intolerance and one discontinued MTX because of hypersensitivity hepatitis.

Kremer and Lee (1986) studied 29 patients receiving a mean dose of 12.4 mg/week for a mean duration of 29.1 months. Two patients (7%) achieved complete remission of their arthritis, and maximum response to MTX seemed to occur at approximately 6 months. Ninety percent of the patients experienced toxicity at some time during therapy; however, most reactions were mild or moderate and did not require discontinuation of therapy. Sequential liver biopsies showed little change in baseline abnormalities, although elevations in liver function tests were common. The authors concluded that methotrexate is an effective drug for long-term treatment of RA; however, long-term toxicities must still be investigated.

Fehlauer et al. (1989) followed 124 patients for 2 years during low-dose MTX therapy. At the 12th week of therapy, 83% of patients showed clinical improvement. After 2 years of therapy, 48% of the initial patients were able to continue MTX therapy. During 2 years of therapy, MTX was discontinued because of adverse drug reactions in 38 patients (31%), lack of clinical benefit in 15 (12%), and for miscellaneous reasons in 11 (9%). Adverse drug reactions were reported by 93% of patients during drug treatment with the greatest number of toxicities occurring within the first year. The authors concluded that long-term use of MTX is limited more by the development of adverse drug effects than by lack of efficacy.

It is clear from these trials that both MTX and SASP are efficacious in the treatment of RA. However, toxicity remains an important factor limiting their long-term usefulness.

FOLATE STATUS OF PATIENTS RECEIVING ANTIFOLATE THERAPY FOR NONNEOPLASTIC DISEASES; COMPARISON WITH UNTREATED PATIENTS AND CONTROLS

Inflammatory Bowel Disease

A depressed folate status has been seen in patients taking SASP for inflammatory bowel disease (IBD). Pounder et al. (1975) evaluated red blood cell morphology in 50 patients with ulcerative colitis (UC) receiving SASP, 50 normal controls, and 10 patients with UC not receiving SASP. Twenty-two percent of SASP-treated patients had elevated mean corpuscular volume (MCV), a classic indicator of folate deficiency, and 4% of SASP-treated patients had frank folate deficiency (as indicated by serum folate less than 2.5 ng/ml and an elevated MCV). Swinson et al. (1981) evaluated folate status and folate absorption in patients with IBD taking SASP. Twenty-two percent of the patients taking SASP had macrocytic red cells, while macrocytosis was not observed in the control group not taking SASP. Forty-two percent of the patients in the SASP-treated group had an increased reticulocyte count compared to 7% in the untreated group. In addition, folate absorption was generally imparied in patients with UC and was further impaired by SASP administration. Macrocytosis, however, may be a poor indicator of impaired folate status in SASP-treated patients since hemolysis and reticulocytosis frequently occur. Folate deficiency can be a significant problem in patients taking SASP, especially if dietary folate intake is inadequate.

Longstreth and Green (1983) studied patients with chronic colitis taking SASP and compared these to patients with colitis not given SASP. In both groups, disease symptomatology was mild and diets were not restricted. The groups did not differ from each other in hemoglobin, MCV, or final folate levels. However, only in the SASP-treated group was there an inverse correlation between drug dose and MCV. Folate depletion may not be inevitable in patients taking SASP; however, subclinical depletion of folates can occur with doses of SASP greater than 2 g/day.

Halsted et al. (1981) examined patients with UC by performing jejunal perfusion studies and determining folate status. Seven patients were taking SASP and 10 patients were not treated with SASP. Folic acid absorption was significantly lower in the SASP-treated patients. Also the serum folate levels were found to be low in four of seven patients taking SASP. The authors concluded that there was a clear relationship between SASP use and folate deficiency. In addition, the jejunal hydrolysis of polyglutamyl folates by conjugase and disappearance of polyglutamyl and monoglutamyl folates from the gut lumen was inhibited more than 50% by concentrations of SASP of more than 1 mM. Folate malabsorption and depletion of folate stores are therefore likely consequences of SASP administration.

Psoriasis and Other Skin Disorders

The folate status of patients with skin diseases such as psoriasis was examined by Shuster et al. (1967). Thirty-three patients not taking antifolates with erythroderma, psoriasis, or eczema were evaluated for formiminoglutamic acid (FIGLU) excretion after an oral histidine load. Vitamin B_{12} and serum folate levels were also determined. Sixty-three percent of the patients had increased

FIGLU excretion (an indicator of folate deficiency), and 75% of the patients had low serum folate concentrations (<5 ng/ml). One patient had a low serum vitamin B_{12} level (<100 pg/ml). The authors concluded that folate deficiency is a common finding in patients with chronic skin disease.

The folate status of 20 patients on long-term MTX therapy for psoriasis and of 17 patients with psoriasis not receiving MTX was studied (Hendel and Nyfors, 1985). Erythrocyte folate levels were significantly lower in the MTX-treated patients. Also, the plasma levels of folate, as determined by an isotope-binding assay, increased significantly after MTX therapy was instituted. This finding is suggestive of leakage from an intracellular site, or displacement, as described by Johns and Plenderleith (1963). There may therefore be a potential for intracellular folate depletion during long-term MTX therapy for psoriasis.

Rheumatoid Arthritis

Gough et al. (1964) surveyed patients with RA and controls and measured serum levels of folate and vitamin B_{12}, and urinary excretion of FIGLU after an oral histidine load. Serum folate levels were significantly lower in the RA group. Seventy-three percent of the RA patients with low folate levels excreted excessive amounts of FIGLU in the urine. None of the controls excreted abnormal amounts of FIGLU. Thus, many patients with RA may have an unsatisfactory folate status, even without the use of antifolate drugs.

Omer and Mowat (1968) evaluated folate metabolism in patients with RA and found that 65% of RA patients had subnormal RBC folate values (<130 ng/ml) and 37% had a reduced plasma folate (<2.6 ng/ml) while none of a control group had abnormal values. In 46% of the deficient group, the folate levels fell within the range found in individuals with megaloblastic anemia, a folate deficiency syndrome. Megaloblastic bone marrow changes were found in 22% of cases and the authors concluded that patients with RA are at particular risk for folate deficiency.

The anemia found in RA patients receiving SASP has been investigated by Grindulis and McConkey (1985). They studied RA patients receiving either SASP (2 g/day or more) or penicillamine (500 mg/day). The MCV increased significantly only in patients taking SASP, while serum and RBC folate levels did not change significantly in either group. The authors concluded that the increased MCV is related to hemolysis, but a dose of SASP higher than 2 g/day may precipitate folate deficiency.

The folate status of RA patients taking low-dose methotrexate was recently examined by Morgan et al. (1987). The folate status of 29 controls with no serious medical illnesses, 20 RA patients not taking MTX, and 16 patients taking low-dose MTX for RA was evaluated by determining the activity of a folate-dependent metabolic pathway in peripheral blood mononuclear cells (PBMCs). This pathway of one-carbon metabolism measures the rate of radiolabeled serine formation from [^{14}C] formate and excess glycine, and is termed the "C_1 index." In control subjects, the C_1 index was found to be positively correlated with folate levels in PBMCs as measured by *Lactobacillus casei* assay. The activity of the C_1 index in the MTX-treated RA group was approximately half of the non-MTX-treated RA group or normal controls (Fig. 1). There was no difference in dietary intake of folate between the three groups, indicating that MTX was responsible for the decreased activity. This observation is believed to be one of the first demonstrations of functional metabolic differences in mononuclear/lymphoid cells due to MTX treatment in RA patients. The C_1 index may prove useful in monitoring function of folate-dependent reactions since it obviates problems such as inhibition of growth of microbiological assay organisms by MTX.

In addition, Weinblatt and Fraser (1989) showed in a retrospective analysis

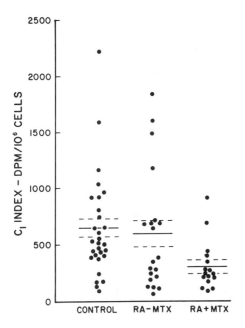

Figure 1   The C_1 index in 29 control subjects, 20 rheumatoid arthritis patients treated with drugs other than methotrexate (RA − MTX), and 16 patients treated with drugs other than methotrexate (RA + MTX). Means and standard errors are indicated by solid and dashed lines, respectively. Each point represents the mean of triplicate assays.

of 23 rheumatoid arthritis patients taking MTX that there is an association between increasing mean corpuscular volume (MCV), folate deficiency, and hematological toxicity. This report also indicates that folate status, as manifested by an increasing MCV, worsens during MTX therapy.

MECHANISM OF ANTIFOLATE ACTIVITY

Sulfasalazine

Sulfasalazine interferes with folate metabolism as several different anatomical and biochemical sites. It inhibits intestinal absorption of folate in human subjects and laboratory animals and inhibits the cleavage of folylpolyglutamates by conjugase (Franklin and Rosenberg, 1973; Halsted, 1980; Halsted et al., 1981; Reisenauer and Halsted, 1981). Sulfasalazine has also been shown to inhibit dihydrofolate reductase, serine transhydroxymethylase, and methylene tetrahydrofolate (THF) reductase in cell-free preparations and in cultured lymphocytes (Selhub et al., 1978; Halsted, 1980; Baum et al., 1981).

Methotrexate

The mechanism of action of MTX is complex. It is an inhibitor of dihydrofolate reductase (DHFR), so that in the presence of active synthesis of thymidylate, recycling of dihydrofolate is blocked, causing depletion of tetrahydrofolate pools necessary for the synthesis of purines and thymidylate (Chabner et al., 1986). Polyglutamylation of MTX occurs intracelluarly and favors retention of the drug. The additional glutamyl residues markedly increase the affinity of the inhibitor for enzymes such as aminoimidazole carboxamide ribotide transformylase (AICAR T'ase), glycinamide ribotide transformylase (GAR T'ase), and thymidylate synthase (TS) (Baugh et al., 1973; Kamen et al., 1981; Baggott et al., 1986; Chabner et al., 1986). Dihydrofolate polyglutamates, which accumulate rapidly after MTX administration, are also strong inhibitors of 5,10-methylenetetrahydrofolate reductase, TS, and AICAR T'ase. Marked and complex changes in the balance and distribution of intracellular folate pools are then produced, resulting in multiple inhibitions of folate-mediated reactions (Chabner et al., 1986).

Experiments in rats have also suggested that there is increased scission of the folate molecule following doses of MTX (Barford et al., 1980; Saleh et al., 1981) and diminished intestinal folate absorption (Barford et al., 1980). Increased catabolism and impaired absorption of folates observed in laboratory animals could explain the low hepatic and erythrocyte folate levels observed in MTX-treated patients (Kamen et al., 1981; Kremer et al., 1986).

TOXICITY OF ANTIFOLATE DRUGS; COMPARISON WITH NUTRITIONAL FOLATE DEFICIENCY

The toxic and biological effects of MTX and SASP are similar, but not identical, to the signs and symptoms of nutritional folate deficiency. Jackson (1984) observed: "It is sometimes stated that the biological effects of antifolate drugs resemble those of folate deficiency, and this analogy appears to be justifiable, at least to a first approximation." The effects of nutritional folate deficiency include diarrhea, sore tongue, anorexia, weight loss, megaloblastic anemia, leukopenia, and thrombocytopenia, all of which have been reported during antifolate therapy.

Toxicity of Sulfasalazine

The major adverse effects of SASP include nausea and vomiting, anemia, leukopenia, agranulocytosis, skin rash, hepatotoxicity, male infertility, and lung disease (Pullar and Capell, 1984). Das et al. (1973) estimated the overall incidence of adverse side effects of SASP therapy to be 15–70%.

Toxicity of Methotrexate

Toxicity has generally been reported in 30–90% of MTX-treated patients and is felt to be the major drawback to long-term treatment of RA (Gispen et al., 1987; Alarcón et al., 1989; Fehlauer et al., 1989). Tugwell et al. (1987) estimated that the most commonly occurring side effects of low-dose MTX therapy in RA are gastrointestinal intolerance (including nausea, vomiting, anorexia, and diarrhea), stomatitis, hematological effects (including leukopenia, anemia, and thrombocytopenia), and alopecia. Hepatotoxicity and pulmonary toxicity have also been reported.

The toxic manifestations of MTX and SASP overlap to a considerable extent, having gastrointestinal intolerance, megaloblastic anemia, leukopenia, agranulocytosis, hepatotoxicity, and pulmonary toxicity in common. While some of the toxicities also occur in nutritional folate deficiency, nutritional folate deficiency is biochemically different from the altered folate state induced by antifolate drugs. Specifically, during MTX therapy, there is an accumulation of dihydrofolates and MTX polyglutamates which does not occur in nutritional folate deficiency. In addition, a folate antagonist may affect different enzymes at different rates, so that the *presence* of an inhibitor is not the same as the *absence* of a cofactor. Therefore, it is reasonable that the signs and symptoms of nutritional folate deficiency will not be identical with those of MTX toxicity.

Combined antifolate therapy (e.g., MTX and trimethoprim-sulfamethoxazole therapy) and antifolate therapy in folate-depleted patients should have a synergistic effect on both desirable and undesirable end points. The high incidence of pancytopenia and other toxic manifestations in patients receiving MTX in combination with trimethoprim-sulfamethoxazole supports this concept (Thomas and Gutterman, 1986; Maricic et al., 1986; Frain, 1987; Thomas et al., 1987). Studies by Hellman et al. (1963) found that low-normal pretreatment serum folate levels were correlated with higher toxicity in patients following treatment with MTX for tumors of the head and neck.

QUANTITATION OF TOXICITY; DEVELOPMENT OF A SCORING SYSTEM

Some of the major problems in assessing and reporting drug toxicity are the lack of uniform terminology (Barker, 1985), lack of uniformity of patient follow-up, and variations in length of studies (Furst and Kremer, 1988). The incidence of discontinuation of the drug ("drop-out" rates) is often used as an indicator of serious toxicity (Barker, 1985). However, the dropout rate is not without flaws, since minimal rates are encountered among stoical patients with aggressive physicians, while maximal rates occur with anxious patients and cautious physicians. Thus, using only dropout rates to establish drug toxicity may be misleading.

A numerical scoring system has been developed to take into account the variables of duration, intensity, and clinical severity of disease and patient-weeks on the protocol (Morgan et al., 1990). The scoring system, based on clinical experience, distinguishes mild and marginal toxic symptoms (e.g., alopecia) from the severe and medically important ones (e.g., cytopenias which may be life threatening). The score reflects toxic events in terms of duration, intensity, importance, and multiplicity. It also incorporates the time on protocol at which the toxic manifestation first appears. The duration of the toxic event was placed in the numerator of the toxicity score in order to quantitatively emphasize persistent morbidities while minimizing the contribution of transitory morbidities and spurious abnormal laboratory values. The system permits the summation of scores calculated separately for different toxic manifestations, e.g., gastrointestinal, hematological. The formula for calculating the toxicity score is as follows:

$$\text{Toxicity score} = \sum \left[\frac{(\text{duration of toxic event [weeks]}) \times (\text{intensity}) \times (\text{clinical severity factor})}{\text{weeks on protocol}} \right]$$

Intensity is scored as:

1 = mild
2 = moderate
3 = severe

Clinical severity factors are as follows:

1 = alopecia, pruritus, nausea, anorexia, pyrosis, cramps, general GI intolerance
2 = vomiting, diarrhea, stomatitis, rash
3 = elevated liver enzymes, elevated serum creatinine
4 = cytopenias, documented infections, pulmonary toxicity

Abnormal liver function tests were defined as a transaminase and/or alkaline phosphatase value greater than two times baseline; cytopenias were defined as WBC $< 3.5 \times 10^9$/liter, or a platelet count $<150 \times 10^9$/liter; a serum creatinine was defined as elevated if >1.5 mg/dl (>133 μmol/liter); pulmonary toxicity was defined as evidence of new interstitial pulmonary infiltrates from the baseline chest radiograph with evidence of restrictive changes in pulmonary function tests. These included vital capacity $<80\%$ of predicted, normal expiratory flow rates, normal maximal voluntary ventilation, and diffusion capacity $<70\%$ of normal. Infection was defined as a documented viral, bacterial, or fungal infection which significantly compromised the patient and/or required hospitalization, and/or the administration of systemic antibiotics or antifungal agents. Any abnormality in transaminase, alkaline phosphatase, WBC, platelet count, or documented infections or pulmonary toxicity was given an intensity of 3 (severe).

FOLATE SUPPLEMENTATION OF METHOTREXATE-TREATED PATIENTS AND A CONTROLLED CLINICAL TRIAL OF FOLIC ACID SUPPLEMENTATION IN METHOTREXATE-TREATED RHEUMATOID ARTHRITIS PATIENTS

Many clinicians have concluded that toxicity is the major factor limiting prolonged antifolate therapy (Gispen et al., 1987). It is not surprising, therefore, that efforts have been made to minimize toxic effects through the use of folic acid or folinic acid supplements in association with MTX and SASP therapy. These efforts have been based on the theory that a mass action effect of folic acid could partially overcome the action of reductase inhibitors, or that folinic acid (which is already in the tetrahydro form) would bypass the metabolic block. Clinicians were hampered in the past by a lack of objective biochemical indicators to assess nutritional status in drug-treated patients. In part this is due to lack of procedures to measure blood levels of antifolate drugs in treated subjects. Another major consideration is the fact that standard microbiological assays for folic acid activity in blood and urine are unreliable because growth of test organisms is inhibited by MTX. Some of the difficulties in status assessment may be overcome by use of the C_1 index as described. This procedure reflects the functional status of several folate-dependent enzymes in viable cells generally regarded as important to immune mechanisms.

There is one report of folic acid supplementation of a patient taking SASP for IBD. Kane and Boots (1977) reported that megaloblastic anemia developed in a patient who had been taking 2.5 g/day of SASP for chronic proctitis. After a month of 5 mg/day of folic acid, the hematological picture cleared, while the IBD remained stable. There was no evidence that the dietary folate intake of this patient was low and no evidence that folic acid supplementation reduced the efficacy of SASP.

There is some evidence that folate supplementation will reduce the toxicity of MTX therapy for psoriasis. Roenigk et al. (1969) used 4–8 mg of folinic acid (leucovorin) intramuscularly (IM) 2 hr after a weekly IM dose of MTX and eliminated drug-induced mouth ulcers without reducing the efficacy of MTX. Ive and De Saram (1970) treated patients with severe psoriasis with a weekly IM dose of at least 3 mg folinic acid for every 5 mg of MTX. A number of MTX-induced abnormalities resolved, including mouth ulcers, nausea, vomiting, macrocytosis, neutropenia, thrombocytopenia, and elevated serum transaminases. Two of the 25 patients receiving leucovorin supplements along with MTX showed a relapse in the control of their skin disease, while four patients showed a slight improvement. However, the authors reported that this group of patients was receiving up to 63 mg of folinic acid for every 5 mg of MTX. This study suggested that this relatively large dose of folinic acid compromised the efficacy of MTX. Burkhart (1980) briefly reported that an oral folinic acid supplement given 4 hr after an oral dose of MTX reduced side effects with no reduction of therapeutic benefit. However, no dose levels of either MTX or leucovorin were reported.

There is also evidence that oral folate supplementation reduces the toxicity of MTX therapy of RA. Wilke and Krall (1984) reported a relatively low incidence of toxicity when a weekly dose of up to 12.5 mg of MTX was followed 5 days later by an oral dose of 6–9 mg of folic acid. For example, nausea was reported in only 1 of 87 patients in contrast with an expected frequency of about 10% (as estimated by Tugwell et al., 1987). This supplement of folic acid does not affect efficacy. Tishler et al. (1988) reported that 45 mg/week of oral folinic acid, beginning 4–6 hr after a 7.5- to 12.5-mg weekly IV dose of MTX, eliminated the nausea reported by four of seven RA patients. However, during folinic acid supplementation, a significant worsening of the disease occurred as judged by Richie articular index, grip strength, erythrocyte sedimentation, and subjective clinical assessment. Thus, a relatively large ratio of the folinic acid supplement to MTX (up to sixfold) markedly reduced the efficacy of the drug. Hanrahan and Russell (1988) conducted a double-blind, placebo-controlled study of 13 RA patients currently receiving 5–25 mg/week (mean 18.5 mg) of IM MTX. The patients received either 20 mg oral doses of folinic acid each week or a placebo. At the end of a 4-week trial, there was a trend toward less nausea in the folinic acid arm of the study. There was also a trend toward worsening of the disease as measured by the tenderness and swelling indices. Buckley et al. (1988) conducted a double-blind, placebo-controlled, crossover study of 24 RA patients using 1 mg of folinic acid per mg of MTX. Patients had received MTX for 6–8 weeks prior to beginning the study. During the 24-week study, there was a trend toward less stomatitis and gastrointestinal upset in the folinic acid arm of the study with no loss of therapeutic effectiveness. The authors stated that folinic acid did not alter the effectiveness of MTX.

In summary, it is apparent that MTX toxicity can be reduced through the use of folic or folinic acid supplements, but not without loss of therapeutic effectiveness under some conditions. A critical consideration for reducing toxicity of MTX therapy is the ratio of the folate supplement to the MTX dose. It is clear from the studies of Ive and De Saram (1970) and Tishler et al. (1988) that a high folate/MTX ratio may reduce the efficacy of the drug. Another consideration is the nature of the folate supplement (i.e., folinic acid or folic acid). Folinic acid is likely to have a narrow useful dose range because it bypasses DHFR and provides cells with a readily available supply of metabolically active coenzyme. In contrast, the oxidized vitamin (i.e., folic acid) has different properties and may enter a larger pool of metabolic reactions. Therefore, folic acid supplementation may have a more predictable effect on the efficacy of MTX.

MTX administration not only inhibits a number of folate-requiring enzymes but also produces a well-documented depletion of cellular folate (Kamen et al., 1981; Saleh et al., 1981; Kremer et al., 1986). These two mechanisms could have synergistic effects in the production of toxicity in MTX-treated RA patients. It may be possible to correct the systemic depletion of cellular folate by the administration of folic acid without substantially affecting the MTX inhibition of certain folate-requiring enzymes in target tissue. Based on this rationale, a randomized, double-blind, placebo-controlled trial was developed to evaluate whether folic acid supplements would significantly lessen toxic manifestations during MTX administration (Morgan et al., 1990).

Patients with RA, who were beginning MTX therapy and had failed to respond to other remittive agents, were entered into the trial. Patients were excluded from the protocol if they had a serious concomitant medical illness, or laboratory evidence of hepatic or renal dysfunction. Subjects were asked to stop any vitamin supplementation containing folic acid. Subjects were randomized to take 1 mg of folic acid (pteroylglutamic acid) or one identical placebo capsule per day. Randomization criteria included age, sex, RA serology, prednisone use, and previous folate-containing supplement use (Table 2).

Patients were evaluated at baseline and the following laboratory tests were performed: a complete blood count with differential, rheumatoid factor titer, liver function tests including transaminases and alkaline phosphatase, a joint count for pain/tenderness and swelling, joint indices, a 1-day dietary recall and mea-

Table 2 Clinical and Demographic Characteristics of RA Patients Receiving MTX and Either a Folate Supplement or Placebo

	Folate, $n = 16$	Placebo, $n = 16$	p value
Age, mean ($\pm$ S.D.)	52.0 (14.6)	50.9 (13.5)	NS
M/F (n)	3/13	3/13	NS
Previous use of folate-containing vitamins (n) (mean 400 µg folate/day)	5	2	NS
Disease duration (years), mean ($\pm$ S.D.)	8.7 (5.5)	15.3 (11.0	<0.05
Rheumatoid factor positive (n) %	15	16	NS
Initial serum folate ng/ml, mean ($\pm$ S.D.)	8.0 (5.0) range 2.0–20.9	8.5 (6.0) range 1.3–23.1	NS
Initial RBC folate ng/ml, mean ($\pm$ S.D.)	355.9 (222.8) range 101–539	361.3 (193.4) range 146–772	NS
Concurrent NSAID/aspirin use (n)	14	16	NS
Concurrent prednisone use (n)	9	8	NS
Anatomical stage, AGC,[a] mean $\pm$ S.D.	3.6 $\pm$ 1.3	3.9 $\pm$ 1.1	NS
CMC ratio,[a] mean ($\pm$ S.D.)	0.50 (0.03)	0.51 (0.03)	NS

[a] AGC is the anatomical grading criteria and CMC is the carpometacarpal ratio (Trenthan and Masi, 1976; Alarcón and Koopman, 1985).
Source: Reprinted from *Arthritis and Rheumatism*, Copyright 1990. From Morgan et al. (1990).

surement of blood vitamins (including vitamins A, C, thiamin, riboflavin, pyridoxine, plasma and RBC folate, beta-carotene, and vitamin B_{12}). The C_1 index was also determined (see above).

Patients were seen after 3 (2nd visit) and 6 (3rd visit) months. Identical laboratory studies were repeated and a list of toxic manifestations was made. In addition, patients were contacted by telephone every 3 weeks to assure compliance and to update any reported side effects. The investigators, the patients, and the treating rheumatologist were not aware of the capsule assignments until the study was completed.

The clinical demographic characteristics of the study population were similar, except for a longer duration of disease among those randomly assigned to receive the placebo (Table 2). Data analysis showed that the cumulative MTX doses at the follow-up visits were not different between the folic acid (FA)– and placebo-treated groups. The median weekly MTX doses for both groups was 7.5 mg. In addition, the dietary intakes of folate and vitamin B_{12} were not different between groups, as estimated by three 24-hr dietary recalls.

The patient response to treatment is shown in Table 3. The therapeutic response is similar in the placebo- and folate-supplemented groups; chi-square analysis revealed no significant differences. These results indicate that concomitant FA supplementation does not detract from the efficacy of MTX treatment for RA under the conditions of the experiment.

The table indicates the results of patient improvement in joint indices, categorized as marked improvement, moderate improvement, no change, or worsening. Marked improvement in the joint swelling index and in the joint tenderness/pain index is defined as a decrease of 50% or more in their values at visits 2 and 3, compared to their values at entry. Moderate improvement is defined as a decrease of 30–49% in these indices, no change means that the values for an index remained with plus or minus 30%, and worsening was a greater than 30% increase. Improvement and worsening in the physician and patient assessment of disease activity represent changes of at least two integers in their five-point scales (Williams et al., 1985).

Table 3 Patient Response to Treatment[a]

Variable and treatment	Number of patients with improvement		None	Worsening
	Marked	Moderate		
Swelling index				
Folate 2nd visit	6	3	5	0
Placebo 2nd visit	5	2	5	2
Folate 3rd visit	7	3	4	1
Placebo 3rd visit	3	5	3	1
Pain/tenderness index				
Folate 2nd visit	5	1	5	3
Placebo 2nd visit	7	1	2	4
Folate 3rd visit	5	3	4	3
Placebo 3rd visit	7	2	0	3
Physician assessment				
Folate 2nd visit		1	13	0
Placebo 2nd visit		0	11	1
Folate 3rd visit		2	11	0
Placebo 3rd visit		0	10	0
Patient assessment				
Folate 2nd visit		3	11	0
Placebo 2nd visit		4	8	2
Folate 3rd visit		3	12	0
Placebo 3rd visit		2	10	0

[a] See text for explanation of responses.
Source: Reprinted from *Arthritis and Rheumatism*, Copyright 1990. From Morgan et al. (1990).

Table 4 Mean Percent Change in the C_1 Index

Group	Visit 2 vs. 1	Visit 3 vs. 1
All patients	-41** (26)	-12 (24)
Folate-supplemented	-18 (12)	$+5$ (12)
Placebo	-65** (14)	-34* (24)

(n) Indicates number of observations with respect to visit 1 used to calculate the mean; *$p < 0.05$, **$p < .01$.
Source: Reprinted from *Arthritis and Rheumatism*, Copyright 1990. From Morgan et al. (1990).

Table 4 shows the drop in folate-dependent enzyme activity (as reflected in the C_1 index) during the trial. There was a statistically significant drop in the C_1 index only in the placebo-treated group at both time points.

Figure 2 shows an analysis of toxicity in the two groups using a clinical toxicity score for each patient (previous section). As seen in Fig. 2, the mean toxicity score is significantly lower in the folate-supplemented group than in the placebo-treated group. There were four dropouts in the placebo group due to the MTX toxicity, and none in the supplemented group. The decision to discontinue the protocol was made by the treating rheumatologist without knowledge as to placebo or supplement status of the subject. The toxic manifestations observed were the following (n = placebo group/folate group), nausea (8/5), elevations in liver enzymes (3/0), cytopenias (1/1), anorexia (2/0), alopecia (0/2), constipation/ bloating (1/0), pyrosis (1/0), stomach cramps (0/1), stomatitis (0/1), and elevated creatinine (1/0). The following toxic manifestations were observed in the four subjects with high toxicity scores: persistently elevated liver enzymes (3), severe nausea (2), cytopenias, anorexia, and elevated creatinine (1 each).

Poor folate status, as measured by plasma and RBC folate levels in the placebo-treated group proved to be predictive of future toxicity. Figure 3 (A and B) shows that low initial level of folate in plasma or red blood cells is associated with more toxicity. The acceptable or desirable level of folate is regarded to be >6.0 ng/ml in plasma and >200 ng/ml in red blood cells.

Figure 4 shows the change in mean corpuscular volume (MCV) over the study period in both groups. There is a trend toward a greater increase in MCV over the treatment period in the placebo group than in the folate-supplemented group. The placebo group had a statistically significant increase in MCV, while the increase in the folate group was not significant.

Table 5 shows the relationship between the drop in folate-dependent enzyme activity, C_1 index, and toxicity. There was a statistically significant drop in the C_1 index only in the placebo-treated group at both time points. When measures of efficacy and toxicity are combined in patients who had improvement, greater

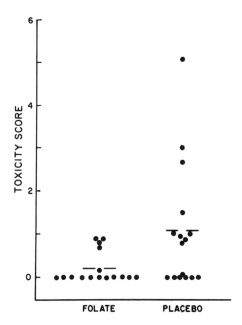

Figure 2 Toxicity scores of the folate-supplemented and placebo groups. The mean toxicity scores of the placebo and folate-supplemented groups are 1.06 and 0.21, respectively
($p = 0.027$).

than 50% decreases in the C_1 index are associated with toxicity, while less than
25% decreases are associated with minor (i.e., toxicity score <0.2) or no toxicity.
These findings indicate that moderate antagonism of folate-dependent reactions
is correlated with efficacy, while excessive antagonism is correlated with toxicity,
affirming the importance of folate metabolism in the mechanisms of efficacy/
toxicity.

The results of this trial indicate that folic acid supplementation can ameliorate
some of the toxicity of MTX therapy for RA during the first 6 months of therapy.
It should be noted that the optimum ratio of folic acid to MTX which will achieve
maximum clinical efficacy with minimum toxicity has not been established.

SUMMARY AND CONCLUSION

Antifolate drugs such as SASP and MTX are now used to treat a wide variety
of nonneoplastic diseases. The folate body pool of patients with psoriasis, IBD,
or RA is often marginal or frankly depleted even in the pretreatment state. When

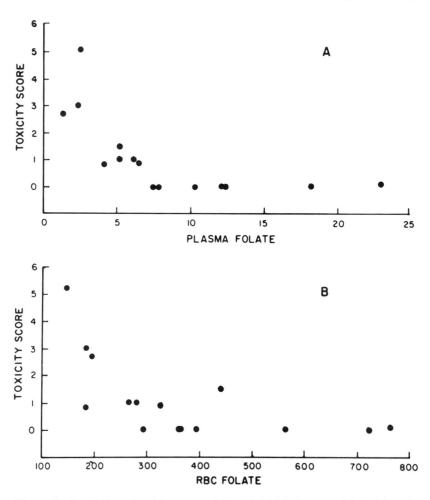

Figure 3   Correlation of toxicity scores (TS) with initial plasma and RBC folates in the placebo group. Spearman's rank correlation coefficient (r_s) was -0.84 ($p < 0.01$) and -0.66 ($p < 0.01$) for Fig. 3A and B, respectively.

an antifolate, such as MTX or SASP, is added for the management of disease, it is not uncommon for toxicities to develop. Many of the toxic manifestations such as weight loss, diarrhea, and cytopenias are the same as those seen in uncomplicated nutritional folate deficiency. Even though the impaired folate status caused by antifolate therapy is biochemically different from nutritional folate deficiency, folate administration has been shown to be useful in lessening drug

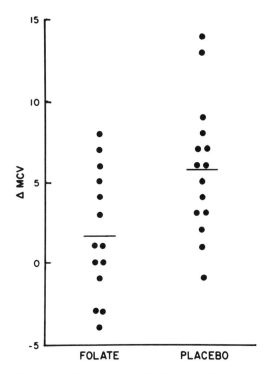

Figure 4 The changes in MCV from visit 1 to visit 3 are shown. Mean changes in MCV in the folate-supplemented and placebo groups are 2.9 (NS) and 5.8 ($p < 0.05$), respectively. Mean change in MCV is also statistically higher in the placebo group when compared to the folate-supplemented group ($p < 0.01$).

toxicity. Specifically, lowered drug toxicity with folate supplementation was seen during SASP therapy for IBD and during MTX therapy for RA and psoriasis.

Using a numerical estimate of toxicity, a randomized, placebo-controlled trial of 1 mg/day of folic acid supplementation in MTX-treated RA patients resulted in a significantly lower mean toxicity score when compared to nonsupplemented patients. This level of folic acid supplementation did not alter the efficacy of a median dose of MTX of 7.5 mg/week. Use of a functional test, the C_1 index, to measure the status of one-carbon metabolism in white blood cells may prove to be an important and useful biochemical indicator of toxicity and efficacy during MTX or other antifolate therapies.

Table 5 Relationship of C_1 Index to Toxicity and
Clinical Response

	Visit 2 plus 3	
Minor (TS < 0.2) or no toxicity	0	(30)
Moderate toxicity	−54**	(20)
Swelling index improved and		
Minor or no toxicity	−24	(17)
Moderate toxicity	−60*	(11)
Pain/tenderness improved and		
Minor or no toxicity	−16*	(17)
Moderate toxicity	−51*	(8)
Swelling index		
Improved	−42**	(28)
Not improved	+5	(22)
Pain/tenderness index		
Improved	−31**	(25)
Not improved	−23	(25)

Note: Improvement in the joint indices is defined as a decrease
greater than 30% from visit 1. The (*n*) indicates the number
of observations with respect to visit 1 used to calculate the
mean. TS, toxicity score. *$p < 0.05$, **$p < 0.01$.
Source: Reprinted from *Arthritis and Rheumatism*, Copyright
1990. From Morgan et al. (1990).

ACKNOWLEDGMENTS

Supported by NIH grants 5P01-CA-28103-10 and 5P60-AR-20614. Dr. Morgan
is the recipient of a Future Nutrition Leader's Award from the International Life
Sciences Institute/Nutrition Foundation (1986–1988).

REFERENCES

Alarcón GS, Koopman WJ. The carpometacarpal ratio: a useful method for assessing
disease progression in rheumatoid arthritis. J Rheumatol 1985; 12:846.

Alarcón GS, Tracy IC, Blackburn WD, Jr. Toxic effects as the major factor in limiting
long-term treatment. Arth Rheum 1989; 32:671.

Andersen PA, West SG, O'Dell JR, Via CS, Claypool RG, Kotzin BL. Weekly pulse
methotrexate in rheumatoid arthritis. Ann Intern Med 1985; 103:489.

Arnett FC, Whelton JC, Zizic TM, Stevens MB. Methotrexate therapy in polymyositis.
Ann Rheum Dis 1973; 32:536.

Baggott JE, Vaughn WH, Hudson BB. Inhibition of 5-aminoimidazole-4-carboxamide
ribotide transformylase, adenosine deaminase, and 5'-adenylate deaminase by poly-

glutamates of methotrexate and oxidized folates and by 5'-aminoimidazole-4-carbox-amide riboside and ribotide. Biochem J 1986; 236:193.

Barford PA, Blair JA, Malghani MAK. The effect of methotrexate on folate metabolism in the rat. Br J Cancer 1980; 41:816.

Barker EF. Assessment of adverse reactions to NSAID'S: pre- and post-marketing. In: Velo GP, Rainsferd D, eds. Side-effects of anti-inflammatory drugs, Part I. Lancaster, UK: MTP Press LTD, 1987, 37–46.

Baugh CM, Krumdieck CL, Nair MG. Polygammaglutamyl metabolites of methotrexate. Biochem Biophys Res Commun, 1973; 52:27.

Baum CL, Selhub J, Rosenberg IH. Antifolate actions of sulfasalazine on intact lymphocytes. J Lab Clin Med 1981; 97:779.

Bird HA, Dixon JS, Pickup ME, Rhind VM, Lowe JR, Lee MR, Wright V. A biochemical assessment of sulphasalazine in rheumatoid arthritis. J Rheumatol 1982; 9:36.

Black RL, O'Brien WM, VanScott EJ, Auerbach R, Eisen AZ, Bunim JJ. Methotrexate therapy in psoriatic arthritis. Double-blind study on 21 patients. J Am Med Assoc 1964; 189:743.

Bleyer WA. The clinical pharmacology of methotrexate. Cancer 1978; 41:36.

Braunwald E, Isselbacher KJ, Petersdorf RG, Wilson JD, Martin JB, Fauci AS. Harrison's principles of internal medicine. New York: McGraw-Hill, 1987, 1287.

Buckley LM, Cooper SM, Vacek PM. The use of leucovorin after low-dose methotrexate in patients with rheumatoid arthritis. Arthr Rheum 1988; 31:(Suppl) R3.

Burkhart CG. Treatment of psoriasis with methotrexate and folinic acid. J Am Acad Dermatol 1980; 3:207.

Butterworth CE, Tomura T. Folic acid safety and toxicity: A brief review, Am J Clin Nutr 1989; 50:353.

Capizzi RL, Bertino JR. Methotrexate therapy of Wegener's granulomatosis. Ann Intern Med 1971; 75:74.

Chabner BA, Allegra CJ, Baram J. Chemistry and biology of pteridines. In: Antifolates: Expanding horizons in 1986. Walter de Gruyter, 1986, 945.

Das KM, Eastwood MA, McManus JPA, Sitcus W. The metabolism of salicylazosulfapyridine in ulcerative colitis. Gut 1973; 14:631.

Edmundson WF, Guy WB. Treatment of psoriasis with folic acid antagonists. Arch Dermatol 1958; 78:200.

Farber S. Some observations on the effect of folic acid antagonists on acute leukemia and other forms of incurable cancer. Blood 1949; 4:160.

Farber S, Diamond LK, Mercer RD, Sylvester RF, Wolff JA. Temporary remissions in acute leukemia in children produced by folic acid antagonist, 4-aminopteroylglutamic acid (aminopterin). N Engl J Med 1948; 238:787.

Fehlauer CS, Carson CW, Cannon GW, Ward JR, Samuelson CO, Williams HJ, Clegg DO. Methotrexate therapy in rheumatoid arthritis: 2-year retrospective followup study. J Rheumatol 1989; 16:307.

Frain JB. Methotrexate toxicity in a patient receiving trimethoprim-sulfamethoxazole. J Rheumatol 1987; 14:176.

Franklin JL, Rosenberg IH. Impaired folic acid absorption in inflammatory bowel disease: Effects of salicylazosulfapyridine (azulfidine). Gastroenterology 1973; 64:517.

Furst DE, Koehnke R, Burmeister LF, Kohler J, Cargill I. Increasing methotrexate effect with increasing dose in the treatment of resistant rheumatoid arthritis. J Rheumatol 1989; 16:313.

Furst DE, Kremer JM. Methotrexate in rheumatoid arthritis. Arthr Rheum 1988; 31:305.

Giannini M, Callen JP. Treatment of dermatomyositis with methotrexate and prednisone. Arch Dermatol 1978; 115:1251.

Gispen JG, Alarcón GS, Johnson JJ, Acton RT, Barger BO, Koopman WJ. Toxicity to methotrexate in rheumatoid arthritis. J Rheumatol 1987; 14:74.

Gough KR, McCarthy C, Read AE, Mollin DL, Waters AH. Folic-acid deficiency in rheumatoid arthritis. Br Med J 1964; 1:212.

Grindulis KA, McConkey B. Does sulphasalazine cause folate deficiency in rheumatoid arthritis? Scand J Rheumato 1985; 14:265.

Gubner R. Therapeutic suppression of tissue reactivity. I. Comparison of the effects of cortisone and aminopterin. Am J Med Sci 1951; 221:169.

Gubner R, August S, Ginsberg V. Therapeutic suppression of tissue reactivity. II. Effect of aminopterin in rheumatoid arthritis and psoriasis. Am J Med Sci 1951; 221:176.

Halsted CH. Intestinal absorption and malabsorption of folates. Ann Rev Med 1980; 31:79.

Halsted CH, Gandhi G, Tamura T. Sulfasalazine inhibits the absorption of folates in ulcerative colitis. N Engl J Med 1981; 305:1513.

Hanno R, Gruber GG, Owen LG, Callen JP. Methotrexate in psoriasis. Acad Dermatol 1980; 2:171.

Hanrahan PS, Russell AS. Concurrent use of folinic acid and methotrexate in rheumatoid arthritis. J Rheumatol 1988; 15:1078.

Hellman S, Iannotti AT, Bertino JR. Serum folate activity in patients with tumors of the head and neck treated with methotrexate. Proc Am Cancer Res 1963; 4:27.

Hendel J, Nyfors A. Impact of methotrexate therapy on the folate status of psoriatic patients. Clin Exp Dermatol 1985; 10:30.

Hirschberg J, Paulus HE. Immunomodulators and other disease modifying antirheumatic drugs. In: Paulus HE, Furst DE, Dromgoole SH, eds. Drugs for rheumatic disease. 1987, 189–193.

Ive FA, De Saram CFW. Methotrexate and the citrovorum factor in the treatment of psoriasis. Trans St Johns Hosp Dermatol Soc 1970; 56:45.

Jackson RC. Biological effects of folic acid antagonists with antineoplastic activity. Pharm Ther 1984; 25:61.

Johns DG, Plenderleith IH. Folic acid-displacement in man. Biochem Pharmacol 1963; 12:1071.

Kamen BA, Nylen PA, Camitta BM, Bertino JR. Methotrexate accumulation and folate depletion in cells as a possible mechanism of chronic toxicity to the drug. Br J Haemato 1981; 49:355.

Kane SP, Boots MA. Megaloblastic anaemia associated with sulphasalazine treatment. Br Med J 1977; 2:1287.

Kaplan MM, Arora S, Pincus SH. Primary sclerosing cholangitis and low-dose oral pulse methotrexate therapy. Ann Intern Med 1987; 106:231.

Kaplan MM, Knox TA, Arora S. Low-dose oral pulse methotrexate in the treatment of primary biliary cirrhosis (PBC): Resolution of symptoms and improvement in biochemical tests of liver function. Gastroenterology 1988; 94:A552.

Kozarek RA, Patterson DJ, Gelfand MD, Botsman VA, Ball TJ, Wilske KR. Methotrexate induces clinical and histologic remission in patients with refractory inflammatory bowel disease. Ann Intern Med 1989; 110:353.

Kremer JM, Galivan J, Streckfuss A, Kamen B. Methotrexate metabolism analysis in blood and liver of rheumatoid arthritis patients. Association with hepatic folate deficiency and formation of polyglutamates. Arthr Rheum 1986; 29:832.

Kremer JM, Lee JK. The safety and efficacy of the use of methotrexate in long-term therapy for rheumatoid arthritis. Arthr Rheum 1986; 29:822.

Lacher MJ. Spontaneous remission or response to methotrexate in sarcoidosis. Ann Intern Med 1968; 69:1247.

Longstreth GF, Green R. Folate status in patients receiving maintenance doses of sulfasalazine. Arch Intern Med 1983; 143:902.

Maricic M, Davis M, Gall EP. Megaloblastic pancytopenia in a patient receiving concurrent methotrexate and trimethoprim-sulfamethoxazole treatment. Arthr Rheum 1986; 29:133.

Malaviya AN, Many A, Schwartz RS. Treatment of dermatomyositis with methotrexate. Lancet 1968; 2:485.

McConkey B, Amos RS, Durham S, Forster PJG, Hubball S, Walsh L. Sulphasalazine in rheumatoid arthritis. Br Med J 1980; 280:442.

McCullough JL, Weinstein GD. Folate antagonists in psoriasis. In: Folate antagonists as therapeutic agents, Vol. 2. New York: In: Academic Press 1984, Chap. 9.

Morgan SL, Baggott JE, Altz-Smith M. Folate status of rheumatoid arthritis patients receiving long-term, low-dose methotrexate therapy. Arthr Rheum 1987; 30:1348.

Morgan SL, Baggott JE, Vaughn WH, Young PK, Austin JV, Krumdieck CL, Alarcón GS. The effect of folic acid supplementation on the toxicity of low-dose methotrexate treatment of rheumatoid arthritis. Arthr Rheum 1990; 30:9.

Mullarkey MF, Blumenstein BA, Andrade P, Bailey GA, Olason I, Wetzel CE. Methotrexate in the treatment of corticosteroid-dependent asthma. N Engl J Med 1988; 318:603.

Omer A, Mowat A.G. Nature of anaemia in rheumatoid arthritis. Ann Rheum Dis 1968; 27:414.

Owen EJ, Cohen ML. Methotrexate in Reiter's disease. Ann Rheum Dis 1979; 38:48.

Pinals RS, Kaplan SB, Lawson JG, Hepburn B. Sulfasalazine in rheumatoid arthritis. Arthr Rheum 1986; 29:1427.

Pounder RE, Craven ER, Henthorn JS, Bannatyne JM. Red cell abnormalities associated with sulphasalazine maintenance therapy for ulcerative colitis. Gut 1975; 16:181.

Pullar T, Hunter JA, Capell HA. Sulphasalazine in rheumatoid arthritis: a double-blind comparison of sulphasalazine with placebo and sodium aurothiomalate. Br Med J 1983; 287:1102.

Pullar T, Capell HA. Sulphasalazine: A "new" antirheumatic drug. Br J Rheumatol 1984; 23:26.

Pullar T, Hunter JA, Capell HA. Sulphasalazine in the treatment of rheumatoid arthritis: relationship of dose and serum levels to efficacy. Br J Rheumatol 1985; 24:269.

Rees RB, Bennett JH, Bostick WL. Aminopterin for psoriasis. Arch Dermatol 1955; 72:133.

Rees RB, Bennett JH. Methotrexate vs. aminopterin for psoriasis. Arch Dermatol 1961; 83:970.

Reisenauer AM, Halsted CH. Human jejunal brush border folate conjugase: characteristics and inhibition by salicylazosulfapyridine. Biochim Biophys Acta 1981; 659:62.

Roenigk HH, Jr, Fowler-Bergfeld W, Curtis G. Methotrexate for psoriasis in weekly oral doses. Arch Dermatol 1969; 99:86.

Saleh AM, Pheasant AE, Blair JA. Folate catabolism in tumor-bearing rats and rats treated with methotrexate. Br J Cancer 1981; 44:700.

Sauberlich HE. Comparative studies with the natural and synthetic citrovorum factor. J Biol Chem 1952; 195:337.

Selhub J, Dhar GJ, Rosenberg IH. Inhibition of folate enzymes by sulfasalazine. J Clin Invest 1978; 61:221.

Shuster S, Marks J, Chanarin I. Folic acid deficiency in patients with skin disease. Br J Dermatol 1967; 79:398.

Swinson CM, Perry J, Lumb M, Levi AJ. Role of sulphasalazine in the aetiology of folate deficiency in ulcerative colitis. Gut 1981; 22:456.

Thomas DR, Dover JS, Camp RDR. Pancytopenia induced by the interaction between methotrexate and trimethoprim-sulfamethoxazole. J Am Acad Dermatol 1987; 17:1055.

Thomas MH, Gutterman LA. Methotrexate toxicity in a patient receiving trimethoprim-sulfamethoxazole, J Rheumatol 1986; 13:440.

Tishler M, Caspi D, Fishel B, Yaron M. The effects of leucovorin (folinic acid) on methotrexate therapy in rheumatoid arthritis patients. Arthr Rheum 1988; 31:906.

Trentham DE, Masi AT. Carpometacarpal ratio: A new quantitative measure of radiological progression of wrist involvement in rheumatoid arthritis. Arthr Rheum 1976; 19:939.

Tugwell P, Bennett K, Gent M. Methotrexate in rheumatoid arthritis. Ann Intern Med 1987; 107:358.

Weinblatt ME, Coblyn JS, Fox DA, Fraser PA, Holdsworth DE, Glass DN, Trentham DE. Efficacy of low-dose methotrexate in rheumatoid arthritis. N Engl J Med 1985; 312:818.

Weinblatt ME, Fraser P. Elevated mean corpuscular volume as a predictor of hematologic toxicity due to methotrexate therapy. Arthr Rheum 1989; 32:1592.

Weinstein A, Marlowe S, Korn J, Farouhar F. Low-dose methotrexate treatment of rheumatoid arthritis: long-term observations. Am J Med 1985; 79:331.

Wilke WS, Krall PL. Resistant rheumatoid arthritis. What to do when conservative therapy doesn't work, Postgrad Med 1985; 75:69.

Wilke WS, MacKenzie AH. Methotrexate therapy in rheumatoid arthritis. Curr Status Drugs 1986; 32:103.

Williams HJ, Ward JR, Dahl SL, Clegg DO, Willkens RF, Oglesby T, Weisman MH, Schlegel S, Michaels RM, Luggen ME, Polisson RP, Singer JZ, Kantor SM, Shiroky JB, Small RE, Gomez MI, Reading RC, Egger MJ. A controlled trial comparing sulfasalazine, gold sodium thiomalate, and placebo in rheumatoid arthritis. Arthr Rheum 1988; 31:702.

Williams HJ, Willkens RF, Samuelson CO, Jr, Alarcón GS, Guttadauria M, Yarboro C, Polisson RP, Weiner SR, Luggen ME, Billingsley LM, Dahl SL, Egger MJ, Reading JC, Ward JR. Comparison of low-dose oral pulse methotrexate and placebo in the treatment of rheumatoid arthritis: A controlled clinical trial. Arthr Rheum 1985; 28:721.

16

Micronutrients and Age-Related Cataracts

Paul F. Jacques and Allen Taylor

*U.S. Department of Agriculture Human Nutrition
Research Center on Aging, Tufts University
Boston, Massachusetts*

INTRODUCTION

Senile cataracts are a major cause of disability in the elderly. Although amenable to treatment, senile cataracts remain one of the leading causes of blindness in the United States and the leading cause of preventable blindness throughout the world (Dawson and Schwab, 1981; Steinkuller, 1983). Approximately 400,000 persons develop cataracts each year (*Vision Research*, 1983). Senile cataracts with accompanying visual impairment are estimated to be present in approximately 45% of all Americans over age 75 and in 20% of those between 65 and 75 years (Kahn et al., 1977a). If early lens changes are also included in the calculation, the estimated prevalence of cataract is doubled (Kahn et al., 1977a). In addition, cataract surgery is the most frequently performed surgical procedure reimbursed by Medicare, representing 12% of the Medicare budget (Stark and Sommer, 1989). It has been suggested that a 10-year delay in cataract formation could cut the need for lens extraction in half (*Vision Research*, 1983). Clearly, identifying determinants of senile cataracts can have a significant impact both on the well-being of the elderly and on the associated health costs.

HYPOTHESES REGARDING CATARACT FORMATION

Structural and Biochemical Basis of Cataract Formation

The lens of the human eye is an avascular, transparent organ (Figs. 1 and 2), and must remain transparent to function properly. The lens surface is covered with a collagenous capsule. Beneath the anterior capsule is a single layer of epithelial cells which is the major site of metabolic activity in the lens (Fig. 3). Near the lens equator, the epithelial cells form a germinative zone of dividing cells. As these epithelial cells migrate toward the equator, they differentiate and elongate to form fiber (cortical) cells. Throughout life, new fibers are formed at the equator and migrate inward. As these fiber cells mature and differentiate, they lose their nuclei and organelles. The old fibers are not lost, but become more dehydrated and compressed in the nucleus or center of the lens.

The function of the lens is to transmit and focus light rays on the photosensitive retina. There are two major factors that permit the lens to transmit rather than scatter light. First, there are few physical obstacles to the passage of light (such

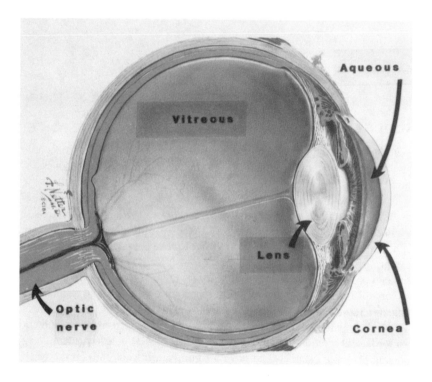

Figure 1   Diagram of the human eye.

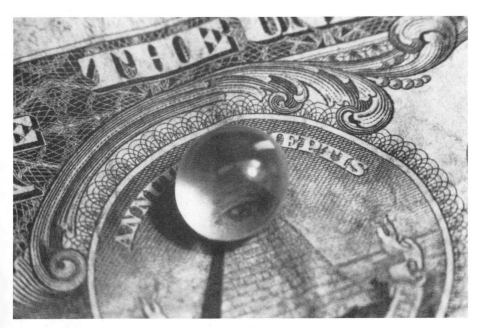

Figure 2 Clear mammalian lens.

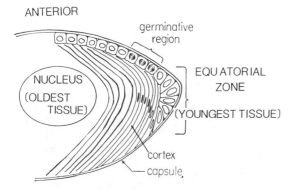

Figure 3 Diagram of the adult mammalian lens. The lens is surrounded by an external noncellular capsule. The lens epithelial cells are found beneath the capsule on the anterior side. The peripheral, equatorial zone is the region of transition where epithelial cells begin to elongate and differentiate into fiber cells. The fiber cells which are newly laid down constitute the cortex; fiber cells laid down during the early growth period of the lens compose the nucleus of the adult lens.

as blood vessels, cell nuclei, and mitochondria). Second, approximately 35% of the lens is protein and the remainder is essentially water. This protein-water mixture forms a gelatin-like medium which has an index of refraction with little variation relative to the wavelength of visible light (Benedek, 1971; Delaye and Tardieu, 1983). The cell membranes and interfaces also transmit rather than scatter light (Trokel, 1962). Changes within the lens producing variations in the refractive index cause increased light scattering and opacification of the lens (Fig. 4). Any opacity occurring in the lens is referred to as a cataract. (For human lenses, a distinction is often made between any lens opacity and a cataract referring to a lens opacity with accompanying visual loss. Although this distinction may serve a clinical function, it is not useful in classification of lens opacities for the purposes of research.)

The proteins in the lens exist in situ for decades. Exposure to light, oxygen, products of normal aging, and environmental factors subject the proteins of the lens to myriad and extensive postsynthetic modifications including (photo)oxidation, racemization, and enzymatic and nonenzymatic glycosylation (Harding, 1981; Hoenders and Bloemendal, 1981; Thomson et al., 1985). Such modifications result in aggregation, polymerization and precipitation of proteins (for reviews, see Taylor and Davies, 1987; Taylor, 1989). Protein aggregation and subsequent precipitation are associated with increased levels of water-in-

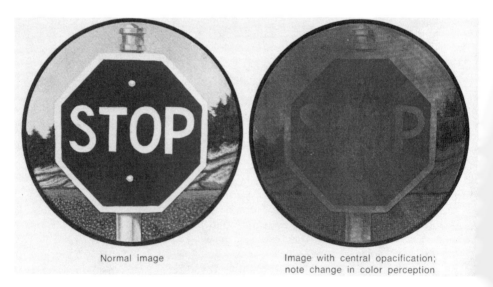

Normal image   Image with central opacification; note change in color perception

Figure 4 View through a clear lens (left) and a cataractous lens (right).

soluble protein in the aged and cataractous lens (Zigman et al., 1976; Anderson et al., 1979; Taylor et al., 1989), and the process of insolubilization appears to be accelerated in cataract formation (Garner and Spector, 1978; Taylor et al., 1989).

Etiology of Senile Cataract

Certain metabolic disorders, such as diabetes (Prchal et al., 1980; Ederer et al., 1981; Klein et al., 1985), galactosemia (Cordes, 1960; Kinoshita, 1965; Beutler et al., 1973), trauma (Harding and Crabbe, 1984), as well as corticosteroids (Skalka and Prchal, 1980), and other drugs (Clayton et al., 1982; Hollwich et al., 1975), are known or suspected to increase the risk of cataract. However, the vast majority of lens opacities fall into a category called senile cataract. This category includes those opacities with unknown etiology occurring in adults. Such opacities are strongly associated with aging but should not be considered to be an inevitable result of aging. Although every aging person develops morphological lens changes, not all progress to visually disabling cataracts. In addition, among those developing senile cataracts, the age of occurrence and rate of development vary greatly. Thus, it is reasonable to assume that certain behavioral or environmental factors may modify the aging process of the lens and increase the risk of cataract.

There are many suspected risk factors for development of senile lens opacities. Epidemiological studies have implicated ultraviolet (solar) radiation in senile cataract formation (Hiller et al., 1977; Zigman et al., 1979; Taylor, 1980; Hollows and Moran, 1981; Taylor et al., 1988). An injurious role for ultraviolet light has been corroborated by experiments demonstrating the formation of cataract-like protein aggregates in lens preparations exposed to ultraviolet light (Harding and Crabbe, 1984; Blondin et al., 1986; Varma, 1987). Infrared (Lydahl and Philipson, 1984a,b), ionizing (Hanna, 1975), and microwave (Cleary and Pasternack, 1966; Aurell and Tengroth, 1973; Hollows and Douglas, 1984; Stewart-DeHann et al., 1985) radiation; and diarrhea and dehydration (Harding, 1982; Minassian et al., 1984) have also been suggested as possible causes of senile cataracts. It has been proposed that aspirin (Cotlier, 1981; Crompton et al., 1985; Gupta et al., 1984; Rao et al., 1985), can delay the onset and retard the progression of cataracts. Gender, blood pressure, blood sugar, education, occupation, vital capacity, and other demographic and biological parameters have been correlated with risk of senile cataracts (Cleary and Pasternack, 1966; Kahn et al., 1977b; Clayton et al., 1980; Hiller et al., 1983; Hollows and Douglas, 1984; Lydahl and Philipson, 1984a,b).

Evidence is accumulating for a relationship between nutritional status and senile cataract in human populations. A few reports relate general undernourishment with cataractous lens changes. Included among these are case reports relating cataract formation with anorexia nervosa (Miller, 1958; Stigmar, 1965; Archer, 1981). Low consumption of protein has been suggested as a factor that may account for the high prevalence of senile lens changes seen in the Punjab region of India (Chatterjee et al., 1982). Abundant experimental evidence exists on specific amino acid deficiency and cataract in many animal species (Hall et al., 1948; von Sallmann et al., 1959; Poston et al., 1977; Bunce et al., 1978, 1984; Ohrloff et al., 1978). However, the majority of relevant experimental and epidemiological evidence relates micronutrients to cataract formation.

Lens Antioxidant Defense Mechanisms

Oxidation of lens proteins is highly correlated with cataract. In aged and cataractous lenses there are high levels of water-insoluble protein aggregates which are formed in part by oxidative processes (e.g., disulfide bond formation, etc.) (Giblin and Reddy, 1978; Garner and Spector, 1980). Protein disulfides in the insoluble protein fraction of cataractous lenses are found to be greatly increased over normal lenses of similar ages (Truscott and Augusteyn, 1977; Anderson et al., 1979; Hoenders and Bloemendal, 1981; Takemoto and Hansen, 1982).

Several biological reactions are known to produce highly reactive intermediates such as superoxide, hydroperoxides, or hydroxyl radicals, and the less reactive hydrogen peroxide (Fridovich, 1984). Photooxidation may also occur in the lens either indirectly through photosenitizers or directly through absorption of radiation (usually by the aromatic amino acids tryptophan or tyrosine) (Lerman and Borkman, 1978; Zigman, 1981). In young lenses, these oxidants are usually maintained at harmless levels by the antioxidant defense mechanisms of the lens. However, a decrease in the activity of any of these defense mechanisms with age may result in the oxidation of lens protein with subsequent cataract formation (Spector, 1985). In addition, lens protein may be more susceptible to accumulated damage than proteins in other tissues due to the low turnover of lens fiber protein (Jahngen et al., 1986, 1989; Taylor and Davies, 1987).

The lens has a number of defense mechanisms to protect it from the effects of oxidation. The major defense mechanisms include three enzyme systems: the glutathione (GSH) redox cycle, the superoxide dismutases, and catalase (Fig. 5). These enzyme systems function in concert with nonenzymatic systems. Proteases may also be considered part of the lens defense system as they aid in selective removal of damaged proteins (Jahngen et al., 1982, 1990; Taylor and Davies, 1987). Reduced activity of each of these components is believed to play some role in cataract formation.

The GSH redox cycle is composed of three compoents: the tripeptide GSH, the enzyme glutathione peroxidase, and the enzyme glutathione reductase (Fig. 6). GSH, which is present at much higher levels in the lens than in other tissues

$$2O_2^- + 2H^+ \xrightarrow[\text{dismutase}]{\text{superoxide}} H_2O_2 + O_2$$

$$2H_2O_2 \xrightarrow{\text{catalase}} 2H_2O + O_2$$

$$H_2O_2 + 2GSH \xrightarrow[\text{peroxidase}]{\text{glutathione}} 2H_2O + GSSG$$

Figure 5 Enzymatic antioxidant defense mechanisms of the lens. H_2O_2 = hydrogen peroxide; GSH = reduced glutathione; GSSG = oxidized glutathione.

(Kuck, 1975), acts as a substrate for glutathione peroxidase, an enzyme which eliminates hydroperoxides. As a result of this process GSH is oxidized, but it can be restored by the enzyme glutathione reductase coupled with the NADPH-regenerating systems. GSH metabolism may contribute significantly to detoxification of hydrogen peroxide in the lens (Giblin et al., 1982). The aqueous humor is known to contain a significant level of hydrogen perioxide and this level in cataract patients has been observed to be almost three times that of patients with normal lenses (Spector and Garner, 1981).

GSH also can act directly as a free radical scavenger and a reducing agent to prevent the oxidation of proteins and disulfide bond formation (Augusteyn, 1979; Rathbun, 1980). As indicated above, cataracts may result from the formation of disulfide bonds. Human cataract formation is known to be accompanied by a progressive decrease in the level of GSH (Harding, 1970; Rawal et al., 1978; Rogers and Augusteyn, 1978).

Other constituents of the lens, either directly or indirectly, influence this enzyme system (Fig. 6). Selenium is a cofactor for the enzyme glutathione peroxidase and riboflavin is a cofactor for the enzyme glutathione reductase. Ascorbate and tocopherol have apparent sparing effects on the GSH redox cycle (Wefers and Seis, 1988).

The superoxide dismutases (SOD) protect the lens from superoxide, producing hydrogen peroxide in the process. Decreased activity of SOD accompanies the formation of cataracts in human lenses (Fecondo and Augusteyn, 1983; Ohrloff and Hockwin, 1984). Catalase may also protect the lens from hydrogen peroxide (Varma et al., 1982).

MICRONUTRIENT INVOLVEMENT IN CATARACT FORMATION

Because of the role of oxidation in cataract formation, research on nutritrion and cataracts has emphasized the micronutrients with direct or indirect antioxidant

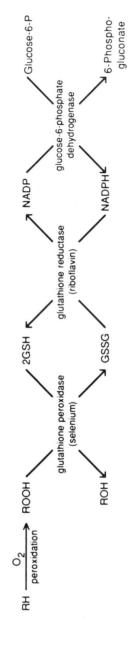

Figure 6 The glutathione peroxidase system. RH = polyunsaturated fatty acid; ROOH = fatty acid hydroperoxide; ROH = hydroxy fatty acid; GSH = reduced glutathione; GSSG = oxidized glutathione.

capabilities. Most of the data presented herein describe the relationship between specific micronutrients and cataracts. The effects of interactions among these nutrients on cataract risk have not been extensively studied.

Ascorbate

Experimental Evidence

Ascorbate is probably the most effective, least toxic antioxidant identified in mammalian systems (Seib and Tolbert, 1982; Frei et al., 1988). Interest in the function of ascorbate in the lens was prompted by teleological arguments based on the observation that lens ascorbate concentration can be as much as 30 times greater than that of plasma (Varma, 1987; Berger et al., 1988, 1989) and aged and cataractous human lens ascorbate concentrations are lower than in the normal lens (Wilczek, 1968; Rawal et al., 1978). In the lens nucleus, the oldest part of the lens and the region of origin of most senile cataracts, the concentration of ascorbate is 25% of that in the surrounding cortex (Nakamura and Nakamura, 1935). Furthermore, ascorbate levels in the lens are significantly lower in old guinea pigs than in young animals with the same dietary intake of ascorbate (Berger et al., 1989).

In vivo studies using guinea pigs, one of the few species for which ascorbic acid is an essential nutrient, indicate that dietary ascorbate may retard or delay the development of galactose-induced cataracts (Kosegarten and Maher, 1978). Dietary ascorbate also reduced the progression of galactose-induced cataracts in rats (Vinson et al., 1986). Treatment of chick embryos with glucocorticoid is known to decrease GSH levels and promote cataract formation. Administration of ascorbate to chick embryos after glucocorticoid treatment reduced the loss of GSH and prevented lens opacification (Nishigori et al., 1985). High dietary ascorbate intakes have been shown to delay UV-induced protein damage in extracted guinea pig lenses (Blondin et al., 1986). In vitro studies of rat lenses demonstrated that light-induced damage to the lens from photochemically produced superoxide was prevented in the presence of ascorbate levels comparable to that of the aqueous humor (Varma et al., 1979, 1982). Blondin et al. (1987) demonstrated that rabbit lens preparations with enhanced ascorbate were better able to withstand photooxidative changes in lens proteins and proteases than unsupplemented preparations.

Epidemiological Evidence

Two epidemiological studies have reported an inverse association between ascorbate status and cataract risk. In a case control study with 175 cases with advanced cataract and 175 controls, Robertson et al. (1989) compared the risk of senile cataracts among regular (daily) ascorbic acid supplement users (who consumed on average 300–600 mg/day) to the risk among persons who did not consume ascorbic acid supplements on a regular basis (Table 1). The risk of senile cataract among the supplement users are only 30% of that seen in non-supplement users.

In a smaller case control study, Jacques et al. (1988a) classified subjects into three plasma ascorbate categories: low (below 40 μmol/liter), moderate (40–90 μmol/liter), and high (greater than 90 μmol/liter). The risk of cataracts for subjects with high plasma ascorbate was about 30% of the risk for subjects with levels below 40 μmol/liter; however, this difference in risk was not statistically significant (Table 2). The risk of cataract for persons with plasma ascorbate between 40 and 90 μmol/liter was comparable to the risk for subjects with ascorbate levels below 40 μmol/liter. The magnitude of the reduction in risk was similar to that seen by Robertson et al. (1989). The relationship between plasma ascorbate and risk of cataract in the posterior subcapsular region of the lens was also considered. Persons with high ascorbate had only one-tenth of the risk observed among persons with ascorbate levels below 40 μmol/liter.

Data from a large case control study conducted in India indicate that the risk of combined posterior subcapsular and nuclear cataract increased about 90% for an increment in plasma ascorbate of 1 SD (Mohan et al., 1989). However, this same study reported that lower levels of an antioxidant index based in part on plasma ascorbate were associated with increased combined posterior subcapsular and nuclear cataract risk (see section, "Antioxidant Nutrient Indices"). Possible reasons which could account for the increased cataract risk with increasing plasma ascorbate were not addressed by the authors.

Tocopherol

Experimental Evidence

The relationship between tocopherol and senile cataract has also received substantial attention. Whereas ascorbate is water-soluble, tocopherol is lipid-soluble and is the major lipid-soluble antioxidant (Machlin and Bendich, 1987). In vitro studies indicate that tocopherol prevents photoperoxidation of lens lipids (Varma

Table 1 Risk of Senile Cataract in Consumers of Vitamin C and E Supplements Relative to Nonconsumers of Supplements

Supplement	Relative risk	Significance (*p* value)
Vitamin C	0.30	0.05
Vitamin E	0.44	<0.01
Vitamin C and E	0.32	0.05

Source: Robertson et al. 1989.

Table 2 Risk of Senile Cataract in Persons with Low and Moderate Plasma Nutrient Levels Relative to Persons with High Plasma Nutrient Levels

Nutrient	Cataract location[b]	Relative risk by plasma nutrient levels[a]		
		Low	Moderate	High
Vitamin C	ANY	1	1.09	0.29
	CX	1	0.91	0.27
	PSC	1	0.73	0.09[c]
Vitamin E	ANY	1	1.00	0.83
	CX	1	0.90	0.84
	PSC	1	1.10	0.33
Riboflavin	ANY	1	0.63	0.54
	CX	1	0.51	0.55
	PSC	1	0.57	0.21
Carotenoids	ANY	1	0.25	0.18[c]
	CX	1	0.22	0.14[d]
	PSC	1	0.11	0.18

[a] See text for definitions of high, moderate, and low.
[b] ANY = any cataract; CX = cortical cataract; PSC = posterior subcapsular cataract.
[c] $0.05 < p < 0.10$.
[d] $p < 0.05$.
Source: Jacques et al., 1988a.

et al., 1982). Like other cells, lens cells have lipid-containing cell membranes, and the integrity of such membranes must be preserved to maintain transport and other critical functions. In vivo protective effects of tocopherol appear to be due to its ability to stabilize cell membranes (Libondi et al., 1985). Tocopherol may also help maintain reduced glutathione levels in the lens and aqueous humor (Costagliola et al., 1986).

Tocopherol is reported to retard the development of cataract-like lens changes in vitro by a number of cataractogenic agents including glucose (Creighton and Trevithick, 1979; Trevithick et al., 1981), galactose (Creighton et al., 1985), sorbitol (Creighton et al., 1985), ionizing radiation (Ross et al., 1983a), heat (Stewart-DeHann et al., 1981), steroids and other cataractogenic drugs (Creighton et al., 1982, 1983). There is also in vivo evidence that tocopherol delays the development of galactose-induced (Bhuyan et al., 1983) and aminotriazol-induced cataracts in rabbits (Bhuyan and Bhuyan, 1984).

Epidemiological Evidence

The relationship between senile cataract risk and tocopherol has been examined in the aforementioned studies of Robertson et al. (1989) and Jacques et al. (1988a).

Robertson et al. reported that subjects taking an average of 400 IU of tocopherol daily in the form of supplements had 40% of the risk of senile cataract as persons not consuming tocopherol supplements (Table 1). Jacques et al. failed to note any difference in the risk of senile cataract between individuals with low (<21 μmol/liter), moderate (21–35 μmol/liter), and high (>35 μmol/liter) plasma tocopherol levels (Table 2). However, it should be noted that only a small percentage (5%) of subjects in this latter study had supplemental intakes at the level of 400 IU per day.

Riboflavin

Experimental Evidence

It is proposed that riboflavin status is linked to cataract formation through its influence on the GSH redox cycle. Riboflavin is a precursor for flavin adenine dinucleotide (FAD), which is a cofactor for glutathione reductase. Through its role in the GSH redox cycle, riboflavin could indirectly influence lens antioxidant capabilities. Recent research by Horwitz et al. (1987) indicates that lens epithelia of patients taking riboflavin supplements or thyroxine showed higher glutathione reductase activity than did lens epithelia of nonconsumers of these substances. Thyroxine enhances glutathione reductase activity by stimulating the enzymatic conversion of riboflavin to FAD. Although laboratory studies have indicated that riboflavin is necessary to maintain lens clarity (as reviewed in Bunce and Hess, 1988), a correlation between riboflavin status and senile cataract has not been firmly established for human populations.

Epidemiological Evidence

Shalka and Prchal (1981) measured riboflavin deficiency in cataract cases and controls with clear lenses. They observed that 34% of the 56 cataract cases over 50 years of age were riboflavin-deficient compared with none of the 16 older controls. No differences in riboflavin status were observed between cases and controls less than 50 years of age. Bhat (1987) observed riboflavin deficiency in 81% of patients with cataract and only 12% of controls. However, thiamine and pyridoxine deficiency were more prevalent in controls than in cataract cases. Both groups appeared to be severely malnourished. Jacques et al. (1988a) measured riboflavin status by in vitro stimulation of erythrocyte glutathione reductase activity expressed as an activity coefficient (AC) and showed no significant differences in cataract risk between the low (AC > 1.22), moderate (AC = 1.02–1.22), and high (AC < 1.02) categories of riboflavin status. However, only 6.5 % of the cases and 3% of the controls in this study were classified as deficient.

Epidemiological evidence cited above suggests that riboflavin deficiency may increase the risk of senile cataract. However, in populations where riboflavin status is adequate, there is no evidence to suggest that riboflavin supplementation can provide any additional protection against cataract.

Carotenoids

Experimental Evidence

There is no experimental evidence relating carotenoids to cataract formation. This is somewhat surprising given the emphasis placed on the antioxidant hypothesis of cataract formation. Beta-carotene demonstrates good radical-trapping and antioxidant behavior at partial pressures of oxygen as low as 15 torr (Burton and Ingold, 1984). The partial pressure of oxygen in the lens is approximately 20 torr (Kwan et al., 1972). In theory, beta-carotene and other carotenoids could play an important role in prevention of cataracts.

Epidemiological Evidence

In the only study to date that examined the relationship between carotenoids and senile cataracts, Jacques et al. (1988a) observed that the risk of cataract among persons with moderate plasma carotenoid levels (1.7–3.3 μmol/liter) was less than 25% of that among persons with carotenoids below this level (Table 2). Higher plasma carotenoid levels (greater than 3.3 μmol/liter) did not offer a substantially lower risk of cataracts.

Antioxidant Nutrient Indices

Jacques et al. (1988b) created a micronutrient antioxidant index for plasma ascorbate, tocopherol, and carotenoids. Subjects in the highest quintile for any two of these nutrients and not in the lowest quintile for the third were assigned to the high antioxidant index category. Subjects with at least one nutrient in the lowest quintile and none of the nutrients in the highest quintile were assigned to the low antioxidant index category. All other were assigned to the moderate category. The results indicate a dose-dependent relationship between antioxidant micronutrient status and risk of senile cataract (Table 3). The risk for subjects with high index scores was only one-fifth of that for persons with low index scores.

Table 3 Relative Risk of Senile Cataract by Plasma Nutrient Antioxidant Status

Antioxidant status[a]		
Low	Moderate	High
1	0.6	0.2[b]

[a] See text for description.
[b] $p < 0.05$ (relative to low).
Source: Jacques et al., 1988b.

The data of Robertson et al. (1989) indicate that supplementation with either ascorbate or tocopherol protect against senile cataract formation; supplementation with both nutrients provided no further protection (Table 1).

Mohan et al. (1989) developed antioxidant indices similar to those described by Jacques et al. (1988b). One of the indices, derived from ascorbate, tocopherol, glutathione peroxidase, and glucose-6-phosphate dehydrogenase levels, demonstrated a strong inverse relationship with combined posterior subcapsular and nuclear cataract risk. Subjects with high index values had approximately one-tenth the cataract risk as subjects with low index values.

Selenium

Experimental Evidence

Selenium is a cofactor for the enzyme glutathione peroxidase, an integral component of the GSH redox cycle. Thus, it would appear that selenium may be required for protection against oxidative insult. However, both deficiency (Sprinker et al., 1971; Lawrence et al., 1974) and excess (McLaren, 1980) of selenium have been associated with elevated risk of experimental cataract.

Epidemiological Evidence

The epidemiological evidence relating selenium and senile cataract formation is limited. The only available data indicate that persons with serum selenium levels greater than 1.27 μmol/liter had a fourfold increased risk of cataract relative to persons with serum selenium levels less than this value (Jacques et al., 1988a). However, this association was only marginally significant ($p < 0.10$). Selenium levels in this study were not unusually high. Only four cases and no controls had elevated serum levels of selenium.

Other Micronutrients

There is scanty evidence relating other micronutrients to cataract formation. Folate intake has also been reported to be significantly lower in cataract patients relative to normal controls (Jacques et al., 1987). The relationship between folate and cataract has not been examined in experimental studies.

There are data linking calcium to cataract formation, although the nature of any relationship and the potential relevance to senile cataract in humans is unclear. Calcium is present in low levels in young lenses and is seen to increase with age (Kuck, 1975). Calcium is known to accumulate in cataractous human lenses (Kuck, 1975) and in experimental cataracts (Bunce et al., 1984). It is uncertain whether this accumulation is a consequence of or cause of cataractous changes. Rabbits maintained on low-calcium diets develop lens changes (Delamere et al., 1981). However, cultures of clear human lenses in calcium-enriched medium resulted in formation of opacities while control lenses remained transparent (Hightower and Farnum, 1985). Cataractogenic effects of calcium may involve alterations in regulating lens cell permeability (Jacob and Duncan, 1981), or in transglutaminase activity (Lorand et al., 1985) and in proteolysis (David and Shearer, 1984; Hightower et al., 1987).

CONCLUSIONS

Senile cataracts are a major cause of disability in the elderly. Although very common, senile cataracts are not inevitable as is evidence by those elderly with insignificant opacities and the wide range of age at onset of senile opacification. Biochemical lens changes associated with cataracts appear to be in part the result of oxidative damage to the lens proteins.

Experimental studies suggest that antioxidant nutrients can delay cataract-like insults to the lens, and the existing epidemiological data corroborate the experimental evidence. These epidemiological data relating the risk of senile cataract and micronutrients, particularly ascorbate, carotenoids, and tocopherol, provides a firm foundation and direction for future work in this area.

RECOMMENDATIONS

It has been known for over 50 years that nutrient deficiency can increase risk of experimental cataract in a number of animal models. Only recently have investigators begun to examine the effects of nutritional status on the risk of human senile cataract. The early results are promising, but data are still limited. These results should be corroborated by prospective studies. In addition, little is known regarding possible effects of nutrient interactions on cataract risk.

In the absence of more data, we recommend a diet consisting of a variety of fruits and vegetables each day. There are not yet enough data to focus our attention on only one or two nutrients. Supplements may be used as nutritional insurance but should not be consumed in place of a prudent diet.

REFERENCES

Anderson EI, Wright DD, Spector A. The state of sulfhydryl groups in normal and cataractous human lens protein. II. Cortical and nuclear regions. Exp Eye Res 1979; 29:233–243.

Archer AG. Cataract formation in anorexia nervosa, Br Med J 1981; 282:274.

Augusteyn RC. On the possible role of glutathione in maintaining human lens protein sulphydryls. Exp Eye Res 1979; 28:665–671.

Aurell E, Tengroth B. Lenticular and retinal changes secondary to microwave exposure, Acta Ophthalmol 1973; 51:764–771.

Benedek GB. Theory of transparency of the eye. Appl Opt 1971; 10:459–473.

Berger J, Shepard D, Morrow F, Sadowski J, Haire T, Taylor A. Reduced and total ascorbate in guinea pig eye tissues in response to dietary intake. Curr Eye Res 1988; 7:681–686.

Berger J, Shepard D, Morrow F, Taylor A. Relationship between dietary intake and tissue levels of reduced and total vitamin C in the guinea pig. J Nutr 1989; 119:1–7.

Beutler E, Matsumoto F, Kuhl W, Krill A, Levy N, Sparkes R, Degnan M. Galactokinase deficiency as a cause of cataracts. N Engl J Med 1973; 288:1203–1206.

Bhat KS. Nutritional status of thiamine, riboflavin and pyridoxine in cataract patients. Nutr Rep Int 1987; 36:685–692.

Bhuyan DK, Podos SM, Machlin LJ, Bhagavan HN, Choudbury DN, Soja WS, Bhuyan KC. Antioxidant in therapy of cataract: II. Effect of all-rac-alpha tocopherol (vitamin E) in sugar-induced cataract in rabbit. Invest Ophthalmol Vis Sci 24(suppl):74.

Bhuyan KC, Bhuyan DK. Molecular mechanism of cataractogenesis. III. Toxic metabolites of oxygen as initiators of lipid peroxidation and cataract. Curr Eye Res 1984; 3:67–81.

Blondin J, Baragi V, Schwartz E, Sadowski JA, Taylor A. Delay of UV-induced eye lens protein damage in guinea pigs by dietary ascorbate. J Free Rad Bio Med 1986; 2:275–281.

Blondin J, Taylor A. Measures of leucine aminopeptidase can be used to anticipate UV-induced age-related damage to lens proteins: Ascorbate can delay this damage. Mech Aging Dev 1987; 41:39–46.

Bunce GE, Hess JL, Fillnow GM. Investigation of low trypotophan induced cataract in weanling rats. Exp Eye Res 1978; 26:399–405.

Bunce GE, Hess JL, Batra R. Lens calcium and selenite-induced cataract, Curr Eye Res 1987; 3:315–320.

Bunce GE, Hess JL, Davis D. Cataract formation following limited amino acid intake during gestation and lactation. Proc Soc Exp Biol Med 1984; 176:485–489.

Bunce GE, Hess JL. Cataract: What is the role of nutrition in lens health. Nutr Today 1988; 23:6–12.

Burton GW, Ingold KU. Beta-carotene: An unusual type of lipid antioxidant. Science 1984; 224:569–673.

Chatterjee A, Milton R.C, Thyle S. Prevalence and etiology of cataract in Punjab. Br J Ophthalmol 1982; 66:35–42.

Clayton RM, Cuthbert J, Phillips CI, Bartholomew RS, Stokoe NL, Ffytche T, Reid J McK, Duffy J, Seth J, Alexander M. Analysis of individual cataract patients and their lenses: A progress report. Exp Eye Res 1980; 31:553–566.

Clayton RM, Cuthbert J, Duffy J, Seth J., Phillips CI, Bartholomew RS, Reid J McK. Some risk factors associated with cataract in S.E. Scotland: A pilot study. Trans Ophthalmol Soc UK 1982; 102:331–336.

Cleary SF, Pasternack BS. Lenticular changes in microwave workers. Arch Environ Health 1966; 12:23–29.

Cordes FC. Galactosemia cataract: A review. Am J Ophthalmol 1960; 50:1151–1158.

Costagliola C, Ivliano G, Menzione M, Rinaldi E, Vito P, Auricchhio G. Effect of vitamin E on glutathione content in red blood cells, aqueous humor and lens of humans and other species. Exp Eye Res 1986; 43:905–914.

Cotlier E. Senile cataracts: Eividence for acceleration by diabetes and deceleration by salicylate. Can J Ophthalmol 1981; 16:113–118.

Creighton MO, Trevithick JR. Cortical cataract formation prevented by vitamin E and glutathione. Exp Eye Res 1979; 29:689–693.

Creighton MO, Trevithick JR, Sanford SE, Dutees TW. Modeling cortical cataractogenesis. IV. induction by Hygromycin B in vivo (swine) and in vitro (rat lens). Exp Eye Res 1982; 34:467–476.

Creighton MO, Sanwal M, Stewart-DeHaan PJ, Trevithick JR. Modelling cortical cataractogenesis: V. Steroid cataracts induced by solumedrol partially prevented by vitamin E in vitro. Exp Eye Res 1983; 37:65–75.

Creighton MO, Ross WM, Stewart-DeHaan PJ, Sanwal M, Trevithick JR. Modelling cortical cataractogenesis: VII. Effects of vitamin E treatment on galactose-induced cataracts. Exp Eye Res 1985; 40:213–222.

Crompton M, Rixon KC, Harding JJ. Aspirin prevents carbamylation of soluble lens proteins and prevents cyanate-induced phase separation opacities in vitro: A possible mechanism by which aspirin could prevent cataract. Exp Eye Res 1985; 40:297–311.

David LL, Shearer TR. Calcium-activated proteolysis in the lens nucleus during selenite cataractogenesis. Invest Ophthalmol Vis Sci 1984; 25:1275–1283.

Dawson CR, Schwab IR. Epidemiology of cataract: A major cause of preventable blindness. Bull WHO 1981; 59:493–501.

Delamere NA, Paterson CA, Holmes DL. Hypocalcemic cataract. I. An animal model and cation distribution study. Metab Pediatr Ophthalmol 1981; 5:77–82.

Delaye M, Tardieu A. Short-range order of crystallin in proteins accounts for lens transparency. Nature 1983; 302:415–417.

Ederer FE, Hiller R, Taylor HR. Senile lens changes and diabetes in two population studies. Am J Ophthalmol 1981; 91:381–395.

Fecondo JV, Augusteyn RC. Superoxide dismutase, catalase and glutathione peroxidase in the human cataractous lens. Exp Eye Res 1983; 36:15–32.

Frei B, Stocker R, Ames BN. Antioxidant defenses and lipid peroxidation in human blood plasma. Proc Natl Acad Sci USA 1988; 85:9748–9752.

Fridovich I. Oxygen: Aspects of its toxicity and elements of defense. Curr Eye Res 1984; 3:1–2.

Garner WH, Spector A. Racemization in human lens: Evidence of rapid insolubilization of specific polypeptides in cataract formation. Proc Natl Acad Sci USA 1978; 75:3618–3620.

Garner WH, Spector A. Selective oxidation of cysteine and methionine in normal and senile cataractous lenses. Proc Natl Acad Sci USA 1980; 77:1274–1277.

Giblin FJ, Reddy VN. High molecular weight protein aggregates in x-ray-induced cataract: Evidence for the involvement of disulfide bonds. Interdis top Gerontol 1978; 12:94–104.

Giblin FJ, McCready JP, Reddy VN. The role of glutathione metabolism in the detoxification of H_2O_2 in rabbit lens. Invest Ophthalmol Vis Sci 1982; 22:330–335.

Gupta PP, Pandey DN, Pandey DJ, Sharma AL, Srivastava RK, Mishra SS. Aspirin in experimental cataractogenesis. Indian J Med Res 1984; 80:703–707.

Hall WK, Bowles LL, Sydenstricker VP, Schmidt HL. Cataracts due to deficiencies of phenylalanine and of histidine in the rat. A comparison with other types of cataracts. J Nutr 1948; 36:277–296.

Hanna C. Radiation cataract. In: Bellows JG, ed. Cataract and abnormalities of the lens. New York: Grune and Stratton, 1975, 217–223.

Harding JJ. Free and protein-bound glutathione in normal and cataractous human lenses. Biochem J 1970; 117:957–960.

Harding JJ. Changes in lens proteins in cataract. In: Bloemendal H, ed. Molecular and cellular biology of the eye lens. New York: John Wiley & Sons, 1981, 327–365.

Harding JJ. Cataract: Sanitation or sunglasses? Lancet 1982; 1:39.

Harding JJ, Crabbe JC. The lens: Development, proteins, metabolism and cataract. In: Dawson H, ed. The eye. New York: Academic Press, 1984, 207–492.

Hightower KR, Farnum R. Calcium induces opacities in cultured human lenses. Exp Eye Res 1985; 41:565–568.

Hightower KR, David LL, Shearer TR. Regional distribution of free calcium in selenite cataract: Relation to calpain. II. Invest Ophthalmol Vis Sci 1987; 28:1702–1706.

Hiller R, Giacometti L, Yuen K. Sunlight and cataract: An epidmiologic investigation. Am J Epidemiol 1977; 105:450–459.

Hiller R, Sperduto RD, Ederer F. Epidemiologic associations with cataract in the 1971–1972 National Health and Nutrition Examination Survey. Am J Epidemiol 1983; 118:239–249.

Hoenders HJ, Bloemendal H. Aging of lens proteins. In: Bloemendal, eds. Molecular and cellular biology of the eye lens. New York: John Wiley & Sons, 1981, 279–326.

Hollows F, Moran D. Cataract: The ultraviolet risk factor. Lancet 1981; 2:1249–1250.

Hollows FC, Douglas JB. Microwave cataract in radiolinemen and control. Lancet 1984; 2:406–407.

Hollwich F, Boateng A, Kolck B. Toxic cataract. In: Bellows JG, ed. Cataract and abnormalities of the lens. New York: Grune and Stratton, 1975, 230–243.

Horwitz J, Dovrat A, Strattsma BR, Revilla PJ, Lightfoot DO. Glutathione reductase in human lens epithelium: FAD-induced in vitro activation. Curr Eye Res 1987; 6:1249–1256.

Jacob TJC, Duncan G. Calcium controls both sodium and potassium permeability of the lens membranes. Exp Eye Res 1981; 33:85–93.

Jacques PF, Phillips J, Chylack LT, Jr, McGandy RB, Hartz SC. Vitamin intake and senile cataract. J Am Coll Nutr 1987; 6:435.

Jacques PF, Hartz SC, Chylack LT, Jr, McGandy RB, Sadowski JA. Nutritional status in persons with and without senile cataract: Blood vitamin and mineral levels. Am J Clin Nutr 1988a; 48:152–158.

Jacques PF, Chylack LT, Jr, Hartz SC, McGandy RB. Antioxidant status in persons with and without senile cataract. Arch Ophthalmol 1988b; 106:337–340.

Jahngen JH, Hass AL, Ciechanover A, Blondin J, Eisenhauer D, Taylor A. The eye has an active ubiquitin-protein conjugation system. J Biol Chem 1986; 261:13760–13767.

Jahngen JH, Lipman RD, Eisenhaur DA, Jahngen EGE, Taylor A. Aging and cellular maturation causes changes in ubiquitin-eye lens protein conjugates. Arch Biochem Biophys 1990; 276:32–37.

Kahn HA, Leibowitz HM, Ganley JP, Kini MM, Colton T., Nickerson RS, Dawber TR. The Framingham Eye Study. I. Outline and major prevalence findings. Am J. Epidemiol 1977a; 106:17–32.

Kahn HA, Leibowitz HM, Ganley JP, Kini MM, Colton T, Nickerson RS, Dawber TR.

The Framingham Eye Study. II. Association of ophthalmic pathology with single variables previously measured in the Framingham Heart Study. Am J Epidemiol 1977b; 106:33–41.

Kinoshita JH. Cataracts in galactosemia. Invest Ophthalmol 1965; 4:786–799.

Klein BEK, Klein R, Moss SE. Prevalence of cataracts in a population-based study of persons with diabetes mellitus. Ophthalmology 1985; 92:1191–1196.

Kosegarten DC, Maher TJ. Use of guinea pig as a model to study galactose-induced cataract formation. J Phar Sci 1978; 67:1478–1479.

Kuck JFR, Jr. Composition of the lens. In: Bellows JG, ed. Cataract and abnormalities of the lens. New York: Grune and Stratton, 1975, 69–96.

Kwan M, Niinikoski J, Hunt TK. In vivo measurement of oxygen tension in the cornea, aqueous humor, and the anterior lens of the open eye. Invest Ophthalmol 1972; 11:108–114.

Lawrence RA, Sunde A, Schwartz GL, Noekstra WG. Glutathione peroxidase activity in rat lens and other tissues in relation to dietary selenium intake. Exp Eye Res 1974; 18:563–569.

Lerman S, Borkman R. Ultraviolet radiation in the aging and cataractous lens: A survey. Acta Ophthalmologica 1978; 56:139–149.

Libondi T, Menzione M, Auricchio G. In vitro effect of alpha-tocopherol on lysophosphatidylcholine-induced lens damage. Exp Eye Res 1985; 40:661–666.

Lorand L, Conrad SM, Velasco PT. Formation of a 55000-weight cross-linked β-crystallin dimer in the Ca^{2+}-treated lens. A model for cataract. Biochemistry 1985; 24:1525–1531.

Lydahl E, Philipson B. Infrared radiation and cataract. I. Epidemiologic investigation of iron- and steel-workers. Acta Ophthalmol 1984a; 62:961–975.

Lydahl E, Philipson B. Infrared radiation and cataract. II. Epidemiologic investigation of glass workers. Acta Ophthalmol 1984b; 62:976–992.

Machlin LJ, Bendich A. Free radical tissue damage: Protective role of antioxidant nutrients. FASEB J 1987; 1:441–445.

McLaren DS. Nutritional Ophthalmology, 2nd ed. London: Academic Press, 1980.

Miller D. A case of anorexia nervosa in a young woman with development of subcapsular cataract. Trans Ophthalmol Soc UK 1958; 78:217–222.

Minassian DC, Mehra V, Jones BR. Dehydrational crises from severe diarrhea or heatstroke and risk of cataract. Lancet 1984; 1:751–753.

Mohan M, Sperduto RD, Angra SK, Milton RC, Mathur RL, Underwod BA, Jaffery N, Pandya CB, Chhabra VK, Vajpayee RB, Kalra VK, Sharma YR. India-US case-control study of age-related cataracts. Arch Ophthalmol 1989; 107:670–676.

Nakamura B, Nakamura O. Uber das vitamin C in der Linse und dem Kammerwasser der menschlichen Katarakte. Graefes Arch Klin Exp Ophthalmol 1935; 134:197–200.

Nishigori H, Hayashi R, Lee JW, Maruyama K, Iwatsuru M. Preventive effect of ascorbic acid against glucocorticoid-induced cataract formation of developing chick embryos. Exp Eye Res 1985; 40:445–451.

Ohrloff C, Stoffel G, Koch H, Wefers U, Bours J, Hockwin O. Experimental cataracts in rats due to tryptophan-free diet. Albrecht V Graefes Arch Klin Exp Ophthalmol 1978; 205:73–79.

Ohrloff C, Hockwin O. Superoxide dismutase (SOD) in normal and cataractous human lenses. Graefe's Arch Clin Exp Ophthalmol 1984; 222:79–81.

Poston HA, Riis RC, Rumsey GL, Ketola HG. The effect of supplemental dietary amino acids, minerals and vitamins on salmonids fed cataractogenic diets. Cornell Vet 1977; 67:472–509.

Prchal J, Skalka H, Clement RS, Bradley EL, Conrad ME. Diabetes and risk of cataract development. Met Pediatr Ophthalmol 1980; 4:185–189.

Rao GN, Lardis MP, Cotlier E. Acetylation of lens crystallins: A possible mechanism by which aspirin could prevent cataract formation. Biochem Biophys Res Commun 1985; 128:1125–1132.

Rathbun WB. Biochemistry of the lens and cataractogenesis: Current concepts. Vet Clin NA (Small Anim Pract) 1980; 10:377–398.

Rawal WM, Patel US, Desai RJ. Biochemical studies on cataractous human lenses. Indian J Med Res 1978; 67:161–164.

Robertson J McD, Donner AP, Trevithick JR. Vitamin E intake and risk fo cataracts in humans. Ann NY Acad Sci 1989; 570:372–382.

Rogers KM, Augusteyn RC. Glutathione reductase in normal and cataractous human lenses (letter). Exp Eye Res 1978; 27:719–721.

Ross WM, Creighton MO, Inch WR, Trevithick Jr. Radiation cataract formation diminished by vitamin E in rat lenses in vitro. Exp Eye Res 1983; 36:645–653.

von Sallmann L, Reid ME, Grimer PA, Collins EM. Tryptophan-deficiency cataract in guinea pigs. Arch Ophthalmol 1959; 62:662–672.

Seib PA, Tolbert BM, eds. Ascorbic acid: Chemistry, metabolism and uses. Washington, DC: American Chemical Society, 1982.

Skalka HW, Prchal JT. Effect of corticosteroids on cataract formation. Arch Ophthalmol 1980; 98:1773–1777.

Skalka HW, Prchal JT. Cataracts and riboflavin deficiency. Am J Clin Nutr 1981; 34:861–863.

Spector A, Garner WH. Hydrogen peroxide and human cataract. Exp Eye Res 1981; 33:673–681.

Spector A. Aspects of cataract biochemistry. In: Marsel H, ed. The ocular lens. New York: Marcel Dekker, 1985, 405–438.

Sprinker LH, Harr JR, Newberne PM, Whanger PD, Weswig PH. Selenium deficiency lesions in rats fed vitamin E supplement rations. Nutr Rep Int 1971; 4:335–340.

Stark WJ, Sommer A. Changing trends in intraocular lens implantation (editorial). Arch Ophthalmol 1989; 107:1441–1444.

Steinkuller PG. Cataract: The leading cause of blindness and vision loss in Africa. Soc Sci Med 1983; 17:1693–1702.

Stewart-DeHaan PJ, Creighton MO, Sanwal M, Ross WM, Trevithick JR. Effects of vitamin E on cortical cataractogenesis induced by elevated temperature in intact rat lenses in medium 199. Exp Eye Res 1981; 32:51–60.

Stewart-DeHaan PJ, Creighton MO, Larsen LE, Jacob JH, Sanwal M, Baskerville JC, Trevithick JR. In vitro studies of microwave-induced cataract: Reciprocity between exposure duration and dose rate for pulsed microwave. Exp Eye Res 1985; 40:1–13.

Stigmar G. Anorexia nervosa associated with cataract. Acta Ophthalmol 1965; 43:787–788.

Takemoto LJ, Hansen JS. Intermolecular disulfide bonding of lens membrane proteins during human cataracto-genesis. Invest Ophthalmol Vis Sci 1982; 28:336–342.

Taylor A, Davies KJA. Protein oxidation and loss of protease activity may lead to cataract formation in the aged lens. Free Rad Biol Med 1987; 3:371–377.

Taylor A. Associations between nutrition and cataract. Nutr Rev 1989; 47:225–234.

Taylor A, Zuliani AM, Hopkins RE, Dallal GE, Treglia P, Kuck JFR, Kuck K. Moderate caloric restriction delays cataract formation in the Emory mouse. FASEB J 1989; 3:1741–1746.

Taylor HR. The environment and the lens. Br J Ophthalmol 1980; 64:303–310.

Taylor HR, West SK, Rosenthal FS, Munoz B, Newland H, Abbey H, Emmett EA. Effect of ultraviolet radiation on cataract formation. N Engl J Med 1988; 319:1429–1433.

Thomson JA, Hum TP, Augusteyn RC. Reconstructing normal alpha-crystallin from modified cataractous protein. Aust J Exp Biol Med Sci 1985; 63:563–571.

Trevithick JR, Creighton MO, Ross WM, Stewart-DeHaan PJ, Sanwal M. Modeling cortical cataractogenesis: 2. In vitro effects on the lens of agents preventing glucose- and sorbitol-induced cataracts. Can J Ophthalmol 1981; 16:32–38.

Trokel S. The physical basis for transparency of the crystalline lens. Invest Ophthalmol 1962; 1:493–501.

Truscott RVW, Augusteyn RC. The state of sulfhydryl groups in normal and cataractous human lenses. Exp Eye Res 1977; 25:139–148.

Varma SD, Kumar S, Richards RD. Light-induced damage to oscular lens cation pump: Prevention by vitamin C. Proc Natl Acad Sci USA 1979; 76:3504–3506.

Varma SD, Srivastava VK, Richards RD. Photoperoxidation in lens and cataract formation: Prevention role of superoxide dismulase, catalase and vitamin C. Ophthal Res 1982; 14:167–175.

Varma SD, Beachy NA, Richards RD. Photoperoxidation of lens lipids: Prevention by vitamin E. Photochem Photobiol 1982; 36:623–626.

Varma SD. Ascorbic acid and the eye with special reference to the lens. Ann NY Acad Sci 1987; 498:280–306.

Vinson JA, Possanza CJ, Drack AV. The effect of ascorbic acid on galactose-induced cataracts. Nutr Rep Int 1986; 33:665–668.

Vision Research: A National Plan. The Report of the Cataract Panel, Vol. 2, Part 3 (1983), US Dept HHS, NIH Publication No. 83-2473.

Wefers H, Seis H. The protection of ascorbate and glutatione against microsomal lipid peroxidation is dependent on vitamin E. Eur J Biochem 1988; 174:353–357.

Wilczek M. Zawartosc witaminy C w roznych typach zacm. Klin Oczna 1968; 38:477–480.

Zigman S, Groff J, Yulo T, Griess G. Light extinction and protein in the lens. Exp Eye Res 1976; 23:555–567.

Zigman S, Datiles M, Torczynski E. Sunlight and human cataract. Invest Ophthalmol Vis Sci 1979; 18:462–467.

Zigman S. Photochemical mechanisms in cataract formation. In: Duncan G, ed. Mechanisms of cataract formation in the human lens. London: Academic Press, 1981, 117–149.

17

Changing American Diets

Susan Welsh and Joanne F. Guthrie

Human Nutrition Information Service, U.S. Department of Agriculture
Hyattsville, Maryland

INTRODUCTION

In the past decade, research has supplied increasing evidence of the link between diet and health. Much of this evidence is based on epidemiological studies of various populations. This investigative approach, with its reliance on population-based research both for identification of diet/health relationships and for assessment of dietary guidance needs, has created a new interest in timely data on the food and nutrient intakes of the American population and important subpopulation groups. The U.S. Department of Agriculture (USDA) has a long history in this area of applied research. Its U.S. Food Supply Series, which reports the amounts of foods and nutrients available for consumption in the U.S. food supply since 1909, is the only source of data on trends in the levels of foods and nutrients in the American diet since the beginning of this century. In addition, since the 1930s, much of the information concerning the diets of Americans at the household and individual levels has come from USDA food consumption surveys. USDA's recent food consumption surveys yield new data on the food consumption trends, eating patterns, and dietary status of Americans which are of special interest to public health professionals, researchers, and clinicians working in nutrition-related areas.

USDA Food Consumption Surveys

USDA's Nationwide Food Consumption Surveys (NFCS), conducted approximately every 10 years, are an important part of the National Nutrition Monitoring System (Life Sciences Research Office, 1989). The Human Nutrition Information Service (HNIS) of USDA conducts these surveys in order to obtain two types of information relating to food consumption: food used by households and food eaten by individuals. The first nationwide survey measuring household food use was conducted in 1936. Since 1965, the Nationwide Food Consumption Surveys have collected data on individual food intake as well as household food use. Data collection for the 1987–1988 NFCS has been completed, and the individual intake data have been released on a documented data tape.*

Continuing Survey of Food Intakes by Individuals (CSFII)

A new type of survey called the Continuing Survey of Food Intakes by Individuals (CSFII) was initiated in 1985 and repeated in 1986. The CSFII provides timely information about the dietary status of the population during the intervals between the large decennial surveys. The 1985 and 1986 CSFII (CSFII-85 and CSFII-86) were designed to assess the food and nutrient intakes of women 19–50 years of age and their 1- to 5-year-old children. These groups were selected because earlier surveys had indicated that they are more likely to be at nutritional risk.

In each year, approximately 1500 women and 550 children were sampled for the basic, all-income sample; separate low-income samples were also collected. Each woman was asked to provide six days of dietary data over a 1-year period for herself and for her participating children. Each day's data were collected at approximately 2-month intervals for each participant, using the dietary recall method. Dietary data include nutrient intakes from food only. Nutrients added to foods (e.g., fortified breakfast cereals) are included, but nutrients obtained from vitamin/mineral supplements are not included in USDA estimates of dietary intakes of nutrients. However, participants are queried on use of vitamin/mineral supplements.

Many participants did not provide data for all 6 days; most, however, reported at least 4 days of dietary intake. USDA has published a series of CSFII reports, using food and nutrient intakes of women and children reporting 1 day or 4 days of information. To develop 4-day data sets, if a woman or child reported 4 days data, all were used; if a woman reported more than 4 days, the first day's data and three of the remaining days, selected randomly, were used. In 1985, data for 1 day's dietary intake were also collected from a national sample of men 19–50 years of age. Reports published from the surveys describe samples and procedures in detail (USDA, 1986b, 1987, 1988).

The CSFII was discontinued during the NFCS 1987–1988 but was resumed

---

* NFCS 1987–1988 data tapes are available from the National Technical Information Service, 5285 Port Royal Rd, Springfield, VA 22161.

in 1989 and will be conducted annually until 1996. In 1989 as well as in future years, the CSFII will include data collected from men and women of all ages. Each year the CSFII will consist of two samples: a sample of individuals in 1500 all-income households and a sample of individuals in 750 low-income households. All household members will provide 3 days of dietary data—a 1-day recall and a 2-day record. The survey has been redesigned to support moving average reporting as a means of providing trend information on the entire population in a timely, cost-effective manner. These data will be reported as 2-year moving averages for women and men 20–49 years of age and 3- to 5-year moving averages for other sex-age groups. Results will be used to provide data on food and nutrient intakes every year, beginning in 1990.

The redesigned CSFII has been modified to accommodate survey modules from HNIS and other agencies that have concerns relative to nutrition monitoring. In 1989, the survey was expanded to include a module on consumer knowledge and attitudes on diet/health and food safety issues which was planned cooperatively with the Food and Drug Administration and USDA's Food Safety and Inspection Service. This Diet and Health Knowledge Survey represents the first time that a nationwide sample will be used to study the relationship between individuals' knowledge and attitudes about foods, nutrition, and food safety, and their actual dietary intake.

Nutrient intake levels for CSFII respondents are calculated using nutrient values obtained from the National Nutrient Data Bank (NDB), which stores, processes, and summarizes data on the nutrient composition of food. The NDB is maintained by HNIS and is used with national food consumption surveys conducted by USDA, the U.S. Department of Health and Human Services (DHHS), and others. Data are included for energy, 28 nutrients, and other food components. Most of the data are based on laboratory analyses. Where analytical data are not available, nutrient values are imputed by food specialists (Perloff, 1989).

FOOD CONSUMPTION TRENDS

Diets reported in the 1985 and 1986 CSFII were very similar, but they differed considerably from diets reported in the 1977–1978 NFCS (USDA, 1983, 1984, 1985a,b, 1986b, 1987, 1988). Some important differences between the food intakes of adult men and women (aged 19–50 years) in 1977 and 1985, based on data for a single day (USDA, 1985b, 1986b), are shown in Table 1. One of the most striking changes was the shift from whole to low-fat and skim milk. Both men and women consumed less whole milk; intakes of low-fat and skim milk, on the other hand, increased greatly. Among women, higher income women used more low-fat milk (see Fig. 1). Only about one-third of the fluid milk intake of lower income women was low fat or skim, while the higher income groups drank one-half to two-thirds of their total milk as low fat or skim. Mean intake of milk and milk products by black women was substantially lower than that for

Table 1 Changes in the Diets of Women and Men: 1977 and 1985 (from NFCS 77–78 and CSFII-85, 1 Day, Spring)

	Percent change	
	Women	Men
More:		
Skim low-fat milk	+ 60	+ 53
Carbonated soft drinks	+ 53	+ 74
Meat mixtures	+ 35	+ 5
Grain products	+ 29	+ 8
Less:		
Whole milk	− 35	− 25
Meat	− 34	− 26
Eggs	− 28	− 26

white women; almost all of the fluid milk drunk by black women was whole milk rather than low-fat or skim milk.

Mean 1-day intakes of cheese and of cream and milk desserts (e.g., ice cream) did not change greatly between 1977 and 1985. However, a higher percentage of men and women reported using cheese and cream and milk desserts during a 1-day period in 1985 compared to 1977. In 1985, 34% of women ate cheese on the survey day, an increase from 28% in 1977. The proportion of men using cheese rose from 26% in 1977 to 33% in 1985. The increase in use of cream and milk desserts was smaller—from 20% in 1977 to 25% in 1985 for women; from 21% in 1977 to 23% in 1985 for men. During the same time period, the percentage of individuals using yogurt in a 1-day period rose from 3 to 5% among women and 1 to 2% among men.

Compared with 8 years earlier, men and women in 1985 consumed less meat as a single item entree and fewer eggs. For decades, surveys have shown, as the 1977 data illustrate, that as income increases, the consumption of meat increases (Fig. 2). In 1985, intakes of meat as a single-item entree were lower than in 1977 for all three income categories of women. Among women, the decrease in meat intake appears to be attributable primarily to decreased intakes of higher fat meats. Popkin et al. (1989) sorted meats (beef/pork) and lunchmeats into categories based on fat content and used USDA data to look at the change between 1977 and 1985 in women's consumption of these items over a 3-day period. They found that intakes of higher fat meats and lunchmeats decreased, while intakes of the lower fat items increased.

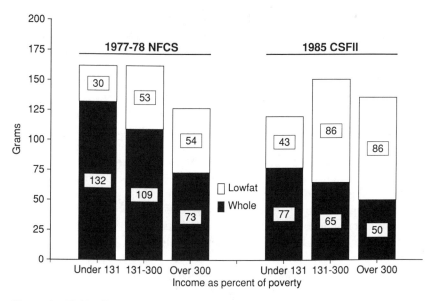

Figure 1 Fluid milk: Mean intakes (g) by women 19–50 years, by income, 1 day, spring 1977 and 1985. (From CSFII-85 and NFCS 77-78.)

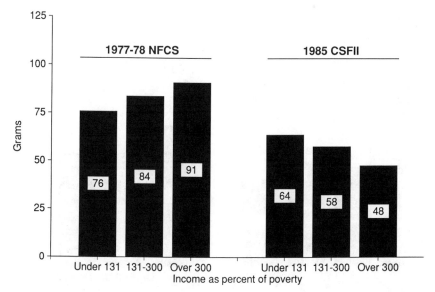

Figure 2 Meat: Mean intakes (g) by women 19–50 years, by income, 1 day, spring 1977 and 1985. (From CSFII-85 and NFCS 77-78.)

The apparent decline in meat intake may or may not be real. In the past decade, women have shifted away from eating meat as a separate item toward eating mixtures that are mainly meat, poultry, or fish. Perhaps rather than eating less meat, women are just changing the way they eat it.

Not only were fewer eggs reported to be consumed; a smaller percentage of individuals reported eating eggs on the survey day. In 1977, 29% of women ate eggs on the survey day; this dropped to 24% in 1985. Among men, the percentages reporting using eggs were 34% in 1977 and 28% in 1985.

Two other trends that are worthy of note are, first, the increase in consumption of mixtures that were mostly grain, and second, the increase in carbonated soft drinks. Grain mixtures include such items as pizza and macaroni-and-cheese. Intakes of total grain products rose between 1977 and 1985, primarily due to the increase in grain mixtures. Larger increases were seen for women than for men.

Soft drink consumption increased substantially between 1977 and 1985. The greatest increase occurred in consumption of low-calorie soft drinks, even though regular soft drinks remained the predominant choice of both men and women. Use of low-calorie soft drinks showed little change from 1977 to 1985 among low-income women, but there were large increases in use among higher income women (Fig. 3).

Consumption trends for other important foods, most notably fruits and vegetables, were more difficult to assess. Data from CSFII-85 (USDA, 1985b, 1986b)

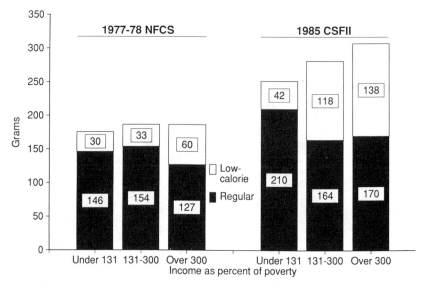

Figure 3 Soft drinks: Mean intakes (g) by women 19–50 years, by income, 1 day, spring 1977 and 1985. (From CSFII-85 and NFCS 77-78.)

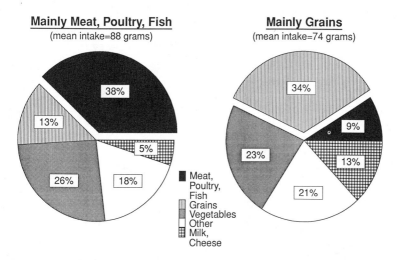

Figure 4 Distribution of mixture ingredients, women 19–50 years, 1 day, 1985. (From CSFII-85.)

indicated a small increase in consumption by men of vegetables eaten separately and a small decrease in intake by women. However, because many meat- and grain-based mixtures (such as casseroles and pizza) include vegetables, some of the vegetables consumed are reported in these categories. Thus, vegetable consumption may be higher than these figures suggest. This is especially likely in 1985, when consumption of meat and grain mixtures was higher than in 1977.

Recently, HNIS developed a methodology for breaking down the food mixtures that people report eating into their component parts. As Fig. 4 illustrates, vegetables are substantial components of both meat- and grain-based mixtures. When vegetables reported as a part of mixtures are combined with vegetables reported separately, a better picture of the trends in vegetable intake emerges. In 1985, again using 1-day data, the vegetables women consumed as part of mixtures represented about one-fifth of all vegetables consumed. Using data on the intake of meat- and grain-based mixtures in 1977–1978, and assuming that vegetables made the same contribution to these mixtures as they did in 1985, HNIS established the intakes of vegetables from mixtures for women at both time points. When the contribution of food mixtures to vegetable intakes is considered, the total intakes of vegetables for women were virtually the same in both periods of time.

Food Selection Patterns

While 1-day data were used to examine food consumption trends over time, food selection patterns are better assessed by looking at several days of data. Using

Table 2 Food Selections of Women (from CSFII-85)

Food	Percent of women using a food or foods from each group	
	Over 1 day	Over 4 days
Legumes, nuts, seeds	22	55
Other vegetables	83	99
White potatoes	44	83
Tomatoes	29	75
Dark green	9	30
Deep yellow	9	29
Fruit	47	81
Citrus	25	56

4-day data from CSFII-85 (USDA, 1987) to look at the proportions of women selecting certain foods provides interesting information regarding eating patterns. Some food groups were almost universally consumed: over the 4 days surveyed, more than 95% of all women chose a food or foods from the milk and milk products group and 99% ate meat, poultry, or fish. However, a sizable proportion of women omitted selections from several important food groups (Table 2). For example, just over one-half of women surveyed ate any legumes, nuts, nut butters, or seeds during the 4 days surveyed; less than one-third ate dark green vegetables, and the same for deep yellow vegetables. A considerable percentage of women— 10–25%, depending on the region of the country—had no fruit or juice during the 4 days. Given that these foods are important sources of several micronutrients, eating patterns that are low in fruits and vegetables are of concern.

Children's Diets

Mean food intakes of children 1–5 years of age for one survey day showed some of the same changes between 1977 and 1985 as were seen in adults. Children consumed more skim and low-fat milk and less whole milk in 1985; they ate more grain products and less meat (consumed as a separate item) and eggs (Table 3). Children's diets, however, showed some changes not seen in those of adults. Young children ate 30% more vegetables and fruits in 1985 than in 1977, while women showed no increase. Children drank smaller amounts of carbonated soft drinks in 1985, while adults drank more.

Changing Meal Patterns

The number and types of meals consumed also changed over the 8 years between 1977 and 1985. Both women and children reported eating more frequently in

Table 3 Comparison of Diet of Children Ages 1–5 Years, 1977 and 1985 (from NFCS 77-78 and CSFII-85, One Day, Spring)

	Percent change
More:	
Skim, low-fat milk	+58
Vegetables/fruit	+30
Grain products	+18
Less:	
Meat	−21
Eggs	−19
Whole milk	−12
Carbonated soft drinks	−12

1985 than in 1977. In 1985, four was the number of meals and snacks reported most often on one survey day, whereas in 1977 three was the usual number. Among men, the number reporting three meals and snacks declined from 37% to 25%, but it was still the most frequently reported response.

Women and children also identified more eating occasions as snacks in 1985 (Fig. 5). In 1977, about 60% of the women and children reported snacking on

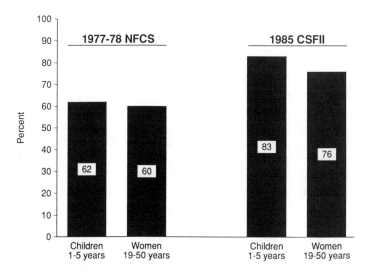

Figure 5 Individuals having snack, 1 day, 1977 and 1985. (From CSFII-85 and NFCS 77-78.)

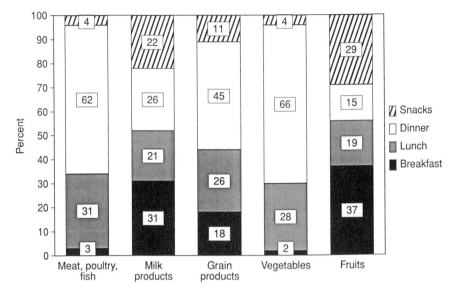

Figure 6 Percentages of food groups consumed by women at meals and snacks, 1985. (From CSFII-85.)

the survey day. This rose to more than 76% on one day in 1985. When responses over four survey days were assessed, essentially all women and children snacked at least once.

The same foods were not selected at meals and snacks (Fig. 6). Over four survey days in 1985, women ate almost all of their meat, poultry, and fish at lunch and dinner (USDA, 1987). The same pattern existed for use of vegetables, with most consumed at lunch and dinner. Among the major food groups, milk and milk products were the most evenly distributed between breakfast, lunch, dinner, and snacks. Women consumed 31% of milk and milk products at breakfast, 26% at dinner, and about 20% at both lunch and snacks. For grain products, almost half were consumed at dinner, with one-fourth eaten at lunch. For fruits, women ate the largest proportion—more than one-third—at breakfast. Snacks were also a popular eating occasion for fruits, with more fruits eaten as snacks than at lunch or dinner.

Almost all women and children reported eating breakfast at least once during the 4 days in 1985. Only 53% of women had breakfast on each of the 4 days; 85% of children had breakfast on each of the 4 days. Fewer black women reported eating breakfast daily: over 4 days throughout the year, twice as many white women as black women (57% vs. 29%) reported eating breakfast every day.

The nutrient contribution of children's breakfast was substantial. Although breakfasts over the 4 days accounted for only 21% of calories and 17% of fat, they provided 30% or more of many important nutrients, including thiamine, iron, vitamin C, calcium, and vitamin A.

Food away from Home

In 1985, adults reported that they consumed 28–33% of their caloric intakes away from home on a single survey day, compared to 22–23% in 1977 (USDA, 1985b, 1986b). Shifts in the eating patterns of women were particularly notable. In 1977–1978, 37% of all adult women aged 19–50 years consumed food only at home over a 3-day period; by 1985, of a comparable group of women, only 14% ate everything at home over three surveyed days (Haines et al., 1988). While in 1977 the eating patterns of the majority of women were dominated by at-home consumption, by 1985 women had developed eating patterns in which away-from-home consumption at eating sites including restaurants, fast-food places, and cafeterias played a much larger role.

Enns and Guenther (1988) analyzed 4-day data from CSFII-85 and found that eating away from home was more common among women at the highest income level than at lower income levels. Away-from-home eating was more common among white than among black women. Women living alone also tended to consume more food energy (calories) away from home than women in larger households.

Foods obtained and eaten away from home differed from those eaten at home. Among all foods and food groups, the proportions that were eaten away from home by women were lowest for fluid milk, cereals and pastas, total milk and milk products, and fruit and fruit juices, and were highest for alcoholic beverages, carbonated soft drinks, and fish and shellfish (Fig. 7).

The effects of away-from-home eating on nutrient intakes varied depending on the nutrient. Food away from home contributed less to vitamin A and vitamin C intakes than to intakes of other nutrients, reflecting the smaller proportions of fruits and vegetables that were eaten away (Fig. 8). It was also found that total fat, fatty acids, and vitamin E had the highest proportions coming from food eaten away.

Guenther and Ricart (1989) also used 4-day data from CSFII-85 to examine the effects of eating at food service establishments (including restaurants, fast-food establishments, and cafeterias) on the nutrient density of women's diets. Higher proportions of calories from food service eating were significantly correlated with lower densities of carbohydrate, vitamin C, fiber, calcium, and iron, as well as with higher densities of alcohol, polyunsaturated fatty acids, saturated fatty acids, and total fat. No statistically significant association was found with protein, cholesterol, vitamin A, or zinc densities.

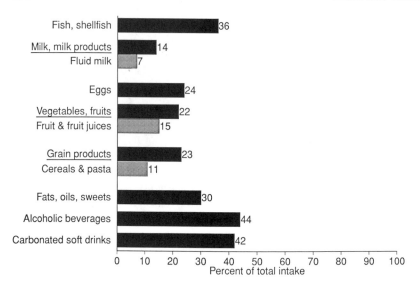

Figure 7 Food eaten away from home as a percentage of total intake by women 19–50 years, four nonconsecutive days, 1985. (From CSFII-85.)

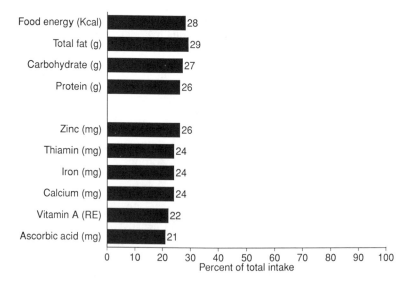

Figure 8 Nutrient contribution of food eaten away from home as a percentage of total intake, women 19–50 years, four nonconsecutive days, 1985. (From CSFII-85.)

DIETARY STATUS

Dietary status, of course, depends on the total intake of nutrients and other food components, whether obtained from meals or snacks, at home or away from home. USDA has used 4-day data to assess the dietary status of women and children rather than 1-day data in order to provide a better approximation of usual intake. Using CSFII-85 data (USDA, 1987), intakes were compared to the Recommended Dietary Allowances or RDAs (Food and Nutrition Board, 1989) for the following nutrients: protein, vitamin A, vitamin E, vitamin C, thiamine, riboflavin, niacin, vitamin B_6, folacin, vitamin B_{12}, calcium, phosphorus, magnesium, iron, and zinc. Tables 4–6 present the mean intakes by women and children (aged 1–3 and 4–5 years) of selected nutrients for which lower-than-recommended intakes by some Americans were noted (Life Sciences Research Office, 1989; USDA, 1987). To illustrate the range of intakes of these micronutrients, intakes at the 25th, 50th, and 75th percentiles for these population groups are also presented. As a point of reference, the RDA for each micronutrient is given.

In Table 4, several nutrients are presented for which the majority of women had intakes below RDA levels. Although mean intakes of vitamin A and folacin were above the RDA, distributions of intake were skewed, and examination of the range of intakes shows that fewer than one-half of all women consumed the recommended levels of these two nutrients. More than three-quarters did not

Table 4 Dietary Status of American Women, Selected Micronutrients and Food Components (from CSFII-85)

| Nutrient | Mean intake | Intake at selected percentiles | | | RDA, 1989 |
		25th	50th	75th	
Vitamin A (RE)	828	389	631	958	800
Vitamin E (alpha-TE)	7.1	4.4	6.2	8.4	8
Vitamin C (mg)	77	39	65	103	60[a]
Vitamin B_6 (mg)	1.16	0.81	1.07	1.42	1.6
Folacin (μg)	189	124	175	234	180
Calcium (mg)	614	378	545	777	800[b]
Phosphorus (mg)	966	718	906	1176	800[b]
Magnesium (mg)	207	153	199	256	280
Iron (mg)	10.1	7.5	9.7	12.0	15
Zinc (mg)	8.6	6.3	8.2	10.3	12

[a] For regular cigarette smokers, the recommended level is 100 mg.
[b] RDA listed is for women 25–50; RDA for women 19–24 is 1200 mg.

Table 5 Dietary Status of American Children, 1–3 Years, Selected Micronutrients and Food Components (from CSFII-85)

Nutrient	Mean intake	Intake at selected percentiles			RDA, 1989
		25th	50th	75th	
Vitamin A (RE)	798	557	730	895	400
Vitamin E (alpha-TE)	5.6	3.6	4.6	6.1	6
Vitamin C (mg)	83	46	67	111	40
Vitamin B_6 (mg)	1.21	0.93	1.18	1.40	1.0
Folacin (μg)	180	133	165	216	50
Calcium (mg)	758	611	740	912	800
Phosphorus (mg)	962	803	942	1111	800
Magnesium (mg)	188	155	188	215	80
Iron (mg)	9.5	7.4	8.9	10.6	10
Zinc (mg)	7.1	5.8	6.7	8.0	10

meet their RDAs for vitamin B_6, iron, zinc, magnesium, and calcium. Among children, there were fewer nutrient intakes below recommended levels (Tables 5 and 6). However, most of the children studied, especially among those 1–3 years old, failed to meet the RDAs for iron, zinc, and calcium.

Among both women and children, mean vitamin E intakes were somewhat lower than recommended levels. Women's mean intake of phosphorus was above

Table 6 Dietary Status of American Children, 4–5 Years, Selected Micronutrients and Food Components (from CSFII-85)

Nutrient	Mean intake	Intake at selected percentiles			RDA, 1989
		25th	50th	75th	
Vitamin A (RE)	790	557	715	966	500
Vitamin E (alpha-TE)	5.4	3.7	4.8	6.6	7
Vitamin C (mg)	86	52	70	120	45
Vitamin B_6 (mg)	1.24	0.89	1.20	1.47	1.1
Folacin (μg)	193	144	182	224	75
Calcium (mg)	821	615	793	966	800
Phosphorus (mg)	1035	830	1014	1147	800
Magnesium (mg)	199	160	193	234	120
Iron (mg)	10.0	8.2	9.6	11.4	10
Zinc (mg)	7.7	6.4	7.6	8.7	10

the RDA level for women aged 25–50 years, but below the higher RDA level for women aged 19–24 years. In the case of vitamin E and phosphorus, however, the available evidence on nutritional status suggests little reason for public health concern (Life Sciences Research Office, 1989). Intakes of the other nutrients examined were found to meet or exceed RDA levels for both women and children.

CSFII-85 also included 1-day intake data on diets of men aged 19–50 years (USDA, 1986b). Among men, mean 1-day nutrient intakes closely approximated or exceeded RDA levels for all of the 15 nutrients which were compared to the RDAs. Energy intake levels of men were higher than those of women; essentially, men fared better than women in their nutrient intakes because they ate more food.

Nutrient intakes below the RDAs do not necessarily mean that intakes are below requirements or that physiological nutrient deficiencies necessarily exist. The RDAs are recommended allowance levels for population groups, not individual requirements, and are set high intentionally to cover the needs of almost everyone in a given sex-age group. Where low nutrient intake levels are of concern, dietary guidance should continue to stress the importance of consuming a varied diet and provide special information about foods which are good sources of nutrients that are relatively low in diets.

Recently, 4-day data from CSFII-85 were used for special analyses into the determinants of women's intake of calcium and iron, two nutrients for which underconsumption has been identified as a current public health issue (Life Sciences Research Office, 1989). After controlling for the effects of all other factors, USDA researchers found that higher calcium intakes were associated with being white or a race other than black (Fig. 9). They also found the following factors to be associated with higher intakes: being younger, having more education, having a higher income, being employed part-time as opposed to being employed full-time or not at all, being a participant in the Food Stamp Program, living in a central city or suburban area as opposed to a nonmetropolitan area, living in the midwest or west as opposed to living in the northeast or south, having a child 1–5 years of age living in the household, being taller, being a regular supplement user. Finally, being pregnant or lactating were also factors associated with higher calcium intakes.

USDA researchers divided the CSFII-85 sample of women into tertiles based on iron intake and found that higher intakes by women were significantly associated with being of a race other than white or black (e.g., Asian or Native American), living alone, presence of a male head of household, previously but no longer smoking, and being pregnant.

Dietary Fat and Cholesterol

One of the most notable changes in the diets of men and women between 1977 and 1985 was the decline in the percentage of calories obtained from fat. Over

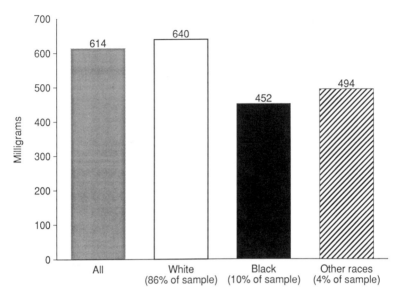

Figure 9   Calcium: Mean intakes (g) by women 19–50 years, by race, 4 non-consecutive days, 1985. (From CSFII-85.)

the 8 years between 1977 and 1985, fat intake decreased from approximately 41% of calories for both men and women to 37% of calories for women and 36% for men (USDA 1985b, 1986b).

Among women, only 12% had fat intakes of no more than 30% of calories over the 4 surveyed days (Harris and Welsh, 1989), the amount recommended by some health authorities (Cronin and Shaw, 1988; Committee on Diet and Health, 1989). Saturated fatty acids provided 13% of calories on the average. Only 10% of women had diets with saturated fatty acids at or below 10% of calories, as suggested by the Food and Nutrition Board's Committee on Diet and Health (1989). However, the Committee's recommendation to limit consumption of dietary cholesterol to 300 mg/day or less was achieved in most of the women's 4-day diets.

In order to better understand the factors associated with different levels of fat intake, USDA researchers divided the CSFII-85 sample of women into quintiles based on their fat intakes as a percentage of calories. The first quintile range in fat intake from 11 to 32% of calories; the second, from 32 to 36%; the third, from 36 to 39%; the fourth, from 39 to 42%; and the fifth, from 42 to 64%.

Analysis of variance revealed significant relationships between quintile of fat intake and intakes of energy and most nutrients. Quintile 1, which had the lowest relative fat intake, also had the lowest mean energy intake and the lowest mean protein consumption. Perhaps surprisingly, the fifth, highest-fat quintile did not show the highest energy intake. This can be attributed to a lower mean carbohydrate intake. Mean fiber intakes were lowest for the first and fifth quintiles.

Thiamine, riboflavin, and vitamin E intakes by quintile of fat intake showed a general pattern of being lowest for the first quintile. Vitamin E intakes were significantly lower within the first quintile than in either the second, fourth, or fifth quintiles—understandable in view of the fact that many foods which are dense sources of vitamin E are also high in fat. Intakes of folacin and vitamin C, two nutrients which are concentrated in fruits and vegetables, were lowest for the fifth quintile of fat intake.

Similarly, mean intakes of most minerals were lowest for the first quintile of fat intake. For iron, they were also low for the fifth quintile. The middle three quintiles had mean intakes of all vitamins and minerals that were either the highest of all the five groups or not significantly different from the highest. The second quintile, which averaged 34% of calories from fat, had relatively good nutrient intakes, combined with lower than average fat intakes.

In women, lower intakes of fat as a percentage of calories were associated with living in the northeast or the south, being a member of a race other than white or black, having less education, being a former smoker or a nonsmoker, and having no children less than 1 year of age. Living in the midwest or the west, being white, having more education, being a current smoker, and having a child less than 1 year of age in the household were all factors associated with an increased probability of having higher fat intakes.

In an analysis of food group sources of fat, Krebs-Smith et al. (1990) used data from four survey days from CSFII-85 to separate mixtures such as sandwiches, casseroles, fried chicken, etc., into their basic food constituents (e.g., bread, meat, and mayonnaise). These food constituents were then regrouped so that the results could be summarized in terms of major food groups (e.g., grains, meats and fats). As Fig. 10 illustrates, when mixtures are separated in this way, less obvious sources of fat, such as fat used in cooking, salad dressings, and sandwich spreads, are identified. This analysis shows that, among these food groups, fats and oils were the primary sources of fat in women's diets in 1985.

Carbohydrate and Fiber

The total amount of carbohydrate in women's diets increased from 41% of calories in 1977 to 46% in 1985, based on 1-day survey data (USDA, 1985b). Among men, the percentage of calories from carbohydrate also increased, from 40% to 45% (USDA, 1986b). Although carbohydrate provided by both starch and sugars has not been measured separately, it is likely that both have increased because the use of certain foods that contain them—such as grain products and soft drinks—has increased. CSFII-85 provided the first national estimates of dietary fiber intakes. Intakes of fiber, based on 1-day data, averaged about 12 g/day for women

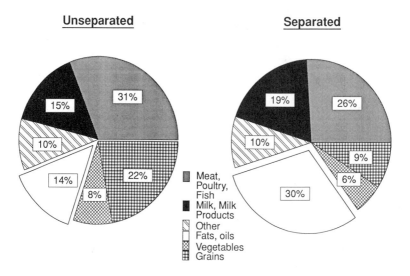

Unseparated

Separated

Figure 10 Total fat: Percent contribution of major food groups when food mixtures are separated vs. unseparated, women 19–50 years, four nonconsecutive days. (From CSFII-85.)

and 18 g/day for men (USDA, 1985b, 1986b). As a point of reference, the National Cancer Institute (Butrum et al., 1988) recommends an intake of 20–30 g/day, not to exceed 35 g/day. Over 4 days, the range in fiber intake was wide for women in 1985—from less than one to just over 40 g/day—but only 5% of the women had intakes greater than 20 g/day.

Using 4-day data from CSFII-85, women were subdivided into tertiles based on their level of fiber intake. Women in the high-fiber tertile had significantly higher intakes of food energy and significantly higher intakes per 1000 kcal of a majority of the vitamins and minerals assessed in CSFII. However, diets higher in fiber were not necessarily lower in fat, saturated fatty acids, and cholesterol. Characteristics found to be significantly positively associated with fiber intake were having a higher level of education, living alone, being a homeowner, being a nonsmoker, and being part of a household in which a male head was present. Race, employment status, and region of residence were also significantly associated with fiber intake. Black women had the highest probability of being placed in the low-fiber tertile, compared to white women and women of other races. Women who worked part time were more likely to be in the high-fiber tertile than either unemployed women or women who worked full time. Women living in the midwest, south, and west were more likely to be in the high-fiber tertile than women living in the northeast.

Relationship of Selected Health Conditions and Health Behaviors to Dietary Status

Pregnancy and Lactation

Pregnancy and lactation are times of special nutritional needs. USDA researchers used 1-day data from the CSFII 1985 and 1986 surveys to compare food and nutrient intakes of pregnant and lactating women with those of nonpregnant, nonlactating women, as well as with current dietary recommendations. Pregnant and lactating women were more likely to use vitamin/mineral supplements than other women: over 80% of pregnant and lactating women used supplements, compared to 53% of other women. The *Dietary Guidelines for Americans* state that certain women who are pregnant or lactating may need a supplement to meet their increased need for some nutrients (USDA/DHHS, 1990).

Pregnant and lactating women also differed from other women in their food selection patterns. They were more likely to use milk products, with fluid milk accounting for the greatest portion of this difference. Among users of milk products, pregnant and lactating women consumed larger amounts than other women; however, intakes were still below recommendations (USDA, 1986a, 1989a). Lactating, but not pregnant, women were more likely to consume both total fruits and juices as well as citrus fruits and juices than were other women. A smaller proportion of pregnant women reported use of regular (caffeine-containing) coffee; only 24% of the pregnant women drank regular coffee vs. 39% of the other women.

Mean dietary intakes of many nutrients were higher among pregnant and lactating women than among other women (Table 7). However, when these nutrient intakes were adjusted for the higher energy intakes by pregnant and lactating women, nutrient intakes per 1000 kcal of pregnant and lactating women were quite similar to those of other women, except for some nutrients, primarily those provided by milk products (Table 8). Compared with diets of other women, diets of both pregnant and lactating women provided more riboflavin, phosphorus, and calcium per 1000 kcal. In addition, lactating women consumed more magnesium and vitamin C per 1000 kcal than did nonpregnant, nonlactating women. Despite their higher mean calcium intake, pregnant women failed to meet their RDA for calcium.

Smoking

Using CSFII-85 1-day data, Larkin et al. (1990) identified several important differences in the food intakes of women smokers and nonsmokers. Consumption of fruits and vegetables by smokers was significantly lower than by nonsmokers, whereas smokers consumed significantly greater amounts of eggs, sugars, regular carbonated soft drinks, coffee, and alcoholic beverages than nonsmokers. After controlling for other health and demographic characteristics, smokers were found

Table 7   Mean Nutrient Intakes of American Women, 19–39 Years, by Physiological Status

Nutrient	Pregnant	Lactating	Other
Energy (kcal)	1947[b]	1989[b]	1629
Protein (g)	76[b]	79[b]	64
Vitamin C (mg)	102	133[b]	83
Thiamin (mg)	1.35[b]	1.50[b]	1.12
Riboflavin (mg)	1.94[b]	2.18[b]	1.40
Vitamin B_6 (mg)	1.60[b]	1.58[b]	1.25
Folacin (μg)	263[b]	299[b]	209
Vitamin B_{12} (μg)	6.2[a]	5.6	4.5
Calcium (mg)	963[b]	1205[b]	637
Phosphorus (mg)	1330[b]	1509[b]	1023
Magnesium (mg)	263[b]	309[b]	217
Iron (mg)	12.9[b]	12.8[a]	10.9
Zinc (mg)	11.0[a]	11.0[a]	9.2

[a] Significantly higher than other women at $p < 0.01$.
[b] Significantly higher than other women at $p < 0.001$.

Table 8   Mean Nutrient Intake per 1000 kcal of American Women by Physiological Status

Nutrient	Pregnant	Lactating	Other
Protein	40	41	41
Vitamin C (mg)	55	71[a]	56
Thiamin (mg)	0.72	0.78	0.70
Riboflavin (mg)	1.02[a]	1.12[b]	0.88
Vitamin B_6 (mg)	0.83	0.84	0.80
Folacin (μg)	143	161	136
Vitamin B_{12} (μg)	3.3	2.9	2.8
Calcium (mg)	500[b]	611[b]	397
Phosphorus (mg)	693[a]	769[b]	642
Magnesium (mg)	137	157[b]	140
Iron (mg)	6.9	6.8	6.8
Zinc (mg)	5.7	5.8	5.8

[a] Significantly higher than other women at $p < 0.01$.
[b] Significantly higher than other women at $p < 0.001$.

Table 9 Percent of Individuals Reporting Use of Supplements (from NFCS 77-78 and CSFII-85, One Day, Spring)

Age groups	1977	1985
Children, all:	47	60
1–3 years	51	61
4–5 years	43	58
Women, all:	39	58
19–34 years	41	56
35–50 years	36	60

to have significantly lower intakes of protein, dietary fiber, vitamin C, and thiamine, and higher cholesterol intakes per 1000 kcal.

Vitamin/Mineral Supplement Use

Not only did food choices change between 1977 and 1985, so did use of vitamin/mineral supplements (1985b). About six out of every 10 women and children reported that they took supplements "every day," "almost every day," or "every so often" (specific frequency of taking supplements not defined) in 1985 (Table 9). This is an increase from four out of 10 women and less than five out of 10 children in 1977. Nutrients obtained from supplements are not included in USDA estimates of dietary intakes of nutrients.

As noted previously, USDA researchers found that supplement users are more likely to have higher calcium intakes from food alone than women who do not use supplements regularly. Although these supplements may or may not include calcium, these results suggest, as other researchers have also noted (Life Sciences Research Office, 1989; Kirinij et al., 1986), that the diets of supplement users provide higher levels of intake of many nutrients from food alone than do the diets of nonusers of supplements.

IMPLICATIONS FOR DIETARY GUIDANCE

While Americans generally are eating nutritious diets, USDA survey data indicate that there is room for improvement. In addition to its food consumption surveys, HNIS conducts applied research on dietary guidance needs and nutrition education strategies. USDA research reaffirms the public's desire for consistent, reliable dietary advice from the federal government.

In order to meet that need, the USDA and the Department of Health and Human Services (DHHS) jointly issued *Nutrition and Your Health, Dietary Guide-*

lines for Americans (USDA/DHHS, 1980; 1985 2nd ed., 1990, 3rd ed.). These guidelines are a statement of federal nutrition policy. The Surgeon General's Report on Diet and Health (DHHS, 1988) provides the scientific basis for these guidelines. As federal policy, the guidelines are the basis of federal nutrition education programs. The guidelines are seven principles for healthful eating: eat a variety of foods; maintain healthy weight; choose a diet low in fat, saturated fat, and cholesterol; choose a diet with plenty of vegetables, fruits, and grain products; use sugars and sodium only in moderation; and if you drink alcoholic beverages, do so in moderation. They are directed to all Americans over the age of 2 years who are not on special diets because of diseases or conditions that interfere with normal nutritional function. This policy and practice helps to ensure that federal agencies "speak with one voice" when issuing dietary guidance to the public.

The first two guidelines—"eat a variety of foods" and "maintain healthy weight"—form the framework of a good diet. The first guideline recommends eating a variety of foods because this is the best way to obtain needed nutrients. Large-dose supplements of nutrients can be harmful. Vitamin and mineral supplements at or below the RDA are safe but are rarely needed if you eat a variety of foods. There are a few exceptions in which use of a supplement under a doctor's guidance may be considered: women in their childbearing years may need an iron supplement to help replace iron lost in menstrual bleeding; women, when they are pregnant or breastfeeding, require more of some nutrients; elderly people who are very inactive and eat little food may need supplements; persons including the elderly, who take medicines that interact with nutrients may need supplements; young children, under some circumstances, may need supplements, especially of iron. The other five guidelines describe characteristics of a good diet—eating plenty of fruits, vegetables, and grain products, and avoiding too much fat, saturated fatty acids, cholesterol, sugar, sodium, and alcohol.

A new Dietary Guidelines Advisory Committee jointly sponsored by USDA and DHHS began work in January 1989 to review the 1985 edition of the *Dietary Guidelines for Americans*. While the Committee agreed that the central messages in the 1985 *Dietary Guidelines* remain sound advice, the new guidelines include more emphasis on translating the guidelines into appropriate food choices. The third edition of the *Dietary Guidelines* was released in the fall of 1990.

REACHING THE CONSUMER WITH DIETARY GUIDANCE

To be truly effective in improving diets, dietary guidance information must reach the consumers who need it; they must understand it and be convinced of its importance and relevance to themselves; and they must know how to apply the information to their own diet. Preliminary results from the new Diet and Health Knowledge Survey indicate that, while many consumers are aware of diet/health relationships, they lack some of the practical knowledge that would help them implement dietary recommendations. Much of USDA's nutrition education research focuses on ways of communicating dietary guidance messages that are understandable and usable to the consumer. Our findings have been applied to the development of a number of new consumer publications.

USDA and DHHS have distributed approximately 12 million copies of the booklet *Dietary Guidelines for Americans* (USDA/DHHS, 1980, 1985, 1990). USDA also published a set of seven short bulletins, *Dietary Guidelines and Your Diet* (USDA, 1986a), which provide information intended to help people put the guidelines into practice. A Dietary Guidelines Teaching Kit was developed in 1988 for junior and senior high-school home economics teachers which contained the *Dietary Guidelines* bulletin, the seven bulletins on the *Guidelines,* and a curriculum guide to help teachers get the *Guidelines* message to this important age group. A similar curriculum guide for high-school health teachers is currently in development. HNIS also provides black-and-white reproducibles and color negatives that allow interested individuals to print their own copies of the *Dietary Guidelines* booklet and support materials.

In July, 1989, HNIS launched a new consumer nutrition education campaign called "Eating Right—The Dietary Guidelines Way." The purpose of this ongoing campaign is to increase awareness of the *Dietary Guidelines for Americans* and to help people put the guidelines into action in their lives. Four new, colorful bulletins were released as part of the *Dietary Guidelines and Your Diet* series. They focus on using all of the *Guidelines* together in particular food-related activities—*Preparing Foods and Planning Menus*; *Making Bag Lunches, Snacks and Desserts*; *Shopping for Food and Making Meals in Minutes*; *and Eating Better When Eating Out* (USDA, 1989a-d).

HNIS developed a new food guide in the early 1980s to provide more specific information that would help people plan diets that follow the *Dietary Guidelines for Americans*. It was first presented as part of a nutrition course developed in cooperation with the American Red Cross (1984), and it has been featured in the USDA series *Dietary Guidelines and Your Diet* (USDA, 1986a, 1989a). The research base for development of the Food Guidance System has been published in an article in the *Journal of Nutrition Education* (Cronin et al., 1987).

The USDA Food Guide is a strategy for planning the total daily food intake. The nutritional objectives for the system are to meet nutrient needs at various calorie levels while avoiding too much fat, saturated fatty acids, cholesterol, sugar, and sodium. It differs from earlier guides because it suggests the total number of servings for all food for the day's intake rather than only the foundation for a day's intake, as earlier guides suggested. There is a clear emphasis on reducing fats, sugars, and sodium, while consuming a diet that contains recommended levels of essential nutrients. The framework of the Food Guide is a core of major groups of nutrient-bearing foods. Special emphasis is put on selected

Table 10 Food Guide Food Groups and Recommended Servings

Food group	Recommended daily servings	Serving size[a]

Fruits
  Citrus, melon, berries
  Other fruits
	2–4.	An average piece of whole fruit, a melon wedge, 6 oz fruit juice, $\frac{1}{2}$ cup berries or sliced or cooked fruit, $\frac{1}{4}$ cup dried fruit

Vegetables
  Dark green and deep yellow
  Starchy, including dry beans and peas
  Other vegetables
	3–5. Include all types regularly. Choose servings of dark green and of dry beans and peas several times a week.	$\frac{1}{2}$ cup cooked or raw, except 1 cup of raw leafy vegetables.

Meat, fish, poultry, and eggs	2–3. A total of 5–7 oz lean daily.	
Milk, yogurt, and cheese	2–3 servings; women who are pregnant or nursing, teenagers, and young adults to age 24 need 3 servings.	1 cup milk, 8 fluid oz yogurt, $1\frac{1}{2}$ oz natural cheese, 2 oz processed cheese

Grains, breads, and cereals
  Whole-grain
  Enriched
	6–11. Included several servings of whole grain products daily.	1 slice of bread, 2 large or 4 small crackers, $\frac{1}{2}$ cup cooked cereal, rice, or pasta; 1 oz ready-to-eat cereal, 1 small roll, muffin, or biscuit. A medium-size roll or muffin is equal to about $1\frac{1}{2}$ servings; a whole English muffin, bagel, hamburger bun, or large roll is equal to 2 servings.

Fats, sweets, alcohol	Fats and sweets in moderation; alcohol, none or in moderation.	

[a] Smaller servings are recommended for young children for all food groups except the milk group; the equivalent of two cups per day from this group is recommended.
Source: Cronin et al., 1987.

subgroups of foods within the major groups which are particularly good sources of nutrients of public health concern. To determine appropriate ranges of servings for different age-sex groups, the nutrient content of diets with different numbers of servings from the major food groups and subgroups were compared with the guidance objectives. The major food groups and subgroups with their corresponding serving recommendations are shown in Table 10. HNIS has just released a new publication that focuses entirely on this food guide called *USDA's Eating Right Pyramid* (USDA, 1991).

To further assist consumers in selecting a nutritionally adequate diet, HNIS recently released a new series of fact sheets entitled *Good Sources of Nutrients* (USDA, 1990b). The 17 fact sheets help consumers select foods that contribute important amounts of vitamins, minerals, and dietary fiber. Other new publications include a revised edition of the popular pocket calorie guide entitled "Calories and Weight: The USDA Pocket Guide (USDA, 1990a)." Currently in production are several materials that focus on the needs of special population groups, e.g., materials adapted for use with low-literacy audiences. HNIS is conducting a project in cooperation with the National Institute of Aging to develop materials to help healthy older Americans implement the *Dietary Guidelines*.

CONCLUSIONS

USDA food consumption survey data show dramatic changes in the diets of Americans between 1977 and 1985. Some of the most notable changes include the shift to consumption of low-fat milk compared to whole milk and the increased consumption of meat mixtures and decreased consumption of meat as a single-item entree. Other changes include a decrease in egg consumption, increased consumption of grain products, and increased consumption of soft drinks. Levels of fruit and vegetable consumption did not change appreciably over the 8-year period between surveys, and food selection patterns indicate that many Americans do not routinely include recommended numbers of servings of fruits and vegetables in their diet.

Eating patterns changed, showing a shift to more frequent eating, with women and children reporting higher average numbers of eating occasions in 1985 compared to 1977. In 1985, individuals also consumed a higher proportion of their food intake away from home. In women's diets, higher proportions of food service eating were significantly correlated with lower densities of some nutrients, such as vitamin C, calcium, and iron, and higher densities of other food components, such as total fat, saturated fatty acids, and polyunsaturated fatty acids.

In 1985, the majority of women 19–50 years of age failed to consume recommended amounts of calcium, iron, zinc, magnesium, vitamin B_6, vitamin A, and folacin. Most children aged 1–5 years failed to meet the RDAs for iron, zinc, and calcium. While nutrient intakes below the RDAs do not necessarily mean that intakes are below individual requirements, low nutrient intake levels indicate the need for dietary guidance stressing the importance of consuming a varied diet and emphasizing foods which are good sources of nutrients low in the diet.

Between 1977 and 1985, the mean percentage of calories obtained from fat in the diets of men and women declined, whereas the percentage of calories from carbohydrates increased. However, fat intake is still in excess of that recommended by some health authorities (Cronin and Shaw, 1988; Committee on Diet and Health, 1989). In 1985, for the first time, national survey data included estimates of dietary fiber intake. Mean intakes of dietary fiber were estimated to be 12 g/day for women and 18 g/day for men, levels below National Cancer Institute recommendations (Butrum et al., 1988).

The emerging evidence connecting nutrition with health in subtle ways, moderated by genetic and behavioral factors (Bloch, 1987), shows the continuing importance of national nutrition-monitoring activities. USDA will continue to play a major role in nutrition monitoring via its U.S. Food Supply Series, its system of Nationwide Food Consumption Surveys, and the new Diet and Health Knowledge Surveys. Survey results will be used to study factors determining food consumption patterns; to target at-risk population groups for nutrition intervention programs; and to develop research-based dietary guidance programs and materials based on actual food intake patterns.

REFERENCES

American College of Obstetricians and Gynecologists (ACOG). Guidelines for perinatal care. Washington, DC, 1988.

American Red Cross. Better eating for better health. Washington, DC, 1984.

Bloch K. Concepts and approaches to scientific inquiry. Am J Clin Nutr 1987; 45:1054–1059.

Butrum RR, Clifford CK, Lanza E. NCI dietary guidelines. Am J Clin Nutr 1988; 48 (Suppl.):888–895.

Committee on Diet and Health, Food and Nutrition Board, National Academy of Sciences. Diet and health: Implications for reducing chronic disease risk. Washington, DC: National Academy Press, 1989.

Cronin FJ, Shaw AM. Summary of dietary recommendations for healthy Americans. Nutr. Today 1988; Nov/Dec:26–34.

Cronin FJ, Shaw AM, Krebs-Smith SM, Marsland PM, Light L. Developing a food guidance system to implement the Dietary Guidelines. J Nutr Educ 1987; 19:281–302.

Enns CW, Guenther PM. Women's food and nutrient intakes away from home, 1985. Family Econ Rev 1988; 1:9–12.

Food and Nutrition Board, Subcommittee on the Tenth Edition of the RDAs, Commission on Life Sciences, National Research Council. Recommended dietary allowances, 10th ed. Washington, DC: National Academy Press, 1989.

Guenther PM, Ricart G. Effect of eating at food service establishments on the nutritional quality of women's diets. Topics in Clin Nutr 1989; 4:41–45.

Haines PS, Popkin BM, Guilkey DK. Dietary status and eating patterns. Prepared for the U.S. Department of Agriculture under Cooperative Agreement No. 53–3198–6–58.

Harris S, Welsh S. How well are our food choices meeting our nutrition needs? Nutr Today 1989; Nov/Dec:20–28.

Kirinij N, Klebanoff MH, Graubard BI. Dietary supplement and food intake in women of childbearing age. J Am Diet Assoc 1986; 86:1536–1540.

Krebs-Smith SM, Cronin FJ, Haytowitz DB, Cook DA. Food group sources of energy-yielding nutrients, cholesterol, and fiber in diets of women: Effect of method of categorizing food mixtures. J Am Diet Assoc 1990; 90:1541–1546.

Larkin FA, Basiotis PP, Riddick HA, Sykes KE, Pao EM. Dietary patterns of women smokers and nonsmokers. J Am Diet Assoc 1980; 90:230–237.

Life Sciences Research Office, Federation of American Societies of Experimental Biology. Nutrition monitoring in the United States—An update report on nutrition monitoring. Prepared for the U.S. Department of Agriculture and the U.S. Department of Health and Human Services. DHHS Publication No. (PHS) 89–1255. GPO# 017–022–01085–2. Washington, DC: U.S. Government Printing Office, 1989.

Perloff BP. Analysis of dietary data. Am J Clin Nutr 1989, 50:1128–1132.

Popkin BM, Haines PS. Reidy KC. Food consumption trends of U.S. women: Patterns and determinants between 1977 and 1985. Am J Clin Nutr 1989; 49:1307–1319.

U.S. Department of Agriculture (USDA). Food intakes: Individuals in 48 states, Year 1977–78. Nationwide Food Consumption Survey 1977–78. NFCS, Report No. I-1. Hyattsville, MD: U.S. Department of Agriculture, 1983.

U.S. Department of Agriculture (USDA). Nutrient intakes: Individuals in 48 states, Year 1977–78. NFCS, Report No. I-2. Hyattsville, MD: U.S. Department of Agriculture, 1984.

U.S. Department of Agriculture (USDA). Food and nutrient intakes: Individuals in four regions, 1977–78. NFCS, Report No. I-3. Hyattsville, MD: U.S. Department of Agriculture, 1985a.

U.S. Department of Agriculture (USDA). Nationwide Food Consumption Survey Continuing survey of food intakes by individuals, Women 19–50 years and their children 1–5 years, 1 Day, 1985. NFCS, CSFII Report No. 85–1. GPO# 001–000–04458–3. Hyattsville, MD: U.S. Department of Agriculture, 1985b.

U.S. Department of Agriculture (USDA). Dietary Guidelines and your diet. Home and Garden Bulletin Nos. 232–1–7. GPO# 001–000–04467–2. Hyattsville, MD: U.S. Department of Agriculture, 1986a.

U.S. Department of Agriculture (USDA). Nationwide Food Consumption Survey: Continuing survey of food intakes by individuals, Men 19–50 years, 1 Day, 1985. NFCS, CSFII Report No. 85–3. GPO# 001–000–04498–2. Hyattsville, MD: U.S. Department of Agriculture, 1986b.

U.S. Department of Agriculture (USDA). Nationwide Food Consumption Survey: Continuing survey of food intakes by individuals, women 19–50 years and their children 1–5 years, 4 days, 1985. NFCS, CSFII Report No. 85–4. Hyattsville, MD: U.S. Department of Agriculture, 1987.

U.S. Department of Agriculture (USDA). Nationwide Food Consumption Survey: Continuing survey of food intakes by individuals, women 19–50 years and their children 1–5 years, 4 days, 1986. NFCS, CSFII Report No. 86–3. GPO# 001–000–04526–1. Hyattsville, MD: U.S. Department of Agriculture, 1988.

U.S. Department of Agriculture (USDA). Preparing foods and planning menus using the Dietary Guidelines. Home and Garden Bulletin 232–8. GPO# 125-W. Hyattsville, MD: U.S. Department of Agriculture, 1989a.

U.S. Department of Agriculture (USDA). Making bag lunches, snacks, and desserts using the Dietary Guidelines. Home and Garden Bulletin 232–9. GPO# 124-W. Hyattsville, MD: U.S. Department of Agriculture, 1989b.

U.S. Department of Agriculture (USDA). Shopping for food and making meals in minutes using the Dietary Guidelines. Home and Garden Bulletin 232–10. GPO# 126-W. Hyattsville, MD: U.S. Department of Agriculture, 1989c.

U.S. Department of Agriculture (USDA). Eating better when eating out using the Dietary Guidelines. Home and Garden Bulletin 232–11. GPO# 123-W. Hyattsville, MD: U.S. Department of Agriculture, 1989d.

U.S. Department of Agriculture (USDA). Calories and weight: The USDA pocket guide. Agriculture Information Bulletin 364. GPO# 178-W. Hyattsville, MD: U.S. Department of Agriculture, 1990a.

U.S. Department of Agriculture (USDA). Good sources of nutrients. GPO# 171-W. Hyattsville, MD: U.S. Department of Agriculture, 1990b.

U.S. Department of Agriculture (USDA). USDA's eating right pyramid. Home and Garden Bulletin 249. Hyattsville, MD: U.S. Department of Agriculture, 1991.

U.S. Department of Agriculture (USDA) and U.S. Department of Health and Human Services (DHHS). Nutrition and your health: Dietary Guidelines for Americans. Home and Garden Bulletin No. 232. Hyattsville, MD: U.S. Department of Agriculture, 1980.

U.S. Department of Agriculture (USDA) and U.S. Department of Health and Human Services (DHHS). Nutrition and your health: Dietary guidelines for Americans, 2nd ed. House and Garden Bulletin No. 232. GPO# 420-W. Hyattsville, MD: U.S. Department of Agriculture, 1985.

U.S. Department of Agriculture (USDA) and U.S. Department of Health and Human Services (DHHS). Nutrition and your health: Dietary guidelines for Americans, 3rd ed. House and Garden Bulletin 232. Hyattsville, MD: U.S. Department of Agriculture, 1990.

U.S. Department of Health and Human Services, Public Health Service. The Surgeon General's report on nutrition and health. DHHS (PHS) Publication No. 88–50210. Washington, DC: U.S. Government Printing Office, 1988.

18

Fruit and Vegetable Consumption: National Survey Data

Blossom H. Patterson and Gladys Block

Division of Cancer Prevention and Control, National Cancer Institute
National Institutes of Health
Bethesda, Maryland

INTRODUCTION

The U.S. Department of Agriculture has long recommended that vegetables and fruit be included in the daily diet because of their vitamin and mineral content and also because they are a good source of fiber. A Daily Food Plan, developed in 1957, suggested four or more servings daily as essential to an adequate diet (U.S. Department of Agriculture, 1957). The 1979 Hassle-Free Guide to a Better Diet (U.S. Department of Agriculture, 1979) suggested eating more fruits and vegetables (again four or more servings daily) as positive steps toward reducing chronic disease incidence. The U.S. Departments of Agriculture and Health and Human Services recommend in their food guidance system that the daily diet include two to three servings of fruits and three to five servings of vegetables (U.S. Department of Agriculture, 1980; Cronin et al., 1987).

Diet and nutrition have been the focus of two recent major reports on the health of the American public. Addressing the role of diet in the prevention of chronic diseases, such as coronary heart disease, some types of cancer, stroke, diabetes mellitus, and atherosclerosis, *The Surgeon General's Report on Nutrition and Health* (U.S. Department of Health and Human Services, 1988) concluded that Americans consume too many foods high in fats, often at the expense of foods high in complex carbohydrates and fiber that may be more conducive to health. The report recommends reducing consumption of fat and increasing consumption of vegetables and fruits. Based on a comprehensive review of the literature, the National Academy of Sciences (NAS) concluded that high fat intake influences the risk of atherosclerotic cardiovascular diseases and possibly certain forms of cancer, while diets high in plant foods are associated with a lower occurrence of coronary heart disease and cancers of the lung, colon, esophagus, and stomach (Committee on Diet and Health, 1989). The NAS recommended eating daily at least five servings of a combination of fruit and vegetables, especially citrus fruits and green and yellow vegetables.

In this chapter, national survey data are examined in an effort to characterize the actual diet of adult Americans with respect to these foods. These surveys are the Second National Health and Nutrition Examination Survey (NHANES II), conducted by the National Center for Health Statistics (NCHS) between 1976 and 1980; the Nationwide Food Consumption Survey (NFCS), conducted by the U.S. Department of Agriculture (USDA) between 1977 and 1978; the Continuing Survey of Food Intakes by Individuals (CSFII), conducted by the USDA in 1985 and 1986; and finally, the Cancer Supplement of the National Health Interview Survey (HIS), conducted in 1987 by the NCHS and the National Cancer Institute. Twenty-four-hour recall, food records, food frequency and diet history data are used. Comparisons are made between the most recent USDA/DHHS recommendations and actual fruit and vegetable consumption, despite the fact that these surveys were conducted when four (or more) daily servings of these foods (rather than five or more) were recommended for an adequate diet. These data thus do not address the impact of the most recent dietary guidelines, but rather may serve as a standard against which to describe the diet.

Other sources of data on fruit and vegetable consumption, such as case control studies and disappearance data, will not be covered here. Dietary information from case control studies typically characterize a particular population group and cannot be generalized to the whole population. Data on the availability of foodstuffs in the marketplace (disappearance data) do not represent actual intakes of individuals because they do not adequately control for wastage.

The focus of this chapter is on actual foods reported rather than on the nutrients contained in them. A large number of epidemiological studies which have compared consumption of either fruits and vegetables or nutrients found in these foods (e.g., beta-carotene, vitamin C, and fiber) have found a protective effect for several cancer sites (Peto et al., 1981; Micozzi, 1989; Block, 1991). However, it is not currently known whether the protective effect found in the majority of these studies derives from the specific nutrient studied, or from some other component or combination of components in the foods eaten.

The various methods of dietary assessment and the problems and advantages of each are discussed. Data by demographic subgroups are presented on the proportions consuming fruits and vegetables, with discussion of the types of these foods consumed. Finally, some health implications of these findings are evaluated.

METHODS OF DIETARY ASSESSMENT

The goal of dietary assessment methods used in surveys is to characterize the diet of groups. Different methods provide different representations of the diet. The surveys discussed in this chapter used the following methods of dietary assessment: 24-hr dietary recall, food records, food frequency and diet history questionnaires. To enhance understanding of the data provided below, these methods of assessment are briefly described and compared. For a more extensive discussion, see Block and Hartman (1989).

24-Hour Recalls

The respondent is asked to report his complete dietary intake of all foods and beverages for the previous 24 hr. The strength of this method lies in its ability to capture very precise and detailed information on the foods consumed. Portion size is often obtained through the use of food models. The 24-hr recall requires a highly trained interviewer and takes about 20–30 min to administer. While this type of data does not provide valid estimates of the usual diet of individuals, it can be used to characterize mean intake for groups (National Center for Health Statistics, 1983). Twenty-four-hour recall data reflect the season during which they are collected; this is particularly important for fruits and vegetables, which are more affected by seasonality than most foods.

Food Records

In this method, respondents are asked to record their diet (typically listing foods eaten and an estimate of portion size) as they are consuming it, frequently for more than a single day. This method requires that respondents be reasonably literate and sufficiently committed to the goals of the survey to record conscientiously all their intake. It requires as well that respondents be instructed in filling out the records by a nutritionist. Multiple days of data, preferably nonconsecutive, provide a measure of habitual intake. The accuracy of records taken on consecutive days was found to decline after the first 2 days (Gersovitz et al., 1978) and to provide less representative data than would an equal number of nonconsecutive days (Hartman et al., 1990). Like 24-hr recall data, consecutive day data reflect seasonality, an effect which can be mitigated when diet recording periods are scattered over the course of a year.

Food Frequency and Diet History Questionnaires

In both of these methods, the respondent is asked to indicate his usual frequency of consumption of each food, or food group, on a list of foods. Food frequency questionnaires ask about frequency of consumption of a list of foods, and diet histories elicit information on portion size as well. A time frame frequently chosen is the previous year, a period sufficiently long to take into account seasonal variation. Information that can be gathered is typically more limited and/or less detailed than that obtained in a 24-hr recall. Responses involve the reporting of patterns of eating behavior (e.g., ''I eat apples about three times a week'') rather than the memory and reporting of specific eating occasions. Both types of questionnaires can be administered by nonnutritionist interviewers or can be self-administered.

Comparison of Dietary Assessment Methods

All methods of dietary assessment have strengths and weaknesses. The 24-hr recall is not a good estimate of an individual's long-term usual diet because dietary intake and food choices vary substantially from day to day. It does, however, provide a reasonably accurate report of foods that were actually consumed on the day of the survey. While it does not categorize *individuals* well with respect to their usual intake, it does provide a useful picture of the food consumption of *groups*. Twenty-four-hour recall data can be used to describe with considerable accuracy the average food intake of Americans, or of subgroups by sex, race, or age, for example.

A quantified food frequency or diet history provides a reflection of an individual's usual intake, since it refers to a longer time period than a single day. It is thus more appropriate for epidemiological studies on the relationship between usual dietary intake and disease. Both methods describe the *distribution* of intakes better than a 24-hr recall, and can provide information about the proportion of the population which may consume certain foods very frequently or very infrequently. However, the estimates of consumption are imprecise because of errors in an individual's report of frequency of consumption and because of methodological features of the instrument itself. Almost invariably, when respondents are presented with a long list of individual vegetables or fruits on a questionnaire, the sum of all the individual frequencies is more than the true overall frequency of consumption of vegetables or fruits. Conversely, a food list which contains too few meat items, for example, may underestimate the true consumption of protein sources.

Data from many types of instruments are presented here. It is not possible or appropriate to compare them directly, or to draw conclusions regarding time trends in intake from different types of instruments used at different time points. However, each method is internally consistent and may be used to compare subgroups within the same survey.

DESCRIPTION OF SURVEYS

The survey data presented below are from nationally representative samples. The NHANES II survey obtained a representative sample of the U.S. population ages 6 months to 74 years (National Center for Health Statistics, 1981). The Health Interview Survey likewise is a representative sample of the U.S. population, but through age 99. This form of sampling permits generalization of the survey results to the U.S. population. Both the NFCS and the CSFII data are based on a probability sample of households (as opposed to individuals), so results from these surveys can be generalized to U.S. households.

Second National Health and Nutrition Examination Survey

The Second National Health and Nutrition Examination Survey (NHANES II) was conducted between 1976 and 1980. A highly stratified multistage design was used to obtain a representative sample of the civilian noninstitutionalized U.S. population. Dietary interviews included both a 24-hr recall and a brief food frequency questionnaire. The interviews were conducted by persons with a knowledge of food preparation methods and nutrient composition. For the 24-hr recall portion, the interviewer recorded the quantity of each food or drink consumed during the previous day, using three-dimensional models to improve portion size quantification. Almost all recall days were weekdays. For the food frequency portion, respondents were asked the frequency with which they consumed foods in various food groups during the preceding 3 months in an effort to ascertain the usual pattern of food consumption. Examination locations were scheduled in the south in the cooler seasons and the north in the warmer seasons, possibly introducing some bias into the reporting of fruit and vegetable consumption.

The NHANES II data presented below are for 10,313 white and 1335 black adults aged 19–74 years, representing about 132 million individuals. Respondents of "other" races were omitted because of small numbers, as were imputed, unreliable, or surrogate data. Data are presented by demographic group. Further, to study the effect of income on fruit and vegetable consumption, the population is divided into thirds by poverty index ratio (PIR), a measure of income status that takes into account total family income, number of persons in the household, and the total income necessary to maintain the family on a nutritionally adequate food plan (U.S. Bureau of Census, 1979).

Data from the NHANES II 24-hr recall (National Center for Health Statistics, 1982) are presented in two ways. First, following Patterson and Block (1988), the proportions of persons in the weighted sample that reported eating *any* amount of a fruit or vegetable, however large or small, on the recall day are given; this provides a "snapshot" of fruit and vegetable consumption on any given day. This approach provides an answer to the question: what proportion of the U.S.

adult population includes fruits and vegetables in the *daily* diet? Second, the proportions eating specific numbers of *servings* of fruit and of vegetables are estimated, as described in Patterson et al. (1990). This approach answers the question: how many servings of fruits and vegetables does the U.S. adult population consume on any given day? The number of servings was estimated as follows. The USDA defines a serving of a vegetable as one-half cup of a vegetable, cooked or raw, and a serving of fruit, as an average piece of whole fruit, or 6 oz of fruit juice (Cronin et al., 1987). An examination of a sample of actual 24-hr recall food records showed that some reported amounts of fruits or vegetables, such as a slice of onion on a hamburger, or lemon juice added to tea, were too small to be considered a serving, while some portions were so large that they should be considered as more than a single serving. A serving was defined as at least 1 oz of either a fruit or a vegetable, or at least 2 oz of fruit juice. A small lower limit was chosen so as not to exclude individuals with small appetites. To take into account very large portions eaten on a single eating occasion, the weight of an "average" piece of whole fruit and the approximate weight of a half-cup serving of vegetables were determined using weights given in Agricultural Handbook No. 456 (U.S. Department of Agriculture, 1975) for the most popular (Patterson and Block, 1988) fruits and vegetables. Any single portion of vegetables exceeding 150 g was defined as two servings, as was any portion of fruit exceeding 240 g. Twelve to eighteen ounces of fruit juice were defined as two servings, and 18 oz or more, (558 g or more) as three servings.

Estimates from NHANES II given below are based on weighted data, permitting generalization to the total U.S. adult population. Standard errors were calculated using software appropriate for complex sample surveys (Shah, 1981).

National Health Interview Survey

The National Health Interview Survey (HIS) is a personal interview survey conducted by the NCHS. The HIS uses a stratified multistage probability sample of the civilian, noninstitutionalized population of the United States (Kovar et al., 1985). Dietary data are from the Cancer Control Supplement to the 1987 HIS. This supplement was conducted in collaboration with the National Cancer Institute. Data for this supplement were collected from a person randomly selected from each family. The dietary data were assessed by means of a quantified diet history questionnaire, whose development and validation have been described elsewhere (Block et al., 1986, 1990). Sixty-three food items were selected on the basis of the importance of their contribution to intake of a wide range of nutrients in the American diet (Block et al., 1985). The respondent was asked how often each food was usually eaten over the past year. Responses were transformed to number of times eaten per week, and to form groups of foods, the frequency of consumption of the foods in the group was summed. For example, a respondent indicating that he eats oranges 16 times a month and drinks orange juice 8 times a month would be coded as consuming citrus products 6 times per week. Results presented below are based on weighted data, and standard errors were calculated using appropriate software (Shah, 1981).

Nationwide Food Consumption Survey and the Continuing Survey of Food Intakes by Individuals

To obtain information on U.S. food intake, the U.S. Department of Agriculture (USDA) conducts a large national food consumption survey, the Nationwide Food Consumption Survey (NFCS) (Human Nutrition Information Service, 1983) approximately every 10 years, and smaller, more frequent surveys, the CSFII, or Continuing Survey of Food Intakes by Individuals. Both surveys use a stratified probability sample of households in the 48 coterminous states.

To examine trends in the consumption of fruit and vegetables, we compare 24-hr recall data on adults 19–50 years of age from both the NFCS and the CSFII (Human Nutrition Information Service, 1985, 1986, 1987b). These data were obtained by personal interview in the spring or summer quarters. In both surveys, a Food Instruction Booklet was used by the interviewers to assist respondents in describing both the foods and the amounts eaten, and standard measuring utensils were also used to help in estimating amounts of both food and beverages consumed. Differences in data collection procedures and probing techniques between the surveys probably had no significant effects on the data reported below, so that comparisons across surveys and over time are valid. The data reflect the use of sample weights by the USDA to adjust for nonresponse. Sample sizes given below are unweighted counts, with the exception of counts for NFCS 24-hr recall data, where only weighted counts are available. Standard errors were not reported by the USDA and so are not presented here.

Nationwide Food Consumption Survey

The Nationwide Food Consumption Survey was conducted by the U.S. Department of Agriculture from April 1977 to March 1978. NFCS respondents were selected from a sample that included 14,930 households of all incomes and individuals of all ages. A stratified multistage design was used. Data were collected over the course of a year, with approximately one-fourth of the households sampled each quarter. Interviewing took place on all days of the week. A trained interviewer recorded the previous day's food intake as recalled by each eligible household member who was present, and then instructed respondents on how to keep a written record of intake for the day of the interview and the following day. Twenty-four-hour recalls were obtained on all individuals in the household ages 19 and over during the spring of 1977 and on half of them during the remaining three-quarters. For the latter quarters, each individual recall has twice the weight, or importance, in the data as those individual recalls collected in the first quarter.

We present 24-hr recall data on 1778 men and 2228 women ages 19–50 and three-consecutive-day data on 6138 men and 8550 women ages 19–74. The percentage of individuals using foods in food groups discussed below during the three-consecutive-day period was obtained by dividing the number of individuals in the sex-age groups who reported the food at least once during the 3 days by the total number of individuals in that sex-age group (Human Nutrition Information Service, 1983).

Continuing Survey of Food Intakes by Individuals

Data from the Continuing Survey of Food Intakes by Individuals (CSFII) are collected by the USDA to complement the NFCS. CSFII data were collected on women ages 19–50 in 1985 (Human Nutrition Information Service, 1985, 1987a) and 1986 (Human Nutrition Information Service, 1987b) and on men ages 19–50 in 1985 (Human Nutrition Information Service, 1986). A single 24-hr recall was collected by personal interview. Some 95% of the interviews were conducted in July, August, and September. For the women, three additional nonconsecutive days of recall data, collected by telephone, were reported as well. In 1985, 24-hr data were collected on some 1459 women and 658 men; 4 days of data were reported on 1032 women. In 1986, data from a single 24-hr recall are available for 1451 women. While dietary information was collected on all races, the data on food intake were not reported by race.

In 1985, information was presented for women 19–50 by income level in relation to poverty guidelines defined by the U.S. Department of Health and Human Services (Human Nutrition Information Service, 1987a). These guidelines are specific to household size; e.g., in 1985, for a household of one, the poverty level was an income of $5250, and for a household of four, an income of $10,650. Each household's (self-reported) income was expressed as a percentage of the poverty guideline in 1985.

FRUIT AND VEGETABLE CONSUMPTION DATA

Introduction

Fruits and vegetables are major contributors of carotenoids, vitamin C, and fiber in the U.S. diet (Block et al., 1985) as well as of folate, vitamin E, and other nutrients (Subar et al., 1989; Murphy et al., 1990), although there are other sources of these nutrients, such as fortified cereal and supplements. Fruits and vegetables are not good sources of many nutrients, among them, vitamins B_6 and B_{12}, omega-3-fatty acids, heme iron, and zinc; these must be obtained from other foods. However, as is apparent in the data presented below, the fruit and vegetable food group appears to need greater emphasis in the U.S. diet.

Roughly 10% of U.S. adults have no fruits, fruit juice, or vegetables on any given day (Tables 1 and 2). Eleven percent had no servings of these foods on the NHANES II recall day; 8% of males and 10% of females ages 19–50 had

Table 1 Proportions (standard error) of Persons Ages 19–74 and Numbers in Sample, by Numbers of Servings of Fruit and Vegetables Consumed: Estimates Based on 24-Hr Dietary Recall Data from NHANES II, 1976–1980

Servings of fruit[a]	Servings of vegetables[b]				
	0	1	2	3+	All
0	0.11 (<.01)	0.11 (<.01)	0.11 (<.01)	0.11 (<.01)	0.45 (<.01)
	1,306	1,244	1,233	1,247	5,030
1	0.05 (<.01)	0.07 (<.01)	0.07 (<.01)	0.07 (<.01)	0.26 (<.01)
	633	814	804	847	3,098
2	0.03 (<.01)	0.04 (<.01)	0.04 (<.01)	0.05 (<.01)	0.15 (<.01)
	325	450	486	562	1,823
3+	0.02 (<.01)	0.03 (<.01)	0.04 (<.01)	0.04 (<.01)	0.14 (<.01)
	261	403	481	552	1,697
All	0.22 (.01)	0.26 (.01)	0.26 (.01)	0.27 (.01)	1.000
	2,525	2,911	3,004	3,208	11,648

[a] Whole fruit and fruit juices.
[b] Potatoes, salad, dried peas and beans, all other vegetables (denoted "garden"; see text).

Table 2 Proportions of Persons Ages 19–50 Using Selected Foods: 24-Hr Dietary Recall Data from NFCS, 1977–1978, and CSFII, 1985 and 1986

Food	Males[a]		Females		
	1977	1985	1977	1985	1986
Fruits					
All	0.44	0.43	0.50	0.47	0.50
Citrus fruits and juices	0.25	0.23	0.31	0.25	0.29
Noncitrus juices and nectars	0.04	0.02	0.04	0.06	0.04
Apples	0.07	0.07	0.09	0.11	0.10
Bananas	0.06	0.07	0.05	0.09	0.10
Dried fruits	<0.01	<0.01	0.09	0.02	0.02
Other fruits[b]	0.18	0.20	0.18	0.16	0.15
Vegetables					
All	0.89	0.85	0.84	0.83	0.81
White Potatoes	0.53	0.51	0.44	0.44	0.41
Tomatoes	0.35	0.42	0.27	0.29	0.31
Dark green	0.05	0.04	0.06	0.09	0.11
Deep yellow	0.07	0.06	0.07	0.09	0.11
Other vegetables[c]	0.72	0.69	0.70	0.66	0.65
Vegetables and fruit (all)	0.92	0.91	0.90	0.90	0.89

[a] CSFII data were not collected on males in 1986.
[b] Includes mixtures which are mainly fruit.
[c] Includes mixtures which are mainly vegetable.

no foods in these food groups on the NFCS recall day. More recent data from the CSFII do not indicate any change in these numbers: 9% of males and 10% of females had neither fruits nor vegetables on the recall day. Food frequency data, although not directly comparable to 24-hr data, present a similar picture: 12% of NHANES II respondents reported eating fruits and/or vegetables less often than daily (Table 3). Only 75% of black males and 85% of black females reported eating foods in this group daily, compared to 87% of white males and 91% of white females.

In contrast to the five or more recommended servings, zero or one serving of a food in the fruit/vegetable food group might be considered to be clearly inadequate. Estimates based on NHANES II 24-hr recall data show that in each demographic group, a large proportion had at most one serving of a fruit or a vegetable (Table 4); overall, this proportion was 28%. More black adults (35%) than white adults (27%) fell into this category. Proportions were somewhat smaller among older than among younger adults.

Fruit Consumption

Number of Servings

Despite minor differences in the composition of the fruit and juice groups (see Appendix), data from both the NCHS and the USDA present a consistent picture

Table 3 Proportions (standard error) of Persons Consuming Foods in the Fruit and Vegetable Group, by Frequency of Consumption, Sex, and Race: Food Frequency Data from NHANES II, 1976–1980

	Whites		Blacks		
Fruits and vegetables	Males	Females	Males	Females	All
All[a]					
1–6/week	0.13(0.01)	0.09(0.01)	0.24(0.03)	0.14(0.02)	0.11(0.01)
Daily	0.87(0.01)	0.91(0.01)	0.75(0.03)	0.85(0.02)	0.88(0.01)
High in provitamin A[a]					
Never	0.06(0.01)	0.06(<0.01)	0.03(0.01)	0.02(0.01)	0.06(<0.01)
<1/week	0.34(0.01)	0.30(0.01)	0.25(0.02)	0.24(0.03)	0.32(0.01)
1–6/week	0.56(0.01)	0.59(0.01)	0.66(0.03)	0.68(0.02)	0.59(0.01)
Daily	0.03(0.01)	0.04(0.01)	0.05(0.01)	0.07(0.01)	0.04(<0.01)
High in vitamin C[a]					
Never	0.04(0.01)	0.04(<0.01)	0.06(0.02)	0.04(0.01)	0.04(<0.01)
<1/week	0.15(0.01)	0.13(0.01)	0.14(0.02)	0.14(0.02)	0.14(0.01)
1–6/week	0.45(0.01)	0.41(0.01)	0.47(0.03)	0.42(0.02)	0.43(0.01)
Daily	0.36(0.01)	0.42(0.01)	0.33(0.03)	0.40(0.02)	0.39(0.01)

[a] See Appendix for list.

Table 4 Proportions (standard error) of Persons Ages 19–74 Consuming at Most a Single Serving of a Fruit or Vegetable, by Race, Sex, and Age Group: Estimates Based on Data from NHANES II, 1976–1980

Age group (years)	Whites		Blacks		
	Males	Females	Males	Females	All
19–29	0.32(0.01)	0.32(0.02)	0.35(0.04)	0.33(0.03)	0.32(0.01)
30–54	0.27(0.01)	0.29(0.01)	0.36(0.05)	0.40(0.04)	0.29(0.01)
55–74	0.22(0.01)	0.20(0.01)	0.36(0.04)	0.30(0.04)	0.22(0.01)
All ages	0.27(0.01)	0.27(0.01)	0.36(0.03)	0.35(0.02)	0.28(0.01)

with respect to the striking inadequacy of fruit consumption by U.S. adults. Forty-five percent had no servings of fruit or fruit juice on the NHANES II recall day and NFCS data show only 44% of men and 50% of women reporting consuming any of these foods on any given day (Tables 1 and 2). During the three-consecutive-day period reported by the NFCS, 28% of whites and 41% of blacks did not have even a single serving of fruit or juice, suggesting that for many fruit consumption is not even frequent (Table 5).

Table 5 Proportions of Persons Reporting Eating Foods in Selected Food Groups in 3 Consecutive Days: Data from NCFS, 1977–1978

Food	Whites		Blacks	
	Males	Females	Males	Females
Fruits				
All	0.70	0.74	0.53	0.62
Citrus fruits and juices	0.45	0.48	0.38	0.47
Noncitrus juices and nectars	0.07	0.09	0.06	0.08
Apples	0.24	0.25	0.16	0.12
Bananas	0.17	0.16	0.08	0.08
Dried fruits	0.03	0.04	0.01	0.01
Other fruits[a]	0.35	0.39	0.16	0.21
Vegetables				
All	0.99	0.98	0.99	0.98
White Potatoes	0.84	0.76	0.66	0.67
Tomatoes	0.52	0.52	0.38	0.38
Dark green	0.16	0.17	0.33	0.32
Deep yellow	0.21	0.24	0.19	0.17
Other vegetables[b]	0.94	0.94	0.91	0.90

[a] Includes mixtures which are mainly fruit.
[b] Includes mixtures which are mainly vegetable.

Table 6   Proportions (standard error) of Persons Aged 19–74 Who Met (or Exceeded) the USDA Guidelines, by Race, Sex, and Age Group: Estimates Based on 24-Hr Dietary Recall Data from NHANES II, 1976–1980

	Age group			
	19–29	30–54	55–74	All ages
Fruit[a] *and vegetable*[b] *guidelines (2 + fruits and 3 + vegetables)*				
White males	0.08(0.01)	0.09(0.01)	0.12(0.01)	0.09(0.01)
Black males	0.05(0.01)	0.08(0.02)	0.08(0.02)	0.07(0.01)
White females	0.05(0.01)	0.08(0.01)	0.15(0.01)	0.09(<0.01)
Black females	0.04(0.02)	0.03(0.01)	0.08(0.02)	0.05(0.01)
All	0.06(0.01)	0.08(0.01)	0.13(0.01)	0.09(<0.01)
Fruit guidelines (2 or more servings)				
White males	0.21(0.02)	0.25(0.01)	0.35(0.01)	0.26(0.01)
Black males	0.16(0.03)	0.24(0.03)	0.22(0.03)	0.21(0.02)
White females	0.24(0.02)	0.28(0.01)	0.47(0.02)	0.32(0.01)
Black females	0.24(0.05)	0.20(0.03)	0.32(0.05)	0.24(0.02)
All	0.22(0.01)	0.26(<0.01)	0.40(0.01)	0.29(<0.01)
Vegetable guidelines (3 or more servings)				
White males	0.32(0.01)	0.31(0.01)	0.31(0.01)	0.31(0.01)
Black males	0.22(0.04)	0.20(0.04)	0.23(0.05)	0.21(0.02)
White females	0.21(0.01)	0.25(0.01)	0.28(0.01)	0.25(0.01)
Black females	0.15(0.03)	0.18(0.04)	0.20(0.03)	0.18(0.02)
All	0.25(0.01)	0.27(0.01)	0.28(0.01)	0.27(0.01)

[a] Whole fruit and fruit juice.
[b] Potatoes, salad, dried peas and beans, all other (denoted "garden") vegetables.

About a quarter of the adult population had a single serving of fruit or fruit juice on the recall day, based on estimates using NHANES II data. Only 29% had the two or more servings recommended by the USDA. Proportions meeting these "fruit guidelines" were markedly higher among those in the 55- to 74-year age group than in the 19- to 29-year age group, yet even in this older group fewer than 50% had the recommended number of servings (Table 6). More whites than blacks met these guidelines; only 16% of young black males had two or more servings of fruit on the recall day.

Despite the issuance of guidelines since the NHANES II and NFCS surveys were conducted, these appears to be little or no change in the proportions consuming fruit or juice on a daily basis. In fact, the proportions of both men and women consuming fruit or juice on the recall day were virtually unchanged between 1977 and 1985 for men, and between 1977 and 1986 for women (Table 2).

Table 7 Average Frequency of Intake per Week (standard error) for Persons Ages 19–99: Data from the National Health Interview Survey, 1987

Food	Whites		Blacks	
	Males	Females	Males	Females
All fruit	8.91(0.11)	10.30(0.11)	9.83(0.39)	11.12(0.28)
All vegetables	13.02(0.10)	13.08(0.09)	12.02(0.35)	11.99(0.22)
Garden vegetables	5.85(0.06)	6.32(0.06)	6.20(0.22)	6.45(0.14)
Potatoes	4.45(0.05)	3.68(0.04)	3.92(0.16)	3.35(0.09)
Salad	2.75(0.04)	3.07(0.03)	1.91(0.09)	2.19(0.07)
Dried peas and beans	1.00(0.02)	0.72(0.01)	1.30(0.06)	1.02(0.05)

Individuals interviewed in the 1987 HIS reported consuming fruit (including juice) more frequently, about nine or 10 times per week (Table 7); juice alone constituted approximately half of these servings (data not shown). These frequencies, which are based on the sum of individual frequencies for individual fruits, may overestimate true consumption, a possibility mentioned in the discussion of methods of dietary assessment. However, this level still falls short of the suggested two or more servings per day. While the list of fruits included in the food history questionnaire (see Appendix) was of necessity not all-inclusive, the data reported here include the most popular fruits and juices.

Types of Fruit

Of the 55% of U.S. adults having at least one serving of fruit or juice on the NHANES II recall day, 27% had juice only and 45% had whole fruit only (data not shown). According to USDA data, citrus fruits and juice are the most popular fruits (Tables 2 and 5). However, only about a fourth of the adult respondents had any on the recall day, and over the 3-day NFCS survey period, more than half of the adult population did not have even a single serving. Apples and bananas, easily included in bag lunches and convenient snacks, were more popular among whites than blacks, but were eaten by fewer than a quarter of the population during this period. Dried fruits, also readily portable and nonperishable as well, were eaten by fewer than 5%. Other fruits, including mixtures such as fruit salad, were reported by 37% of whites and 19% of blacks.

Fruits high in carotenoids and vitamin C, along with vegetables rich in these nutrients, were examined as a separate group in the NHANES II survey. Beta-carotene, found in many fruits and vegetables, can be converted to vitamin A, but this and other carotenoids have biological effects unrelated to their activity as vitamin A precursors. There are also other carotenoids that can be sources of vitamin A. This composite group will be discussed following the section on vegetable consumption.

Table 8 Proportions (standard error) of Persons Ages 19–74 Consuming Foods in Selected Food Groups, by Race and Poverty Index Ratio (PIR)[a] Tertile: 24-Hour Dietary Recall Data from NHANES II, 1976–1980

Food	Whites			Blacks		
	Low	Mid	High	Low	Mid	High
All Fruits	0.51(0.01)	0.59(0.01)	0.65(0.01)	0.50(0.02)	0.59(0.04)	0.70(0.04)
Fruits and vegetables						
High in carotenoids	0.18(0.01)	0.20(0.01)	0.22(0.01)	0.24(0.02)	0.27(0.04)	0.32(0.05)
High in vitamin C	0.24(0.01)	0.27(0.01)	0.31(0.01)	0.31(0.02)	0.36(0.03)	0.42(0.06)
Vegetables						
All	0.80(0.01)	0.84(0.01)	0.87(0.01)	0.73(0.02)	0.78(0.03)	0.83(0.05)
Garden	0.46(0.01)	0.51(0.01)	0.57(0.01)	0.46(0.03)	0.46(0.03)	0.53(0.06)
Cruciferous	0.14(0.01)	0.18(0.01)	0.20(0.01)	0.22(0.02)	0.23(0.02)	0.26(0.06)
Deep yellow	0.10(0.01)	0.10(0.01)	0.12(0.01)	0.08(0.01)	0.09(0.02)	0.12(0.03)

[a] Poverty Index Ratios (PIR) for tertiles: low: ≤1.92, mid: 1.93–3.20, high: >3.20.

Table 9 Proportions of Women Ages 19–50 Eating Foods in Selected Food Groups at Least Once in 4 Nonconsecutive Days, by Income Group: Data from CSFII, 1985

Food	Under 131% poverty	131–300% poverty	Over 300% poverty	All
Fruits				
All	0.69	0.84	0.88	0.81
Citrus fruits and juices	0.42	0.59	0.65	0.56
Noncitrus juices and nectars	0.11	0.13	0.17	0.15
Apples	0.21	0.30	0.36	0.30
Bananas	0.14	0.26	0.33	0.25
Dried fruits	0.02	0.05	0.04	0.04
Other fruits[a]	0.28	0.45	0.57	0.46
Vegetables				
All	0.97	1.00	1.00	0.99
White Potatoes	0.80	0.82	0.85	0.83
Tomatoes	0.60	0.78	0.79	0.75
Dark green	0.22	0.30	0.34	0.30
Deep yellow	0.19	0.33	0.33	0.29
Other vegetables[b]	0.89	0.97	0.98	0.95

[a] Includes mixtures that are mainly fruit.
[b] Includes all other vegetables not explicitly listed, as well as vegetable juices and soups and mixtures that are mainly vegetable.

Income and Fruit Consumption

Available data point to a marked relationship between income and fruit consumption (Tables 8 and 9). Among those in the lowest one-third of the population on income in the NHANES II 24-hr recall data, only about 50% had *any* fruit on the recall day, compared with 65% of whites and 70% of blacks in the highest third. NFCS data present a similar picture: for those earning less than $6000 per year, only 66% consumed any fruit or juice in a three-consecutive-day period, compared with 76% of those earning $16,000 or more (data not shown). In 1985, 69% of women in households with annual incomes in the lowest category (under 131% of poverty) ate fruit at least once in four nonconsecutive days, compared with 88% in the highest (over 300% of poverty).

Vegetable Consumption

The vegetable groups discussed below, and given in the Appendix, differ somewhat in their composition, so that data from the various surveys are not directly comparable. Briefly, the "vegetable" category used in the NHANES II analyses includes potatoes, green salad, and dried peas and beans, in addition to yellow, green, and other vegetables. The USDA definition of "all vegetables" includes all of these except dried peas and beans and includes as well vegetable juices, vegetable condiments such as catsup, and soups and mixtures that are mainly vegetable. The vegetable group designated "all" from the HIS is not inclusive of all vegetables, but does include major contributors such as salad, potatoes, and green and yellow vegetables such as carrots, tomatoes, and cabbage. This group excludes dried peas and beans.

Number of Servings

While U.S. adults have a greater number of servings of vegetables than of fruits on any given day, most fall short of the recommended number of three or more servings. Twenty-two percent had no servings of vegetables on the NHANES II recall day, and 14% had none on the NFCS recall day (Tables 1 and 2). This difference may be due in part to differences between the vegetable groups, the NFCS including condiments and soups, as noted above.

Twenty-six percent of U.S. adults had one serving of a vegetable on the NHANES II recall day, and 26% had two servings. Proportions meeting the recommendation of three or more servings of vegetables daily were extremely small over all age-sex groups for both blacks and whites (Table 6). Overall, only 27% met the "vegetable guidelines." Greater proportions of males than females and of whites than blacks met the guidelines; deficits were especially notable among black females, only 18% of whom fell in this category. Slightly greater proportions in the older age group met the guidelines than did those in the younger, but this trend was less striking than that observed for fruit consumption. Virtually all adults had a vegetable at least once during the 3-day NFCS survey period (Table 5).

Vegetable consumption appears to have declined slightly between the mid-1970s and the mid-1980s (Table 2). In 1985, 85% of men ages 19–50 reported eating a vegetable on the recall day, compared to 89% in 1977. A similar decrease was seen for females; 81% consumed a vegetable on the study day in 1986, 83% in 1985, compared to 84% in 1977, perhaps reflecting a decrease in proportions eating potatoes and tomatoes.

In the 1987 HIS survey, adults reported eating about 12–13 servings of vegetables a week (Table 7). As with consumption of "all fruits," this may represent an overestimate of actual consumption. As mentioned above, this group includes salad and potatoes as well as many yellow and green vegetables.

Types of Vegetables

The various national surveys provide information on the popularity of many vegetables. The types of vegetables eaten by those who had a single serving of a vegetable and by those who had exactly two servings of vegetables on the NHANES II recall day are shown in Fig. 1, and Table 10 gives estimated

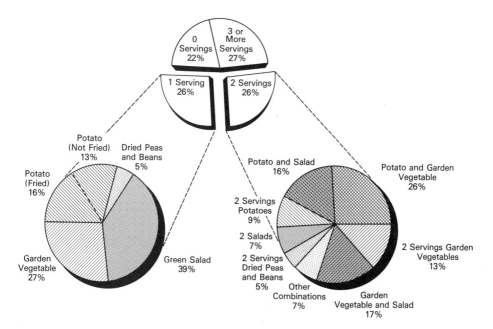

Figure 1 (Top) Estimated percentages of individuals consuming zero, one, two, or three or more servings of vegetables on the NHANES II recall day. (Lower left) The type of vegetable consumed by those who had a single serving of a vegetable. (Lower right) The types of vegetables consumed by those who had exactly two servings of a vegetable.

proportions consuming various vegetables on that day. More detailed information on the most popular, as well as some of the less popular, vegetables consumed on the recall day is given in Table 11; these data reflect the numbers per 10,000 populations who had *any* amount, however small, of the foods listed. Popkin et al. (1989) examined food group consumption of women ages 19–50 using 3 days of data from the 1977–1978 NFCS and the 1985 CSFII. They looked at changes both in the percentages using foods and in the grams per user per day for food groups determined, in part, by fat and dietary fiber content. In this subsection, demographic differences, trends, and associations with income for various groups of vegetables as well as for a few individual vegetables are discussed.

Potatoes. The potato is the single most popular vegetable. Between a third and half of all adults have one or more servings of potato on any given day (Tables 2 and 10). Among those who had only one serving of a vegetable (26% of the population) on the NHANES II recall day, that vegetable was a potato for almost a third (Fig. 1). Among the 26% of the population having exactly two servings

Table 10 Proportions (standard error) of Persons Consuming Various Vegetables, by Race, Sex, and Type of Vegetable: Estimates Based on 24-hour Dietary Recall Data from NHANES II, 1976–1980

Type of vegetable	Whites		Blacks		All
	Males	Females	Males	Females	
Garden[a]	0.42(0.01)	0.44(0.01)	0.41(0.03)	0.44(0.02)	0.43(0.01)
Cruciferous[b]	0.17(0.01)	0.18(0.01)	0.20(0.03)	0.25(0.02)	0.18(0.01)
Deep yellow[b]	0.09(0.01)	0.11(0.01)	0.08(0.02)	0.09(0.01)	0.10(<0.01)
Potatoes[a]					
Fried[a]	0.22(0.01)	0.13(0.01)	0.15(0.02)	0.10(0.01)	0.16(<0.01)
Not fried[a]	0.28(0.01)	0.26(0.01)	0.20(0.02)	0.20(0.02)	0.26(0.01)
All[a]	0.46(0.01)	0.37(0.01)	0.33(0.03)	0.30(0.03)	0.40(0.01)
Salad[a]	0.39(0.01)	0.40(0.01)	0.19(0.02)	0.24(0.02)	0.37(0.01)
Dried peas and beans	0.11(0.01)	0.08(0.01)	0.13(0.02)	0.10(0.02)	0.10(0.01)

[a] Proportions consuming one or more servings.
[b] Proportions consuming *any* (see text).

Table 11 Selected Vegetables, by Number of Times Reported and Nutritional Characteristics: 24-Hr Dietary Recall Data from NHANES II, 1976–1980

Vegetable	Numbers consuming (per 10,000)	Cruciferous	Deep yellow	Fibrous	High in carot.[a]	High in vit C[b]
Potatoes	4171	.	.	.	.	.
Green salad	4030	.	.	.	.	.
Tomatoes (raw and cooked)	2552	.	.	.	.	.
Dried peas and beans	1070	.	.	X	.	.
Green beans	992	.	.	.	.	.
Cole slaw, cabbage	944	X	.	.	.	.
Corn	852	.	.	X	.	.
Carrots	811	.	X	.	X	.
Green peas	553	.	.	.	.	.
Onions	385	.	.	.	.	.
Broccoli	249	X	.	.	X	X
Greens (collards, etc.)	244	X	.	.	X	X
Spinach	237	.	.	.	X	.
Sweet potatoes	158	.	X	.	X	.
Cooked green peppers	129	.	.	.	.	X
Cauliflower	125	X	.	.	.	X
Winter squash	63	.	X	.	X	.
Turnips	42	X	.	.	.	X
Brussels sprouts	38	X	.	.	.	X

[a] Average portion contains at least 2500 IU of provitamin A carotenoids.
[b] Average portion contains at least 30 mg.

of vegetables, potatoes constituted at least one of those servings for 54%. Potatoes are less popular among blacks than among whites, and among females than among males. Both races report eating potatoes about four times per week (Table 7).

Potatoes can indirectly add to the fat in the diet because they are often eaten fried or with butter or margarine. On the NHANES II recall day, for adult males, almost half of the servings of potatoes were eaten fried, compared to about a third for females. Popkin et al. (1989) found that the percentage of women using "higher fat" potatoes (french fries, potato salad, and hash browns) increased from 39.2 to 46.1 between 1977 and 1985, while the grams per user per day declined slightly.

Garden Vegetables. The NAS stresses the importance of green and yellow vegetables in the daily diet (Committee on Diet and Health, National Research Council, 1989). Following Patterson and Block (1988), garden vegetables are defined as those vegetables that might be thought of as "vegetables" in a "meat, potatoes, and vegetable" dinner. Examples include peas, beans, carrots, and corn, and this broad group includes subgroups of interest in cancer prevention such as the cruciferous and dark green leafy and deep yellow vegetables.

On the NHANES II recall day, only 43% of the adult population had one or more servings of a garden vegetable, and there was little difference in consumption across race and sex groups (Table 10). A little more than a quarter of adults having a single serving of a vegetable had a garden vegetable, and vegetables in this group were eaten by almost 60% of those having two servings (Fig. 1). According to data from the HIS, vegetables in this broad group are eaten about six times per week (Table 7).

Cruciferous and Dark Green Vegetables. Cruciferous and dark green vegetables are two overlapping groups that have been linked with disease prevention in such major health statements as *Diet, Nutrition, and Cancer* (National Research Council, 1982) and the *Surgeon General's Report on Nutrition and Health* U.S. Department of Health and Human Services, 1988). The American Cancer Society recommends including cruciferous vegetables in the diet (American Cancer Society, 1984), and the National Cancer Institute suggests choosing several servings of these vegetables each week (National Cancer Institute, 1985). Cruciferous vegetables include broccoli, cauliflower, cabbage, brussels sprouts, and southern greens (e.g., kale, collards, mustard and turnip greens). Dark green vegetables, which are good sources of carotenoids, include broccoli and dark green leafy vegetables such as spinach and southern greens. Only 18% of white adults had any vegetable in the cruciferous family on the NHANES II recall day, compared with 23% of blacks. The most popular cruciferous vegetable was cabbage, eaten by almost one-tenth of the adult population; half was eaten as cole slaw. Broccoli was eaten by only 249 persons per 10,000 (Table 11); consumption was even lower for cauliflower (125 per 10,000) and for brussels sprouts (only 38 per 10,000). Among both blacks and whites, there was a positive association between proportions consuming these vegetables and income (Table 8).

Dark green vegetables were eaten by only 5% of males and 6% of females on the NFCS recall day (Table 2). More recent CSFII 24-hr recall data showed almost a doubling in the proportion of women using these vegetables, while the proportion of men using them remained unchanged. NFCS data showed that about 17% of whites and a third of blacks had dark green vegetables at least once during a period of three consecutive days (Table 5). As with cruciferous vegetables, there is a positive association between consumption and income. CSFII data for 1985 show that a third of women in the highest income group used vegetables in this group at least once in four nonconsecutive days, compared to about a fifth in the lowest income group (Table 9).

Deep Yellow Vegetables.   Like dark green vegetables, deep yellow vegetables (e.g., carrots, winter squash) are a rich source of beta-carotene. Vegetables in this group are consumed by a very small percent of the adult population (6–11%) on any given day (Tables 2 and 10). Fewer than a quarter had a vegetable in this category during a three-consecutive-day period (Table 5). As with cruciferous and dark green vegetables, larger proportions of those in the higher than in the lower income groups ate vegetables in this group (Tables 8 and 9). CSFII data showed a third of the women in the middle- and high-income groups using vegetables in this group at least once in 4 days, as compared to only 19% of those in the lowest group.

Dried Peas and Beans.   Dried peas and beans, such as baked beans and black-eyed peas, are eaten on any given day by roughly 10% of the population. These vegetables are somewhat more popular among blacks than whites (Table 10). This difference is reflected in the HIS data (Table 7), where the average frequency of intake per week is 1.0 for white and 0.7 for white females, compared to 1.3 for black males and 1.0 for black females.

Salad and Tomatoes.   About 40% of whites ate one or more servings of green salad (lettuce, raw tomatoes, and other salad ingredients, such as cucumbers) on the NHANES II recall day. Salad was eaten by far fewer blacks, only 22% (Table 10). Salad, like potatoes, is very popular; among those having a single serving of a vegetable, for about 40% that serving was salad (Fig. 1). Similarly, among those having two servings, about 40% had at least one serving of salad. White males report eating salad 2.7 times a week, and white females, 3.1 times (Table 7). Intakes for blacks is lower—1.9 times a week for males, and 2.2 times for females. Popkin et al. (1989) examined changes in the consumption of a group of "lower fiber" vegetables that included lettuce, tomatoes, onions, cucumbers, and slaw. They found that the percentage of women using these foods at least once in a 3-day period increased slightly between 1977 and 1985, from 79 to 82%, but that the grams per user per day decreased.

Tomatoes can be a good source of vitamin C. About 25% had some tomatoes (raw or cooked) on the NHANES II recall day (Table 11). The USDA presents data on a comprehensive group of tomatoes (raw and cooked) and tomato products (tomato juices, sauces, catsup, and tomato mixtures). Over a 3-day period, 52% of white adults had tomatoes or tomato products at least once, compared to 38% of blacks (Table 5). Among women surveyed on four nonconsecutive days in 1985 (Table 9), tomatoes were more popular among those with incomes over 130% of poverty (almost 80% had some at least once) than among those under this level (only 60% reported having any).

Vegetables Rich in Vitamins A and C.   The American Cancer Society recommends including foods rich in vitamins A and C in the daily diet (American Cancer Society, 1984). The consumption of vegetables falling in these two categories has been investigated in NHANES II 24-hr recall data (Patterson and

Block, 1988) and food frequency questionnaire data. The list of foods included in these two separate studies of consumption (see Appendix) differs in that the first, which is based on individual portions containing a proportion of the U.S. RDAs for these foods is more restrictive than the second, which includes many more foods, some meeting a smaller proportion of the U.S. RDAs than those included in the former group.

Only 21% of the adult population had any fruits or vegetables high in carotenoids on the recall day and 28% any rich in vitamin C. The proportions eating any of these foods increased with age (data not shown), and larger proportions of blacks than of whites had foods in both groups (Table 8). Consumption was far higher among those in the highest one-third of the population on income, and this trend was especially prominent for blacks. Fruits and vegetables in both groups were consumed by a third more blacks in the highest tertile than in the lowest.

Many reported eating fruits and vegetables in these categories infrequently. In NHANES II, roughly 5% reported *never* eating these foods, and more than a quarter of blacks and almost a third of whites said they eat fruits and vegetables high in carotenoids less than once a week (Table 3). About 60% reported eating these foods one to six times per week. Because vitamin C is water-soluble and not stored appreciably in the liver, sources of this nutrient must be consumed frequently to maintain adequate levels in the body. About a seventh of U.S. adults reported eating fruits and vegetables rich in this important vitamin less than once a week, and only about 40% said they eat foods in this category daily.

DISCUSSION

The data presented in this chapter are striking in their consistency and disturbing in the picture they present of the adult American diet. Not only did fewer than 10% consume the recommended five or more servings of fruits and vegetables on any given day, but large numbers had diets clearly deficient in these foods. About 10% had *neither* on any given day, as evidenced by both USDA and NHANES II 24-hr recall data and by food frequency data from NHANES II. Twenty-eight percent had at most a single serving of a fruit *or* a vegetable on the NHANES II recall day.

Dietary recommendations stress the importance of a varied diet including both fruits and vegetables. Yet, on the recall day, roughly *half* of U.S. adults had no servings of fruit or fruit juice and 22% had no serving of a vegetable. Almost half of the adult population had at most a single serving of a vegetable. Three-consecutive-day data show that consumption of fruit and garden vegetables was not a routine feature of the U.S. diet. Low levels of consumption of dark green and deep yellow vegetables suggests a lack of appreciation of the possible importance of these vegetables to a nutritious diet.

Differences in consumption between various sex, race, and age groups may be indicative of different lifestyle and generational eating habits, education, and economic status. The markedly low consumption of fruits and vegetables by the poor, in particular, may reflect both lack of availability and lack of the wherewithal to purchase these sometimes costly foods.

While the dietary recommendations discussed in this chapter were not issued until after NHANES II and the NFCS were conducted, fruit and vegetable consumption has been a mainstay of dietary recommendations for decades. Earlier recommendations were issued with an eye to maintaining good nutrition, while some of those issued in the early 1980s, such as the Surgeon General's Report and that of the National Academy of Sciences, have related diet to the prevention of chronic disease as well. Despite the appearance of these guidelines and evidence of the relationship of diet to heart disease, atherosclerosis, and some types of cancer, the most recent national survey data do not suggest any change in fruit and vegetable consumption. Indeed, the proportions reporting consuming these foods have either stayed constant or declined slightly.

A first step in achieving population behavior change is recognition, not only by nutrition policymakers and educators, but also by health professionals and by the general public, of the extent of the failure to meet the dietary guidelines. The data presented here show deficiencies in the numbers of fruits and vegetables in the diets of virtually all demographic groups. For some types of these foods, and for some population groups, the deficiencies are substantial. The "food/ health connection" seems to be vague in the public's mind; further, the public seems unsure of what constitutes a good diet (Crawford, 1988). The promulgation of nutrition recommendations alone appears to be ineffective in influencing people to change their diets. Many may not actually hear the message at all; those who do hear it appear to perceive it as little more than a "good idea." A vigorous, active campaign akin to the cholesterol education campaign is needed. Such a campaign should have several goals: (1) to emphasize the National Academy of Sciences finding that "diets high in plant foods . . . are associated with a lower occurrence of coronary heart disease and cancers of the lung, colon, esophagus, and stomach" (Committee on Diet and Health, 1989); (2) to change the public perception of diet so that daily consumption of fruits and vegetables comes to be seen as something that *defines* a good diet; and (3) to examine and perhaps even modify economic and regulatory policies, so that these foods become more economically accessible.

APPENDIX: FOOD GROUPS

A summary of individual food items included in selected food categories is given in this appendix; more detailed lists are given in the references indicated throughout. Items included in one survey but excluded in others are noted. Self-explanatory food group names are omitted here.

    I.   National Center for Health Statistics Surveys.

        A.   The Second National Health and Nutrition Examination Survey

1. Food Frequency (Diet History) Questionnaire Data
   Food groups designated by the National Center for Health
   Statistics (1982).
   a. Fruits and vegetables
      Includes all kinds, fresh, canned, frozen, cooked or raw,
      as well as juices, including Tang and fruit drinks
   b. Fruits and vegetables rich in provitamin A carotenoids
      Includes cantaloupe, mango, apricots, papaya, peaches,
      and watermelons; carrots; greens such as collards, kale,
      mustard or turnip, pumpkin, spinach, sweet potato, win-
      ter squash, broccoli
   c. Fruits and vegetables rich in vitamin C
      Includes avocado, cantaloupe, grapefruit, lemon, lime,
      oranges, and strawberries; brussels sprouts, broccoli,
      cauliflower, green pepper, tomato, lightly cooked greens
      such as collards, kale, mustard, or turnip
2. Twenty-four-hour recall data
   Food groups specified by Patterson and Block (1988) and
   Patterson et al., 1990). Mixtures are not included.
   a. Fruits
      1) All
         Includes whole fruits and fruit juices (excludes Tang
         and fruit "drinks")
      2) Fruit juice
         Includes citrus and other fruit juices (excludes Tang
         and fruit "drinks")
   b. Vegetables
      1) All
         Includes white and sweet potatoes, garden vegeta-
         bles (see below), salad, dried peas and beans (e.g.,
         black-eyed peas, navy beans). Excludes mixtures
         that contain vegetables such as vegetable soup, cat-
         sup, pickles, relishes
      2) Garden vegetables
         Includes all vegetables *except* potatoes, salad, dried
         peas and beans. Examples are broccoli, green
         beans, carrots
      3) Deep yellow vegetables
         Includes carrots, winter squash, sweet potatoes
      4) Cruciferous vegetables
         Includes broccoli, cauliflower, brussels sprouts, cab-
         bage, turnips, collards, kale, mustard greens, turnip
         greens, kohlrabi, watercress, radishes

    5) Salad
        Includes lettuce, raw tomatoes, cucumbers, and
        other vegetables (e.g., cucumbers) typically found
        in green salad (excludes raw broccoli, cauliflower,
        etc.)
    c. Fruits and vegetables high in carotenoids*
        Includes apricots, cantaloupe, watermelon, carrots, spin-
        ach, mustard greens, turnip greens, collards, kale, mis-
        cellaneous greens, broccoli, winter squash, sweet pota-
        toes, mixed vegetables
    d. Fruits and vegetables high in vitamin C†
        Includes oranges, orange juice, strawberries, grapefruit,
        cantaloupe, miscellaneous fruit drinks (including forti-
        fied fruit drinks), mangos, papayas, muskmelons, plan-
        tains, mustard greens, turnip greens, collards, kale, mis-
        cellaneous greens, broccoli, cauliflower, brussels
        sprouts, sweet peppers, hot peppers
B. National Health Interview Survey
    1. Vegetables
        a. All
            Includes white and sweet potatoes, tomatoes, carrots,
            mixed vegetables containing carrots, broccoli, spinach,
            southern greens, cabbage
        b. Garden
            Includes tomatoes, carrots, broccoli, spinach, southern
            greens, cole slaw
        c. Potatoes
            Includes white and sweet potatoes
        d. Salad (green)
        e. Dried peas and beans
            Includes all, such as baked, kidney beans, or beans in
            chili. Excludes green beans

    2. Fruit (All)
        Includes oranges, grapefruit, cantaloupe, apples, applesauce,
        orange juice, other fruit juices and fortified fruit drinks.
II. U.S. Department of Agriculture Surveys
    Food categories include mixtures that consist mainly of the food or
    foods comprising the category (e.g., "all vegetables" includes
    mixtures that are mainly vegetables).

---

* Average portion size provides at least 2500 IU (one-half of the recommended daily allowance of
vitamin A) from provitamin A carotenoids.
† Average portion size provides at least 30 mg (one-half of the recommended daily allowance)

A. Nationwide Food Consumption Survey (USDA, 1984: pp. 564–566) and Continuing Survey of Food Intakes by Individuals (USDA, 1985: pp. 140–141): Food groups for these surveys are the same.

    1. Fruit

        a. All

        Includes citrus fruits and juices, dried and other fruits, and juices. Excludes citrus fruit drinks and ades such as lemonade

        b. Citrus fruits, juices

        Includes oranges and other citrus fruits, orange juice, other citrus juices, mixtures of citrus and other fruit juices. Excludes citrus fruit ades such as lemonade

        c. Apples, bananas

        Includes raw and cooked

    2. Vegetables

        a. All

        Includes white potatoes, tomatoes, dark green and deep yellow vegetables, other vegetables and mixtures that are mainly vegetable

        b. White potatoes

        Includes all white potatoes, potato chips, and mixtures mainly potato

        c. Tomatoes

        Includes raw and cooked tomatoes; tomato juice and soup; catsup, chili sauce, and other tomato sauces

        d. Dark green vegetables

        Includes raw and cooked greens (chard, collards, escarole, mustard and turnip greens, kale); spinach; broccoli

        e. Deep yellow vegetables

        Includes raw and cooked carrots, pumpkin, winter squash, sweet potatoes

        f. Other vegetables

        Includes vegetables not listed above; vegetable juices and soups, pickles, olives, relishes, and salads

REFERENCES

American Cancer Society. Nutrition and Cancer: Cause and Prevention. CA 1984; 34:121.

Block G. Ascorbic acid in cancer prevention: The epidemiologic evidence. Am J Clin Nutr 1991; 53:2705.

Block G, Hartman AM, Naughton D. A reduced dietary questionnaire: Development and validation. Epidemiology 1990; 1:58.

Block G, Dresser CM, Hartman AM, Carroll MD. Nutrient sources in the American diet: Quantitative data from the NHANES II survey. Am J Epidemiol 1985; 122:13.

Block G, Hartman A. Dietary assessment methods. In: Moon TE, Micozzi MS, eds. Nutrition and cancer prevention. New York: Marcel Dekker, 1989, 159.

Block G, Hartman AM, Dresser CM, Carroll MD, Gannon J, Gardner L. A data-based approach to diet questionnaire design and testing. Am J Epidemiol 1986; 124:453.

Committee on Diet and Health, Food and Nutrition Board, Commission on Life Sciences, National Research Council. Diet and health: Implications for reducing chronic disease risk. Washington, DC: National Academy Press, 1989.

Crawford P. The nutrition connection: Why doesn't the public know? Am J Public Hlth 1988; 78:1147.

Cronin FJ, Shaw AM, Krebs-Smith SM, Marsland PM, and Light L. Developing a food guidance system to implement the dietary guidelines. J Nutr Educ 1987; 19:281.

Gersovitz M, Madden JP, Smiciklas-Wright H. Validity of the 24-hour dietary recall and seven-day record for group comparisons. J Am Diet Assoc 1978; 73:48.

Hartman AM, Brown CB, Palmgren J, Pietinen P, Verkasalo M, Naughton D, Virtamo J. Variability in nutrient and food intakes among older middle-aged men: Implications for design of epidemiologic and validation studies using food recording. Am J Epidemiol, in press.

Human Nutrition Information Service. Food Intakes: Individuals in 48 States, Year 1977–78. Nationwide Food Consumption Survey 1977–78, Report No. I–1, United States Department of Agriculture, Hyattsville, Maryland, 1983.

Human Nutrition Information Service. Nationwide Food Consumption Survey, Continuing Survey of Food Intakes by Individuals, Women 19–50 Years and Their Children 1–5 Years, 1 Day, 1985. United States Department of Agriculture, Hyattsville, Maryland, NFCS, CSFII Report No. 85–1, 1985.

Human Nutrition Information Service. Nationwide Food Consumption Survey, Continuing Survey of Food Intakes by Individuals, Men 19–50 Years, 1 Day, 1985. United States Department of Agriculture, Hyattsville, Maryland, NFCS, CSFII Report No. 85–3, 1986.

Human Nutrition Information Service. Nationwide Food Consumption Survey, Continuing Survey of Food Intakes by Individuals, Women 19–50 Years and Their Children 1–5 Years, 4 Days, 1985. United States Department of Agriculture, Hyattsville, Maryland, NFCS, CSFII Report No. 85–4, 1987a.

Human Nutrition Information Service. Nationwide Food Consumption Survey, Continuing Survey of Food Intakes by Individuals, Women 19–50 Years and Their Children 1–5 Years, 1 Day, 1986. United States Department of Agriculture, Hyattsville, Maryland, NFCS, CSFII Report No. 86–1, 1987b.

Kovar MG, Poe GS. The National Health Interview Survey design, 1973–84, and procedures, 1975–83. National Center for Health Statistics. Vital Health Statistics 1, 1985.

Micozzi MS. Foods, micronutrients, and reduction of cancer. In: Moon TE, Micozzi MS. eds. Nutrition and cancer prevention: Investigating the role of Micronutrients. New York: Marcel Dekker, 1989, 213.

Murphy SP, Subar AF, Block G. Vitamin E intakes and sources in the United States. Am J Clin Nutr 1990; 52:361.

National Cancer Institute. Diet, nutrition and cancer prevention: A guide to food choices.

United States Department of Health and Human Services. Washington, DC: U.S. Government Printing Office, NIH Publication No. 85–2711, 1985.

National Center for Health Statistics. Plan and operations of the Second National Health and Nutritional Examination Survey, 1976–1980. Vital and Health Statistics Series 1, No. 15. DHEW Publication No.(PHS) 81–1317. Washington, DC: U.S. Government Printing Office, 1981.

National Center for Health Statistics. Public use data tape documentation. Total nutrient intake, food frequency, and other related dietary data tape. Tape Number 5701. National Health and Nutrition Examination Survey, 1976–80. Hyattsville, Maryland: U.S. Department of Health and Human Services, 1982.

National Center for Health Statistics. Dietary intake source data: United States, 1976–80. Vital and health statistics, Series 11. No. 231. Washington, DC: U.S. Government Printing Office, DHHS Publication No. 83–1681, 1983.

National Research Council, Committee on Diet, Nutrition and Cancer, Assembly of Life Sciences. Diet, nutrition and cancer. Washington, DC: National Academy Press, 1982.

Patterson BH, Block G. Food choices and the cancer guidelines. Am J Public Hlth 1988; 78:282.

Patterson BH, Block G, Rosenberger WR, Pee D, Kahle LL. Fruit and vegetables in the American diet: Data from the NHANES II survey. Am J Public Hlth, 1990; 80:1443.

Peto R, Doll R, Buckley J, Sporn M. Can dietary beta-carotene materially reduce human cancer rates? Nature 1981; 290:201.

Popkin BM, Haines PS, Reidy KC. Food consumption trends of U.S. women: Patterns and determinants between 1977 and 1985. Am J Clin Nutr 1989; 49:1307.

Shah BV. SESUDAAN: Standard Errors Program for Computing of Standardized Rates from Sample Survey Data. Research Triangle Institute, Research Triangle Park, NC., 1981.

Subar AF, Block G, James, LD. Folate intake and food sources in the U.S. population. Am J Clin Nutr 1989; 50:508.

U.S. Bureau of the Census. Money Income and Poverty Status of Families and Persons in the United States: 1978. (Advance Report), Current Population Reports, Series P-60, No. 120. Washington, DC: U.S. Government Printing Office, 1979.

U.S. Department of Agriculture, Agricultural Research Service. Nutritive value of American foods, in common units. Agriculture Handbook No. 456. Washington, DC: U.S. Government Printing Office, 1975.

U.S. Department of Health and Human Services, Public Health Service. The Surgeon General's report on nutrition and health. DHHS (PHS) Publication No. 88–50210. Washington, DC: U.S. Government Printing Office, 1988.

U.S. Department of Agriculture, Agricultural Research Service. Essentials of an adequate diet—Facts for nutrition programs. Home Economics Research Report No. 3. Washington, DC: U.S. Government Printing Office, 1957.

U.S. Department of Agriculture. Science and Education Administration. Food. The Hassle-Free Guide to a Better Diet. Davis CA, Home and Garden Bulletin no. 228. Washington, DC: U.S. Government Printing Office, 1979.

U.S. Department of Agriculture, U.S. Department of Health and Human Services. Nutrition and Your Health: Dietary Guidelines for Americans, Home and Garden Bulletin No. 232, Washington DC: U.S. Government Printing Office, 1980.

CRITICAL ISSUES

19

Safety of Vitamin and Mineral Supplements

John N. Hathcock

Food and Drug Administration, Washington, D.C.

INTRODUCTION

The safety of vitamin and mineral supplements depends on (1) the inherent toxicodynamic potency of the specific vitamin or mineral, (2) the chemical form of the vitamin or mineral, (3) daily dosage, (4) duration of supplementation at the chemical form–dosage level combination under consideration, and (5) biological characteristics of the person consuming the supplement (Hathcock et al., 1990; Hathcock and Rader, 1990).

The vitamins and essential minerals, like all substances, can be toxic at sufficiently high intakes. Safety evaluation for a nutrient requires careful specification of the intake level under consideration and a data base on the types of adverse effects and the dose-response relationships for excessive intakes of that nutrient.

Because of ethical proscriptions on the experimental evaluation of toxicity of vitamins and minerals, the levels at which credible reports indicate adverse effects must be used in safety evaluation. The pharmacological therapeutic index (median toxic dose divided by median effective dose) may be modified to a nutrient safety index (minimum toxic intake divided by recommended intake) (Hathcock, 1985). The recommended intake can be specifically identified as the Recommended Dietary Allowance (RDA) or the upper limit of the Estimated Safe and Adequate Daily Dietary Intake (ESADDI) (NRC, 1989), or any other recommendation

---

This chapter was written by John N. Hathcock in his private capacity. No official support or endorsement by the Food and Drug Administration is intended or should be inferred.

under consideration. Identification of the minimum toxic intake, however, is problematic, i.e., it requires either the acceptance of the lowest reported toxic intake as the minimum toxic intake or the identification of the intake that would generate a socially acceptable level of risk identified through a probability approach (NRC, 1986; Hathcock, 1989a,b).

This chapter will use the lowest reported levels for adverse effects by selected nutrients because data on nutrient toxicities in humans do not support detailed application of the probability approach.

VITAMIN SAFETY

Generally, fat-soluble vitamins are much more toxic than those that are water-soluble because of extensive tissue storage and slow rate of metabolism (Hathcock, 1989b). It does not follow, however, that all fat-soluble vitamins present equal toxic hazard or that all water-soluble vitamins are innocuous. There are large differences in inherent toxic potency within each category.

Vitamin A

Among the vitamins, vitamin A is one of few for which substantial numbers of human cases of intoxication have been reported (Bauernfiend, 1980; Miller and Hayes, 1982; Bendich and Langseth, 1989; Hathcock et al., 1990). The intake associated with acute intoxications is usually several hundred thousand international units (IU) per day (Bauernfiend, 1980; Bendich and Langseth, 1989). Chronic intoxication has been attributed to intakes of approximately 25,000 IU/day (Bauernfiend, 1980; Miller and Hayes, 1982; Hathcock et al., 1990). Most toxicities at relatively low intakes have been in people whose liver function has been compromised by drugs, viral hepatitis, or protein-energy malnutrition (Hathcock et al., 1990). Common symptoms of chronic toxicity include elevated cerebrospinal fluid pressure (pseudotumor cerebri), dermatitis, and sometimes liver disease. Apparently related characteristic birth defects may be temporally associated with maternal vitamin A intakes of about 25,000 IU/day (Bauernfiend, 1980; Underwood, 1986; Hathcock et al., 1990). In general, present recommendations are to limit vitamin A intakes for pregnant women to 8000–10,000 IU/day (Kizer et al., 1990; Hathcock et al., 1990). A recent report suggests that slight vitamin A toxicity in elderly individuals was caused by prolonged supplementation of 5000–10,000 IU/day (Krasinski et al., 1989).

Beta-Carotene

The scientific literature indicates a high order of safety for beta-carotene (Bendich and Langseth, 1989; Hathcock et al., 1990). Adverse effects associated with consumption of foods rich in beta-carotene (Frumar et al., 1979; Kemmann et al., 1983; Vakil et al., 1985) have not been observed in tests of equivalent or greater amounts of crystalline beta-carotene (Mathews-Roth, 1975). No effects other than carotenemia were observed in volunteers given 180 mg beta-carotene/day for 10 weeks (Mathews-Roth, 1983).

Vitamin E

Vitamin E is usually considered relatively innocuous with no side effects at intakes of up to 300 IU/day (10 times the U.S. RDA) (Miller and Hayes, 1982) and few side effects at intakes as high as 3200 IU/day (Bendich and Machlin, 1988). Headaches, nausea, fatigue, and diplopia have occurred in people taking more than 300 IU/day (King, 1949). The side effect of vitamin E therapy that occurs at the lowest dosage levels is elevation of serum lipids, especially of triglycerides, HDL, and HDL cholesterol (Bendich and Machlin, 1988). Although these effects may be associated with intakes as low as 600 IU/day (Briggs, 1974; Tsay et al., 1978; Hermann et al., 1979; Howard et al., 1982), it is unclear whether they should be considered adverse. High intakes of vitamin E antagonize vitamin K activity (March et al., 1973; Rao and Mason, 1975) and therefore vitamin E supplements are contraindicated for persons taking drugs which are vitamin K antagonists (Roe, 1982).

Pyridoxine

For most of the time since their discovery, water-soluble vitamins usually have been considered virtually nontoxic because of their solubility and rapid excretion. The toxic effects of pyridoxine proved such assumptions to be unjustified. This vitamin is neuroactive; its deficiency produces neurological symptoms, possibly through disturbances in L-dopa metabolism, and its toxicity produces a sensory neuropathy of uncertain etiology (Cohen and Bendich, 1986). Numerous cases of sensory neuropathy apparently caused by excess pyridoxine consumed over periods from a few days to about 5 years have been reported (Cohen and Bendich, 1986). Early evidence of this toxic effect involved intakes of about 2000–6000 mg/day (Schaumberg et al., 1983). Present evidence suggests that the toxicity threshold for sensory neuropathy may be as low as 300–500 mg/day in a significant number of people (Dalton, 1985; Parry and Bredesen, 1985). Observations in one report suggest that adverse effects may result from only 100–200 mg/day over a 3-year period (O'Brien, 1982). The U.S. RDA for pyridoxine is 2 mg/day.

Since sensory neuropathy from excess pyridoxine was first reported, the lowest reported toxic dose has gradually decreased, but the threshold for individual toxicity is still uncertain. Certainly, a probability approach would indicate a decreasing risk of toxicity as the dose is lowered. In a probability analysis of a hypothetical toxicity distribution with a 500 mg/day mean and 20% coefficient of variation, an intake of 100 mg/day would represent 4 SD below the mean and a probability of toxicity of less than 10^{-4}.

Vitamin C

Vitamin C supplementation is very controversial. Both claimed benefits and claimed adverse effects are numerous. Because of the widespread belief that it provides a range of benefits and is virtually nontoxic, vitamin C is often taken in large quantities. One survey indicated that the mean supplemental vitamin C intake by adults was 3.3 times the RDA (3.3 × 60 mg) and the 95th percentile supplemental intake was 28 times the RDA (28 × 60 mg) (Stewart et al., 1985).

Apparently, vitamin C has a low order of toxicity, or intoxications would be common. Although large intakes may cause adverse effects in some individuals, some of the widely reported and often cited adverse effects have little apparent basis. The evidence to support several potential toxic effects is summarized below:

(1) Conditioned scurvy: This phenomenon is widely reviewed and interpreted to result from conditioning in adults who have had large intakes of vitamin C (Danford and Munro, 1980; Alhadef et al., 1984) and in infants whose mothers took vitamin C supplements during pregnancy (Rhead and Schrauzer, 1971; DiPalma and Ritchie, 1977; Danford and Munro, 1980; Alhadef et al., 1984). Careful review of the literature does not substantiate this phenomenon; it provides only a few basic sources. Excessive intake results in faster clearance, but this does not result in blood levels significantly lower than normal (Schrauzer and Rhead, 1973; Tsao and Leung, 1988). A paper commonly cited as demonstrating conditioned scurvy was speculative only and does not support a relation of scurvy in infants to high prenatal ascorbate intake by the mother (Cochrane, 1965).

Conditioned scurvy due to withdrawal from high intakes of vitamin C has been reported (Seigel et al., 1982), but the diagnosis was not confirmed by clinical chemistry or pathology methods. To the contrary, the time for symptom onset was suspiciously short, and no plasma vitamin C values were reported.

(2) Oxalate kidney stones: Reported increased urinary oxalate levels with large vitamin C intakes appear to be due to oxalate production from ascorbic acid in a urinary oxalate analysis procedure that involves heat (Hoffer, 1985). Reports of increased oxalate excretion raised concern about possible kidney stone formation as a result of excessive vitamin C intake, but the predicted clinical effect has not been observed (Ringsdorf, 1981). Some exacerbation of renal stones of other etiology may have occurred.

(3) Vitamin B_{12} destruction: Apparent vitamin B_{12} destruction that was caused by ascorbic acid in a widely used method of cobalamin extraction seems to be an artifact of the method of sample preparation (Miller and Hayes, 1982). There is no present evidence that ascorbic acid has any deleterious effect in people through this mechanism.

(4) Gastrointestinal distress: The most common adverse reactions to high vitamin C intakes are gastrointestinal symptoms such as nausea, abdominal cramps, and diarrhea, which can occur after ingestion of as little as 1000 mg (Miller and Hayes, 1982). The acidity rather than the ascorbate per se seems to cause the distress because the symptoms can be avoided by taking the vitamin as a buffered salt (Barness, 1975).

(5) Increased oxygen demand: The reduction potential of vitamin C can raise oxygen requirements of cells and tissues, which results in loss of high-altitude resistance (Schrauzer et al., 1975). This may increase the risk of hypoxia in people subjected to hypobaric oxygen or to increase oxygen demand, but the clinical importance of this effect is not known.

(6) Erosion of dental enamel: Regular use of several chewable vitamin C tablets per day has led to severe erosion of dental enamel (Guinta, 1983). Measurements of oral pH and rate of enamel erosion from extracted teeth indicated that use of chewable vitamin C preparations may contribute significantly to loss of dental enamel.

(7) Negative copper balance: The effect of dietary ascorbic acid to increase the absorption of nonheme iron is well established. Conversely, high levels of dietary ascorbic acid decrease intestinal copper uptake, which may lead to negative copper balance (National Nutrition Consortium, 1978). As little as 1500 mg/day may pose long-term risk of copper depletion. However, the health significance of copper loss would depend on copper intake and status.

(8) Delayed-type hypersensitivity and allergy: Vitamin C allergy of the delayed type has been reported (Metz et al., 1980). Eczematous skin lesions on the torso, buttocks, and legs appeared during moderate intake of vitamin C in food. The sensitivity to ascorbic acid was established by withdrawal and reestablishment of the symptoms after resumption of the ascorbic acid intake and by skin patch testing. No estimate was given of the vitamin C intake associated with this allergy. The condition appears to be quite rare and not related to dosage.

Folate

Oral folate is considered as having an extremely low order of toxicity, with no convincing reports of adverse effects at intakes below 15 mg/day (Hathcock, 1985; Butterworth and Tamura, 1989). Major considerations for folate toxicity are the possible antagonism of anticonvulsant drugs and inhibition of zinc utilization and function in pregnant women (Butterworth and Tamura, 1989).

Summary of Vitamin Safety

Recommended levels of intake and levels at which adverse effects may occur after chronic consumption of excess vitamin A, vitamin E, vitamin C, and pyridoxine are shown in Table 1. Beta-carotene is not included in the table because

Table 1 Recommended Levels of Intake and Possible
Adverse Effect Levels for Vitamins

Vitamin	Adult male RDA[a]	Possible adverse effect level (chronic)
Vitamin A	1000 RE[b]	—
	(3300 IU)	25,000 IU
Vitamin E	10 TE[c]	—
	(14.9 IU)	400 IU
Vitamin C	60 mg	1,000 mg
Pyridoxine	2.0 mg	300–500 mg
Folate	200 μg	5–15 mg

[a] From NRC, 1989.
[b] RE, retinol equivalent = 1 μg retinol = 3.33 IU.
[c] TE, tocopherol equivalent = 1 mg d-alpha-tocopherol = 1.49 IU.

no generally recognized recommended intake has been established and the level
at which toxic effects might occur could not be identified. For vitamin A the
adverse effect threshold is less than 10 times the RDA. In contrast, the threshold
for adverse effects by pyridoxine seems to be more than 100 times the RDA.
Consequently, more caution is required to prevent adverse effects by vitamin A
than by pyridoxine. Vitamin E and vitamin C are intermediate in this regard.
Even though a large number of multiples of the RDA is needed to produce toxicity
with pyridoxine, limitation of intake is required because a toxic intake is only
a few hundred milligrams, a quantity that can easily be ingested. The degree to
which interactions with other substances, such as food chemicals or drugs, or
with other conditions such as liver or kidney disease may decrease vitamin safety
cannot be estimated for most vitamins. However, liver disease and exposure to
other substances seems to cause substantial increases in the toxic potency of
vitamin A (Hathcock et al., 1990).

MINERAL SAFETY

Zinc

The toxicity of various zinc salts in humans has not been studied systematically.
Individual tolerances for zinc sulfate, for example, vary widely (Hathcock and
Rader, 1990). One to two grams of zinc sulfate is generally an emetic dose.
Although long-term intakes of moderate amounts of zinc are necessary in some
conditions such as zinc malabsorption, chronic ingestion of large doses of supplements may have adverse effects. For example, when 11 healthy adult men
ingested 300 mg zinc daily for 6 weeks, there was a significant impairment in
lymphocyte and neutrophil function and a potentially harmful increase in the

LDL/HDL ratio (Chandra, 1984). Excessive intakes of zinc may aggravate marginal copper deficiency (Beisel, 1982). Because zinc's toxicity depends on intake of copper, iron, and phytate and other dietary factors, it is not possible to generally define the levels of intake associated with toxicity. The adult U.S. RDA is 15 mg/day.

Iron

The relationship between safe iron intake and the effects of iron on resistance to microbial pathogens is complex (Beisel, 1982; Brock and Mainou-Fowler, 1986; Good et al., 1988; Hathcock and Rader, 1990). Enhanced growth of infectious agents is a major concern for iron supplementation in iron-deficient individuals. Significant direct alterations in immune function are also associated with iron overload.

Major causes of increased tissue iron stores include genetic hemochromatosis, chronic transfusion therapy, alcoholic cirrhosis, and excess dietary iron intake. Alterations in neutrophil defense in hemodialyzed patients with iron overload have been reported (Cantinieaux et al., 1988). Excessive production of toxic oxygen species in tissues in response to high cellular iron may contribute to decreased phagocytosis. Decreased natural killer cell activity in response to multiple transfusions in thalassemia patients has also been reported (Akbar et al., 1986).

Clinical experience and nutritional surveys indicate a wide range of differences in ability to withstand iron overdosage. In hereditary or acquired hemochromatosis, the intestine lacks the ability to exclude excess dietary iron and siderosis occurs. People with genetic predispositions to hemochromatosis who consume diets with excess iron are at greater risk of developing iron overload than normal individuals who consume iron-adequate diets. Widespread iron storage disease which developed following chronic consumption of food and beverages prepared in iron vessels has been reported among the Bantus of South Africa. When iron intake (substantially as ferrous acetate) ranges from 100 to 200 mg/day, iron storage disease may occur in about 80% of the population. The chemical form of the iron intake may be critical in these cases. Iron overload in children may occur after consumption of supplements which contain 200–400 mg Fe (McEnery, 1971). The threshold for adverse effects of supplemental iron is not known but is probably dependent on intakes of other minerals, e.g., manganese and zinc, and possibly ascorbic acid and protein. The adult U.S. RDA for iron is 18 mg/day.

Copper

Copper is among the most inherently toxic of the trace elements. Livers of individuals with Wilson's disease, an inherited disorder characterized by a deficiency of the copper-binding plasma protein ceruloplasmin, may accumulate copper to more than 50 times normal levels (National Nutrition Consortium, 1978). Ultimately, the excess copper exceeds the sequestering capacity of intracellular and extracellular proteins and diffuses into the circulatory system. When the copper reaches other tissues, susceptible cells undergo toxic effects. Hepatic necrosis may also occur in response to an excessive level of stored copper. Studies on the cytotoxicity of copper have included consideration of its capacity to generate radicals and peroxides in biological systems. In general, humans are less sensitive to copper intoxication than are some animals, e.g., sheep. The toxicity of specific levels of copper are affected by dietary iron and zinc as well as protein. The adult U.S. RDA is 2 mg/day.

Selenium

Ingestion of excess selenium can cause extensive tissue damage, especially in the tissues that concentrate the element to the greatest extent (National Nutrition Consortium, 1978). Selenium's toxicity also depends on the form ingested. Selenite is generally regarded as the most toxic. Selenoamino acids which are metabolized to higher oxidation states and selenate are also highly toxic forms. Ingested selenium (as selenite) is toxic at intakes of 1–5 mg/kg body weight.

Although the lowest daily dose of selenium that will cause chronic toxicity in humans is not known, severe human intoxications have occurred with extremely high intakes (20–30 mg/day) after a period of a few weeks (McEnery, 1971; Fox and Jacobs, 1986). Some risk of toxicity may be associated with continuous intakes above 1000 μg/day (NRC, 1989; National Nutrition Consortium, 1978). Limitation of selenium supplementation to the RDA (70 μg/day for the adult male) would have little impact on selenium intake in geographic areas with high natural selenium contents of food and water.

Manganese

There are few reports of intoxications from excessive oral intake of manganese. In one episode of subacute poisoning by manganese-contaminated well water (Mn, 14 μg/ml) for 2–3 months, diagnosis was based on neurological symptoms, histopathological changes in brain tissue, and liver manganese levels (National Nutrition Consortium, 1978). Consumption of 1.5 liters/day of the contaminated well water would contribute an intake of 21 mg/day, a level that some reports suggest may not be safe. A report on the effects of manganese in drinking water (Kondakis et al., 1989) indicates a correlation between increasing manganese levels in drinking water and neurological symptoms. This report indicates significant neurological symptoms in the lowest intake area (3.6–14.6 μg/ml). To the contrary, levels of less than 50 μg/ml are common and generally believed to be safe (NRC, 1977). The lowest adverse effect level for dietary manganese cannot be identified from present data.

Because anemic animals fed excess manganese do not regenerate hemoglobin

Table 2 Recommended Levels of Intake and Possible Adverse Effect Levels for Minerals

Element	Adult males		Possible adverse effect level (chronic)
	RDA[a] (mg)	ESADDI[a] (mg)	
Fe	10	—	100–200 mg/day
Zn	15	—	>100 mg/day
Cu	—	1.5–3.0	>0.5 mg/kg/day (>35 mg/day)
Mn	—	2.0–5.0	>1 mg/g diet (~700 mg/day)
Se	0.07		>0.2 mg/day

[a] From NRC, 1989.

as rapidly as do normal animals, it has been postulated that manganese interferes with iron absorption and thereby may contribute to one of the most common nutritional deficiencies. Thus, individuals with low iron status may be more at risk from excess manganese than those with adequate iron status.

Summary of Mineral Safety

Table 2 shows recommended intakes and levels at which adverse effects may occur after chronic consumption of elevated amounts of zinc, iron, copper, manganese, and selenium. Deficiencies may develop from inadequate dietary intake or indirect causes. Excesses may occur through self-administration of supplements of single or multiple nutrients, contamination of foods, or accumulation during chronic dialysis or transfusions. Deficiencies of iron, vitamin A, and zinc often coexist with protein-energy malnutrition. New considerations about dosage and combinations of vitamins and trace elements for the optimum development and function are complicated by the many interactions among essential and nonessential minerals. Research must be able to distinguish the metabolic effect of deficiencies or excesses of a specific element from that of other minerals. Interactions among iron, zinc, and copper, for example, are now widely recognized. Requirements or safe limits for any one of these elements should be established only in conjunction with an awareness of its interaction with the others.

REFERENCES

Akbar AN, Fitzgerald-Bocarsly PA, DeSousa M, Giardina PJ, Hilgartner MW, Grady RW. Decreased natural killer cell activity in thalassemia major: A possible consequence of iron overload. Immunology 1986; 136:1635–1640.

Alhadef L, Gualtieri CT, Lipton M. Toxic effects of water-soluble vitamins. Nutr Rev 1984; 42:33–40.

Barness LA. Safety considerations with high ascorbic acid dosage. Ann NY Acad Sci 1975; 258:523–528.

Bauernfiend JC. The safe use of Vitamin A. A report of the International Vitamin A Consultative Group (IVACG). Washington, DC: The Nutrition Foundation, 1980.

Beisel WR. Single nutrients and immunity. Am J Clin Nutr 1982; 35 (Feb. Suppl.):417–468.

Bendich A, Langseth L. Safety of vitamin A. Am J Clin Nutr 1989; 49:358–371.

Bendich A, Machlin LJ. Safety of oral intake of vitamin E. Am J Clin Nutr 1988; 48:612–619.

Briggs MH. Vitamin E in clinical medicine. Lancet 1974; 1:220.

Brock JH, Mainou-Fowler T. Iron and immunity. Proc Nutr Soc 1986; 45:305–315.

Butterworth CE, Tamura T. Folic acid safety and toxicity: A brief review. Am J Clin Nutr 1989; 50:353–358.

Cantinieaux B, Boelaert J, Hariga C, Fondu P. Impaired neutrophil defense against Yersinia enterocolitica in patients with iron overload who are undergoing dialysis. J Lab Clin Med 1988; 111:524–528.

Centers for Disease Control. Selenium intoxications—New York. MMWR 1983; 33:157–158.

Chandra RK. Excessive intake of zinc impairs immune responses. J Am Med Assoc 1984; 252:1443–1446.

Cochrane WA. Overnutrition in prenatal and neonatal life: A problem? Can Med Assoc J 1965; 93:893–899.

Cohen M, Bendich A. Safety of pyridoxine—A review of human and animal studies. Toxicol Lett 1986; 34:129–139.

Dalton K. Pyridoxine overdose in premenstrual syndrome. Lancet 1985; 1:1168–1169.

Danford DE, Munro HN. Water-soluble vitamins. In: Gilman AG, Goodman A, Gilman A, eds. Pharmacological basis of therapeutics, 6th ed. New York: Macmillan, 1980, 1560–1582.

DiPalma JR, Ritchie DM. Vitamin toxicity. Ann Rev Pharmacol Toxicol 1977; 17:133–148.

Fox MRS, Jacobs RM. Human nutrition and metal ion toxicity. In: Sigel H, ed. Metal ions in biological systems. New York: Marcel Dekker, 1986.

Frumar AM, Meldrum DR, Judd HL. Hypercarotenemia in hypothalmic amenorrhea. Fertil Steril 1979; 32:261–264.

Good MF, Powell LW, Halliday JW. Iron status and cellular immune competence. Blood Rev 1988; 45:43–49.

Guinta JL. Dental erosion resulting from chewable vitamin C tablets. J Am Dent Assoc 1983; 107:253–256.

Hathcock JN. Quantitative evaluation of vitamin safety. Pharmacy Times 1985; 51:104–113.

Hathcock JN. High nutrient intakes—The toxicologist's view. J Nutr 1989a; 119:1779–1784.

Hathcock JN. Risk/benefit for vitamin supplements. In: Hathcock JN, ed. Nutritional toxicology, Vol. 3. Orlando: Academic Press, 1989b.

Hathcock JN, Rader JI. Micronutrient safety. Ann NY Acad Sci 1990; 587:257–266.

Hathcock JN, Hattan DL, Jenkins MY, McDonald J, Sundaresan PR, Wilkening V. Evaluation of vitamin A toxicity. Am J Clin Nutr 1990; 52:183–202.

Hermann WJ, Ward K, Faucett J. The effect of tocopherol on high-density lipoprotein cholesterol. Am. J. Clin Pathol 1979; 72:848–852.

Hoffer A. Ascorbic acid and kidney stones. Can Med Assoc J 1985; 132:320.

Howard DR, Rundell CA, Batsakis JG. Vitamin E and serum lipids: A non-correlation. Am J Clin Pathol 1982; 77:243–244.

Kemman E, Pasquale SA, Skaf R. Amenorrhea associated with carotenemia. J Am Med Assoc 1983; 249:296–299.

King RA. Vitamin E in Dupuytren's contracture. J Joint Surg 1949; 31B:443.

Kizer KW, Fan A, Bankowska J, Jackson RJ, Lyman D. Vitamin A—A pregnancy hazard alert. Western J Med 1990; 152:78–81.

Klevay LM. The ratio of zinc to copper in diets in the United States. Nutr Rep Int 1975; 11:237–242.

Kondakis XG, Makris N, Leotsinidis M, Prinou M, Papapetropoulos T. Possible health effects of high manganese concentration in drinking water. Arch Environ Health 1989; 44:175–178.

Krasinski SD, Russell RM, Otradovec CL, Sadowski JA, Hartz SC, Jabob RA, McGandy RB. Relationship of vitamin A and vitamin E intake to fasting plasma retinol, retinol binding protein, retinyl esters, carotene, alpha-tocopherol, and cholesterol among elderly and young adults: Increased plasma retinyl esters among vitamin A-supplemented users. Am M Clin Nutr 1989; 49:112–120.

March BE, Wong E, Seier L, Sim JB. Hypervitaminosis E in the chick. J Nutr 1973; 103:371–377.

Mathews-Roth MM. Amenorrhea associated with carotenemia. J Am Med Assoc 1983; 250:731.

McEnery JT. Hospital management of acute iron ingestion. Clin Toxicol 1971; 4:603–616.

Metz J, Hundertmark U, Pevny I. Vitamin C allergy of the delayed type. Contact Dermatitis 1980; 6:172–174.

Miller DR, Hayes KC. Vitamin excess and toxicity. In: Hathcock JN, ed. Nutritional toxicology, Vol. 1. New York: Academic Press, 1982.

National Nutrition Consortium. Vitamin-mineral safety. Chicago: The American Dietetic Association, 1978.

National Research Council. Drinking Water and Health. Washington, DC: National Academy of Sciences, 1977.

National Research Council. Nutrient adequacy. Washington, DC: National Academy Press, 1986.

National Research Council. Recommended Dietary Allowances, 10th ed. Washington, DC: National Academy Press, 1989.

O'Brien P. The premenstrual syndrome: A review of the present status of therapy. Drugs 1982; 24:140–151.

Parry GJ, Bredensen DE. Sensory neuropathy with low-dose pyridoxine. Neurology 1985; 35:1466–1468.

Rao GH, Mason KE. Antisterility and antivitamin K activity of D-alpha-tocopherol hydroquinone in the vitamin E-deficient female rat. J Nutr 1975; 105:495–498.

Rhead WJ, Schrauzer GN. Risks of long term ascorbic acid overdose (letter). Nutr Rev 1971; 29:262–263.

Ringsdorf WM, Cheraskin E. Nutritional aspects of urolithiasis. South Med J 1981; 74:41–46.

Roe DA. Handbook: Interactions of selected drugs and nutrients in patients, 3rd ed. Chicago: The American Dietetic Association 1982.

Schaumberg H, Kaplan J, Windebank A, Vick N, Rasmus S, Pleasure D, Brown MJ. Sensory neuropathy from pyridoxine abuse. N Engl J Med 1983; 309:445–448.

Schrauzer GN, Rhead WJ. Ascorbic acid abuse: Effects of long term ingestion of excessive amounts on blood levels and urinary excretion. Int J Vit Nutr Res 1973; 43:201–211.

Schrauzer GN, Ishmael D, Kiefer GW. Some aspects of current vitamin C usage: Diminished high-altitude resistance following overdosage. Ann NY Acad Sci 1975; 258:377–381.

Seigel C, Barker B, Kunstadter M. Conditioned oral scurvy due to megavitamin C withdrawal. J Peridontol 1982; 53:453–455.

Stewart ML, McDonald JT, Levy AS, Schucker RP, Henderson DP. Vitamin/mineral supplement use: A telephone survey of adults in the United States. J Am Diet Assoc 1985; 85:1585–1590.

Tsao CS, Leung PY. Urinary ascorbic acid levels following withdrawal of large doses of ascorbic acid in guinea pigs. J Nutr 1988; 118:895–900.

Tsay AC, Kelley JJ, Peng B, Cook N. Study on the effect of megavitamin E supplementation in man. Am J Clin Nutr 1978; 31:831–837.

Underwood BA. The safe use of vitamin A by women during the reproductive years. Washington, DC: International Life Sciences Institute/Nutrition Foundation, 1986.

Underwood EJ. Trace elements in human and animal nutrition, 4th ed. New York: Academic Press, 1977.

Vakil DV, Ayiomamitis A, Nizami N, Nizami RM. Hypercarotenemia: A case report and review of the literature. Nutr Res 1985; 5:911–917.

20

Role of the Physician in Nutrition Education

Lillian Langseth and Donald H. Gemson

Columbia University School of Public Health
New York, New York

INTRODUCTION

In the early part of the 20th century, the need to educate physicians-in-training about nutrition was obvious. Nutritional deficiency diseases were important public health problems, and new scientific knowledge about the nutrients that could prevent these diseases was growing rapidly. Today, all of the vitamins have long since been identified and most of the classic deficiency disease have become rare curiosities in the United States. Nevertheless, a knowledge of nutrition is still crucial for the practicing physician because nutrition is important in both the prevention and treatment of the chronic degenerative diseases that are today's most pressing health problems. In the words of the 1988 *Surgeon General's Report on Nutrition and Health* (DHHS, 1988):

> *For the two out of three adult Americans who do not smoke and do not drink excessively, one personal choice seems to influence long-term health prospects more than any other: what we eat. . . . The quantity of current animal, laboratory, clinical, and epidemiologic evidence that associates dietary excesses and imbalances with chronic disease is substantial and, when evaluated according to established principles, compelling.*

Nutritional factors are implicated in the etiology of six of the 10 leading causes of death in the United States: heart disease, cerebrovascular disease, cancer, adult-onset (type II) diabetes, arteriosclerosis, and alcohol-induced cirrhosis

(DHEW, 1979; DHHS, 1983). The role of diet in cardiovascular disease, the leading cause of death among American adults (DHHS, 1984), is particularly significant. Nutritional factors are important in the prevention and control of two risk factors strongly associated with cardiovascular disease: high blood cholesterol levels and high blood pressure (Levy and Moskowitz, 1982; Harland et al., 1984; Harland and Stross, 1985; NCEP, 1988). Obesity is a major health problem in the United States. Eighteen percent of U.S. men and 24% of U.S. women are 20% or more above their ideal weight (Abraham et al., 1983). Obesity is associated with elevated risks of high blood pressure, high blood lipid levels, diabetes, complications of pregnancy, osteoarthritis, and other ailments (Stewart and Brook, 1983). In order for physicians to help their patients avoid these consequences of obesity, they need to be trained in the prevention and treatment of overweight. While many Americans choose to tackle their weight problems without medical assistance, the involvement of physicians and other health professionals is desirable. The *Surgeon General's Report* recommends professional guidance "because many popular means to reduce weight may themselves pose risks to health and because unsupervised efforts to control obesity usually fail over the long term" (DHHS, 1988).

Physicians also need a knowledge of nutrition to help patients reduce their risks of several other major diet-related health problems common in this country. These include low birth weight, a major cause of infant mortality that is often associated with poor maternal nutrition during pregnancy (Brandt, 1984); osteoporosis, a major cause of bone fractures and invalidism among the elderly (Avioli, 1984); and some types of cancer, which may be associated with high-fat diets or other nutrition-related risk factors (NRC, 1982; ACS, 1984; NCI, 1984).

Nutrition plays a critical role in disease treatment as well as prevention. Diet is used in the management of diabetes (Bierman, 1985), gastrointestinal disorders (Inglett and Falkehag, 1979), kidney disorders (DHHS, 1988), eating disorders (Schwabe et al., 1981; Halmi et al., 1981), severe catabolic states such as major burns or surgery (Thompson et al., 1984), and inborn errors of metabolism (Palmer and Zeman, 1983), among other conditions.

Nutrition also plays an important role in optimum health care for the well person, particularly those individuals in vulnerable stages of the life cycle, including infancy, childhood, pregnancy, lactation, and aging. The 1988 *Surgeon General's Report* recommends that "health care programs for individuals of all ages should include nutrition services," and makes extensive, specific recommendations for including nutrition services in the care of healthy older adults and healthy mothers and children (DHHS, 1988).

Finally, physicians need a knowledge of nutrition in order to support their patients' efforts to take greater responsibility for their own health by modifying their lifestyles. Although the increased interest of the American public in diet and health is generally beneficial, physicians need to be knowledgeable enough to counsel patients about potential medical risks involved in such practices as indiscriminate micronutrient supplementation (Raven, 1981; NRC, 1980), self-prescribed weight reduction regimens (Dwyer, 1980), scientifically invalid dietary treatments for serious chronic diseases (DHHS, 1988), and poorly planned vegetarian diets (Herbert, 1983).

BACKGROUND

Concern over Nutrition Education for Physicians

Education of physicians about nutrition should begin in medical school, but "medical schools are following, not leading, the trend of increased interest in nutrition" (Health Values, 1989). While specific improvements in medical school education have been documented, numerous studies have shown that nutrition education at this stage of a physician's career is likely to be inadequate.

Concerns about the attention given to nutrition in the medical school curriculum have been raised since at least the early 1960s. In 1961, the American Medical Association (AMA) Council on Foods and Nutrition stated that nutrition was receiving "inadequate recognition, support and attention" in medical education (White et al., 1961). A 1963 national conference sponsored by the AMA and the Nutrition Foundation confirmed this conclusion and called for expansion and improvement of nutrition teaching in both undergraduate and postgraduate medical education (NME, 1985).

At the White House Conference on Food, Nutrition, and Health held in 1969 in response to testimony given earlier in the year to a Senate Select Subcommittee on Nutrition and Human Needs (U.S. Congress, 1969), concerns were expressed over the lack of nutrition in the medical school curriculum (White House Conference, 1969). In 1971, a survey of second-year medical students revealed an inadequate knowledge of essential nutrition concepts, as defined by the White House Conference (Phillips, 1971). Even 20 years after the conference, one of the two most urgent future needs cited at an anniversary symposium was the inclusion of nutrition as a mandatory part of the curricula in medical and dental schools and allied health sciences programs (Goldberg and Mayer, 1990).

Although some medical schools improved their nutrition programs in the late 1960s and early 1970s, surveys conducted by the AMA in 1976 and 1978 showed that less than 20% and 25% of them, respectively, required a course in nutrition (Cyborski, 1977; Geiger, 1979). Many other schools reported teaching nutrition topics within the framework of other courses and offering elective courses in nutrition, but the amount of nutrition training actually provided in these ways could not be determined.

In the late 1970s, the teaching of nutrition in medical schools became a public policy issue. At congressional hearings in 1979, the General Accounting Office

(GAO) reviewed the federal government's efforts to improve nutrition training for medical students and stated that in spite of its importance to health, nutrition was not taught adequately in many medical schools (GAO, 1980). *Healthy People: The Surgeon General's Report on Health Promotion and Disease Prevention* also noted the importance of the physician's role in advising patients about prevention. The report said that "training in nutrition for physicians and other health professionals should have high priority" (DHEW, 1979).

In the same year, a congressional committee looked at the nutrition-related questions on the 1978 National Board examinations for physicians and concluded that the quantity of questions on nutrition was low, the quality poor, and the topical distribution inappropriate (U.S. Congress, 1979).

At a National Workshop on Nutrition in Health Professions Schools held in 1981, the statement was made that "it is likely that the most prevalent nutritional deficiency in the United States today is the deficiency of nutrition information" (Weinsier, 1982).

More recently, the same message was reiterated in the *Surgeon General's Report on Nutrition and Health* (DHHS, 1988), which stated:

> *Improved nutrition training of physicians and other health professionals is needed. Training should emphasize basic principles of nutrition, the role of diet in health promotion and disease prevention, nutrition assessment methodologies and their interpretation, therapeutic aspects of dietary intervention, behavioral aspects of dietary counseling, and the role of dietitians and nutritionists in dietary counseling of patients.*

This report particularly emphasized that health professionals should be able to guide patients in dietary means of reducing blood cholesterol levels and should be able to provide counseling on maternal and child nutrition. The report specifically called for expanded training opportunities in these two areas for health professionals.

Medical Student Education in Nutrition

One major source of criticism of nutrition education in medical schools has been medical students themselves. Of more than 40,000 medical students who completed graduation questionnaires in 1981–1984, more than 60% reported that the instruction time devoted to nutrition was inadequate (AAMC, 1981–1984).

In a 1985 statement prepared for the Food and Nutrition Board of the National Research Council (NRC), the American Medical Students Association (AMSA) observed:

> *Nutrition is not well taught, if taught at all, in most medical schools. . . . Most nutrition in the formal curriculum is incorporated into other courses. . . . Too often in such courses, nutrition is touched on briefly, with*

the primary emphasis on the major discipline. It is quite possible to finish such a course and not even realize that nutrition was covered (AMSA, 1985).

The students' conclusion that nutrition is most effectively taught as a separate course is consistent with the findings of Cohen et al. (1981), who reported that students who take a separate course in nutrition acquire more knowledge than those taught nutrition integrated in another course.

The American Medical Students Association also stated the following:

Generally, patients should be able to expect physicians to have at least a minimum level of knowledge and skill in the area of nutrition. . . . Unfortunately, very few physicians have this level of expertise, and if they do, it has been generally acquired outside the traditional medical school curriculum (AMSA, 1985).

The students' group said that preclinical instruction in nutrition should emphasize the application of nutrition principles to current major public health problems, rather than focusing only on metabolism.

There are several sources of information on nutrition education in medical schools in the 1980s. One source is a curriculum questionnaire sent annually to all U.S. medical schools by the Joint Liaison Committee on Medical Education (LCME), composed of representatives of the AMA and the Association of American Medical Colleges (AAMC). For the academic years 1979–1980 through 1983–1984, the responses to this survey indicated that 24–37% of all medical schools had a required nutrition course, 51–66% of the schools lacking such a course incorporated nutrition into some other course, and 54–65% offered nutrition electives (AAMC, 1980–1984).

These findings would seem to indicate that a substantial proportion of U.S. medical schools do not teach nutrition at all. However, the accuracy of these survey results has been questioned by an NRC committee that undertook its own comprehensive investigation of nutrition education in medical schools (CNME, 1985). The NRC committee noted that the LCME curriculum questionnaires are often completed by administrative personnel who may be unfamiliar with details of the curriculum. In many cases, these individuals do not check the data with those faculty members who are responsible for the teaching of nutrition.

The 1985 NRC survey was designed to obtain more detailed qualitative information on the teaching of nutrition in medical schools. The survey, limited to 46 medical schools, was directed at the faculty member responsible for teaching nutrition at each of these schools and was followed up with telephone interviews in many cases. Responses from 39 schools showed that most medical schools teach some nutrition; however, only two-thirds teach it in the first academic year, along with the other basic preclinical sciences, and only 18% teach it as a separate, required course. Many schools also offer nutrition clerkships and electives, but only a small number of students take advantage of them.

There is great variation in the number of classroom hours devoted to nutrition in medical schools. The NRC survey showed that an average of 21 hours of instruction was devoted to nutrition, but that 60% of schools taught less than 20 hours and 20% taught less than 10 hours. Thirty percent taught 30 or more hours. The NRC committee stated that 25–30 classroom hours is needed for adequate coverage of the core concepts of nutrition (CNME, 1985).

The NRC survey showed considerable variation in the scope of topics taught in nutrition courses. Some key concepts, such as energy balance and obesity, are covered in almost all medical schools, but other topics important in medical practice, such as nutrient-drug interactions, nutrition in adolescence, renal disease, allergies, nutrition and cancer, prevention of dental disease, cultural variations in dietary habits, and effects of nutrition on the immune response and the central nervous system, are taught in 50% or fewer of the surveyed schools.

On the basis of its survey findings, plus a review of previous research and detailed interviews with faculty members at several medical schools, the NRC committee reached the following conclusions:

1. The teaching of nutrition in most U.S. medical schools is inadequate.
2. Nutrition is not taught as a separate subject—the most effective presentation—in the majority of schools.
3. Some medical schools do not teach important nutrition topics.
4. Many schools do not devote sufficient classroom hours to nutrition.
5. The success of a nutrition program depends heavily on the willingness of faculty to commit time to initiate and develop such a program. There is a specific need for faculty members who can demonstrate the application of nutrition to clinical practice, i.e., clinically active physicians rather than researchers who hold doctorate degrees.
6. There is "a distinct lack of organizational structure and administrative support for nutrition programs" in medical schools.
7. Resources, such as textbooks, available for teaching nutrition in medical schools are insufficient or inappropriate.

It should perhaps be pointed out that the publication of a guide to materials for use in teaching clinical nutrition in medical, dental, and public health schools (Read, 1983) was met with a very positive response, prompting the publication of a supplement 3 years later (Read et al., 1987).

In 1984, a collaborative effort of the medical schools in Alabama, Florida, Georgia, and South Carolina resulted in the establishment of the Southeastern Regional Medical-Nutrition Education Network (SERMEN) to enhance nutrition education in this part of the United States. Required hours in nutrition at SERMEN schools ranged from a high of 56 hours (in a separately identifiable course) to zero hours. Results of an examination voluntarily taken by 21% of senior medical students at 10 of the SERMEN schools showed significant variation in nutrition knowledge levels (Weinsier et al., 1986). Eighty-five percent of seniors examined were dissatisfied with the quantity and 60% with the quality of their medical-nutrition education. Knowledge scores correlated with the students' assessments with r values of 0.28 and 0.35, respectively.

Other, cross-sectional studies of volunteer SERMEN students at three stages in their training revealed that only 13% of preclinical students perceived nutrition as important to their careers, compared with 74% of entering and 59% of graduating students (Weinsier et al., 1988). Upperclassmen's scores were higher than freshmen's and varied with the amount of required nutrition teaching, suggesting that nutrition knowledge can be increased through preclinical course work and that the knowledge level can be maintained through the clinical years.

The two factors critical to the successful development of a medical nutrition program at the University of Alabama at Birmingham appear to be revelance of the course material to medical practice and the presence of a strong, positive role model as a physician-nutritionist (Weinsier, 1982). A 58-hour required nutrition course can be an effective way to introduce basic and clinical nutrition with good retention of knowledge in subsequent years (Morgan et al., 1989), enhanced by the availability of nutrition support service activities throughout medical training. Basic science courses such as biochemistry, in which 37 hours is devoted to nutrition-related topics, cannot be relied on to add significantly to nutrition knowledge (Morgan et al., 1989).

To aid in the establishment of a consensus on core content for a medical school curriculum, the Committee on Medical/Dental School and Residency Nutrition Education of the American Society for Clinical Nutrition surveyed medical school nutrition educators and medical school curriculum planners and conducted a workshop of 100 participants (Weinsier et al., 1989). Responses of 178 medical school nutrition educators and 40 medical school curriculum planners showed close agreement on the importance ratings of 41 nutrition topics and on the number of hours of nutrition course work that medical schools should provide (44 vs. 37 hours, respectively). The highest priority topics identified were body weight, body composition, and energy balance; proteins and amino acids; carbohydrates, fiber; lipids (including cholesterol); vitamins; major minerals; water, electrolytes, and acid-base balance; trace minerals; diet and hypertension; diet, hyperlipidemia, and atherosclerosis.

Nutrition Education Programs for Physicians

In addition to improved medical school education, the lack of clinical training in nutrition may be mitigated by clinical nutrition training programs for physicians, many of whom appear to be interested in such programs. A mail survey of more than 1000 family and general practitioners, internists, and obstetricians/gynecologists in Maryland found that two-thirds were interested in continuing education about nutrition, with the strongest interest found among those who believe a balanced diet and vitamin supplementation are important to promote and maintain the health of the average person (Sobal et al., 1987).

A survey in the *American Journal of Clinical Nutrition* listing medical schools and universities that offer physicians special training in human nutrition (Howard and Bigaouette, 1983) was followed by publication of biennial program listings in the same journal (Heymsfield et al., 1985; Merritt et al., 1988). These researchers urged that the scope of clinical nutrition training programs for physicians be broadened to include a wider range of patient age groups and diseases, and that a program-certifying agency be employed to identify programs that meet certain minimum standards.

Another source of physician information is the registered dietitian. The "professional upgrading of competence" of the dietitian, the increasing use of dietitians by physicians, and the intensified role dietitians play in assessing patients have been noted as major changes in the past 10–15 years (Shils, 1986). Moreover, the Surgeon General's 1988 *Report on Nutrition and Health*, which emphasized the role of diet in the prevention of disease, suggested public policy initiatives that specifically recognized nutritionists and dietitians as important sources of dietary information (Donato, 1988). In addition, the National Cholesterol Education Program Adult Treatment Panel Report (NCEP, 1988) has also recognized nutritionists and registered dietitians as a key source of nutrition information for patients and recommends that physicians refer certain patients to dietitians for more intensive nutrition counseling and education. At least one survey of the general public found that the dietitian is viewed as the most appropriate health provider for nutrition counseling and education, including calculating calorie needs, providing dietary counseling, evaluating nutritional status, and prescribing diets—the latter perception prevailing even though dietitians cannot legally prescribe diets (Koteski and McKinney, 1988).

Communicating Nutrition Information

Nutritional information must be effectively communicated before it can be of use. Effective communication by physicians to patients is dependent on physicians' knowledge, attitude, and skills. As noted in the National Cholesterol Education Program (NCEP) report:

> *The success of dietary therapy will depend to a large extent on the physician's attitudes and skills in motivating the patient, and in organizing a team approach to dietary therapy. The physician can have a major impact on the patient's attitude toward diet modification. A positive attitude on the part of the physician is absolutely vital* (NCEP, 1988).

Studies reveal that many physicians fail to pass on what they know to patients who could benefit. Following are some examples taken from recent survey studies.

In a survey of 64 randomly selected physicians from the University of Minnesota Family Practice Clinical Faculty, almost half the 49 responders gave advice about dietary fat, sodium, or fiber to fewer than 20% of their patients, and only 10% gave such advice to more than 80% of their patients (Kottke et al., 1984). The most common reason given for not counseling patients was the absence of elevated risk factors for cardiovascular disease or nutritional disease. Other reasons cited by these physicians included a perceived lack of patient interest, the expectation of patient noncompliance, and, on occasion, the unpalatability of the diet.

Results of a study conducted by Columbia University researchers showed that of 329 primary care physicians surveyed in New York State, many opted for drug treatment without an adequate trial of diet therapy in the management of patients with high blood cholesterol levels. Of the physicians surveyed 41% said they would initiate drug treatment for a healthy 40-year-old man with total cholesterol of 300 mg/dl either at the initial visit or after only one month of a lipid-lowering diet (Shea et al., 1990). Such an approach is contrary to the NCEP Adult Treatment Panel guidelines, which call for 6 months of dietary therapy before starting drug treatment (NCEP, 1988).

National surveys suggest that many physicians feel poorly prepared to provide dietary counseling or believe that such counseling is not practical in the modern practice setting (Schucker, 1987). While this problem may seem daunting, it may be overcome in some cases by referring the patient to a registered dietitian or qualified nutritionist (U.S. Preventive Services Task Force, 1989).

Physicians also seem to lack confidence in their ability to help patients change their behavior, with studies finding that fewer than 20% of physicians perceive themselves as being very successful in changing unhealthy patient practices (Levine, 1987). In one survey, only 3–8% felt they were very successful in getting patients to make health-enhancing lifestyle changes (Wechsler et al., 1983). Physicians tend to feel less successful in modifying patient behaviors related to drug use, diet, smoking, alcohol use, and stress than in encouraging patients to exercise (Wechsler et al., 1983). Physicians' perceptions of their ability to get patients to change their lifestyle may be a key factor behind their counseling practices (Green et al., 1988).

Physicians who themselves have poor health habits have been found less likely to counsel patients about behavior changes they should make (Lewis et al., 1986), although at least one study was unable to find a relationship between the level of obesity of the physician and the likelihood of patients being advised to lose weight (Adamson et al., 1988). Physicians who were working to improve their own behavior were found to admonish their patients significantly more often than those physicians who were not trying to change their own behavior (Lewis et al., 1986). Consequently, attempts to adopt a healthier way of life among physicians may have a multiplier effect.

Perhaps for good reason, physicians tend to assume that patients are not seeking their advice on lifestyle changes that would promote health (Kottke et al., 1984; Lunin, 1987). In the case of smoking, most physicians feel smokers lack the motivation to stop, and many physicians do not know what to say or lack confidence in their antismoking advice (Fortmann et al., 1985). Nevertheless, physicians seem to feel more confident about counseling patients to stop smoking than they do about providing dietary counseling. One recent study found that 69% of physicians rated themselves as highly competent to counsel patients about smoking, whereas only 32% considered themselves highly competent to provide dietary counseling (Shea et al., 1990).

As noted by Kottke et al. (1984), a lack of confidence in their ability to counsel patients about diet may make physicians reluctant to provide nutrition counseling to *all* patients:

> *We found that most physicians are not averse to initiating nutritional intervention—thus, this is not a barrier to care. However, the majority of physicians use the high-risk strategy to decide who is appropriate to receive care* (Kottke et al., 1984).

Perceived lack of interest and anticipated lack of adherence are also significant barriers to intervention.

> *As with anyone else, it is natural for physicians to avoid practices that are associated with negative reinforcement and perceived to result in failure. It is not surprising that an intervention for which it is so hard to detect an effect and [which] is sometimes unwanted by the patient is avoided* (Kottke et al., 1984).

Nonetheless, there is some evidence that patients may be more motivated than some physicians believe. For example, patients with a low socioeconomic status have been found to have a high level of interest and knowledge about elevated cholesterol as a health risk (Whiteside and Robbins, 1989). In fact, nearly half of the 110 patients in this study said they were making considerable efforts to reduce their fat intake.

Physicians recognize that counseling a patient about behavior change, including dietary change, takes time. One study conducted in The Netherlands found that the best predictor of both the amount of information given during an office visit and the amount of questioning by the patient was the duration of the consultation (Verhaak and van Busschbach, 1988). When a doctor allows his patient more time, the chance of a full explanation is increased, as is the likelihood that the patient will seek the answers he needs. In most cases such counseling is not specifically reimbursed by third-party payers, and insufficient time or inadequate reimbursement is frequently cited by physicians as a barrier to the exchange of health information with patients (Gemson and Elinson, 1986; Lunin, 1987; Nash, 1988; Donato, 1988; Langner et al., 1989; U.S. Preventive Services Task Force, 1989).

Another barrier to dietary counseling may be the seemingly mundane nature of nutritional information. While surveys show that physicians embrace the idea of preventive care, they still tend to be oriented toward curative medicine (Wechsler et al., 1983; Gemson and Elinson, 1986). One physician commented in 1988:

> *The prevention of disease states should represent the highest ideal for the practitioner, yet all too often such efforts are merely given lip service. . . . In my training program, establishing an obscure diagnosis underlying the patient's esoteric signs and symptoms was the Holy Grail we sought. Once this was achieved, vigorous therapy aimed at elimination of the disease was pursued with a singleminded purpose. The patient was then discharged. Any idea of follow-up or preventive care was relegated to the doctors providing ambulatory care. The "real" action was limited to the acutely ill patient on the ward. Most training programs are still crisis-oriented* (Nash, 1988).

Indeed, physicians who counsel their patients most often about nutrition may differ from their colleagues in measurable ways. A study conducted in Quebec found that such physicians have stronger beliefs than others about their role in influencing their patients' eating habits, have greater satisfaction with their medical training in this area, and are more likely to deliver care in the private rather than the public sector (Maheux et al., 1989).

NUTRITION INFORMATION SOURCES USED BY PHYSICIANS

In 1988 a nationwide cross-sectional mail survey of office-based primary care physicians in the United States was conducted to determine sources of nutrition information used by physicians, as well as information on attitudes about nutrition in medicine and use of nutrition information in medical practice (Langseth, 1990).

A total of 464 physicians responded (response rate 31%). Of these, 47% were in family medicine, 33% in internal medicine, and 14% in general practice. Just over half of these physicians (54%) were in solo practice while 46% were in group practice. Over 44% were affiliated with a teaching hospital. The sample was 90% male. Eighty-two percent of the physicians were graduates of medical schools in the United States and Canada. By age, the greatest proportion of respondents were in the 36- to 45-year age group followed by the 56- to 65-year age group. The lowest response rate was among those aged 35 years and under. There was no geographic response bias.

Sources of Information

The questionnaire covered a wide variety of sources of information ranging from professional to popular and included printed information, television and radio sources, as well as other individuals including health professionals, colleagues, friends, and family. The responses by total percentages are shown in tabular form in Table 1 and in graphic form in Fig. 1. These data show that the physicians surveyed relied most on printed professional sources of information and information from nutritionists and dietitians, and somewhat less on information from colleagues.

The four sources of information used most often were medical group literature (33%), medical journal articles (33%), nutritionists and dietitians (30%), and government literature (23%). When the categories of "often" and "sometimes" were combined, the same four sources were used most frequently by the largest percentages of respondents: medical journal articles (87%), medical group literature (86%), government literature (80%), and nutritionists and dietitians (79%).

Despite the fact that there was a clear tendency for the physicians who responded to use professional sources of information most often, other nonprofessional sources of information should not be underestimated. A significant

Table 1 Sources of Nutrition Information Used by Physicians

Source	Often	Sometimes	Combined
Medical group literature	33	52	85
Medical journal articles	33	54	87
Nutritionists/RDs	30	48	78
Government literature	23	57	80
Newspapers	20	44	64
Professional meetings	20	49	69
Medical magazines	18	48	66
News magazines	17	43	60
University newsletters	15	33	48
Ads in medical journals	8	37	45
Drug firm literature	7	40	47
Colleagues	6	49	55
Food firm literature	6	36	42
Popular books	5	24	29
Television	3	32	35
Family	3	21	24
Friends	2	20	22
Radio	2	16	18

Response by % total

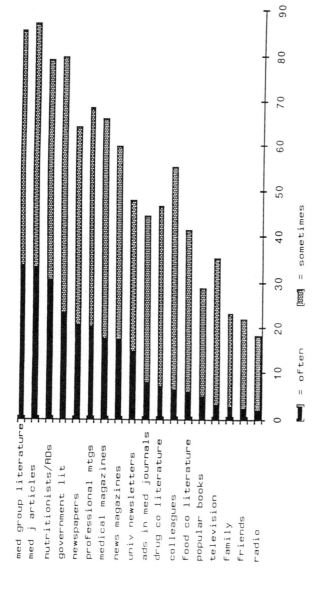

Figure 1 Summary of nutrition information sources used by physicians.

proportion of physicians indicated reliance on the following sources often or sometimes: newspapers (64%), magazines (60%), television (35%), popular books (29%), information from family and friends (24 and 22%, respectively), and radio (18%).

Attitudes about Nutrition in Medicine

A majority of the physicians had positive attitudes about the role of nutrition in medicine and the benefits thereof, and almost 85% indicated that nutrition will become even more important in medicine in the future. Sixty-seven percent also indicated that nutrition counseling should be part of virtually all routine health contacts with primary care physicians. Finally, 70% of physicians agreed that preventive care (such as nutrition counseling) is at least as gratifying as diagnosis and treatment.

A majority of physicians (76%) believed that nutrition counseling was an effective use of physician time and 75% indicated that they saw benefits to patients from nutrition counseling by a physician. An even greater proportion (84%) indicated that nutrition counseling by a nutritionist or dietitian would benefit patients.

Physicians were in agreement about the importance and benefits of nutrition in medicine, and 83% indicated that it was the role of the physician to provide such counseling. However, their perception of their own preparedness and abilities in this area revealed distinct reservations: only 53% indicated that they were prepared to provide nutrition counseling. About 30% felt ill-prepared to provide nutrition counseling and felt that such counseling would be better left to other health professionals.

Physicians were also well aware of their limitations as the major source of nutrition information for patients: 63% indicated that most patient nutrition information was obtained from nonphysician sources and only 46% believed that the physician was the major source of health information for patients. Slightly over 44% indicated that patients decided their own diets, regardless of whether or not they received nutrition counseling, and 70% indicated that dietary compliance was usually poor.

The responses to questions about nutrition education in medical school were predictable based on the percentage of physicians who felt ill-prepared to provide nutrition counseling. Almost half (47%) of the physicians responding to the questionnaire indicated that they did not have "identifiable sections of the curriculum primarily concerned with nutrition" in medical school (and 16% could not remember). Sixty-eight percent indicated that the nutrition education they received in medical school was "inadequate," 19% said it was "adequate," and less than 1% said it was "extensive." Of the physicians surveyed 77% indicated that they wished they had been taught more nutrition when they were in medical school and 86% indicated that more nutrition should be taught in medical school as part of the basic curriculum.

Use of Nutrition Information in Medical Practice

There were 10 questions that probed how physicians use nutrition information in office practice. These questions were designed to determine who initiates discussions of nutrition issues, the kinds of information that is made available to patients, and information on referrals to nutritionists and dietitians. A summary of the responses is shown in tabular form in Table 2 and in graphic form in Fig. 2.

The pattern of referrals is of interest. Sixty-two percent of physicians made counseling referrals to a hospital or clinic, 13% referred to an ''outside professional,'' and about the same percentage provided counseling using in-house staff. Responses to estimates of referral patterns in the future did not substantially change the ratios: 59% expected to use hospital or clinic nutritionists or dietitians, 22% indicated they would handle the counseling in house, and 19% indicated they would refer to outside professionals.

A number of questions also asked for estimates of future counseling trends in general. Of the physicians surveyed 47% expected to do more counseling, 34% said they already counseled most patients, and only 1% expected to do less counseling.

Correlations

Bivariate analysis revealed some correlations of interest relative to sources of information, attitudes, and use of nutrition information:

1. Younger age correlated significantly with using nutrition information and positive attitude toward use of nutrition information in medicine. Younger

Table 2 Use of Nutrition Information in Medical Practice

	Range of responses in percentages[a]			
Question	Often	Sometimes	Rarely	Never
Patients initiate discussion	33	49	17	0
Physician initiates discussion	63	33	3	<1
Provide printed information	49	40	8	3
Printed info in waiting room	31	32	25	12
Recommend group program	46	41	10	2
Refer to nutritionist/RD	34	44	17	4

[a] Row percentages may not add up to 100 due to rounding.

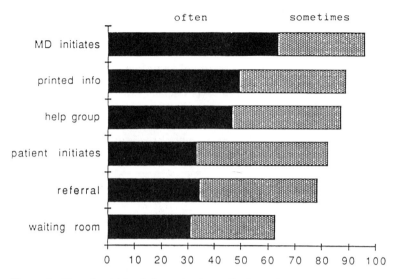

Figure 2   Use of nutrition information in medical practice.

physicians tended to use nutrition information more, and their attitude toward nutrition in medicine was more positive than that of older physicians.

2.   Group practice, compared with solo practice, showed a significant correlation: physicians in group practice were more likely to use nutrition information. At the same time, younger physicians are more likely to be in group practice than are older physicians.

3.   Affiliation with a teaching hospital showed a weak but significant correlation with use of nutrition information.

4.   Total amount of information used showed significant correlations with a positive attitude toward nutrition in medicine and the use of nutrition information in medical practice.

5.   Use of professional sources of information (as compared with all other sources of information) showed the strongest correlations with a positive attitude toward nutrition in medicine and the use of nutrition information in medical practice.

6.   There was a significant correlation between nutrition training received in the medical school curriculum and use of nutrition information in practice. Physicians who received little or no nutrition training in medical school were more likely to minimize the importance of nutrition in medicine and were less likely to incorporate nutrition information into medical practice. Conversely, those physicians who received more nutrition training in medical school were more likely to have a positive attitude about nutrition in medicine and to use nutrition in medical practice, including nutrition counseling.

Conclusions

In summary, total information sources, and nutrition instruction in medical school (Langseth, 1990), were salient factors in explaining both attitude toward nutrition in medicine and use of nutrition in medical practice. Physicians said they used professional sources of information more frequently than other sources, and greater use of professional sources was correlated with a better attitude toward the use of nutrition in medicine. However, while the physicians were more interested in professional sources of information, the significance of "other sources" should not be overlooked. For those physicians less interested or less positive about the role of nutrition in medicine, other sources appear to be more important than professional sources. Information found in newspapers, news magazines, university health and nutrition newsletters, advertisements, and literature from food and pharmaceutical firms provide a significant proportion (35–48%) of information for these physicians.

RECOMMENDATIONS

Physicians can play an important role in providing accurate and timely nutrition information and counseling to patients. Evidence indicates that many physicians are poorly equipped for this role as a result of inadequate training and education in nutrition. Physicians appear interested in learning more about nutrition, however, and medical schools have recently begun to increase their emphasis on it. As the critical role of nutrition in health has become increasingly apparent, so has the need for strongly increased training of physicians in nutrition. If physicians are to provide more appropriate nutrition counseling to patients, there needs to be a greater consensus within the medical community about the role of nutrition in medicine along with a concerted effort to fully integrate nutrition into medical education.

REFERENCES

Abraham S, Carroll MD, Najar MF, Fullwood R. Obese and overweight adults in the United States. Vital and health statistics. Series 11, Number 230. DHHS Publication Number (PHS) 83-1680. National Center for Health Statistics, Public Health Service, U.S. Department of Health and Human Services, Hyattsville, Maryland, 1983.

Adamson TE, Tschann JM, Guillion DS. Patient feedback as a tool to influence physician counseling. Patient Educ Counseling 1988 11:109–117.

American Cancer Society. Nutrition and cancer: Cause and prevention. An American Cancer Society special report. New York: American Cancer Society, 1984, 7–9.

American Medical Students Association. Testimony: Nutrition education in the undergraduate medical curriculum. Appendix F, in: National Research Council, 1985. Nutrition education in U.S. medical schools. Washington, DC: National Academy Press, 1985, 121–126.

Association of American Medical Colleges. Medical student graduation questionnaire survey. Summary report for all schools. Washington, DC: Association of American Medical Colleges, 1981–1984.

Association of American Medical Colleges, The Liaison Committee on Medical Education (LCME) annual medical school questionnaire. Washington, DC: Association of American Medical Colleges, 1980–1984.

Avioli LV. Calcium supplementation and osteoporosis. In: Armbrecht HJ, Prendergast JM, Coe RM. eds. Nutrition intervention in the aging process. Part III. Effect of nutrition on aging—Length of life. New York: Springer-Verlag, 1984, 183–190.

Bierman EL. Diet and diabetes. Am J Clin Nutr 1985; 41:1113–1116.

Brandt EN. Infant mortality—A progress report. Public Health Rep 1984; 99:284–288.

Cohen JD, Hunsley J, Wattler A, Karsten L, Olson RE. Evaluation of a nutrition education program for medical students. J Med Educ 1981; 56:773–775.

Committee on Nutrition in Medical Education, Food and Nutrition Board, National Research Council, National Academy of Sciences. Nutrition education in U.S. medical schools. Washington, DC: National Academy Press, 1985.

Cyborski CK. Nutrition content in medical curricula. J Nutr Educ 1977; 9:17–18.

Department of Health, Education, and Welfare, Public Health Service. Healthy people: The Surgeon General's report on health promotion and disease prevention. DHEW Publication Number 79-55071A. Washington, DC: U.S. Government Printing Office, 1979.

Department of Health and Human Services, Public Health Service. Health in the United States. DHHS Publication Number (PHS) 84-1232. Washington, DC: U.S. Government Printing Office, 1983.

Department of Health and Human Services, Public Health Service. Advance report of final mortality statistics, 1981. Monthly Vital Statistics Report 33(3) Supplement. Washington, DC: National Center for Health Statistics, 1984.

Department of Health and Human Services, Public Health Service. The Surgeon General's report on nutrition and health, DHHS Publication Number 88-50211. Washington, DC: U.S. Government Printing Office, 1988.

Donato KA. New opportunities to expand the role of the dietitian: Can we meet the challenge? J Am Diet Assoc 1988; 88:1369–1372.

Dwyer J. Sixteen popular diets: Brief nutritional analyses. In: Stunkard AJ. ed. Obesity. Philadelphia: WB Saunders, 1980, 276–291.

Fortmann SP, Sallis JF, Magnus PM, Farquhar JW. Attitudes and practices of physicians regarding hypertension and smoking: Stanford Five City Project. Prev Med 1985; 14:70–80.

Geiger CJ. Activities of the department of foods and nutrition of the American Medical Association. Cont Med 1979; 43:655–657.

Gemson DH, Elinson J. Prevention in primary care: Variability in physician practice patterns in New York City. Am J Prev Med 1986; 2:226–234.

General Accounting Office. Greater federal efforts are needed to improve nutrition education in the U.S. medical schools, CED-80-39. Washington, DC: U.S. General Accounting Office, 1980.

Goldberg J, Mayer J. The White House conference on food, nutrition and health twenty years later: Where are we now? J Nutr Ed 1990; 22:47–50.

Green LW, Eriksen MP, Schor EL. Preventive practices by physicians: Behavioral determinants and potential interventions. Am J Prev Med 1988; 4:101–107.

Halmi KA, Falk JR, Schwartz E. Binge-eating and vomiting: A survey of a college population. Psychol Med 1981; 11:697–706.

Harland WR, Stross JK. An educational view of a national initiative to lower plasma lipid levels. J Am Med Assoc 1985; 253:2087–2090.

Harland WR, Hull AL, Schmouder RL, Landis JR, Thompson FE, Larkin FA. Blood pressure and nutrition in adults: The National Health and Nutrition Examination Survey. Am J Epidemiol 1984; 120:17–28.

Health Values. Nutrition education for medical students needs improvement. Health Values 1989; 13:56–57.

Herbert V. Hematology and the anemias. In: Schneider JA, Anderson CE, Coursin DB. eds. Nutritional support of medical practice, 2nd ed. Philadelphia: Harper and Row, 1983.

Heymsfield SB, Howard L, Heird W, Rhoads J. Biennial survey of physician clinical nutrition training programs. Am J Clin Nutr 1985; 42:152–165.

Howard L, Bigaouette J. A survey of physician clinical nutrition training programs in the United States. Am J Clin Nutr 1983; 38:719–729.

Inglett GE, Falkehag SI. eds. Dietary fibers: Chemistry and nutrition. New York: Academic Press, 1979.

Koteski DR, McKinney S. Who does the public think should perform health care tasks? J Am Diet Assoc 1988; 88:1281–1283.

Kottke TE, Foels JE, Hill C, Choi T, Fenderson DA. Nutrition counseling in private practice: Attitudes and activities of family physicians. Prev Med 1984; 13:219–225.

Langner NR, Hasselback PD, Dunkley GC, Corber SJ. Attitudes and practices of primary care physicians in the management of elevated serum cholesterol levels. Can Med Assoc J 1989; 141:33–38.

Langseth L. Nutrition in medicine: A survey of primary care physicians. DrPH dissertation, Columbia University, School of Public Health, New York, 1990.

Levine D. The physician's role in health-promotion and disease prevention. Bull NY Acad Med 1987; 63:950–956.

Levy RI, Moskowitz J. Cardiovascular research: Decades of progress, a decade of promise. Science 1982; 217:121–129.

Lewis CE, Wells KB, Ware J. A model for predicting the counseling practices of physicians. J Gen Intern Med 1986; 1:14–19.

Lunin LF. Where does the public get its health information? Bull NY Acad Med 1987; 63:923–938.

Maheux B, Pineault R, Jacques A, Beland F, Levesque A. Factors influencing physicians' counseling on nutrition, presented at the conference, "Nutrition in Health: The Scientific Challenge for the 21st Century" (Montreal, Canada, August 13–16, 1989), 1989.

Merritt RJ, Heymsfield SB, Howard L, Rombeau J. Biennial survey of physician clinical nutrition training programs. Am J Clin Nutr 1988; 47:911–921.

Morgan SL, Weinsier RL, Boker JR, Brooks CM. Nutrition education for medical students: Evaluation of the relative contribution of freshman courses in biochemistry and nutrition to performance on a standardized examination in nutrition. Nutrition 1989; 5:31–36.

Nash DT. Encouraging physician interest in preventive cardiology. NY State J Med 1988; 88:3–5.

National Cancer Institute. Cancer prevention. National Institutes of Health, Department of Health and Human Services, Bethesda, MD, 1984.

National Cholesterol Education Program (NCEP). Report of the Expert Panel on Diet Evaluation and Treatment of High Blood Cholesterol in Adults. Arch Intern Med 1988; 148:36–39.

National Research Council. Recommended dietary allowances, 9th revised ed. Washington, DC: National Academy Press, 1980.

National Research Council. Diet, nutrition and cancer. Washington, DC: National Academy Press, 1982.

Palmer S, Zeman FJ. Inborn errors of metabolism. In: Zeman FJ. ed. Clinical nutrition and dietetics. Lexington, MA: Collamore Press, 1983.

Phillips MG. The nutrition knowledge of medical students. J Med Educ 1971; 46:86–90.

Raven M. The A,B,Cs of today's competitive marketplace. Drug Topics 1981; 125:45.

Read MS. Guide to materials for use in teaching clinical nutrition in schools of medicine, dentistry, and public health. Am J Clin Nutr 1983; 38:775–794.

Read MS, Bodner J, Sayadi H. Guide to materials for use in teaching clinical nutrition in schools of medicine, dentistry, and public health II. Am J Clin Nutr 1987; 45:643–660.

Schucker B. Change in physician perspective on cholesterol and heart disease: Results from two national surveys. J Am Med Assoc 1987; 258:3521–3526.

Schwabe AD, Lippe BM, Chang J, Pops MA, Yager J. Anorexia nervosa, Ann Intern Med 1981; 94:371–381.

Shea S, Gemson DH, Mossel P. Management of high blood cholesterol by primary care physicians: Diffusion of the National Cholesterol Education Program Adult Treatment Panel Guidelines. J Gen Intern Med 1990; 5:327–334.

Shils ME. An affirmation of our Society's commitment to clinical nutrition. Am J Clin Nutr 1986; 44:576–580.

Sobal J, Muncie HL, Jr, Valente CM, DeForge BR, Levine D. Physicians' beliefs about vitamin supplements and a balanced diet. J Nutr Educ 1987; 19:181–185.

Stewart AL, Brook RH. Effects of being overweight. Am J Public Hlth 1983; 73:171–178.

Thompson JS, Burrough CA, Green JL, Brown GL. Nutritional screening in surgical patients. J Am Diet Assoc 1984; 84:337–338.

U.S. Congress. The food gap: Poverty and malnutrition in the United States. Publication No. 32-571. Ninetieth Congress, Second Session. Hearings before the Select Committee on Nutrition and Human Needs. Washington, DC: U.S. Government Printing Office, 1969.

U.S. Congress. Nutrition education in medical schools. Hearings Before the Subcommittee on Nutrition of the Committee on Agriculture, Nutrition, and Forestry, U.S. Senate, Ninety-Sixth Congress, First Session on Current Status, Impediments, and Potential Solutions, January 30, 1979, Part II. Washington, DC: U.S. Government Printing Office, 1979.

U.S. Department of Health and Human Services. Public screening for measuring blood cholesterol—Issues for special concern. Office of Prevention, Education, and Control. National Heart, Lung, and Blood Institute. National Cholesterol Education Program. Coordinating Committee, October 5, 1987.

U.S. Preventive Services Task Force. Guide to clinical preventive services: An assessment of the effectiveness of 169 interventions. Report of the U.S. Preventive Services Task Force. Washington, DC: U.S. Government Printing Office, 1989.

Verhaak PFM, van Busschbach JT. Patient education in general practice. Patient Educ Counseling 1988; 11:119–129.

Wechsler H, Levine S, Idelson RK, Rohman M, Taylor JO. The physician's role in health promotion—A survey of primary-care practitioners. N Engl J Med 1983; 308:97–100.

Weinsier RL. Nutrition education in the medical school: Factors critical to the development of a successful program. J Am Coll Nutr 1982; 1:219–226.

Weinsier RL, Boker JR, Feldman EB, Read MS, Brooks CM. Nutrition knowledge of senior medical students: A collaborative study of southeastern medical schools. Am J Clin Nutr 1986; 43:959–968.

Weinsier RL, Boker JR, Morgan SL, Feldman EB, Moinuddin JF, Mamel JJ, DiGirolamo M, Borum PR, Read MS, Brooks CM. Cross-sectional study of nutrition knowledge and attitudes of medical students at three points in their medical training at 11 southeastern medical schools. Am J Clin Nutr 1988; 48:1–6.

Weinsier RL, Boker JR, Brooks CM, Kushner RF, Visek WJ, Mark DA, Lopez-S A, Anderson MS, Block K. Priorities for nutrition content in a medical school curriculum: A national consensus of medical educators. Am J Clin Nutr 1989; 50:707–712.

White PL, Johnson OC, Kibler MJ. Council on Foods and Nutrition, American Medical Association—Its relation to physicians. Postgrad Med 1961; 30:502.

White House Conference on Food, Nutrition, and Health. Final report. Proceedings of the White House conference on food, nutrition and health. December 2, 1969. Publication Number 0-378-473. Washington, DC: U.S. Government Printing Office, 1969.

Whiteside C, Robbins JA. Cholesterol knowledge and practices among patients compared with physician management in a university primary care setting. Prev Med 1989; 18:526–531.

Young EA. Nutrition in medical education. Nutr News 1988; 51:9–11.

Index